NCLEX-RN™

A Comprehensive Study Guide

5th Edition

JoAnn Zerwekh, EdD, RN, FNP, CS

Executive Director
Nursing Education Consultants
Midlothian, Texas
Online Nursing Faculty
University of Phoenix
Phoenix, Arizona

Jo Carol Claborn, MS, RN, CNS

Executive Director
Nursing Education Consultants
Midlothian, Texas

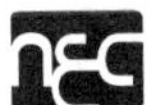

Nursing Education Consultants
Midlothian, Texas

Cover Design: Tim Fennell
Production Coordination: CuleGo, Waxahachie, Texas

✦

✦

Printed in the United States of America

Nursing Education Consultants
P.O. Box 1685
Midlothian, Texas 756065-1685

ISBN 1-892155-04-4, 5th Edition, 2002
Library of Congress Catalog Card Number: 2002-101867

✦

Any procedure or practice described in this book should be applied by the health-care practitioner under appropriate supervision in accordance with professional standards of care used with regard to the unique circumstances that apply in each practice situation. Care has been taken to confirm the accuracy of information presented and to describe generally accepted practices. However, the authors, editors, and publisher cannot accept any responsibility for errors or omissions or for consequences from application of the information in this book and make no warranty, express or implied, with respect to the contents of this book.

The authors and publisher have exerted every effort to ensure that drug selection and dosage set forth in this text are in accord with current recommendations and practice at the time of publication. However, in view of the ongoing research, changes in government regulations, and the constant flow of information relating to drug therapy and drug reactions, the reader is urged to check the package insert of each drug for any change in indications and dosage and for added warnings and precautions. This is particularly important when the recommended agent is a new or infrequently used drug.

This book is written to be used as a review book for the NCLEX-RN™. It is not intended for use as a primary resource for procedures, treatments, medications or to serve as a complete textbook for nursing care.

Copies of this book may be obtained directly from *Nursing Education Consultants.*

Last Digit is the Print Number: 6 5 4 3 2 1

To Tom Gaglione
who has a wonderful sense of humor that warms the heart.
We can always count on you
to bring a smile to our face that brightens our day !
We love you.

Contributors

Sharon Decker, MS, RN
Texas Tech University
Health Science Center
Lubbock, Texas

Alice B. Pappas, PhD, RN
Baylor University School of Nursing
Dallas, Texas

Linda Stevenson, PhD, RN
Baylor University School of Nursing
Dallas, Texas

Tom Gaglione, RN, MN
Nursing Education Consultants
Midlothian, Texas

Susan Priest, RN, MSN, CNS
Alvin Community College
Alvin, Texas

Cathy Rosser, RN, MSN
University of Texas @ Tyler
Tyler, Texas

Joanna Barnes, RN, MS
Grayson County Community College
Denison, Texas

Mary Ann Yantis, RN, PhD
Baylor University School of Nursing
Dallas, Texas

Preface

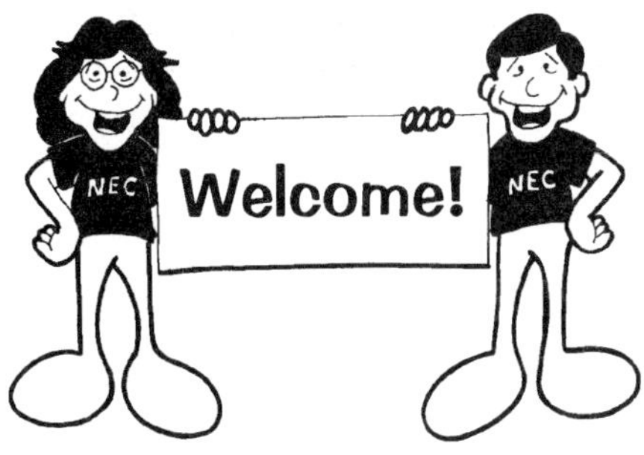

This 5th edition of *NCLEX-RN™: A Comprehensive Study Guide* presents updated information specifically designed to assist you in preparing for the National Council Licensure Examination for Registered Nurses (NCLEX-RN™). This text emphasizes the integrated approach to nursing practice that the NCLEX-RN™ is designed to test. This book's primary purpose is to assist you to thoroughly review facts, principles, and applications of the nursing process. It should alleviate many of the concerns you may have about what, how, and when to study.

We have spent a great deal of time studying the NCLEX-RN™ test format and have incorporated this information into this book. In our review courses which we have taught across the country, we have identified specific student needs and correlated this information with the test plan in order to develop this study guide. Study questions are at the end of each chapter for you to check your reading and comprehension. In addition, there is a practice test at the end of the book and a computer disk of questions.

We have designed graphics that highlight important information to make the book more visually appealing.

NCLEX ALERT: *NCLEX Alert identifies what we feel are frequently tested concepts that we have interpreted from the RN Job Task Analysis from the National Council State Boards of Nursing, Inc.*

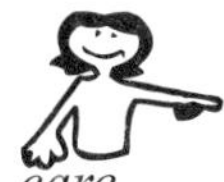

NURSING PRIORITY: *Nursing Priority assists to distinguish priorities of nursing care.*

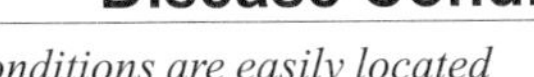

Disease Conditions

Disease conditions are easily located

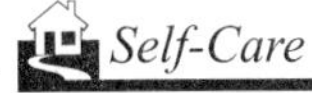

Self-Care

Information on self care can be found under nursing interventions.

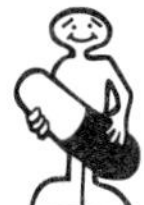

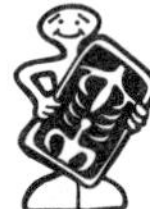

Appendices highlight medications, diagnostic, and nursing procedures in each chapter.

The comments from our review course participants on our fourth edition have helped to shape the development of this fifth edition. We hope this text will prove even more beneficial to nursing faculty, students, and graduate nurses. Thank you for allowing us to be part of your success in nursing.

JoAnn Zerwekh
Jo Carol Claborn

Acknowledgments

We wish to express our appreciation to our children — Tyler and Ashley Zerwekh, Mike Brown, Kimberley Aultman, and Jaelyn Conway for their continuing support as their mothers wrote, rewrote, and put together the fifth edition of this review book. To our parents, Charles Graham and Hazel Cooper, who remain our steadfast, loving support in all that we do. To Lucy Claborn, who continues to amaze us with her youth and vitality. To Robert and Tom, thank you for your tolerance, love, and willingness to continue to share in our hectic professional lives.

The revision of a book offers the opportunity to be responsive to nursing faculty and students who have utilized the book. We appreciate their comments and suggestions for the production of this fourth edition. It is our pleasure to express an appreciation to the individuals who assisted us in the technical preparation and production of this fifth edition. Our sincere appreciation to:

James Halfast, our technical assistant for developing the design and manuscript layout.

Elaine Nokes, our administrative assistant, who keeps everything organized and running smoothly for our business;

Robert Zerwekh, PhD, for developing the software program for our computer disk of test questions;

The staff at CuleGo for their persistence and patience in working with us on the production and printing;

Tim Fennel for his continuing creativity in the production of the cover designs.

Table of Contents

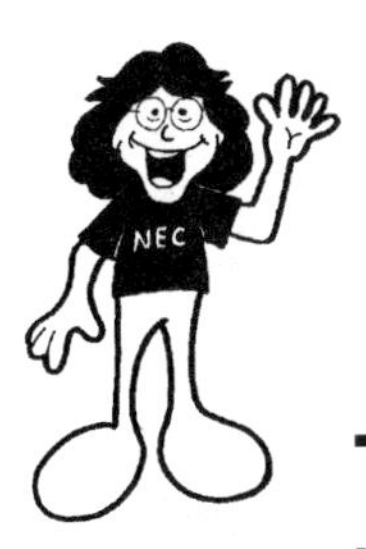

INTRODUCTION & NCLEX-RN™ TESTING STRATEGIES

The first step to being successful on the NCLEX is to understand how it is developed. The National Council of State Boards of Nursing is responsible for the development of the examination. The National Council is composed of members from all of the respective state boards of nursing. The NCLEX-RN™ is used by all of the states to determine entry into nursing practice as a registered nurse. Each state is responsible for the testing requirements, retesting procedures, and entry into practice within that state. Every state requires the same competency level or passing standard on NCLEX, there is no variation in the passing standard from state to state.

Test Plan

The test plan is based on research done by the National Council every 3 years. The purpose of the research is to determine the activities of nurses within a year of completing school and the NCLEX. This research indicates that the majority of graduate nurses are working in an acute care environment and are responsible for caring for adult clients.The exam consists of questions that are designed to test the candidate's ability to apply the nursing process and to determine appropriate nursing responses and interventions in order to provide safe nursing care. The framework of the test plan reflects two components: the nursing process and areas of client needs.

Phases of the Nursing Process

Each question is based on the nursing process and all questions reflect some type of nursing decision or action. All of the questions in the test bank are categorized according to the nursing process. See Table 1-1 for commonly used terms that are incorporated into a question to designate levels of the nursing process. You have had the nursing process since the beginning of school, there is nothing new about the nursing process on NCLEX. The process must go in order - assessment, analysis, planning, implementation and evaluation. You must have adequate assessment data before you can proceed with the process. Frequently questions will be based on obtaining critical assessment data, other questions will present the assessment data in the stem of the question. It is important to keep the steps of the nursing process in mind when critically evaluating an NCLEX question.

Areas of Client Needs

The National Council Examination Committee has identified 4 primary areas of client needs. These areas reflect an integrated approach to the testing content, there are not any predetermined number of questions, or percentage of questions that reflect medical surgical nursing, pediatrics, obstetrics, etc. In Table 1-2, the areas of client needs are listed with the sub categories and specific weights for each subcategory. With each of the sub-categories are *examples* of content to be tested in that area. This table has been adapted and summarized, it does not refect the entire test plan content. National Council Detailed Test Plan for the NCLEX-RN™ Examination may be obtained from the National Council of State Boards of Nursing, Inc. (www.ncsbn.org).

The majority of questions on the NCLEX are written at the level of application and analysis. This means you have to know the facts and understand concepts to be able to apply the nursing process to the client presented in the question.

Table 1-1: DESCRIPTORS FOR STEPS OF THE NURSING PROCESS

Assessment	Planning	Implementation	Evaluation
assess	include	implement	evaluate
determine	plan	teach	monitor
observe	generate	give	question
collect	arrange	administer	repeat
recognize	formulate	document	re-establish
detect	short-term goal is...	inform	consider
find	long-term goal is...	encourage	
gather	patient outcome is...	advise	
describe		explain	
		provide	

Brown, Patricia A., et al (2000). *NCLEX Examination: National Council Detailed Test Plan for the NCLEX-RN ™Examination*, Chicago, National Council of State Boards of Nursing, Inc.

Table 1-2: NCLEX TEST PLAN

Safe, Effective Care and Environment	
Management of Care (7-13%)	Management of nursing care – supervision, delegation, prioritizing, and delivery of safe care; legal and ethical practices; documentation; client rights.
Safety and Infection Control (5-11%)	Prevention of errors and accidents, implementation of standard precautions, asepsis, use of restraints, disaster planning, handling hazardous materials.
Health Promotion and Maintenance	
Growth and Development Across Life Span (7-13%)	Aging process and expected body changes; developmental stages and transitions, ante/intra/post partum, and newborn; family characteristics.
Prevention and/or Early Detection of Disease (5-11%)	Health promotion programs, disease prevention, immunizations, techniques of physical assessment.
Psychosocial Integrity	
Coping and Adaptation (5-11%)	Mental health concepts and interventions, end of life care, coping mechanisms related to change in body image, sensory and perceptual alterations, spiritual influences.
Psychosocial Integrity (5-11%)	Nursing care for acute or chronic mental illness, behavioral interventions/crisis intervention, chemical dependency, domestic violence/abuse.
Physiological Integrity	
Basic Care and Comfort (7-13%)	Assistive devices, mobility, nutrition, elimination, hygiene, comfort care.
Pharmacological and Parenteral Therapies (5-11%)	Medication administration – actions, adverse effects/ contraindications, nursing implications; blood administration, IV therapy, central venous access devices, chemotherapy, pain control, parenteral nutrition.
Reduction of Risk Potential (12-18%)	Pathophysiology, nursing implications for and nursing care to minimize potential complications of diagnostic tests/procedures/surgery, laboratory values, and health alterations. (tubes, pacemakers, hyper/hypoglycemia, specimens, bleeding, immobility, wounds, positions)
Physiological Adaptation (12-18%)	Pathophysiology/alterations in body systems – signs and symptoms of conditions, traction devices, seizures, vascular access for dialysis, assess tube drainage, sign and symptoms of infections, complications of pregnancy, medial emergencies, hemodynamics, respiratory care, infections, fluid and electrolytes, radiation therapy.

Adapted from the National Council Detailed Test Plan for the NCLEX-RN Examination, National Council of State Boards of Nursing, 2001.

NCLEX questions are based on critical thinking concepts which will demonstrate your ability to make decisions and solve problems. NCLEX questions are not fact, recall or memory level questions. Nurses who have taken the NCLEX will be the first to tell you that the questions are not like anything you had on nursing school examinations. The questions and answers have been thoroughly researched and have been tested prior to your examination. This is what is called a "standardized exam". The standardization is important because the NCLEX is used nation wide to determine entry level into practice. This means that regional differences in nursing care will not be a component of the exam. All of the questions have been designed according to the test plan, then researched and documented as entry level nursing behaviors. What was great new information in the last months journals will not be immediately reflected on the NCLEX.

NCLEX ALERT: *The NCLEX-RN is a test that requires application of nursing concepts and principles across the life span.*

Throughout this book are NCLEX-Alerts that call your attention to areas of the test plan. Pay attention to this information and think about how this concept or principle can apply to different types of clients.

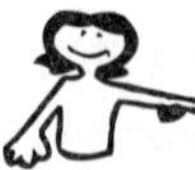

NURSING PRIORITIES: *This is critical information to consider in order to care for a specific client safely.*

Another characteristic of this book is the Nursing Priorities. As conditions are discussed, the nursing priorities call your attention to critical information regarding a client with specific conditions being presented.

What is Computer Adaptive Testing (CAT)?

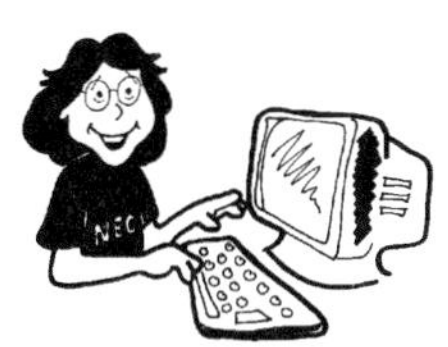

Computer adaptive testing allows for a test to be generated according to each candidates' needs. As a candidate progresses through questions, the computer will select the next question to be presented to provide an opportunity to demonstrate competence. The NCELX-RN™ is graded in a different manner from conventional school exams. It is not based on the number of questions answered correctly, but rather the level of competency. The pass/fail is determined by the competence level based on the level of difficulty of the questions presented.

When each candidate begins their test, a test bank of questions will be loaded into the computer. Different candidates will receive different sets of questions, but all the pools of questions will be based on the same test plan. For example, standard precautions is a critical element of the test plan. There are lots of situations and clients where this concept can be tested, you may receive an obstetrical client, someone else a respiratory client, and still someone else a newborn.

The questions to be presented are determined by your response to the previous question. When you get a question correct, you will get a harder question the next time. The more of the harder questions you answer correctly, the closer you are to passing. You cannot skip questions, or go back to previously answered questions. As you progress through the exam, it is interactively assembled as you go. As long as you answer the questions correctly, you will get a harder question. When you answer a question incorrectly, the computer will select an easier question. The really easy questions are often below the level of competency. The computer will continue to present to you questions that are based on the test plan, and on your level of ability.

Taking the NCLEX

When you begin taking your NCLEX, there will be a tutorial to help you get started and to make sure you understand how to use the computer. You will have a maximum of 5 hours to complete the examination. When you have been testing for 2 hours, there is a mandatory 10 minute break. If you need a break before that time, notify one of the attendants at the testing center.

Your examination will stop when one of the following occurs:

1. You have answered 75 questions and demonstrated minimum competency, or a lack of minimum competency.

2. You have completed the maximum number of 265 questions.

3. You have been testing for 5 hours.

You will receive somewhere between 75-265 questions. The number of questions on your NCLEX is not indicative of your level of competency. A lot of candidates who complete all 265 questions will have demonstrated a level of minimum competency and therefore pass NCLEX. You will use a mouse to select your answers, so you don't have to worry about different computer function keys. There will also be an on screen calculator to use for your math problems. If you have any problems with the environment or with the equipment, there will be someone there to assist you.

When you receive your Candidate Bulletin from the National Council, read it carefully. This will provide you with a lot of information that will give you direction and answer some of the questions you may still have regarding the NCLEX.

Successful Test Taking on NCLEX

NCLEX ALERT: *You must practice testing skills for them to become part of your testing abilities. Practice test-taking is necessary if you are going to be able to fully utilize these skills on the NCLEX-RN™.*

The ability to take an examination is a skill that is developed through practice and experience. Being able to take an examination effectively is almost as important as the basic knowledge required to answer the questions correctly. Everyone has taken an examination only to find in the review of the exam that questions were missed due to poor testing skills. Nursing education provides the graduate with a comprehensive base of knowledge; how you, the graduate, utilize this knowledge will determine your success on the examination.

The NCLEX-RN™ is designed to evaluate minimum levels of competency. The exam is not testing your total knowledge, your knowledge of specialty areas, or any degree of professionalism. It is designed to test whether you have an adequate knowledge base in order to practice nursing safely. On NCLEX, the questions are described as being based on clinical situations common in nursing; uncommon situations are not emphasized. NCLEX questions are not fact, recall or memory level questions, they are questions you are going to have to "critically think" about to answer.

Practice testing is an excellent method of studying for NCELX. However, you have to use the results to determine if you have areas of content you need to review, or if you are missing questions due to poor testing strategies.

NCLEX Testing Strategies

The NCLEX questions are different from those you have had in school. Sometimes the questions are longer than you have had in school. One of the biggest problems graduates encounter is that there appears to be two or more correct answers. Or sometimes, you feel that you want more information. You have got to answer the question as it is presented, no one is going to clarify or answer any questions you may have about the question. Presented here is information that is critical for you to consider when evaluating and answering NCLEX questions.

✎ **The NCLEX Hospital** - What a great place to work! On the NCLEX, all of your clients are being cared for in the NCLEX Hospital. Questions ask for nursing care and decisions based on a situation where everything you need to care for the client in the best possible way is available to you. *NCLEX questions are based on textbook practices, not on the real world.* Clients are going to respond just like the books indicate they will. If you have had a lot of clinical experience, you may find yourself thinking that you cannot do something because you do not have adequate staff, or equipment, or it just is not "realistic" to do it that way. It is in the NCLEX Hospital. This approach is necessary since this is a nationally standardized examination.

✎ **Calling the Doctor (or anyone else)** - Don't pass the responsibility for care of the client to someone else. This is an exam on nursing care, evaluate the question carefully and see what nursing action needs to be taken before consulting or calling someone else. This includes social workers, respiratory therapist, hospital chaplain, as well as the doctor. After carefully evaluating the question, if the client's condition is such that you cannot do anything to resolve the problem, than call the doctor may be the best answer. Frequently there is a nursing action to be taken before contacting the doctor.

✎ **Doctors Orders** - you can assume that you have a doctors order to provide the nursing care in the options presented to you. If the questions asks for administration of a specific medication for the client's problem than consider that you have an order for it. If a question is asking whether or not you need a doctor's order for an action it will be stated as such in the stem of the question. For example the question may request a dependent or independent nursing action.

✎ **Focus on the client** - look for answers that focus on the client. Wrong choices would be those that focus on maintaining hospital rules and policy, or dealing with equipment. Evaluate the status of the client first, than deal with the equipment problems or concerns.

✎ **Laboratory Values** - It is important to know the normal lab values for the most common laboratory tests. It is also important to know what to anticipate the lab values to indicate when a client's condition is improving or when it is getting worse. A guideline here is to look at the lab values that when they are abnormal it will affect the delivery of nursing care. Check table 1.2 for examples of these laboratory tests. For example, when a client's blood sugar is 50mg and he is awake and alert, you are going to find a complex carbohydrate to feed him. If a client has a

Table 1-3: IMPORTANT LAB TESTS

Know These Lab Values:

Serum blood tests:	Prothrombin time
Potassium	Partial thromboplastin time
Glucose (blood sugar)	**Arterial blood gass (ABG's)**
Complete Blood Test	Oxygen (PO2)
Hemoglobin	Carbon dioxide (PCO2)
Hematocrit	pH (acid or alkaline)
Platelets	Bicarbonate (HCO3)
White cell count	**Specific gravity of urine**
Creatinine	
Blood urea nitrogen (BUN)	

Review the normal values, significance of an increase or deccrease, and the specific nursing actions in the respective chapters.

Hgb of 8.5, you don't want him doing any unnecessary physical activities and you will need to keep him warm.

✎ **Positions** - positioning a client tends to appear regularly on the NCLEX, both as a question and as options for you to consider in your implementation of care. If the positioning appears in the stem or the question, than you need to consider if the position is for comfort, for treatment, or to prevent a complication. Evaluate the question - what is it you want to accomplish with the position and why is it important for this client?

Sometimes the position appears in the options. Consider if positioning is important to the care of this client. For example, the semi-Fowlers position is very important to a client who is having difficulty breathing, the supine position or low-Fowlers may be the position of comfort for a client postoperatively. Determine why you are placing a client in a specific position and then determine if this is priority in planning or intervention. Check Appendix 3.1 for a further description of positions.

Management of Client Care

Don't panic and pull out all of your management textbooks to review. As the role of the registered nurse has expanded, this is an area that has become increasingly important over the past few years. There are licensed practical/vocational nurses (LVN/LPN), and unlicenced assistive personnel (UAP) or patient care attendants (PCA) to supervise and direct in the provision of safe nursing care. Frequently this is information you had in class, but did not have the opportunity to apply the principles in the clinical setting. If you will pay attention to some of the rules of delegation and supervision, you should be able to answer these questions. Pay attention to whom you are delegating the care or nursing activity - is it to another RN, or is it to a less qualified person (LVN/LPN or UAP/PCA).

✎ **Don't delegate assessment, evaluation or nursing judgement** - these are levels of the nursing process that must be done by a registered nurse.

✎ **Don't delegate teaching assignments** - this is another area that is the responsibility of the registered nurse.

✎ **Keep in mind the NCLEX Hospital** - you will have all of the staff you need, you don't have to worry about short staffing. You only need to focus on the client or clients in the question - don't worry about what is happening on the rest of the unit.

✎ **Determine your most stable client** - the one who has the most predictable outcome and is least likely to have abrupt changes in his condition that would require critical nursing judgements. These are the clients you can possibly delegate some of their nursing care activities to someone else. When determining the most stable clients, Maslow's Hiearchy of Needs should also be considered (Figure 3-1). Very carefully consider any clients with respiratory compromise, they are most likely the clients you do not want to delegate nursing care.

✎ **Identify your priority client** - this is the client who is mot likely to experience harm, or ill effects if he is not taken care of first. Priority clients would include those with respiratory compromise, those whose condition is unstable. It is not unusual for NCLEX to give you a typical nursing care assignment and ask you what you should do first. You will need to identify your most unstable client, see him first and/or determine what you need to do first for this client.

✎ **Delegate tasks that have specific guidelines** - those tasks that have specific guidelines that are unchanging, and are utilized in the care of a stable client can often be delegated. Bathing, collecting urine sample, feeding, personal hygiene, and ambulating are just a few examples of these activities. Remember you are in the NCLEX Hospital, so reword the question and select an answer that puts the registered nurse making the decisions. Be careful to work through each option and eliminate the incorrect ones, so you are left with the right answer. You cannot predict the answer!

Establishing Nursing Priorities

Almost all nurses will tell you that the NCLEX is full of priority questions. These questions may be worded as: "what is the priority nursing action", "what is the first nursing action", "what is the best nursing action". In other words, the NCLEX wants to know if you can establish what is the most important action for you to take to care for a client in the situation presented. This is frequently where three or four of the answers are correct, however one of them needs to be done prior to the others presented. This is where some critical thinking is needed. There are three areas to consider when determining priority nursing actions - Maslow, the nursing process and client safety.

✎ **Maslow's Hierarchy of Needs** - and you thought this was just for fundamentals! *Always consider Maslow and that physiological needs come first.* When evaluating options identify those that are physiological and psychosocial, most often one of the physiological needs will be the correct answer. You have to take care of a client's physical needs before you can take care of his psychosocial or teaching needs. Also remember the ABC's - airway, breathing, and circulation as the critical physiological needs - and at the base of Maslow. But be cautious, don't always jump on the airway as the best answer - sometime the client does not have an airway problem! Maslow's needs also apply to the psychosocial questions, take care of physical needs first, than focus on the psychosocial needs. (See the section in this chapter regarding answering psychosocial questions)

✎ **Nursing Process** - once again. The first step in the nursing process is assessment, this is frequently the first nursing action as well. Assessment must be done in order to determine what nursing implementation actions are appropriate. Go back to Table 1.2 for words that indicate levels of the nursing process, the term "assess" will not always be used. If the assessment data is provided in the stem of the question, than consider Maslow when selecting the best nursing action or implementation.

✎ **Safety Issues -** this may include situations in the hospital, home or school. The first issue to consider is meeting basic needs of survival - oxygen, nutrition, elimination. Reducing environmental hazards is also a concern. This could be prevention of falls, accidents, or medication errors. The environmental safety would also include the prevention of spread of diseases, this may include how to avoid contagious diseases, importance of immunizations, or even activities such as hand washing. When critically evaluating questions that involve a client's safety and there are multiple options that appear to be correct. Determine what activity will be of most benefit to the client, or what will cause the least harm to the client.

STRATEGIES TO EVALUATE MULTIPLE-CHOICE QUESTIONS

These are testing strategies that will help you during school, as well as on NCLEX. Start practicing them now, and you will increase your testing scores in school as well as being one more step toward success on NCLEX.

Question Characteristics

The majority of questions on the NCLEX, as well as your nursing school exams, are multiple choice. This is a type of testing that most of you are familiar with.

1. **Stem of the question:** states the question that is being asked. This frequently includes a situation with information that describes a clients' conditions, or circumstances and asks the question.
2. **Options**: there are four options from which to choose an answer.
   a. Three options are designed to distract you from the correct answer.
   b. One option correctly answers the question asked in the stem.
   c. There is only one correct response; no partial credit is given for another answer.

1. Read the question carefully before ever looking or considering the options. If you glance through the options you may pick up key words that will affect the way you perceive the question.

This will prevent you from formulating an opinion about the answer before you have read the question. On a paper and pencil test, just cover the answers with your hand or a notecard. If you practice this before NCLEX, than when you get there you will be able to do this without physically covering the answers.

2. Do not read extra meaning into the question. The question is asking for specific information; if it appears to be simple "common sense," then assume it is simple. Do not look for a hidden meaning in a question. (Don't make the client any sicker then he already is!)

Example: *A bronchoscopy was performed on a client at 7 am. He returns to his room and the nurse plans to assist the client with his AM care. The client refuses the care. What is the best nursing action?*

① Encourage the client to take a shower.
② Perform all of his AM care.
③ Postpone the AM care until client is more comfortable and can participate.
④ Cancel all of the AM care since it is not necessary to perform after a bronchoscopy.

The correct answer is # 3. The question is asking for a nursing judgment regarding AM care. Do not read into the question and make it more difficult by trying to put in information relating to respiratory care.

3. Read the stem correctly. Make sure you understand exactly what information the question is asking. Watch for words that provide direction to the question - " the client would need further teaching", "indicates the client understands the preoperative teaching, medication administration ...", "contraindicated", "the client should avoid" Try rewording the question to better understand what it is asking.

These words or phrases change the direction of the question. It may help to rephrase the question in your own words in order to better understand what information is being requested.

Example: *Clients with arteriosclerotic heart disease (ASHD) go through several stages before becoming severely compromised. Which does not occur in the early stages of ASHD?*

① Decreased urine output.
② Dyspnea on exercise.
③ Anginal pain relieved by rest.

④ Increased serum triglyceride levels.

Rephrase the question: In early stages of ASHD, what is not characteristic? It is important that you identify the key point "early stages of ASHD" and the key words "does not occur." If you miss these essential points, you do not understand the question, and chances are you will not choose the correct answer. The correct answer is option # 1: a decrease in urine output occurs when cardiac disease is advanced enough to cause a severe decrease in cardiac output and renal perfusion.

4. Watch where your client is in the disease process or condition he is experiencing. Examples of this are terms such as: "immediately postoperatively", "the first post operative day", "experienced a myocardial infarction this am".

***Example:** A client had a cardiac catheterization using the left femoral artery. During the first few hours after the heart catheterization procedure, which nursing action would be most important?*

Rewording - What is the **most important** nursing care in the **first few hours** after a cardiac catheterization?

① Check his temperature q2h.
② Elevate the head of the bed 90 degrees.
③ Evaluate blood pressure and respiratory status.
④ Check his pedal and femoral pulses q1h x 4.

The correct answer is #4. The phrase, "during the first few hours after the procedure," is important in answering this question correctly. The danger of hemorrhage from the puncture site is greatest during this time. The question also asks for the most important nursing care, which #3 is important to do, however #4 is critical to this particular procedure.

5. Identify the step of the nursing process being tested. Remember, you must have adequate assessment data before you can continue. Identify the steps of the nursing process for each option - than look for the assessment. Look for key words that can assist you in determining what type of information is being tested. (see Table 1-1).

***Example:** An elderly client from a residential facility is brought into the emergency room. There are numerous bruises and abrasions in various stages of healing on the client's face and arms. The attendant from the residential facility explains that the elderly client fell down. What is the priority nursing action?*

① Call the residential facility and ask for an incident report.
② Put ice on the bruises and cover the abrasions with Vaseline gauze.
③ Notify the charge nurse.
④ Determine the extent of injuries.

The correct answer is #4, to determine or assess the extent of injuries. The stem of the question did not present adequate enough information on which to make a nursing judgement. Options #1, #2, and #3 relate to nursing actions that would be done after the injuries are assessed.

6. Before considering the options, think about the characteristics of this condition and critical nursing concepts. What are the nursing priorities in caring for a client with this condition/procedure/medication/problem?

***Example:** A mother who is three days postpartum is complaining of soreness and fullness in her breasts and states that she wants to stop breast feeding her infant until her breasts feel better. What is the best nursing response?*

Think about breast feeding and what are the common discomforts and problems the client encounters. Don't look at the options - think "Is it normal to have fullness and soreness in the breasts during the first three days of lactation?" If you are unsure, go back and reassess the question. Now progress to the options:

① Show the client how to apply a breast binder to decrease the discomfort and the production of milk.
② Tell the client that breast fullness may be a sign of infection and to stop breast feeding.
③ Suggest to the client that she decrease her fluid intake for the next 24 hours to temporarily suppress lactation.
④ Explain to the client that the breast discomfort is normal and that the infant's sucking will promote the flow of milk.

In this question, option #4 is correct. Initially, breast soreness may occur for about 2-3 minutes during each feeding until the let-down reflex is established.

7. Don't focus on predicting a right answer! Frequently the answer you want is not going to be an option! Keep in mind the characteristics and concepts of nursing care for a client with the condition or problem in the situation presented.

***Example:** A client has an ulcer (2 in x 2 in) on the calf of his right leg. It is draining purulent fluid. The vital signs are: P-114, R-22, T-102°. Which order will the nurse implement first?*

Reword the question: The client has an infection in the ulcer on his leg, his temperature is up, so is his pulse - this is a normal response to infection. What nursing actions do I need to do first?

① Ceftrixone (Rocephin), 1 gm, intravensouly q2hours.

② Blood cultures x 2, 20 minutes apart and from different venipuncture sites.

③ Polysporin (Bacitracin) ointment topically to leg ulcer TID.

④ Acetaminophen (Tylenol), 650 mg suppository, q 4h for temp > 101.8° F.

Consider #1 - this is an antibiotic that will begin to fight the infection.

Consider #2 - This is important to do in order to identify the causative bacteria, this is more important now than #1.

Consider #3 - This is treating the infection topically - it will cause a decrease in the bacteria, still need to get the blood cultures first - eliminate it.

Consider #4 - This is treating the symptoms, not the cause of the problem, not as important as # 2, eleminate it.

All of these options are feasible for treating this client, however obtaining the blood culture is the most important. If you had approached this question with a specific answer in mind (give an antibiotic), you would have found that answer, however it would have been wrong.

8. Evaluate all of the options in a systematic manner. After you understand the question, read all of the options carefully. Remember, distracters are plausible to the situation and are designed to "distract" you from the correct answer. *NCLEX Style* - all of the options may be correct, but one is the best answer.

Example: *A client has just returned to his room from the recovery room following a lumbar laminectomy. In considering possible complications the client might experience, what nursing action is important?*

① Monitor vital signs every four hours.

② Assess breath sounds every two hours.

③ Evaluate every two hours for urinary retention.

④ Check when he last had a bowel movement.

In evaluating the options, all are plausible for the situation. However, consider that this is his operative day, and the question is asking for complications he might encounter post lumbar laminectomy. Distracters #1 and #4 are not appropriate at this period of postoperative recovery. Option #2 would be appropriate if respiratory problems were anticipated (don't always jump on respiratory answers). The correct answer is #3, as this is a common problem in the immediate postoperative period after a lumbar laminectomy.

9. As you read the options, eliminate those you know are not correct. This will help narrow the field of choice. When you select an answer or eliminate an option, you should have a specific reason for doing so.

Example: *A 38-year-old client is in her third trimester of pregnancy; she is scheduled for a sonogram. The nurse explains to the client that results of this exam will reveal what information regarding the fetus?*

① Maturity of the fetus's lungs (No, sonogram does not show any evidence of surfactant or maturational level of the lungs.)

② Presence of congenital heart defect (No, sonogram is not specific enough for congenital heart).

③ Gestational age (Yes, sonogram gives overall picture of bone formation, thereby indicating gestational age.)

④ Rh factor antibody level (No, this does not occur until after birth.)

After systematically evaluating the options, option #3 is the correct answer.

10. Identify similarities in the options. Frequently the options will contain similar information but one will be different. The different one may be the correct answer.

Example: *Which foods would meet the requirement for a high protein, low residue diet?*

① Roast beef, slice of white bread.

② Fried chicken, green peas.

③ Broiled fish, green beans.

④ Cottage cheese, tomatoes.

Distracters #2, #3, and #4 all contain a vegetable that has a peeling and is high residue. The correct answer is #1, for both high protein and low residue. NCLEX does not focus on recipes that contain a mixture of foods that you wonder just how they made that dish. There are no special characteristics to the food, if it has a special characteristic it will be stated ("low sodium", or "low fat").

11. Select the most comprehensive answer. All of the options may be correct, but one may include the other three options or need to be considered first.

Example: *The nurse is planning to teach a diabetic client about his condition. Prior to the teaching, what is important for the nurse to evaluate?*

① Required dietary modifications.

② Understanding of the exchange list.

③ Ability to administer insulin.

④ Present understanding of diabetes.

Options #1, #2, and #3 are certainly important considerations in diabetic education. However, they cannot be initiated until the nurse evaluates the client's knowledge of his or her disease state. When two options appear to say the same thing, just in different words, than look for another answer. Options #1 and #2 both refer to the client's understanding of nutrition.

12. After you have selected an answer, reread the question. Does the answer you chose give the information the question is asking for? Sometimes the options are correct but do not give the information the question is asking for.

Example: *An 83-year-old client had a thoracotomy to repair his hiatal hernia. He is three days post-op with a temperature of 102°F. He is complaining of severe chest pain, and his cough is productive with thick yellow mucus. What measures should the nurse take to decrease the client's chest pain?*

① Encourage deep breathing and coughing.
② Teach him to take short, shallow breaths.
③ Support the incisional area with a pillow while he coughs.
④ Administer an analgesic and encourage him to remain in bed.

The question is asking for nursing measures to decrease chest pain. Option #1 is correct for the situation but would increase his chest pain. Option #2 will increase his pulmonary congestion. Option #4 will decrease his pain but will increase his congestion. Therefore, the correct answer is #3. After evaluating all of the distracters, the one that answers the question correctly, based on the situation, is #3. Always recheck your answer to make sure it provides the information requested.

13. Multiple-multiple-choice questions are not utilized on the examination. However, you will find questions in which the options contain several items to consider. After you are sure you understand what information the question is requesting, evaluate each part of the option. Is it appropriate to what the question is asking? If an option contains one incorrect item, the entire option is incorrect. All of the items listed in the option must be correct if it is to be the answer to the question.

Example: *In evaluating the lab data of a client in renal failure, the nurse would identify what findings as indicative of increasing renal failure?*

① Increased BUN, hyperkalemia, decreased creatinine clearance.
② Increased hemoglobin, hyponatremia, increased urine electrolytes.
③ High fasting blood glucose, increased prothrombin time.
④ Increased platelets, increased urine specific gravity, proteinuria.

In a methodical evaluation of the items in the options, you can eliminate items in options #2, #3, and #4. Therefore, option #1 is correct.

14. Multiple-choice mathematical computations will be included in the exam. Mathematical computations may include calculations of IV rate and drip factors; calculations of IM, PO, IV dosages; and conversion of units of measurement. You should be able to apply the appropriate formula to the situation. Some of the questions may call for two computations, as in a dosage question for which you must convert all items to one unit of measurement before calculating the dosage.

Example: *The doctor has ordered ampicillin 250 mg IM. Available is ampicillin 1 gm in 5 cc. How many cc would you administer?*

① 0.25 cc
② 1 cc
③ 1.25 cc
④ 1.5 cc

First, you must convert milligrams and grams to the same unit of measurement. Memorize the formulas necessary to calculate the information. Frequently these questions will contain options that are similar, making guessing hazardous. Correct answer is option #3.

THERAPEUTIC NURSING PROCESS: PRINCIPLES OF COMMUNICATION

Throughout the examination there will be questions requiring utilization of the principles of therapeutic communication. In therapeutic communication questions, don't assume the client is being manipulative, or is in control of how he feels. Psychosocial problems, or mental health problems are not under the conscious control of the client.

NCLEX ALERT: *Listening to a client's concerns and assessing a client's response to illness are two primary areas of the psychosocial component.*

✦ **Situations requiring utilization of therapeutic communication are not always centered around a psychiatric client.** Frequently these questions are centered around the client experiencing stress and anxiety. There will be questions relating to therapeutic communication in the care of clients experiencing stress and anxiety as a result of their physiological problems.

- **Look for responses that focus on the concerns of the client.** Do not focus on the concerns of the nurse, hospital, or of the physician.
- **Watch for responses that are open ended and encourage the client to express how he feels.** Clients frequently experience difficulty in expressing their feelings. Focus on responses that encourage the client to describe how he/she feels. These are frequently open ended statements by the nurse.
- **Eliminate responses that are not honest and direct.** In order to build trust and promote a positive relationship, it is important to be honest with the client. Telling the client "don't worry", or "everything is going to be all right",or "your doctor knows best" will be wrong answers.
- **Look for responses that indicate an acceptance of the client.** Regardless of whether his views or moral values agree with yours, you should respect and accept them. This is not the time to tell the alcoholic that he should quit drinking.
- **Be careful about responses that give opinions or advice on the client's situation.** Don't assume an authoritarian position, you should not insist that the client follow your advice.
- **Do not select responses that block further interaction.** These are frequently presented as closed statements, or encourage a yes or no answer from the client. "Did your family visit today", "Are you feeling anxious about what happened?"
- **Don't tell the client how he should or should not feel.** Look for responses that encourage the client to describe how he feels, response that reflect, restate, or paraphrase feelings expressed.
- **Look for responses that reflect, restate, or paraphrase feelings the client expressed.**
- **Don't ask "why" a client feels the way they do.** Frequently if they understood why they felt the way they do, they would be able to do something about it. The most common answer when a nurse asks a client why he feels this way is "I don't know" and that does not help anyone.
- **Do not use coercion to achieve a desired response.** Don't tell them they can't have their lunch until they get out of bed, or bribe a child to take his medicine by promising him candy.
- **See examples of therapeutic and non-therapeutic communication in Chapter 9.**

Testing Tips for Success

- **Do not indiscriminately change answers.** If you go back and change an answer, you should have a specific reason for doing so. Sometimes you do remember information and realize you answered the question incorrectly. Frequently, students "talk themselves out" of the correct answer and change it to the incorrect one.
- **Watch your timing. Do not spend too much time on one question.** It is very important you practice your timing on the practice exams. This will help you be more comfortable with timing on computer testing. The NCLEX will allow a total of 5 hours to complete the examination. You can plan for about a minute a question. Some questions you will answer quicker, others may take sometime. Don't spend more than 2 minutes on a question. If you don't have a good direction for the right answer in 2 minutes, then you probably don't know the answer. Pick the best one you can and move on. (Remember - you are not supposed to know all of the right answers.)
- **Remember the NCLEX is a nursing competency examination and the correct answer will focus on nursing knowledge and the provision of nursing care.** It does not focus on medical management or making a medical diagnosis.
- **Eliminate distracters that assume the client "would not understand," or "is ignorant" of the situation, or those distractions that "protect them from worry."** For example, "The client should not be told she has cancer because it would upset her too much."
- **There is no pattern of correct answers.** The exam is compiled by a computer, and the position of the correct answers is selected at random. So, don't believe those who say to pick answer C or #3 when you are guessing.

STUDY HABITS

- **Study effectively**

1. **Use memory aids, mind mapping, and mnemonics**. Memory aids and mind mapping are tools that assist in drawing associations from other ideas with the use of visual images (see Figure 1-1). Mnemonics are words, phrases, or other techniques that help you remember information. Images, pictures and mnemonics will

stay with you longer than just reading the information.

2. **Develop 3x5 cards with critical information.** Don't overload the card, put a statement or question on one side, and answers or follow up information on the other side. For example, on one side you might put "low potassium", on the back side you would put the values. Another card might be "nursing care for hypokalemia", on the back list the nursing care. These cards are much easier for you to carry than the load of books or notes. When you have developed your set of cards with priority information, trade them with a friend and see what is on their cards. These can be used whenever you have only 15-20 minutes of quick study time. Take about 20 cards with you to soccer practice, doctor's office, or anywhere you are going to have to sit and wait for a few minutes. This is quick and easy and very effective.
3. **Plan your study time when you are most receptive to learning.** Don't wait until the end of the day when you finish everything else. It is difficulty to get up at 6am, work all day, deal with family activities, and finally get some study time at 10pm.
4. **Set a schedule** - and let everyone know what the schedule. Don't expect your family to leave you alone while you study - this is frequently too much to ask of children and spouse. Go to the library, nursing school, someone's house where there are no disturbances.
5. **Start planning your review and study about 2-3 months prior to the NCLEX.** Do not wait until the week before the exam to start reviewing. Even if you were an "A" student, you need to review.

✦ **Set a study goal.**

1. Decide on a study method.
2. Divide the review material into segments.
3. Prioritize the segments; review first the areas in which you feel you are deficient and/or weak.
4. Identify areas which will require additional review in the review book and in a basic nursing textbook.
5. Establish a realistic schedule and follow it. Planning for 8 hours of studying on your day off does not work. Instead, plan for 2-4 hours each day, and may 4-6 hours on your days off
6. Plan on achieving your study goal several days prior to the examination.

✦ **Group study.**

1. Keep the group limited to four or five people.
2. Group members should be mature and serious about studying.
3. The group should agree on the planned study schedule.

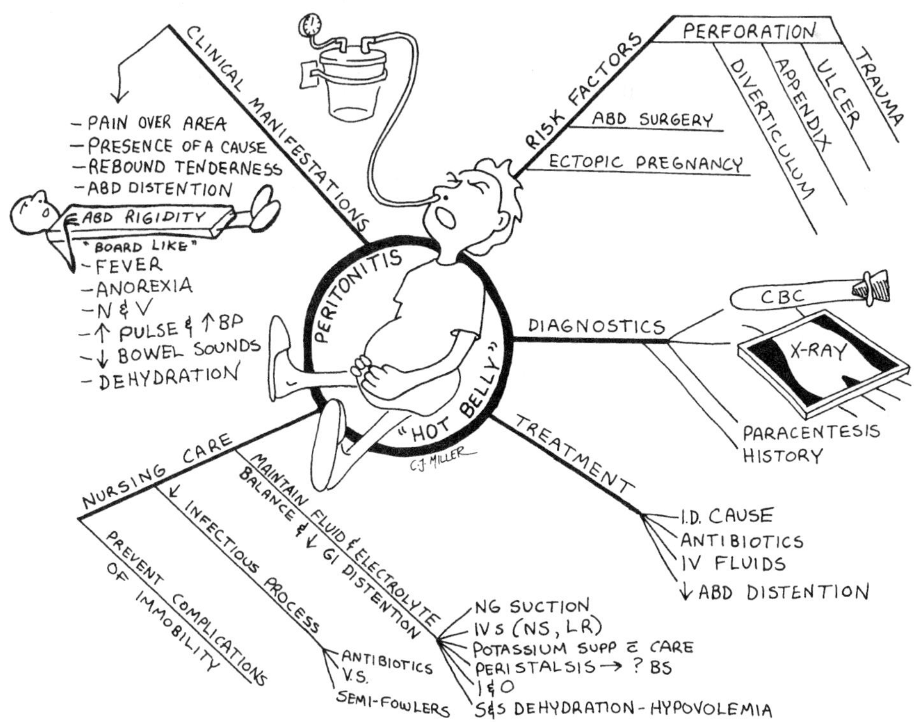

Figure 1-1: Peritonitis "Hot Belly"
Reprinted with permission: Zerwekh, J., Claborn, J., & Miller, C. (1994): Memory Notebook of Nursing, Dallas, TX: Nursing Education Consultants Publishing, Inc., pg. 85.

4. If the group makes you anxious or you do not feel it meets your study needs, do not continue to participate.

✦ **Testing practice.**

1. Include the testing practice in your schedule.
2. Plan for answering one question per minute. This will allow you to evaluate the pace of the exam and keep you on target with your timing as you practice answering test questions.
3. Try to answer the questions as if you were taking the real exam.
4. Utilize the testing strategies in the comprehensive practice test in the back of this book and on the computer disk.
5. Evaluate the practice exam for problem areas.
   a. Testing skills.
   b. Knowledge base.
6. Evaluate the questions you answer incorrectly. Review the rationale for the right answer and understand why you missed it.
7. Utilize the questions at a later point to review the information again.
8. There is a computer disk with additional practice questions in the back of the book. The more questions you practice, the better you will be able to implement your testing strategies.

DECREASE ANXIETY

Your activities the day of the examination strongly influence your level of anxiety. By carefully planning ahead, you will be able to eliminate some anxiety-provoking situations.

1. Visit the examination site prior to the day of the exam. Evaluate travel time, parking, and time to get to the designated area. Get an early start to allow extra time.
2. If you have to travel some distance to the examination site, try and spend the night in the immediate vicinity. Don't cram 4 or 5 people in one room. Each of you needs your own bed!
3. Do something pleasant the evening prior to the examination. This is not the time to "cram"
4. Anxiety is contagious. If those around you are extremely anxious, avoid contact with them prior to the examination.
5. Carefully evaluate if you want to go to the testing site with anyone else. If they finish before you do it will put increased pressure on you to hurry up and finish - you don't need that!
6. Make your meal before the test a light healthy one.
7. Avoid eating highly spiced or different foods. This is not the time for a gastrointestinal upset.
8. Wear comfortable clothes. This is not a good time to wear tight clothing or new shoes.
9. Wear clothing of moderate weight. It is difficult to control the temperature to keep everyone comfortable. Take a sweater or wear clothes that can be removed if you get too warm.
10. Wear soft-soled shoes; this decreases the noise in the testing area.
11. Make sure you have the "Authorization to Test" papers that are required to gain admission to the exam site. Don't forget your photo IDs.
12. Do not take study material to the exam site. You cannot take it into the exam area, and it is too late to study.
13. Do not panic when you encounter a clinical situation you have not heard of. Use good test-taking strategies, select an answer, and continue.
14. Reaffirm to yourself that you know the material. It is not time for any self-defeating behavior or self-talk. **YOU WILL PASS!!** Build your confidence by visualizing yourself in 6 months working in the area you desire. Create that mental picture of where you want to be and who you want to be-RN. Use your past successes to bring positive energy and "vibes" to your NCLEX exam. **WE KNOW YOU CAN DO IT!**

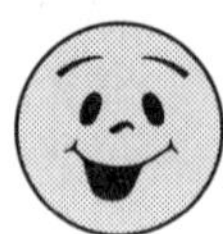

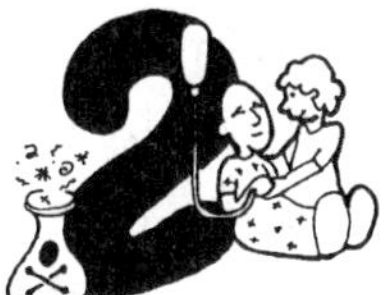

Growth and Development

Normal growth and development progresses in a steady predictable pattern across the life span. From birth to elderly, there are proportional physical change and sensory changes, as well as maturation and decline of systems, development of and loss of fine motor development.

When assessing the growth and development of the child and adult, it is important to consider the characteristics of the developmental stage and that development progresses cephalocaudal (head to tail), proximal to distal, and gross to fine motor skills.

Psychosocial development is also predictable and may be observed in a pattern across the years. The psychosocial, cognitive, moral and spiritual development can be observed to occur in specific patterns as an infant matures to an adult, then from adult to elderly. The developmental age of a client is critical to the planning of care in the hospital. When assessing infants, nurses need to be aware of the major developmental milestones. If an infant displays head lag at 6 months, or cannot sit with support at 9 months, they are demonstrating a significant developemntal lag and need to have further developmental/neurological evaluation.

NCLEX ALERT: *Compare a client's behavioral development to norms, modify approaches to care according to client's development stage; and plan anticipatory guidance for developmental transitions (e.g., puberty, retirement, etc.).*

Anticipatory Guidance for the Family of an Infant

1. Infant car seat, facing backwards.
2. Put the baby on his back or side to sleep.
3. Safety.
   a. Keep one hand on the baby when he is on a high surface - rolls over around 3-4 months.
   b. Never leave baby alone with young children or pets.
   c. Baby-proof home—stairs, cabinets, pool and tub water safety.
   d. Do not recommend use of an infant walker.
4. Immunization schedule.
5. Sibling jealousy.
6. Talk and read to infant, provides visual and auditory stimulation, toys should stimulate hand-eye coordination, as well as sensory stimulation.
7. Bottle tooth decay—do not put infant to bed with a bottle, offer juice in a cup.
8. Colds, fevers, and reaction to immunization—administer infant strength Tylenol for fever, increase fluids, no aspirin products.
9. Separation anxiety is a major stress on hospitalized children through middle infancy through the preschool years.
   a. Protest - loud crying and screaming for parent, refuse attention from anyone else.
   b. Despair - crying stops and there is less activity, child is not interested in play and withdraws.
   c. Detachment (denial) - child appears to have adjusted to hospitalization. Behavior is due to resignation, not a sign of contentment. This is not a positive reaction to hospitalization.

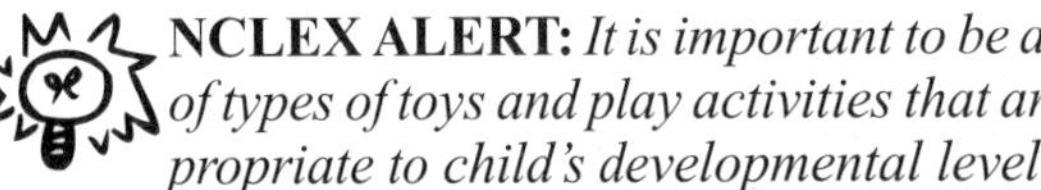

NCLEX ALERT: *It is important to be aware of types of toys and play activities that are appropriate to child's developmental level.*

Anticipatory Guidance for Family of a Toddler

1. Continue to emphasize safety - medications, poisons, car seats, latches on doors, falls.
2. Toilet training usually begins around 2 years, accidents are common.
3. Sibling rivalry is common if there is a new baby in the family.
4. Temper tantrums are attention seeking behavior and not uncommon for a toddler.
5. Need to start regular dental checkups.
6. Establish and maintain consistency in discipline.
7. Enjoys motion toys - pull toys, riding toys, wagons.
8. Finger paints, interlocking blocks, large piece puzzles increase fine motor skills.
9. May regress to previous level of development in time of stress, especially with potty training.
10. Has no concept of death, primary reaction is to separation and loss.
11. See separation anxiety under anticipatory guidance for the infant.

Anticipatory Guidance for Family of a Preschooler

1. Safety—car seat/seat belts, swimming pools, pedestrian and street safety skills, playgrounds.
2. Preschool activities - reading, puzzles, coloring large pictures. Toys include building blocks, cars, dolls.
3. Control time watching TV, screen programs for suitable viewing.
4. Encourage socialization with other children.
5. Household chores—picking up clothes, room, etc.
6. Structured learning environment—Mother's Day Out, Head Start, Sunday school.
7. School readiness (attention span, easy separation from mother)begins around 5 years.
8. Should know full name, address, by age 5.
9. Curious about fire, matches, firearms—keep articles locked.
10. Sees death as temporary and reversible, much like going to sleep. May view death as a punishment, fears the separation and abandonment.
11. Can tolerate brief periods of hospitalization, may trust other significant adults. Stress of illness may cause regression of previously attained levels of behavior and separation anxiety may become an issue.

Table 2-1: GROWTH AND DEVELOPMENT

Birth – 4 months	Consistently gains weight (5-7 oz per week) Posterior fontanel closes Responds to sounds and begins vocalizing Gains head control → lifts chest → rolls over one way Smiles responsively → smiles when spoken to	Teething may begin Coordination progresses from jerky movement to grasping objects Provide toys that increase hand-eye coordination.
4 – 9 months	Doubles birth weight (gains 3-5 oz per week) Teething begins with lower incisors Sits with support Turns over both directions Begins crawling	Reaches for objects and grasps them Begins "stranger anxiety" Begins vocalizing with single consonants Provide brightly colored toys that are easy to grasp. Enjoys noisemakers, and mirrors, plays pat-a-cake
9-12 months	Birth weight triples Head and chest circumference is equal Anterior fontanel begins to close Teething - has 6-8 teeth Sits alone → moves from prone to sitting position Crawling → pulling up → walks holding onto furniture	May stand alone Has developed crude to fine pincer grasp Transfers objects from one hand to another Recognizes own name Enjoys playing alone (solitary) Explores objects by putting them in the mouth.
Toddler (12 - 24 months)	50% of height at 2 years Exaggerated lumbar curve Mobile – walks/runs/jumps Walks up and down stairs-one foot at time. Begins using eating utensils Obeys simple commands Begins to develop vocabulary	Speech becomes understandable Thumbsucking may be at peak Solitary play at 12 months,parallel play at 18 months Beginning to develop bladder and bowel control Attention seeking behavior – temper tantrums Enjoys activities that provide mobility – riding vehicles, wagons, pull toys.
Preschool (3-5 years)	Birth length doubles at 4 years Coordination continues to improve Rides tricycle, throws a ball Walks stairs with alternating feet	Begins self care abilities Knows own name Good verbalization – talks about activities Plays "dress up", cars, dolls, grooming aids.
School Age (6-10 years)	Growth spurts begin Increasingly active Very concerned with body image Need for conformity – rules and ritual	Increasing importance of peer groups Plays with groups of same sex Competes for attention
Adolescence (11 -17 years)	Beginning and completing puberty Girls maturing earlier than boys Very conscious of changes in body Rapid growth	Move from concrete to abstract thinking Increased independence Strong peer group association Increased interest in opposite sex
Young Adult (18-30 years)	Physical maturity Full mental capacity Assumes responsibility for own learning Adult relationship with parents	Launches career Selects a mate, begins own family Begins involvement in community

Table 2-1: GROWTH AND DEVELOPMENT

Adult (30-60 years)	Physiological processes begin slow decline Cognitive skills peak Creativity at maximum Increase in community involvement Increase in concern for future of society	Family tasks Assist children to responsible adulthood Role reversal with aging parents Defines role of grandparenting
Older Adult (60 + years)	Decline of physiological status Demineralization of bones ↓ Cardiac output ↓ Respiratory vital capacity ↓ Glomerular filtration rate ↓ Serum albumin ↓ Glucose tolerance	Maintains reasoning ability and abstract thinking Thinking slows Restructure in family roles Retirement Reorganization of activities Continues with community involvement and politics

Anticipatory Guidance for the Family of a School Aged Child

1. Safety—water, seat belts, skateboard, bicycle.
2. Encourage good dental hygiene habits.
3. Encourage good eating habits.
4. Regular physical activity (group and team activities)—wear protective sports gear.
5. Encourage peer relationships and communication.
6. Maintain consistency in limit setting.
7. Parental role model—using seat belts, avoiding tobacco, eating properly, regularly exercising.
8. Teaching—avoid drugs, alcohol, and tobacco.
9. Age-appropriate sex education materials.
10. Injury prevention—around age 8-10 years may begin to engage in dangerous risk-taking (dares, smoking, drinking).
11. Develop independence—allowance, choice of when to complete household chores, tests rules and questions authority.
12. Avoid high noise levels, (e.g., music headsets).
13. Physical development and puberty changes may begin in the girls as early as 10 years.
14. Strong influence and dependence on peer group.
15. Spends less time with family.
16. In early childhood, begins to see death as irreversible, may interpret it as destructive, scary and/or violent.
17. Later childhood, views death as final and irreversible. May become interested in details regarding biological death and funerals.
18. The hospitalized child fears being away from the family, peers and usual activities. May exhibit feelings of loneliness, boredom, and feel isolated.

Anticipatory Guidance for the Family of an Adolescent

1. Establish realistic expectations for family rules.
2. Minimize criticism, nagging, derogatory comments, and demeaning comments.
3. Respect need for privacy.
4. Recognize positive behavior and achievement.
5. Establish clear limits; curfew, working.
6. Strive for independence from parents and acceptance by peers.
7. Begin to exhibit a mature understanding of death, may deny their own mortality by increase risk taking. May have difficulty coping with death of significant other.
8. Hospitalized adolescents may exhibit rejection, uncooperativeness, or withdrawal due to the loss of control. Are frequently labeled by care givers as difficult, unmanageable clients.

Anticipatory Guidance for Adolescent.

1. Learn techniques to protect self from physical, emotional, and sexual abuse, including rape.
2. Seek help if physically or sexually abused.
3. If sexually active, safe sex information, pregnancy prevention. (e.g., condoms, STDs, etc).
4. Avoid smoking, drugs, and alcohol.

Health Implications and Guidance for Adults and Older Adults

1. Assist to identify health care resources within their community.
2. Encourage health screening and regular physical examination.
3. Encourage health living style - exercise, good nutrition, decrease stress.
4. Response to hospitalization will reflect moral and cultural values.
5. Hospitalization causes increased stress due to family and job responsibilities, as well as threat to their well being.
6. Concepts of death follows common sequence:
   a. Shock, anger, denial, disbelief
   b. Development of an awareness, bargaining, may experience depression.

Box 2-1: Elderly Care Focus
Age- Related Factors Influencing Geriatric Care

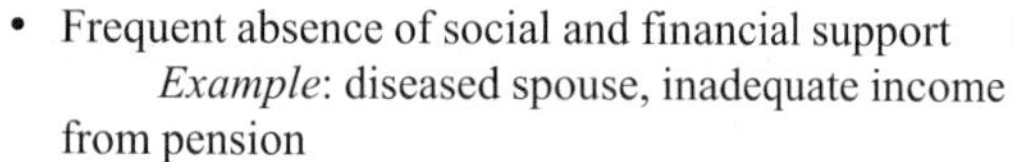

- Frequent absence of social and financial support
  Example: diseased spouse, inadequate income from pension
- Presence of significant concurrent illness
  Example: dementia, COPD, CHF, depression, diabetes
- Altered pain perception
  Example: increased incidence of referred pain.
- Impaired homeostatic mechanisms
  Example: increased problems with dehydration, incontinence, impaired defecation, altered immune status.
- Impaired mobility
  Example: dependent on walkers, need for bed transferring, use of transportation, may have Parkinsonism, degenerative joint disease
- Increased frequency of adverse reactions to drugs
- Impaired equilibrium, resulting in falls

c. Acceptance, reorganization, restitution.

7. Adults age 18 to 65 years tend to have an abstract and realistic concept of death.
8. Geriatric clients (65 and older) tend to have a more philosophical concept of death.

CHILDHOOD DISEASES

Varicella (Chicken pox)

Characteristics

1. Herpes virus—varicella zoster; highly contagious.
2. Maculopapular rash with vesicular scabs in multiple stages of healing.
3. Incubation period: 13-17 days.
4. Transmission: contact, airborne.
5. Communicability: 1-2 days before lesions appear to 4 days after 1st crop of vesicles.

Assessment

1. Prodromal: low grade fever, malaise.
2. Acute phase: red maculopapular rash which turns almost immediately to vesicles, each with an erythematous base; vesicles ooze and crust.
3. New crops of vesicles continue to form for 3-5 days spreading from trunk to extremities.
4. All three stages usually are present in varying degrees at one time; pruritus.
5. Complications: secondary infection may lead to sepsis, abscess, cellulitis, or Reye's syndrome.

Health Care Interventions

1. Preventive—varicella immunization (Table 2-2).
2. Skin care to decrease itching.
   a. Antihistamines, antipruritics, calamine lotion, and Tylenol.
   b. **Acyclovir** and/or zoster immune globulin within 3 days after exposure for immunosuppressed child.
   c. Cool baths without soap; or **Aveeno**.
   d. Paste of baking soda on lesions; no cornstarch.
3. Keep fingernails of child short; apply mittens.
4. Isolate from other children until vesicles have crusted.
5. Provide quiet activities to keep child occupied to lessen pruritus.
6. Avoid use of aspirin.
7. A vericella infection in the first trimester of pregnancy may cause serious birth defects.

Parotitis (Mumps)

Characteristics

1. An acute viral disease characterized by tenderness and swelling of one or both of the parotid glands and/or the other salivary glands.
2. Incubation period: 14-21 days.
3. Transmission: direct contact and droplet.
4. Communicability: one week before swelling and immediately after swelling begins.

Assessment

1. Prodromal: headache, fever, malaise.
2. Acute phase: Swelling of salivary glands (peaks in 3 days) leading to difficulty in swallowing, earache.
3. Complications:
   a. Postinfectious encephalitis.
   b. Meningoencephalitis.
   c. Orchitis, epididymitis.

Health Care Interventions

1. Preventive—mumps, measles, and rubella (MMR) immunization (Table 2-2).
2. Bed rest until swelling subsides.
3. Fluids and soft bland food.
4. Orchitis—warm or cold pack, light support to scrotum.
5. Hot or cold compresses to swollen neck area.

Rubeola (Measles, Hard measles, Red measles)

A. Characteristics.

1. An acute viral disease characterized by fever and a rash.
2. Incubation: 10 to 21 days.

3. Transmission: respiratory droplet and direct contact.
4. Communicability: 4 days before rash to 5 days after rash appears.

Assessment

1. Prodromal: fever, malaise, cold-like symptoms.
2. Koplik's spots—small, irregular red spots noticed on the buccal mucosa opposite the molars; usually appear two days prior to rash.
3. Acute phase: maculopapular rash begins on face and gradually spreads downward-head to feet.
4. Photophobia, conjunctivitis, and bronchitis.
5. Complications: otitis media, pneumonia, laryngotracheitis, and encephalitis.

Health Care Interventions

1. Preventive—MMR immunization (See Table 2-2).
2. Bed rest until fever subsides.
3. Dim lights to decrease photophobia.
4. Tepid baths and lotion to relieve itching.
5. Force fluids to maintain hydration, temperature may spike to 104° F two to three days after rash appears.

Rubella (German Measles, Three-Day Measles)

Characteristics

1. An acute, mild systemic viral disease that produces a distinctive three-day rash and lymphadenopathy.
2. Incubation: 14-21 days.
3. Transmission: contact, air, transplacentally.
4. Communicability: from up to 7 days before rash until 5 days after rash.

Assessment

1. Prodromal: low-grade fever, headache, malaise, and symptoms of a cold.
2. Rash first appears on face and spreads down to neck, arms, trunk, and then legs.
3. Diagnostics: rubella antibody titer; persistent titer of 1:8 usually indicates immunity.
4. Complications: teratogenic effect on fetus.

Nursing Intervention

1. Primarily symptomatic; bed rest until fever subsides.
2. Preventive—MMR immunization (See Table 2-2).
3. Pregnant woman should avoid contact with child who has rubella or who has recently received an MMR.

Roseola Infantum (Exanthema Subitum)

Characteristics

1. A common, acute benign viral infection usually occurring in infants and young children (ages 6 months to 3 years) characterized by a sudden onset of high temperature followed by a rash.
2. Incubation period: usually 5-15 days..
3. Transmission: unknown, probably air.
4. Communicability: unknown.

Assessment

1. Sudden onset of high temperature (103° to 106° F).
2. As fever drops, abrupt appearance of a maculopapular, nonpruritic rash which blanches or fades under pressure; disappears in 1-2 days.
3. Complications: febrile seizures.

Health Care Interventions

1. Symptomatic—tepid baths, offer fluids frequently, cool clothing.

Fifth's Disease (Erythema Infectiosum)

Characteristics

1. A common, benign viral infection which occurs without fever that is characterized by a "slapped cheek" rash appearance.
2. Incubation period: 7-14 days.
3. Transmission: probably respiratory and blood.
4. Communicability: uncertain, symptomatic outbreaks usually subside within 1 to 2 months after onset of rash.

Assessment

1. Rash appears in 3 stages.
   a. Erythema on face especially cheeks—gives a "slapped-cheek" appearance.
   b. Maculopapular red spots appear primarily on the upper and lower extremities; rash progresses from proximal to distal surfaces and may lasts 2-40 days; average 11 days.
   c. Rash generally subsides but may reappear if skin is irritated or traumatized by temperature changes, friction, exercise, or sunburn.
2. Complications: self-limited arthritis and arthralgia.

Health Care Interventions

1. Primarily symptomatic treatment.
2. Child is not isolated; may attend school.

Diphtheria

Characteristics

1. An infection caused by the *Corynebacterium diphtheriae.*
2. Incubation period: 3-6 days.
3. Transmission: direct contact, contaminated articles (fomites).
4. Communicability: variable, usually 2 weeks, but may be longer.

Assessment

1. Nasal discharge, anorexia, sore throat, low-grade fever.
2. Smooth, white or gray membrane over tonsillar region; hoarseness and potential airway obstruction.
3. Often tachypnea, dyspnea, strider, airway obstruction may occur if condition goes untreated.
4. Complications: myocarditis, neuritis.

Health Care Interventions

1. Maintain isolation from other children.
2. Antibiotic and IV diphtheria antitoxin are common medications.
3. Have tracheostomy set available.
4. Provide adequate humidification to allow for liquefaction of secretions.
5. Preventive—DPT immunization (See Table 2-2).

Pertussis (Whopping Cough)

Characteristics

1. An acute inflammation of the respiratory tract caused by the *Bordetella pertussis,* is most severe in children under 2 years of age.
2. Incubation period: 6 to 20 days, average 7 days.
3. Transmission: air droplet.
4. Communicability: highly contagious; greatest during the catarrhal stage before the onset of paroxysms of coughing.

Assessment

1. Catarrhal stage - upper-respiratory infection, fever.
2. Paroxysmal stage.
   a. Cough occurs primarily at night; consists of a series of short rapid coughs followed by a sudden inspiration that is a high-pitched, crowing sound or a "whoop".
   b. Cyanosis, bulging eyes, vomiting.
   c. Paroxysm of coughing may continue until thick mucous plug is expelled.
3. Convalescent stage -paroxysms of coughing are seen less frequently.
4. Diagnostics: culture and sensitivity of nasopharyngeal secretions—identification of organism.
5. Complications: pneumonia, atelectasis, convulsions.

Health Care Interventions

1. Respiratory isolation during catarrhal stage, maintain bed rest as long as fever is present.
2. Administer pertussis immune globulin and antibiotic therapy (erythromycin) to kill organism.
3. Provide oxygen, humidification and observe for signs of increasing respiratory distress.
4. Avoid environmental precipitants of paroxysms of coughing—cold air, smoke, dust, etc.
5. Maintain nutrition by small frequent feedings: O_2, or IV therapy as required.
6. Avoid cough suppressants and sedatives.

Tetanus (Lockjaw)

Characteristics

1. An acute, very serious, potentially fatal disease characterized by muscle spasms and convulsions due to the anaerobic gram-positive bacillus, *Clostridium tetani.*
2. Incubation period: generally from 2 days to 2 months, average is 10 days.
3. Transmission: through a puncture wound that is contaminated by soil, dust, or excreta that contains *Clostridium tetani*, or by way of burns and minor wounds (e.g., infection of the umbilicus of a newborn).

Assessment

1. Progressive stiffness and tenderness in the muscles of the neck and jaw (trismus or lockjaw).
2. Progressive involvement of trunk muscles causes opisthotonos positioning.
3. Paroxysmal contractions occur in response to stimuli (noise, touch, light).
4. Client remains alert; mental status not affected.
5. Complications: laryngospasm and tetany of the respiratory muscle cause contractions that may precipitate atelectasis and pneumonia.

Health Care Interventions

1. Preventive.
   a. Careful cleansing and debridement of wounds.
   b. Immunization—DPT (See Table 2-2).
   c. Stress importance of maintaining active immunization—booster dose tetanus toxoid every 10 yrs.

2. Administration of tetanus immune globulin (TIG) and/or tetanus antitoxin for temporary immunity and protection.
3. Maintain seizure precautions—quiet, nonstimulating environment, monitor VS, muscle tone, etc.

Poliomyelitis

Characteristics

1. An acute, contagious disease affecting the central nervous system.
2. Incubation period: 5 to 35 days; with an average of 7 to 14 days.
3. Transmission: contact (fecal-oral), pharyngeal-oropharyngeal contact.
4. Communicability: virus in throat for 1 week after onset, in feces intermittently for 4-6 weeks.

Assessment

1. Abortive or inapparent type.
   a. Fever, sore throat, headache, malaise, nausea, vomiting, abdominal pain.
   b. Lasts a few hours to a few days.
2. Nonparalytic type—same symptoms as abortive but more severe, with pain and stiffness in the neck, back and legs.
3. Paralytic type—Initial symptoms are similar to nonparalytic poliomyelitis, followed by recovery then signs of CNS paralysis.

Health Care Interventions

1. Preventive—inactivated polio virus vaccine (IPV) (See Table 2-2).
2. Bed rest during acute phase.
3. Assess for complications, teach family early signs of respiratory distress—respiratory assisted ventilation may be necessary due to paralysis.
4. Physical therapy for muscles after acute stage.

Scarlet Fever (Scarletina)

Characteristics

1. Group A *beta-hemolytic streptococcal* infection that occurs most commonly in children ages 2 to 10; often follows acute streptopharyngitis, impetigo, or even a superficial wound infection.
2. Incubation period: 1-7 days, average 3 days.
3. Transmission: direct contact, or droplet.
4. Communicability: variable, approximately 10 days.

Assessment

1. Sudden onset of high fever.
2. Enlarged edematous tonsils covered with exudate, nausea, vomiting, and "strawberry" tongue.
3. Diffuse, fine erythematous rash that blanches on pressure and resembles a sunburn with goose bumps; rash is more intense in folds and joints, but is often absent on the face.
4. Desquamation of the skin which usually begins by end of first week, and is often seen on the palms and the soles of the feet during the convalescent period.
5. Diagnostics: history of a recent streptococcal infection, positive antistreptolysin—O (ASO titer), and a positive throat culture of group A *beta-hemolytic streptococci*.
6. Complications: otitis media, tonsillar abscess, glomerulonephritis.

Health Care Interventions

1. started
2. Administration of a full course of penicillin (or
3. erythromycin in penicillin-sensitive children).
4. Administration of antipyretics and anesthetic throat sprays or gargles to relieve sore throat.
5. Encourage fluids to prevent dehydration during febrile phase.
6. Assess for or teach family to observe for early symptoms of complications.

Infectious Mononucleosis

Characteristics

1. An acute, self-limiting infectious disease caused by the Epstein-Barr virus (EBV); member of the herpes group viruses, occurring most often among young persons between the ages of 12 and 25 years of age; often called the "Kissing Disease".
2. Incubation period: 2 to 6 weeks.
3. Transmission: direct intimate contact; probably oral pharyngeal route.

Assessment

1. Onset of symptoms occurs any time 10 days to 6 weeks following exposure—may be acute or insidious.
2. Malaise, sore throat, fever with generalized lymphadenopathy.
3. Diagnostic: a positive heterophil antibody test (titer of 1-160 is considered diagnostic), positive Monospot test.
4. Complications: hepatic involvement, otitis media, in severe cases cardiac and neurologic involvement.

Health Care Interventions

1. Bed rest, anesthetic throat gargles, antipyretics.

2. Provide adequate nutrition—soft foods, fluids.
3. Penicillin—to prevent secondary beta-hemolytic strep infections.

POISONING

General Principles (Acronym SIRES)

A. Stabilize the client's condition.
   1. Assess the condition and provide respiratory support, obtain IV access site.
   2. Terminate the exposure of the toxic substance—remove pills from mouth, flush eyes, remove contaminated clothing, etc.

B. Identify the toxic substance.
   1. Obtain accurate history and retrieve any available poison.
   2. Notify local poison control center, emergency facility, or physician for immediate care and advice regarding treatment.

C. Remove the substance to decrease absorption.
   1. Shower or wash off substance—radioactive substances.
   2. Antidotes—for heroin or drug overdose.
   3. Ingested substances—emesis, lavage, absorbents (activated charcoal) or cathartics.

D. Eliminate the substance from the client's body.
   1. Induce emesis by administering syrup of ipecac or apomorphine.
   2. Emesis is contraindicated:
      a. If a person is comatose, in severe shock, convulsing or has lost the gag reflex.
      b. If person has ingested low-viscosity hydrocarbons or strong corrosive (acid or alkaloid) substances.

E. Support the client both physically and psychologically.
   1. If intentional overdose or suicide attempt, refer for psychiatric evaluation.
   2. If accidental poisoning with a child, parents often demonstrate guilt, and self-reproach in regard to their parenting role.

Salicylate Poisoning

A. Toxic dose levels: 4.4 grains per kilogram of body weight. For a 30 lb. child (13.6 kg), 12 adult aspirin, or 48 baby aspirin would be toxic.

B. Toxic amounts affect the respiratory center with direct stimulation of the medulla resulting in hyperventilation, loss of carbon dioxide, and precipitating respiratory alkalosis.

C. In severe toxic overdose, there is also an increase in the metabolic activity, this results in an increased consumption of oxygen; increased temperature, and increased production of carbon dioxide. Metabolic acidosis eventually occurs as a result of the change in body processes.

D. Chronic overdose causes a deficiency in platelets leading to bleeding tendencies.

E. Assessment
   1. Clinical manifestations.
      a. Hyperventilation, respiratory alkalosis.
      b. Nausea, vomiting.
      c. Increased temperature.
      d. Tinnitus.
      e. Altered consciousness.
      f. Metabolic acidosis (severe toxicity).
      g. Seizures (severe toxicity).
      h. Diaphoresis and dehydration.
      i. Oliguria
   2. Diagnostics.
      a. Serum salicylate level.
      b. Electrolytes.
      c. Signs of mild salicylate toxicity.
         (1) Ringing in the ears.
         (2) Dizziness.
         (3) Hearing and visual problems.
         (4) Nausea, vomiting, diarrhea.
         (5) Delirium and sweating.

Treatment

1. Induce vomiting with syrup of ipecac or gastric lavage followed by administration of activated charcoal.
2. Administer vitamin K to decrease bleeding tendencies.
3. IV fluids and sodium bicarbonate to treat the acidosis.
4. In severe cases hemodialysis.

Nursing Intervention

✦ *Goal: to provide initial stabilization of the child.*

1. Decrease absorption of salicylate by administering syrup of Ipecac— second dose may be necessary to induce vomiting in children over 1 year. Take precautions to prevent aspiration when using Ipecac.
2. Administer activated charcoal to reduce systemic absorption. Dose of charcoal should be 10X the amount of drug ingested, frequently difficult to get this amount down the child.
3. Administer a cathartic (magnesium sulfate) with charcoal, to hasten elimination of the drug.

Table 2-2: RECOMMENDED CHILDHOOD IMMUNIZATION SCHEDULE — January -December 2002
The shaded areas indicate the acceptable ages for the immunizations.

Vaccine	Birth	1 mos	2 mos	4 mos	6 mos	12 mos	15 mos	18 mos	4-6 yrs	11-12 yrs	14-18 yrs
Hepatitis B	Hep B-#1										
		Hep B-#2			Hep B-#3						
Diphtheria, tetanus, pertussis			DTaP	DTaP	DTaP		DTaP		DTaP	Td	
H.influenzae type b			Hib	Hib	Hib	Hib					
Polio			IPV	IPV	IPV				IPV		
Pneumococcal			PCV	PCV	PCV	PCV					
Measles, mumps, rubella						MMR			MMR		
Varicella zoster virus vaccine						Var					

Source: Adapted from the Centers for Disease Control and Prevention, Advisory Committee on Immunization Practices (ACIP), Recommended childhood immunization schedule, United States, www.cdc.gov/nip/recs/child-schedule.

NCLEX ALERT: *Apply principles of infection control, evaluate client's immunization status.*

4. Ongoing assessment of VS, LOC, and measure urine output.

✦ *Goal: to prevent salicylate poisoning and provide teaching to family.*

1. Educate family regarding safe storage of medications— childproof caps, locked medicine cabinets, etc.
2. Teach parents to read labels on medications; frequently other medications contain salicylate.
3. Parents need to be told that activated charcoal will cause the child's stool to be black.

Acetaminophen Poisoning

A. Range of toxicity in children is 140 mg/kg, or blood level of 150 mg/ml four hours after ingestion.

B. Primary toxic effects are on the liver.

C. No known antidote.

Assessment

1. Clinical manifestations - 4 stages.
   a. Stage 1 (2-4 hours).
      (1) Nausea and vomiting.
      (2) Sweating and pallor
   b. Stage 2 Latent stage 24-36 hours, child improves.
   c. Stage 3 Hepatic involvement
      (1) Right, upper quadrant pain.
      (2) Coagulation defects.
      (3) Jaundice.
   d. Stage 4 recovery if hepatic damage is not severe.
2. Treatment.
   a. Emesis with ipecac at home or activated charcoal in hospital.
   b. N-acetlycysteine (NAC) if the blood levels are toxic.

Nursing Intervention

See Salicylate poisoning.

Lead Poisoning

❑ **An acquired condition (also known as plumbism) in which blood levels of lead are above normal, causing damage first in the hematologic system (disruption of heme synthesis leading to a microcytic, hypochromic anemia), the renal system is less often damaged in children then in adults (damages cells of proximal tubules). Neurological**

system (irreversible damage, causing a fluid shift which results in increased ICP, ischemia, and cellular destruction).

A. Etiology: Ingestion of lead from hand to mouth and lead contaminated dust, eating off of improperly glazed glassware (leaded glass) or Mexican pottery.

B. Increased risk in children because they absorb 40-50% of lead, while adults absorb only 5-10%.

Assessment

1. Clinical manifestations.
   a. Initially are non-specific GI disturbances.
   b. Advanced stage.
      (1) Encephalopathy.
      (2) Drowsiness.
      (3) Ataxia.
      (4) Seizures.
   c. Chronic stage.
      (1) Brain damage.
      (2) Poor school performance.
      (3) Delayed development.
      (4) Blue lead line on gums and "lead lines" on X-rays of the long bones.
2. Diagnostics.
   a. Blood lead blood (BLL) level of 20-44 mg/dL.
   b. Elevated erythrocyte protoporphyrin (EP).

Treatment

1. Chelating agents to prevent absorption and aid in excretion by the kidneys.
   a. Calcium disodium edetate (CaEDTA)—deep IM, frequently used with BAL, do not give in absence of adequate urine output.
   b. Dimercaprol (BAL)—IM, is used in conjunction with CaEDTA for cases of severe toxicity.
   c. Succimer (Chemet) - 10mg/kg, 3x day for 5 days.

Nursing Intervention

✦ *Goal: to identify lead poisoning and assist with the elimination of lead from the body.*

1. Identify high-risk groups related to children who are involved in pica or environment containing old lead based paint.
2. Administer chelating agents and assist with the planning of rotation injection sites for the child (as many as 12 injections may be given daily for 5-7 days).
3. Encourage high fluid intake.

✦ *Goal: to educate parents and child as to the nature of the disease and provide teaching to maintain homeostasis.*

1. Educate parents as to the dangers and sources of lead ingestion.
2. Assist parents to identify measures to prevent occurrence or recurrence of the problem.

LONG-TERM CARE

❑ **Long-term care includes those services provided in institutional settings, such as a nursing home, rehabilitation center, or adult day care program *after the acute phase of the illness* has passed. Often involves restorative care for clients with chronic health care problems.**

A. Types of long-term care facilities.

1. Nursing home—provides services ranging from maintenance to restorative care with skilled nursing, use of certified nursing assistants (CNAs), LPNs, and RNs.
2. Adult day care home—client lives at home during the evening and night and spends the day in a facility that provides a range of care from skilled nursing to restorative care.
3. Hospice care—end of life care provided in both the home and in-patient care settings.
   a. Does not institute life support by extraordinary means.
   b. Emphasis on pain control for client and support of family members through dying process.
4. Respite care—a type of short-term care for the primary care giver (often a family member) to give him/her a rest from the daily responsibilities of taking care of the long-term client.
5. Rehabilitation center—facility that provides multiple services for the client and family to make adjustments to daily living. Assists the client to achieve as much independence as possible in activities of daily living.
6. Home care—nursing care is provided in the home to clients who do not need hospitalization, but do need additional assistance with medical problems.
7. Adult housing or assisted living centers—places where clients can live under minimal supervision; meals and other services are offered to the residents.

CHRONIC HEALTH CARE

❑ **A chronic illness may be defined as an illness or condition that is present for more than three months in a year and interferes with daily function and lifestyle. As medical technology continues**

to increase the life span of individuals with chronic illnesses, there is an increase in the nurse's role to provide initial health care and to assist in planning, as well as providing long term care.

NCLEX ALERT: *Help client and significant others to adjust to role changes; assess a family's emotional reaction to a client's illness; determine ability of family/support system to provide care for client.*

Nursing Considerations

A. The majority of clients with extended health care needs are suffering from at least two chronic health conditions. These conditions may or may not be interrelated.

B. The focus of care for chronically ill clients is on assisting them to control their disease and manage their lifestyle.

1. Prevention and management of medical crises.
2. The control of disease symptoms, which may focus on pain control and comfort measures.
3. The implementation of the prescribed therapeutic regimens.
4. Psychosocial implications and adjustment of lifestyle; frequently requires dealing with social isolation.
5. Adjustments of lifestyle as disease and/or condition changes.
6. Financial strain to pay for medical care and supplies.
7. Coping with strain on marriage and on family structure.

C. The majority of clients with chronic health care needs are over 65 years old. The developmental level of these individuals, according to Erickson, is ego integrity vs despair. The feeling of powerlessness is not uncommon in the elderly.

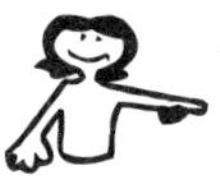

NURSING PRIORITY: *In planning home health care for a client with a chronic disease, it is very important to assist the client to maintain control over his condition and his lifestyle. Frequently, health care providers and family tend to take control of the situation and further the feeling of powerlessness in the individual.*

Chronically Ill Pediatric Client

The diagnosis of a child's chronic illness is a major situational crisis in the family. Support systems, perception of the problem, and coping mechanisms will ultimately determine the resolution of the crisis.

A. Focus care on the child's developmental age rather then the chronological age. Emphasis should be made on the child's strengths rather the on the child's disabilities.

B. Assist the child and the family to return to or establish a normal pattern of living.

C. Promote the child's maximum level of growth and development. Current trend is to return the child to the academic environment with his peer group.

D. Assess the family response to the child's illness and evaluate for parental overprotection. Overprotection by the parents prevents the child from developing self-esteem, independence, and self-control over disease and ADLs. Observe for the following parental characteristics.

a. Inconsistency with discipline; discipline often differs from that of the other children in the family.

b. Attempts to protect the child from every discomfort, both physical and psychosocial. Frequently, restricts play with peers for fear of injury and/or rejection by peers.

c. Makes decisions for the child without involving the child.

d. Does not allow the child the opportunity to learn self care; Frequently, afraid the child cannot handle the requirements for self-care (e.g., encouraging and assisting the diabetic child to become responsible for administration of his own insulin).

e. Continues to do things for the child, even when the child is capable of doing for himself.

f. Self-sacrifice and isolation of family from social interactions.

NCLEX ALERT: *Determine the needs of family regarding ability to provide home care after discharge. A pediatric situation may contain questions regarding the parents' or family response to the child's chronic illness.*

It is frequently the nurse who assesses the family and the client regarding their immediate needs. The appropriateness of the nurse's response depends on the nurse/client/family relationship and the environment. Priorities of care must be established, with goals and nursing interventions to meet the client's immediate health care needs. It is difficult in an acute care environment to even attempt to meet long term needs of the client and his family. It is important to assist them to identify community resources and the availability of counseling and home health care in order to meet the ever changing needs the client and his family will encounter in dealing with a chronic health condition.

REHABILITATION

NCLEX ALERT: *Determine client's ability to perform self-care (ADLS, hygiene, resources); plan with client to meet self-care needs.*

❑ ***Rehabilitation*** **means the restoration of an individual to his optimum level of functioning. This includes physical, mental, social, vocational, and economic parameters.**

A. Rehabilitation: term used when an individual has lost functional ability due to illness or injury.

B. Habilitation: term used to refer to congenital problems or deficiencies.

Goals of Rehabilitation

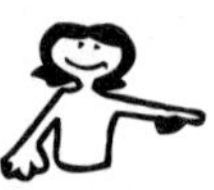

NURSING PRIORITY: *Rehabilitation is an area that affects all levels of nursing care. A primary goal in planning any client's care is to prevent complications.*

In order for the rehabilitation client to achieve the highest level of productivity, the rehabilitation process must begin when the condition becomes evident, or when the disease is diagnosed.

A. Prevention of deformities and complications.
   1. Maintain function and prevent deterioration of unaffected organs or areas.
   2. Prevent further injury to affected area or organ.
   3. Prevent or reduce complications of immobility.

B. Assist client to perform his activities of daily living (ADL) with minimum or no assistance, depending on his or her level of disability.

   Examples of ADLs: eating, dressing, bathing.

C. Assist client with independent activities of daily living (IADL).

   Examples of IADLs: shopping for groceries, paying bills, lawn care.

D. Promote continuity of care when the client is discharged or transferred.
   1. Plan with other rehabilitation team members in determining appropriate placement.
   2. Assist client and family through the transitional process.

NCLEX ALERT: *Client needs to be actively involved in setting goals for his care.*

Psychological Responses to Disability

Not every client will progress through all stages of grief in an orderly fashion. Clients will fluctuate between emotional crises.

A. Initial responses of confusion, disorganization, and denial represent a state of internal conflict..

B. A period of depression may occur as the client mourns for the loss or change in body function.

C. An anger stage may occur as client projects blame and hostility on family and health care providers.

D. Adaptation and adjustment will come as the client begins to redirect his or her energy toward coping with the disability.

E. New situations (going home, new job, etc.) may precipitate emotional outbursts and trauma.

F. Some clients will refuse to accept their disability and will not put forth any effort to adapt to everyday living.

HOME HEALTH CARE

❑ **The provision of health care to clients in the home environment.**

A. Levels of home health care.
   1. Intensive—clients with serious health care problems requiring the expertise of skilled nursing care.
   2. Intermediate—clients with stable health care problems who require professional level of care to promote rehabilitation through restorative nursing.
   3. Maintenance—assistance with ADLs; the underlying health care problem is stable.

B. Guidelines for home health care personnel.
   1. Respect client's religious, cultural, and ethnic background.
   2. As a care giver/guest in the client's home, your behavior should reflect sensitivity to the client and family —a pleasant attitude and sense of humor are helpful.
   3. Develop family members and significant others as your advocates.

Table 2-3: VITAMINS AND MINERALS

Name	Function	Food Sources	Nursing Implications
Vitamins - Fat Soluble			
Vitamin A Retinol	Vision adaptation, night vision, normal bone and tooth formation	liver, whole milk, egg yolk, yellow/green vegetables	If child eats excessive amounts of yellow vegetables, he will develop yellow skin color. Important in preterm infants. Children with reduced fat absorption may have deficiency (CF, hepatitis, etc.)
Vitamin D Cholecalciferol	Promotes normal absorption of calcium and phosphorus	Fish, direct sunlight, , enriched foods - milk products, cereals	May need supplement in breast fed babies. Expose infant to short periods of mild sunlight.
Vitamin E Tocopherol	Production of normal red blood cells, antioxident	Milk, meat, egg yolk, whole grains, legumes, spinach, broccoli	Preterm infant may need supplement
Vitamin K Aqua-mephyton	Necessary for production of clotting factors	Pork, liver, green leafy vegetables, tomatoes, egg yolks, cheese	Administer prophylactically to newborns. Intake may be decreased in clients receiving warfarin and dicumarol anticoagulants.
Vitamins - Water Soluble			
Vitamin B_1 Thiamine	Necessary for healthy nervous system; coenzyme for carbohydrate metabolism	Pork, beef, legumes, whole grains, enriched cereals, green vegetables	Clients with increased metabolic rate need increased B_1 - fever, pregnancy, long term IV therapy. Increase intake in alcoholic clients.
Vitamin B_6 Pyridoxine	Stimulates heme production for red cells, necessary for antibody formation	Organ meats, wheat and corn cereal grains, soybeans, tuna, chicken, salmon	Be aware of drug induced deficiencies - isoniazid, oral contraceptives.
Vitamin B_{12} Cobalamin	Formation of normal red cells, nerve function.	Meat, liver, fish, poultry, milk, eggs, cheese,	Supplement necessary for clients with gastric resection, must have intrinsic factor for normal absorption.
Vitamin C Ascorbic acid	Increases absorption of iron for hemoglobin formation, necessary for collagen formation, antioxidant.	Citrus fruits, tomatoes, strawberries, potatoes, cabbage, broccoli, melons, spinach	Cook vegetables with a lid and minimum water added. Clients on aminoglycocides, and anticoagulants need increased intake. Increased need during growth, or conditions which cause an increase in metabolism.
Minerals			
Iron (Fe)	Normal formation of hemoglobin, essential part of enzymes	Liver - pork, beef; red meat, poultry, beans, whole grains, enriched infant formula, enriched cereals and bread	Administer iron between meals, administer with Vit.C, avoid use of antacids, stool will be black. Increase iron intake with iron deficiency anemias - vegetarian diets, pregnancy, excessive milk consumption in infants.
Calcium (Ca)	Normal formation of bone and teeth, muscle contraction - especially the heart, clotting factors, normal nerve conduction	Dairy products, egg yolk, dark green leafy vegetables (except spinach).	Adequate intake for normal bone and teeth formation. Administer IV preparations with caution due to effects on heart. Increase supplements during pregnancy, lactation, and after menopause.
Potassium (K)	Acid base balance, nerve conduction, cardiac muscle contraction.	Dried fruits, bananas, citrus fruits.	Supplement when client is on diuretics. Decreased potassium increases effects of digitalis.
Sodium (NA)	Acid base balance, fluid balance.	Table salt, prepared foods	Sodium deficiency is rare, focus is on decreasing intake except in situation with high sodium loss - CF, diaphoresis.

Figure 2-1: Food Pyramid

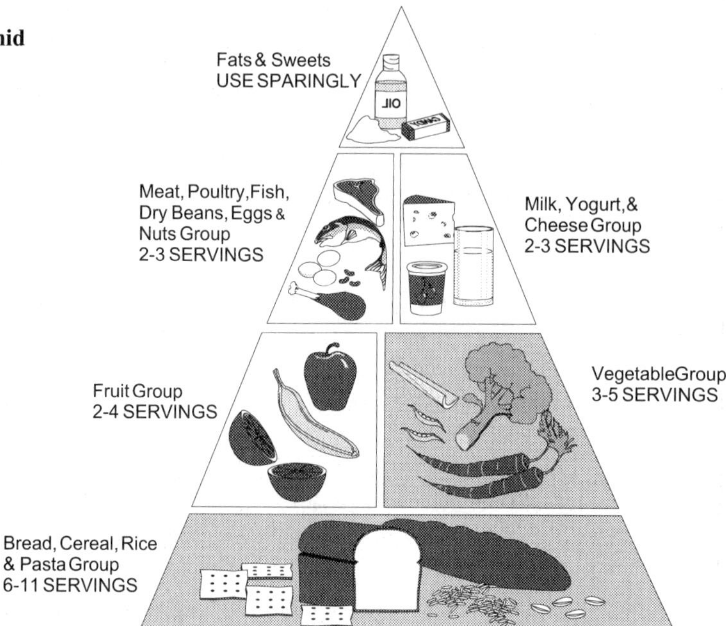

The Food Pyramid emphasizes foods from the five food groups shown in the three lower sections of the pyramid.

Each of these food groups provides some, but not all, of the nutrients you need.

Foods in one group can't replace those in another.

No one food group is more important than another - for good health, you need them all.

4. Communication with other health team members is vital to the maintenance of the client's well-being.
5. Working with more autonomy without immediate hospital support is challenging and requires an increased level of nursing competence for decision making.
6. A Patient Bill of Rights is applicable in the home health setting, (i.e., client has right to disclosure of information concerning his condition and care and has the right to refuse or stop treatment, etc).

NUTRITION

NCLEX ALERT: *Monitor client's nutritional and hydration status.*

DIETARY CONSIDERATIONS THROUGHOUT THE LIFE SPAN

Infant

NURSING PRIORITY*: a newborn infant will lose weight for the first few days, but should not lose more than 10% of its birth weight or take longer than 10-14 days to regain it.*

1. Growth.
   a. Birth weight triples at 1 year.
   b. Infant gains only another 4-6 lbs. until 2 years old.

Example: Birth weight 7½ lbs.; at 4 months 14 lbs.; another 7½ lbs. will be added in the next 8 months.

2. Diet.
   a. Ideal food is breast milk, because it is nutritionally superior to alternatives.
   b. Breast fed infants do not need additional water.

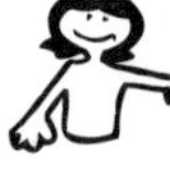

NURSING PRIORITY: *Newborn has a higher fluid requirement in relation to body size than the adult.*

   c. Whole cow's milk, low fat cow's milk or imitation milks are not recommended for infants less then 12 months old.
   d. Cereal, usually rice is the first solid food introduced, recommended around age 6 months. If child is not satisfied with formula, cereal may be introduced earlier.
   e. Strained vegetables and fruits are introduced one at a time to determine infant's tolerance of food.
   f. Chopped foods are introduced at 6-9 months.

NURSING PRIORITY: *Breast-fed infants grow at a slower rate than formula-fed infants.*

   g. Formula consumption.
      (1) 1 month old - up to 22 ounces per day
      (2) 4 month old - up to 30 ounces per day
      (3) 6 months old - up to 28 ounces per day, solid foods are introduced.

Table 2-4: THERAPEUTIC MEAL PLANS

Diet	Purpose/ Use	Foods Allowed	Foods Restricted
Clear Liquid	To begin introduction of food after removal of N/G tube or after GI surgery	Liquids that are clear.	Milk products, juice with pulp, any solid food.
Full Liquid	To begin introduction of food , used after removal of N/G tube or after GI surgery	Any food that is liquid at room temperature	Any solid food
Soft Diet	To progress diet as tolerated, should be easy to chew, and swallow.	Soft, tender foods easy to swallow and digest	Highly seasoned foods, whole grains, fruits, vegetables, nuts, fried foods.
Mechanical Soft Diet	To assist clients who cannot chew effectively	Soft foods easy to chew and to swallow.	Tough foods that are difficult to swallow
Bland Diet	To eliminate foods irritating to the digestive system. Used in clients after GI surgery, peptic ulcer disease, GI inflammatory problems.	Milk, custards, refined cereals, creamed soups, potatoes (baked or broiled). All foods are white – no bright colored food.	Highly seasoned or strong flavored foods. Tea, colas, coffee, fruits, whole grains, raw fruit
Low Residue Diet	Decrease fiber or stool in GI tract. Acute episodes of enteritis, diverticulitis, diarrhea; after GI surgery	Clear liquids, meats, fats, eggs, refined cereals, white bread, peeled white potatoes, small amount milk.	Cheeses, whole grains, raw fruits and vegetables, foods that are high carbohydrate are usually high in residue and fiber.
High Residue Diet	Prevent constipation and acute diverticulitis	Raw fruits and vegetables, whole grains; high carbohydrate foods are high in residue and fiber.	Undigestible fibers – celery, whole corn; seeds such as sesame and poppy, foods with small seeds.
Lactose Free Diet	Used for lactose intolerance	Non milk products, yogurt	Milk and milk products, processed foods may have dried milk as filler.
PKU Diet	To control intake of phenylalanine, an essential acid Affected children cannot metabolize it.	Specially prepared infant formula if not breastfed. Vegetables, fruits, juices, some cereals, and breads. May allow 20-30mg phenylalanine per kg body weight to maintain normal growth needs.	Most high protein foods – meat and dairy products are significantly reduced.
Low Fat/Low Cholesterol Diet	Gall bladder spasms, increased cholesterol, or malabsorption of fat	Skimmed or low fat milk, fruits, vegetables, breads, cereals, reduced amount of red meat.	Egg yolks, whole milk, fried foods, processed cheese, shrimp, avacados.
Low Sodium Diet	Reduce sodium intake to decrease body retention of fluids. Especially in cardiac and or hypertensive clients.	Salt free preparations, fresh fruits, vegetables with no added salt.	Processed foods, smoked or salted meats, prepared foods, frozen/canned vegetables.
High Potassium Diet	Clients on diuretics and/or digitalis, replaces lost potassium	Dried fruits, fruit juices, fresh fruits - bananas, apricots, grapefruit, oranges, and tomatoes	No specific restrictions.
Renal Diet	Control potassium (K), sodium (Na) and protein in clients with renal problems.	High biologic protein (limited intake) – eggs, milk, meat; decreased Na products, and decreased K (cabbage, peas, cucumbers are low K).	High potassium foods, high sodium foods (processed foods), salt substitutes with high potassium.
Low Purine	To decrease serum levels of uric acid used in clients with gout, kidney stones.	Vegetables, fruits, cereals, eggs, fat free milk, cottage cheese.	Glandular meats, fish, poultry, nuts,beans, oatmeal, whole wheat, cauliflower.
Acid Ash Alkaline Ash	Used to prevent formation of renal stones by promoting acid urine.	Meats, cereals, eggs, corn, cranberries, prunes, plums	Fruits, vegetables, limited intake of milk.

(4) 12 months old - up to 23 ounces per day with intake of solid food.

3. Implications for family teaching.

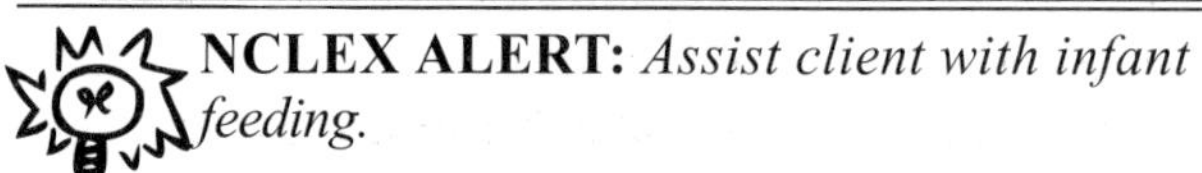

NCLEX ALERT: *Assist client with infant feeding.*

a. Newborns cannot swallow voluntarily until 10-12 weeks of age.
b. Extrusion reflex (pushing food out of mouth with tongue) lasts until 4 months, therefore solids are not introduced until around 6 months.
c. When solids are introduced, offer only one new food per week, avoid multi grain cereals until tolerance is established.
d. Usual progression of food textures is strained to mashed to minced to chopped to cut table foods.
e. Increase the use of small-sized finger foods as pincer grasp develops (9 months).
f. Texture of food becomes increasingly important from 6 months to 1 year, but the food must be easily dissolved, (e.g., crackers or zwieback).
g. Teach parents to not warm frozen breast milk in the microwave.

Toddler

1. Diet.
   a. Needs 16 oz. of milk daily; more than 24 oz. can lead to refusal of other foods and development of a milk anemia (peak incidence at 18 months).
   b. Prefers finger foods, (e.g., vegetables they can pick up, crackers, macaroni).
   c. Tends to refuse casseroles, salads, and mixed dishes.
   d. After two years, a child may be give skim milk, or fat free milk is fat intake is a concern.
   e. Struggle for autonomy may be manifested by refusal of food, mealtime negativism, and ritualism.
   f. Bribery and rewards for eating should be avoided.
   g. Around 18 months old a decreased appetite is normal, toddler may become a very picky eater. Don't mix food on plate, or overfill the plate.
   h. Ritualistic behavior frequently carries over into eating habits - same dish, same spoon, etc..

Preschooler

1. Diet.
   a. *Food jags* are common; may refuse to eat anything except one food at each meal.
   b. Continues to refuse casseroles and mixed food items.
   c. Finger foods remain popular.
   d. Do not bribe children to eat, or make them "clean their plates". Serve smaller portions, if sufficient amounts are not eaten during mealtimes eliminate snacks.
   e. Recognize that refusing to eat is a way to attract attention.

School Age

1. Diet.
   a. Food intake is more varied.
   b. They enjoy most foods, with vegetables being least favorite.
2. Implications for family teaching.
   a. After-school snack: encourage healthy choices -fruits, raw vegetable sticks, and peanut butter sandwiches.
   b. Appetite is usually good, but children often do not want to take the time to eat. Sometimes helpful to spend a specific time at the table (15 to 20 minutes) to prevent the child from forming the habit of gulping food down.
   c. Avoid use of food as reward for behavior.
   d. There is an increased influence of media and peers regarding fast food.
   e. Begin teaching child to recognize high fat foods.

Adolescent

1. Rapid growth rate and maturation changes make them vulnerable to nutritional deficiencies. Diets in general are deficient in calcium and Vitamin C.
2. Girls peak growth between 10 and 14 years old.
3. Boys peak growth between 12-15 years old.
4. Six out of ten girls eat only 2/3 of the nutrients required. Girls tend to be deficient in iron, while boys tend to be deficient in thiamin. (See Table 2-3)

Adult

1. Diet.
   a. Energy requirements decrease with age.

Example: *55-year-old man requires 2400 kcal; at age 76 requires only 2050 kcal.*

Example: *55-year-old woman requires 1800 kcal; at age 76 only requires 1600 kcal.*

   b. Improved financial status during middle adulthood tends to promote an increased intake of rich foods and frequency of dining out.
2. Nursing Implications.
   a. Adherence to a prudent diet pattern.
   b. Promotion and continued maintenance of a regular exercise program.
   c. Reduce sodium intake to 3-6 gm. daily.

d. Maintain serum cholesterol level below 200 mg/dl.

Older Adult

1. Diet.
   a. Encourage a diet low in fat, high in fiber, iron, Vitamin C, thiamin, with adequate sources of calcium.(see Table 2-3)
   b. If confined to bed rest, need fluid intakes as high as 3-4 L/day to prevent kidney stones, providing they have no fluid restrictions, (e.g., CHF).
   c. Since the older adult often has impaired renal function, protein intake should be evaluated.
2. Nursing Implications.
   a. Alteration in taste and reduced digestive function occurs.
   b. Logical sequence of eating food is biting, chewing, and swallowing. New denture wearers should be encouraged to reverse this order—swallow a liquid diet first, then chew soft foods, and last, bite regular foods.
   c. The older adult may intentionally restrict fluids because of nocturia or stress incontinence.
   d. Constipation is a chronic problem secondary to decreased peristalsis, encourage fluids and high fiber diet.
   e. Loneliness and depression are often associated with poor appetite.

GERIATRIC PRIORITY: *Usually it takes more time for an older person to eat and early satiety is reached. Encourage frequent small feedings, rather than 3 meals; providing liquid supplements is beneficial.*

Nutritional Assessment

A. Assess nutrition needs.
B. Client profile—age, sex, height, weight, socioeconomic status, culture.
C. Nutritional status—food habits, observe for physical signs indicative of nutritional status.
D. Determine disease or pathophysiologic process.
E. Be alert to high-risk patients—overweight, underweight, congenital anomalies of G.I. tract, surgery of G.I. tract, problem with ingestion, digestion, absorption, and patients on IV therapy for 10 days or more.

Diet Therapy for High-Level Wellness

A. Food pyramid (See Figure 2-1).
B. Prudent diet.
   1. Increased amounts of fresh fruits, vegetables, and whole grains.
   2. Reduced amounts of animal fats, cholesterol, refined sugar, salt, and alcohol.
   3. Adaptations to the Food Pyramid (Figure 2-1).
      a. Meat—increase amounts of fish, chicken, turkey, and veal; also increase use of legumes, nuts, and seeds as a source of protein; limit egg yolks to 2 or 3 weekly, including those used in cooking.
      b. Milk— adults and older children use low-fat dairy products.
      c. Fruits and Vegetables—increase total intake.
      d. Grains, Breads, and Cereals—select whole grain products and starches as source of carbohydrates.

THERAPEUTIC MEAL PLANS

A therapeutic meal plan or prescription diet is a modification of an individual's normal nutritional needs based on the changes in their physiological needs as a result of an illness or disease state. See Table 2-4.

Study Questions—Health Implications

1. Which behavior indicates that an 18-month-old infant is developing a nonadaptive reaction to the hospitalization?

① Cries when the mother leaves.
② Ignores mother when she arrives to visit.
③ Eats using fingers rather than utensils.
④ Is afraid of the dark.

2. What would the nurse expect to find when exploring a 9-year-old's concept of death?

① Knows that death is a final process.
② Regards death as a temporary state of sleep.
③ Believes death is something that "just happens."
④ Thinks death results from being bad.

3. When obtaining a health history from an older client, which characteristics of the older client must be taken into consideration?

① The older client responds to pain sensation with the same intensity as a young client.
② Auditory acuity is the most common sensory loss in the aged population and may hinder the interview.
③ The older client requires a lot of repetition because the IQ declines with the aging process.
④ An older client's response time to answering a question is just as quick as a young client.

4. The nurse recommends that a 12-month-old infant receive which nutrients for growth?

① Exclude milk from the infant's diet until he begins to like other foods.
② Offer the infant small amounts of meat and vegetables before offering him milk.
③ Withhold desserts from the infant, until he has eaten his vegetables.
④ Mix strained meat and vegetables into the milk given to the infant.

5. What are appropriate toys for an 18-month-old infant to have for play while in a croup tent?

① Rattles.
② Stacking rings.
③ Crayons and coloring book.
④ Soap bubbles.

6. Which food choices provide the highest calcium intake and are consistent with a low salt dietary program for hypertension?

① Cheese and macaroni, fresh fruit, milk shake.
② Cottage cheese, glass of skim milk, orange slices.
③ Roast beef with whole wheat bread, potato, and a vegetable salad.
④ Cheeseburger, french fries, milk shake.

7. The nurse is serving a diet tray to a client who has glomerulonephritis and azotemia. Which food selection would the nurse question?

① Bread and rice.
② Dried peaches and apricots.
③ Bran muffin and eggs.
④ Apples and cucumbers.

8. In late adulthood, how may death be viewed?

① A romanticized situation.
② A time of disassociation.
③ As a part of life.
④ A time of denial

9. Immunization for infants should start at what age?

① four months.
② three months.
③ two months.
④ one month.

10. Varicella zoster vaccination should be administered at what age?

① at birth
② 1 month
③ 6 months
④ 12 months

11. Chicken pox (varicella) is characterized by which symptoms?

① Vesicles that rupture with clear fluid.
② Erythematous, fine macular rash on the trunk.
③ Pustules that are filled with pus.
④ Papules that are confined to the face and trunk.

12. A client comes to the emergency room with a deep penetrating wound he received in his garden. What is the best nursing action?

① Rinse the wound with antibiotic solution.
② Administer gamma globulin intramuscularly.
③ Anticipate notifying poison control for plant toxicology.
④ Determine when client received last tetanus injection.

Answers and rationales to these questions are in the section at the end of the book entitled "Chapter Study Questions: Answers & Rationales."

Appendix 2-1:
DEVELOPMENTAL TASKS

Stageof Development	Erickson's Developmental Tasks	Play/Social Activities	Health Promotion/ Maintenance
INFANCY (Birth to 1 year)	Trust versus mistrust. Parent-child bonding is crucial to the foundation for building a basic sense of trust. It is essential that primary needs are gratified promptly.	Involved in solitary play activities. Provide toys which are soft, cuddly, and colorful; mobiles are very popular.	Encourage routine immunizations. Teach safety precautions related to burns, poisonings, accidents, and drowning.
TODDLER (1 year to 3 years)	Autonomy versus shame and *doubt.* Child relies heavily upon parental responses for support.	Toilet training is the major developmental accomplishment. Involved in parallel play activities. Provide toys which can be pulled, stacked together.	Continue to monitor safety by "childproofing" the home. Increased incidence of respiratory and ear infections.
EARLY CHILDHOOD (3 years to 6 years)	*Initiative versus guilt.* Child uses imagination and creativeness.	Follows rules, compares self to others.	Progresses from solitary play to a more cooperative play with others in a group.
MIDDLE CHILDHOOD (6 years to 12 years)	*Industry versus inferiority.* "Chum" period, progresses from self-centered to more other-directed behavior. Reality testing improving.	Younger child plays by assuming roles as a fireman, doctor, nurse, teacher, etc. Older child involved with bicycle riding, table games, sports, etc.	Respiratory infections are a common illness as child goes to school. Booster immunizations are important.
ADOLESCENCE (12 years to 18 years)	*Identity versus role diffusion.* Completion of previous tasks successfully will lead to a secure sense of self.	Peer groups are most important with behavior being defined more by group members. Social activities include dating.	Mood swings common. Accidents associated more with driving cars and motorcycles.
YOUNG ADULTHOOD (18 years to 44 years)	Intimacy versus isolation. Disturbances in sex role identity may occur due to inadequate resolution of identity crisis.	Involvement with social network of peers from community, work, etc. Appraisals by others affects sense of identity and self.	Stress related illness, drug and alcohol abuse are common during this period. Another health issue is pregnancy.
MIDDLE ADULTHOOD (45 years to 64 years)	*Generativity versus stagnation.* Reassessment of life goals. Mutuality among peers.	Leisure time becomes more of a concern. Key socializing agents are lovers, spouses, and close friends. Retirement occurs.	Menopause occurs, along with chronic health problems, (i.e. diabetes, cancer).
OLDER ADULTHOOD (65 years and older)	*Ego integrity versus despair.* If viewed life as worthwhile will be better equipped to deal with aging.	Central process is introspection with the favorable outcome of wisdom along with a detached yet active concern with life in the face of death.	Safety concerns reoccur due to impaired sensory input. Alterations in all major body systems occurs.

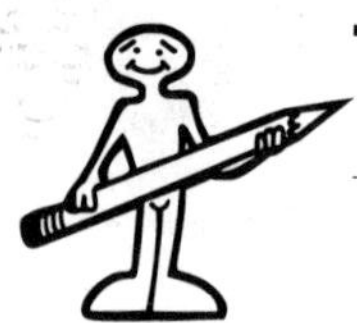

Notes

CONCEPTS OF NURSING PRACTICE

BASIC HUMAN NEEDS

A. Maslow's Hierarchy of Basic Human Needs.
   1. Human behavior is motivated by a system of needs.
   2. Clients will focus or attempt to satisfy needs at the base of the pyramid before focusing on those higher up (Figure 3-1).
   3. Human needs are *universal*; however, some may be modified by cultural influence.
   4. The Nursing Process is always concerned with physiological needs first - then progressing to teaching, decreasing anxiety, etc. This is also true for the client with psychosocial needs - his physiological needs must be met before he can progress to the next level.

Self-Actualization
Needs for Esteem and Self-Respect
Needs for Belongingness and Affection
Needs for Safety and Security
Physiological Needs - Oxygen, Food, Water, Rest, Elimination

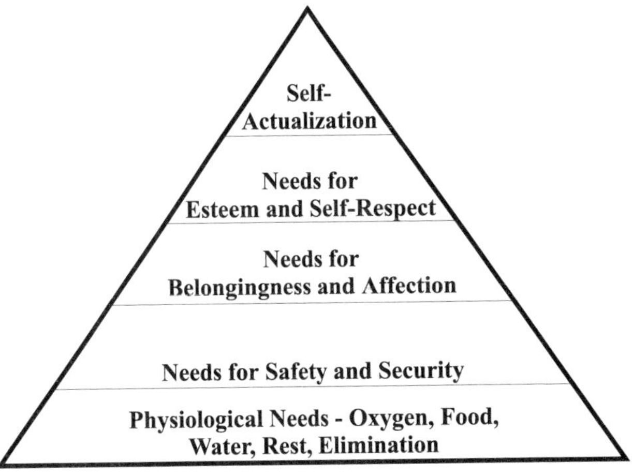

Figure 3-1: Maslow's Hierarchy Of Needs

NCLEX ALERT: *Maslow's Hierarchy is very useful in answering test questions related to setting priorities. Always remember the physiological needs at the base of the pyramid must be satisfied in order to focus on other needs and that oxygenation is always first physiological need or priority.*

STEPS OF THE NURSING PROCESS

❑ **The nursing process information correlates with the activity statements as outline in the NCLEX-RN Job Task Analysis.**

NCLEX ALERT: *Always remember to apply the steps of the nursing process in chronological order when answering test questions. You must assess before you plan or implement.*

Assessment

- Gather and organize data.
- Collect physical assessment data.
- Obtain client data from client's family or significant others.
- Ask client to describe his/her symptoms.

Analysis

- Determine impact of results of laboratory diagnostic tests on client.
- Identify client's unmet needs.
- Determine cause of client's symptoms.
- Identify client's potential problems.
- Determine client's strengths and weaknesses.
- Formulate nursing diagnosis.

Planning

- Set priorities for client care.
- Develop individualized plan of care.
- Plan measures to minimize anticipated symptoms.
- Consult with client/family in developing a plan of care.

Implementation

- Implement a plan of care.
- Report significant changes in client's condition.
- Document provision of client care.
- Communicate client's needs to others.
- Utilize client's strengths to achieve goals of care.

Evaluation

- Revise goals/plan of care to accommodate client's values, customs, or habits.
- Compare client's response to expected outcomes.
- Gather data to indicate effectiveness of each intervention.
- Determine impact of therapeutic interventions on client.
- Determine if goals of care are being achieved.
- Identify need for change in approach to client care.

- Revise approach to care in order to meet client's specific needs.

HEALTH ASSESSMENT

Subjective Health Assessment

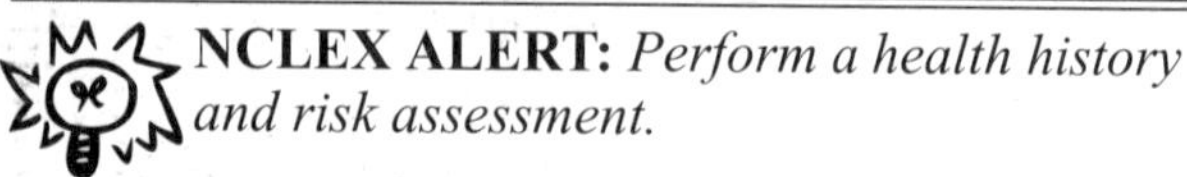
NCLEX ALERT: *Perform a health history and risk assessment.*

Health History

A. Demographic data.
   1. Name, address, phone, age, sex, marital status.
   2. Race, religion, usual source of medical care.

B. Chief Complaint/reason for visit.
   1. Chief complaint (CC)—main reason client sought health care.
   2. CC is recorded in client's own words.

   Example: "I have been vomiting blood since this morning."

C. History of the present illness.
   1. Chronologic narrative.
   2. Contains *eight areas of investigation* to evaluate the symptom.
      a. Sequence and chronology.
      b. Frequency.
      c. Bodily location and radiation.
      d. Character of the complaint.
      e. Intensity or severity.
      f. Setting.
      g. Associated phenomena or manifestations.
      h. Aggravating or alleviating factors.
   3. Includes relevant family history.

D. Medical history.
   1. Perception of illness.
   2. Previous Illnesses
      a. Hospitalization.
      b. Surgery
      c. Chronic illnesses.
   3. Allergies.
   4. Immunizations.
   5. Accidents and injuries.
   6. Current medications.
   7. Prenatal, labor and delivery, or neonatal history (recorded for all children under age of 5 and older children with a congenital or developmental problem).
   8. Psychosocial history.
      a. Sources of stress.
      b. Coping mechansims.
   9. Activities of daily living
      a. Nutrition.
      b. Elimination.
      c. Rest/sleep.
      d. Personal habits (alcohol, smoking, etc).
   10. Developmental level - school/education, work, family activities, social activities,

E. Review of Systems (ROS).

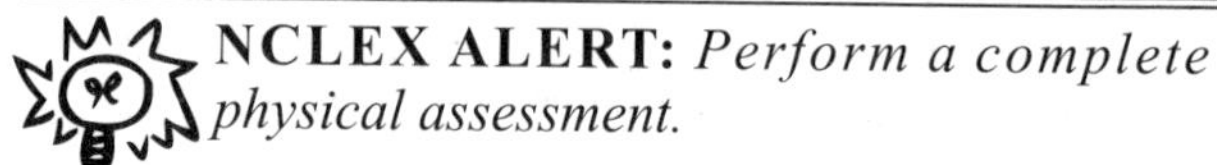
NCLEX ALERT: *Perform a complete physical assessment.*

1. Brief account from the client regarding any recent signs or symptoms associated with the body systems.
2. Contains subjective data given by the client; *does not* contain information from the physical examination.
3. When a symptom or problem is encountered in the ROS, the following information should be determined:
   - Location: what area of the body does the symptom occur.
   - Character: quality of the problem, feeling, or sensation, is it sharp, dull, constant, intermittent.
   - Intensity: severity of symptoms or feeling, does it interfere with activities of daily living.
   - Timing: when does the problem occur, onset, duration, frequency, does anything precipitate the problem.
   - Aggravating/alleviating factors: what activities make the problem better or worse.
4. Review of systems progress is from head to toe. The pertinent information to include is located in the assessment section at the beginning of each system.

Nursing Assessment

Comprehensive Physical Assessment

A. General guidelines.
   1. Good lighting is essential.
   2. If examiner is right-handed, examine from the right side of the bed.
   3. Position bed or examining table to appropriate height.

4. Assure a quiet, private environment.
5. Adequately expose areas being examined.
6. Explain to client as examination proceeds.

B. Techniques of physical assessment.

1. Inspection.
   a. Careful examination and observation of area is an important part of the assessment.
   b. Each anatomical area is inspected *before* it is touched by examiner's hands or instruments.
2. Palpation.
   a. Uses the sense of touch.
   b. Evaluates the size and shape of organs or masses, mobility, tenderness, swelling, surface temperature, muscle rigidity or spasm.
   c. Parts of the hand used during palpation.
      (1) Fingertips for fine, tactile discrimination, lymph nodes, skin texture.
      (2) Dorsa of hands for skin temperature (dorsal skin is thinner and more sensitive).
      (3) Palmar and ulnar surfaces for vibratory sensation.
      (4) Grasping position (pinching) of fingers for tissue consistency.
   d. Light palpation identifies areas of tenderness and muscle resistance.
   e. Deep palpation essentially same as light palpation, however, examiner uses two hands to press deeper into the client's abdomen.
3. Percussion.
   a. Technique of striking body surface lightly but sharply to produce sounds.
   b. Indirect percussion.
      (1) Middle finger of the non-dominant hand (*pleximeter*) is placed against the body surface with palm and other fingers raised off the skin. Tip of middle finger of dominant hand (*plexor*) strikes the base of the distal phalanx of the pleximeter in a quick, sharp stroke.
   c. Direct percussion.
      (1) Gentle direct striking of the body with one or more fingers or with the ulnar surface of the clenched fist.
      (2) Useful in assessing sinuses, kidneys, or the liver.
   d. Percussion sounds.
      (1) Resonance: loud, low note heard over normal lung tissue.
      (2) Hyper resonance: louder, lower, and longer note heard over emphysematous lung.
      (3) Tympany: loud, musical note with drum-like quality, heard over air-filled viscera (i.e., stomach or bowel).
      (4) Flat: soft, high-pitched, short note heard over the thigh, for example.
      (5) Dull: medium-pitched note of intensity and duration heard over the liver.
4. Auscultation.
   a. Use of a stethoscope to evaluate sounds arising from the lungs, abdomen, and cardiovascular systems.
   b. Bell of stethoscope is used for low-pitched sounds such as murmurs and bruits.
   c. Diaphragm of stethoscope is used for high-pitched sounds such as wheezes and crackles.

Table 3-1: SEQUENCE OF PHYSICAL EXAMINATION

CLIENT POSITION	AREAS ASSESSED
Supine, seated, and standing	Blood pressure and other vital signs
Seated	Head, face, eyes, ears, nose, mouth, neck, chest, breasts, and hands
Supine	Breasts, heart, abdomen, inguinal region, anus and rectum, female genitourinary system (lithotomy position), hips, knees, ankles, feet
Seated	Reflexes, hands, arms, shoulders (muscle strength), cerebellum (rapid, alternating movements, sensory function (stereognosis)
Standing	Spine, ROM, varicose veins, cerebellum, gait, male genitourinary system

C. Sequence of the physical examination (Table 3-1).

D. When a client indicates a problem or symptom during the physical examination, that area should be investigated (see ROS).

E. Detailed assessment findings for each body system are discussed at the beginning of each chapter.

Focused Assessment

A. An assessment that is limited to the particular need, health care problem, or health risk the client is experiencing.

B. Frequently utilized for bedside assessments.

1. Assess the specific characteristics of the problem.
2. Determine if and what type of nursing intervention is necessary
3. When should the intervention be done - immediate, later in shift, prior to client's discharge, etc.

C. An ongoing assessment is frequently focused on client's current health problems. This type of assessment is most often done at the beginning of each shift by the nurse responsible for the care of the client.

1. Focuses on client's current status, determine if it correlates with the report the nurse received.
2. Monitor or determine the client's response to previous nursing interventions.
3. Evaluate client's response to current plan of care and determine if any changes are necessary.
4. Evaluate for any evidence of development of complications.
5. Determine if there are any other problems the client is experiencing that have not been addressed.

HEALTH PROMOTION

Levels of prevention

❑ **Preventive health care is more dynamic than health maintenance; focuses on health enhancement and health promotion, whereas health maintenance is concerned with maintaining the status quo.**

A. Primary—prevention of disease

1. Goal is to achieve maximum functioning in each health potential area.
2. Examples: Stop smoking, practice safe sex, maintain body weight, limit alcohol intake, follow a regular exercise program, and healthy diet.

B. Secondary—early diagnosis and treatment.

1. Emphasis is determining intervention priorities.

Examples: Screening for tuberculosis, yearly glaucoma, pap smear, breast self-examination and testicular self-examination.

C. Tertiary—prevention of complications.

1. Focus is on the prevention of complication and rehabilitation after the disease or condition has already occurred.

Examples: Have CBC drawn before chemotherapy, speech therapy after a CVA, cardiac rehabilitation.

NCLEX ALERT: *Teach client actions to maintain health and prevent disease.*

Nursing Intervention

1. Providing health education programs.
2. Enhancing behavior change.
   a. Encourage motivation by identify client's needs.
   b. Focus on factors which motivate client.
   c. Realize resistance is a healthy, normal response to threat and change.
3. Role modeling (the nurse) healthy lifestyle choices.

HEALTH TEACHING

Principles of Client Education

NCLEX ALERT: *Consider client's background and culture when preparing teaching materials and determine when client is ready to learn.*

A. Common characteristics of the adult learner.

1. Self-directed.
2. Client's background of experience, skills, and attitudes and culture form the base for any new information received.
3. Level of psychosocial development affects the readiness to learn. If a client is in a mid-life transition, it may be very difficult for him to learn new attitudes and skills which threaten his self image.

Example: a man in his early 40s may have difficulty accepting any education regarding his colostomy.

4. Wants to apply the learning immediately.

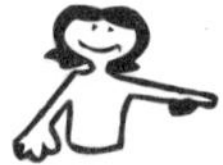
GERIATRIC PRIORITY: *Elderly clients tend to be solitary learners, the nurse needs to consider ill health and sensory deficits that tend to occur, (e.g., large-type books for reading).*

B. Factors contributing to the teaching-learning process.

1. Readiness to learn.
   a. Must feel the material is relevant.
   b. Must have the mental capacity to learn and physical ability to perform the skills.
   c. Must have his physical and safety needs met.
   d. Comfort.
      (1) Physical comfort—discomforts such as pain, nausea, hunger, need to void, are distracters to the learning process.

(2) Psychological comfort—anger, frustration, fear, and guilt severely hamper the learning process.

NURSING PRIORITY: The first step in the education process is to make sure the client's physiological needs are met then determine what the client already knows about his condition.

e. Client and nurse need to discuss and agree on specific long-and short-term goals.

C. Factors relating to the presentation.

NCLEX ALERT: *Choose appropriate teaching techniques and strategies*

1. State the specific objective of each teaching session; identify exactly what the client is to gain.
2. Use vocabulary and terminology appropriate to client's understanding and to his or her developmental level. Utilize correct terms for body parts.
3. Try to stimulate as many senses as possible. Utilize charts, handouts, and pieces of equipment when appropriate.
4. Repetition is an integral part of learning.
5. More active the client is in the process, the better he/she will retain the information.
6. Plan short sessions; do not overwhelm the client with too much information at one time.
7. Actively involve the family and significant others when appropriate.
8. Be generous with positive reinforcement.

D. Pediatric factors influencing the learning process.

1. Intellectual development moves from the concrete to the abstract.
2. Nurse needs to assess the developmental level of the child before planning the educational approach.

NURSING PRIORITY: A typical "No" response from a toddler when being taught a new activity (e.g., combing hair) is usually an assertion of his independence, and not that he will not learn.

a. Preschooler.

(1) Frequently experience fears of body injury.

(2) Explanations should be simple.

(3) Need to know how a procedure will affect them.

(4) If under four years, generally do not benefit from anatomy and physiology information.

(5) If under four years, need clarification of reality and fantasy.

(6) If under four years, separation anxiety is a problem; include parents in teaching session.

(7) Preschool children are aware of the physical and mechanical causes of problems they can see; unaware of physical and mechanical forces they cannot see.

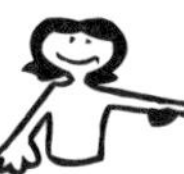

NURSING PRIORITY: It is important to emphasize to the preschooler that treatment is not punishment.

b. School age.

(1) Benefit from tours, drawings, anatomical dolls.

(2) Cooperate with treatment and express feelings in words.

(3) Learn well from role-playing and puppets.

(4) Need to include parents in teaching session for reinforcement and consistency.

c. Adolescent.

(1) Needs to be as independent as possible in management of health problem.

(2) Present information with a scientific rationale rather than by giving specific directions.

(3) Needs assistance in coping with loss of independence and self-direction.

(4) Focus programs to deal with changes in body image and in maintaining ego.

E. Special needs of the older client.

1. Determine their functional losses (i.e., hearing or vision impairment, memory loss).

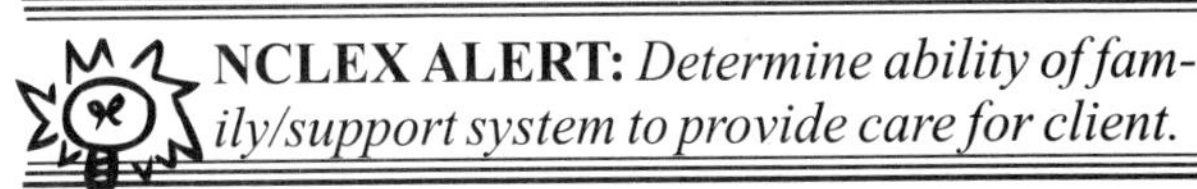

NCLEX ALERT: *Determine ability of family/support system to provide care for client.*

2. Identify social support to aid the older adult; this often increases compliance with information being taught.

BASIC NURSING SKILLS

Body Alignment and Range of Motion

A. Characteristics of correct body alignment in bed.

1. Head up with eyes looking straight forward.
2. Neck and back straight.

3. Arms relaxed and supported at sides.
4. Legs parallel to hips with knees slightly flexed.
5. Feet separated and parallel to the legs with the toes pointed upward and slightly outward.

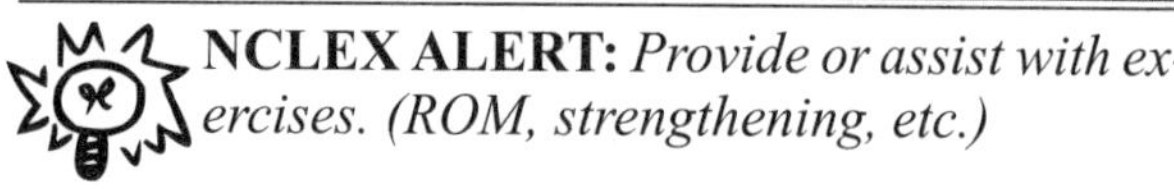

NCLEX ALERT: *Provide or assist with exercises. (ROM, strengthening, etc.)*

B. Range of motion (ROM)
1. Active ROM
a. Client performs exercise without assistance.
b. Used for client who independently performs activities of daily living (ADLs), but for some reason is immobilized or limited regarding activity.
c. Goal is to maintain or increase muscle strengthen and prevent muscle atrophy.
2. Passive ROM
a. Client can not actively move.
b. Cannot contract muscles, therefore muscle strengthening *cannot* be accomplished.
c. Goal is to maintain joint flexibility.

C. Principles of ROM exercises.
1. Stretch muscles by moving the body part; avoid movement to the point of discomfort.
2. Perform ROM at least twice daily on immobile clients, with a minimum of 4-5 repetitions of each exercise.
3. Always support extremity above and below the joint when doing passive ROM on extremities.
4. Involve the client in planning their exercise program.

D. Client positions (see Appendix 3-1).

Asepsis

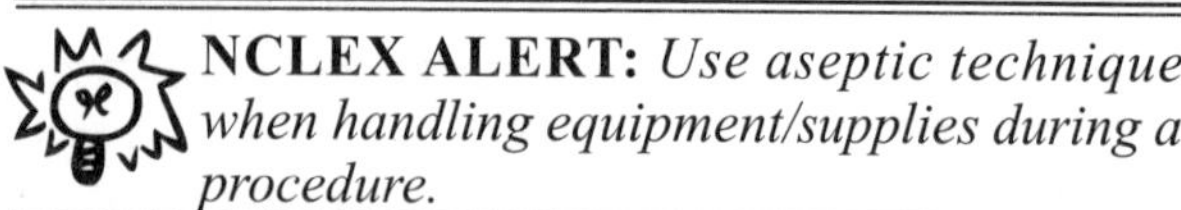

NCLEX ALERT: *Use aseptic technique when handling equipment/supplies during a procedure.*

A. Medical asepsis.
1. Designed to reduce the number of pathogens in an area and decrease the likelihood of their transfer, (e.g., hand washing).
2. Often referred to as *clean technique*, wash hands between each client.
3. Administration of oral medications, enemas, tube feedings, daily hygiene practices fall under this category.

B. Surgical asepsis.
1. Designed to *not* just simply reduce the number of pathogens, but to make the object free of all microorganisms.
2. Also known as *sterile technique.*
3. Surgical asepsis is reserved primarily for sterile dressing changes, performing sterile catheterizations, and surgical procedures in the operating room (Table 3-2: Sterile Technique: Procedures and Guidelines).

NCLEX ALERT: *Set up a sterile field.*

Wound Care

❑ **A wound is a disruption in normal tissue caused by traumatic injury or surgically created.**

NCLEX ALERT: *Promote the progress of wound healing (e.g., turning, hydration, nutrition, skin care, etc.).*

A. Major goals.
1. Promote healing.
2. Prevent further damage.
3. Prevent infection.

B. Wound Healing.
1. Black wounds.
a. Necrotic devitalized tissue, high risk for infection.
b. Frequently requires sharp or surgical debridement of tissue for healing to occur.
2. Yellow wounds.
a. Contains devitalized tissue, requires cleaning for healing to occur.
b. Mechanical debridement requires irrigations and dressings. A 19F IV catheter on a 30cc syringe provides safe pressure to irrigate and remove devitalized tissue.
c. Wet to dry dressings, wet to moist dressings, wound packing and enzymatic debridement may be used to cleanse the yellow wound.
d. Moisture retention dressings.
3. Red wounds.
a. Require protection of fragile granulation tissue.
b. Topical antibiotic ointment and nonadhering dressings may be used on shallow wounds.
c. Wound should be kept moist (moisture retention dressings), dry dressings will damage the new granulation tissue.

Table 3-2: STERILE TECHNIQUE: PROCEDURES GUIDELINES

PROCEDURES REQUIRING STERILE TECHNIQUE

- Surgical procedures in the operating room, (i.e., TURP, appendectomy)
- Biopsies in the operating room, treatment room or client's room
- Catheterizations of the heart, bladder, or other body cavities
- Injections: IM, SQ, Intradermal
- Infusions: IV, instillations or infusions of medication or radioactive isotopes into body cavities
- Dressing changes:
  Usually, first postoperative dressing change is done using sterile technique
  Dressings over catheters inserted into body cavities, (i.e., Hickman catheter, subclavian lines, dialysis access sites)
  Dressings of clients with burns, immunologic disorders, and skin grafts

GUIDELINES FOR STERILE FIELD

- Never turn your back on a sterile field.
- Avoid talking.
- Keep all sterile objects within view, (i.e., below waist is not within sterile field).
- Moisture will carry bacteria across/through a cloth or paper barrier.
- Open all sterile packages away from the sterile field to prevent crossover and contamination.

C. Wound healing affected by:

1. Nutritional status.
2. Circulation to the wound.
3. Characteristics of the wound.
4. Presence of existing disease, (i.e., diabetes).
5. Location and approximation of wound.

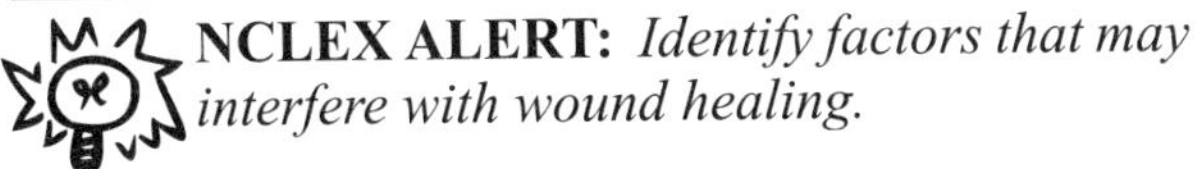

NCLEX ALERT: *Identify factors that may interfere with wound healing.*

D. Nursing intervention.

1. Cleansing of wound.
   a. Horizontal wound — cleansed from center of incision outward, then laterally.
   b. Vertical wound — cleansed from top to bottom, then laterally.
   c. Drain or a stab wound — cleansed in a circular motion.

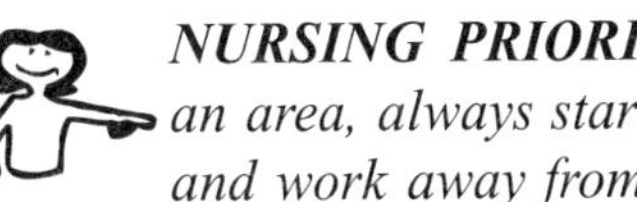

NURSING PRIORITY: *When cleansing an area, always start at the cleanest area and work away from that area. Never return to an area you have previously cleaned; be sure to discard cleansing swab after each horizontal or vertical stroke.*

2. Drain — inserted into open wound to prevent the accumulation of secretions and exudate.
   a. Safety pins are inserted into Penrose drains to prevent them from slipping back into the wound.
   b. Frequent dressing changes are preferable to reinforcing the same dressing.

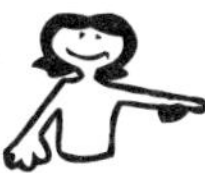

NURSING PRIORITY: *Avoid pooling of excessive drainage under saturated dressing; this can lead to skin irritation and infection.*

3. Montgomery straps — used when frequent dressing changes are needed, helps to prevent skin irritation from tape removal.
4. Elasticized abdominal binders.
5. Jackson-Pratt catheter or drainage system — bulb must be compressed to allow air to escape and then is re-capped to maintain suction.
6. Hemovac— evacuator must be compressed at least every four hours to provide suction; be sure to empty drainage from pouring spout.

NCLEX ALERT: *Monitor effective function of portable wound suction devices. Empty and re-establish negative pressure suction devices.*

7. Wet-to-dry dressings.
   a. Purpose is to trap necrotic tissue in the dressing as it dries.
   b. Dressing should be moist when applied and allowed to dry for four to six hours.
8. Moisture retention dressing
   a. Maintain moisture to promote healing and to prevent damage to healing tissue.
   b. Dressing is coated with gel, colloids, or antibacterial preparations to prevent skin maceration and to promote healing.
   c. May be used to assist in debridement of wounds, or to protect healthy tissue during healing process.
9. Obtain a specimen of wound drainage.
   a. Gently roll a sterile swab in the purulent drainage.

b. Obtain wound specimen before any medication or antimicrobial agent has been applied to wound area or administered to client.

NCLEX ALERT: *Manage wound care - irrigation, dressings, wound drainage devices.*

Specimen Collection

A. General principles.

1. Use sterile equipment.
2. Use the correct container for each specimen—preservatives, anticoagulants, or chemicals may be required.
3. Always observe standard precautions when obtaining specimens—keep outside of container clean to prevent contamination in transfer to the laboratory.
4. Properly label the specimen. Collect the correct amount at the correct time.

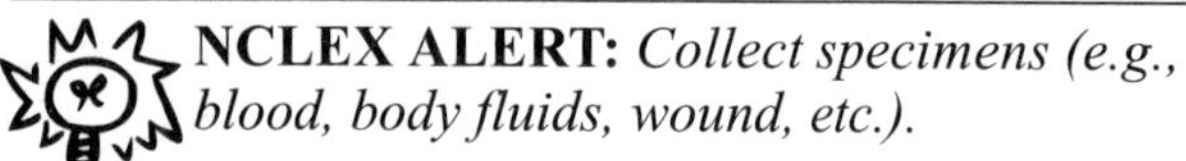

NCLEX ALERT: *Collect specimens (e.g., blood, body fluids, wound, etc.).*

B. Types of specimen (Refer to appendices in chapters listed).

1. Urine (Chapter 23).
2. Stool (Chapter 18).
3. Sputum, throat or nasopharyngeal (Chapter 15).
4. Blood (Chapter 14).
5. Wound specimen.

Heat and Cold Applications

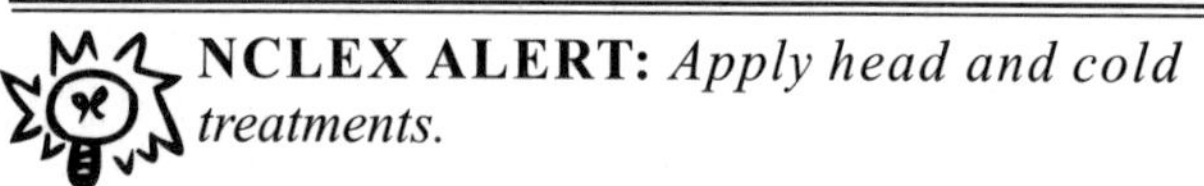

NCLEX ALERT: *Apply head and cold treatments.*

A. Heat applications.

1. Purpose—soften exudate, increase vasodilatation, promote healing, decrease pain.
2. General principles.
   a. Moist heat penetrates deeper than dry heat.
   b. Unless a physician orders continuous heat applications, treatment time is usually 20-30 minutes.
3. Types of heat application.
   a. Moist heat pack.
   b. Aquamatic or Aqua K-pad—circulates warmed water through the pad to distribute dry heat to body parts.
   c. Heat lamp or heat cradle.
   d. Sitz bath.

B. Cold applications.

1. Purpose—promote vasoconstriction, decrease edema or temperature, stop bleeding, or stop pain by numbing pain receptors.
2. Types of cold applications.
   a. Ice bag, ice collar, or ice glove.
   b. Cold compress or cold pack.
   c. Hypothermia blanket.
3. Reduces edema, if applied immediately after an injury.

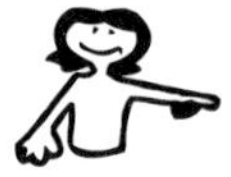

NURSING PRIORITY: *Do not use cold applications with conditions of impaired circulation, (i.e., peripheral vascular disease or diabetes).*

Self-Care

1. Self-locking plastic sandwich bags can be used for cold packs; wrap in a lightweight towel before applying to client.
2. Large plastic trash bags can be used to protect bedding while soaks or wet compresses are in place.
3. Use lower settings when warming washcloths or other linens in a microwave oven.
4. Caution client regarding hot baths and vasodilating effect that may cause postural hypotension.

Vital Signs

NCLEX ALERT: *Determine if vital signs are abnormal (e.g., hypotension, hypertension, bradycardia, etc.). Know the range of normal for vital signs at different age levels. This is critical in identifying abnormal as well as evaluating response to treatment and specific criteria for medication administration.*

A. Normal values (see Table 3-3: Normal Vital Signs).

B. Assessment.

1. Respirations.
   a. Evaluate an infant's respiratory pattern prior to stimulating him.
   b. Check thoracic cavity for symmetrical excursion.

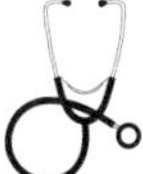

Table 3-3: NORMAL VITAL SIGNS

Neonate:	
Respiration	30 to 60
Pulse	120 to 160
Child 2 to 4 years:	
Respiration	24 to 32
Pulse	90 to 130
Child 6 to 10 years:	
Respiration	15 to 26
Pulse	75-120
Blood Pressure	80/40 to 110/60
Adult:	
Respiration	12 to 18
Pulse	60 to 100
Blood Pressure	100/60 to 140/90

c. Breath sounds—evaluate with adult client in sitting position.

d. d. Compare breath sounds on each side of client's chest.

2. Pulse.

a. Irregular radial pulse, weak volume, or low rate should be assessed by taking an apical pulse for a full minute.

b. Apical pulse—auscultated at the fifth intercostal space at the mid-clavicular line (point of maximal impulse — PMI).

c. Apical-radial pulse—determined by two people counting both the apical and the radial at the same time; provides the *pulse deficit*, which is the difference in the two values.

d. Weak peripheral pulse—evaluate by Doppler ultrasound.

3. Temperature.

a. Temperature affected by mouth-breathing and temperature of oral intake.

b. Oral temperature is taken unless otherwise indicated.

4. Blood pressure assessment (See Table 3-4).

IMMOBILITY

❑ **Immobility is the therapeutic or unavoidable restriction of a client's physical activity.**

A. Causes of restricted movement.

1. Spinal cord injury or neurological damage.

2. Presence of severe pain—arthritis, surgery, or injury.

B. Therapeutic reasons for restricted movement.

1. To decrease pain.

2. To immobilize a wound.

Table 3-4: BLOOD PRESSURE ASSESSMENT

Procedure:
The inflatable cuff is wrapped tightly around the upper half of the arm.
The cuff is inflated 20-30 mm Hg above the point at which radial pulsation disappears.
As the cuff is deflated, a sound is produced within the brachial artery just below the cuff and is audible with the stethoscope.
The sounds (Korotkoff sounds) coincide with each pulse beat.
Usually, when the cuff pressure is below diastolic, the sounds will cease or become muffled.

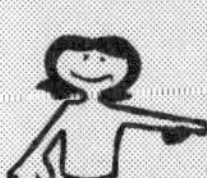

NURSING PRIORITY: *It is important to ascertain and record when the sounds becomes muffled. If there is any doubt, the BP may be recorded as a tripartite pressure (120/70/50) implying that the sound became muffled at 70 mm Hg and disappeared at 50 mmHg.*

Nursing Implications:
Size of cuff should be 20% wider than the diameter of the limb.
If the cuff is too large (i.e., child's arm), the BP obtained will be substantially lower than the true BP. If the cuff is too small (i.e., obese person's arm), the BP obtained will be higher than the true BP.
The difference of BP in right and left arms is normally 5-10 mm Hg.

3. To limit exercise and activity—clients with cardiac problems.

4. To reduce effects of gravity on the vascular bed and reduce edema formation.

Adverse Physical Effects of Immobility

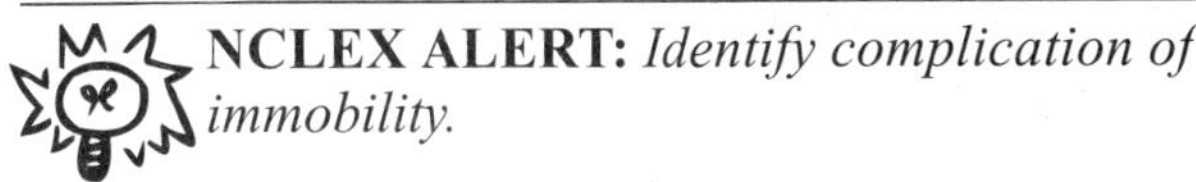

NCLEX ALERT: *Identify complication of immobility.*

✦ *Goal: to prevent complications.*

A. Cardiovascular System.

1. Assessment of physical effects.

a. Orthostatic hypotension.

b. Decrease in cardiac reserve.

c. Venous stasis.

d. d. Formation of thrombi

e. Increase in cardiac workload.

2. Nursing implications.

a. Position body to decrease venous stasis.

b. Change position frequently.

c. Passive and active range of motion.

d. Begin activity gradually; allow client to sit before standing.

e. Utilize bedside commode when possible to decrease effects of Valsalva maneuver.

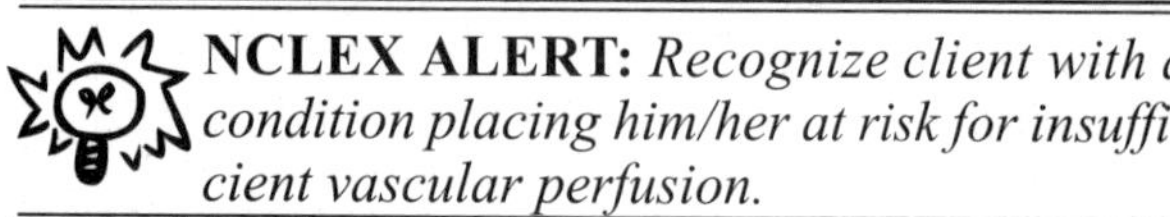
NCLEX ALERT: *Recognize client with a condition placing him/her at risk for insufficient vascular perfusion.*

B. Respiratory System.
1. Assessment of physical effects.
a. Decrease in thoracic excursion.
b. Decrease in ability to mobilize secretions.
c. Decrease in O_2/CO_2 exchange.
d. Increase in pulmonary infections.
2. Nursing implications.
a. Elevate head of bed.
b. Maintain adequate hydration—2400cc/day.
c. Have client turn, cough, and deep breathe at regular intervals (every 2 hours while awake).
d. Promote increase in activity as soon as possible-have client sit up in chair at bedside.
e. Evaluate pulmonary secretions for infection.

C. Urinary System.
1. Assessment of physical effects.
a. Urinary stasis.
b. Increase calcium, stasis, and infection precipitating stone formation.
c. Urinary tract infections.
2. Nursing implications.
a. Have client sit to void if possible.
b. Increase fluid intake.

D. Musculoskeletal System.
1. Assessment of physical effects.
a. Demineralization of bones-decrease in bone strength.
b. Muscle weakness and atrophy.
c. Loss of motion in joints leads to fibrosis and contractures.
2. Nursing implications.
a. Perform range of motion exercises.
b. Active contraction and relaxation of large muscles.
c. Position body to maintain proper alignment.
d. Encourage daily weight bearing when possible.

E. Gastrointestinal System.
1. Assessment of physical effects.
a. Anorexia.
b. Ineffective movement of feces through colon-constipation and impaction.
c. Diarrhea secondary to impaction.
2. Nursing implications.
a. Establish bowel program—every other day, or three times a week.
b. Encourage diet with adequate protein, bulk, and liquids.
c. Check for impaction.

F. Integumentary System.
1. Assessment of physical effects.
a. Decrease in tissue perfusion leading to decubitus ulcer.
b. Decrease in sensation in area of increased pressure.
2. Nursing implications.
a. Maintain cleanliness.
b. Promote circulation through frequent positioning.
c. Protect bony prominence when turning.
d. Prevent pressure areas from tight clothing, cast, braces.
e. Frequent visual inspection of pressure areas.

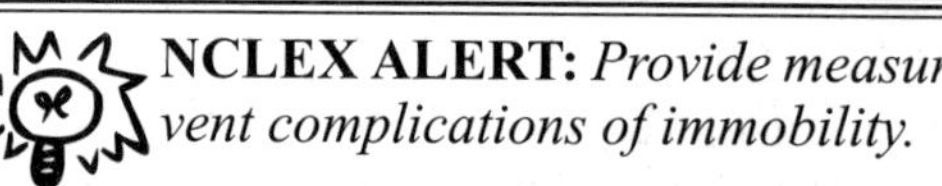
NCLEX ALERT: *Provide measures to prevent complications of immobility.*

Adverse Psychological Effects of Immobility

A. Assessment of psychological effects.
1. Depression, increased anxiety.
2. Feelings of helplessness.
3. Intellectual and sensory deprivation.
4. Change in body image.

B. Nursing implications.
1. Maintain sensory stimulation.
2. Encourage family, social contact.
3. Promote reality orientation.
4. Encourage family to bring items from home—pictures, bed clothes, toys.
5. Encourage verbalization of feelings.
6. Provide opportunities for client to have choices and participate in care.
7. Arrange counseling as appropriate—vocational, sexual, financial.

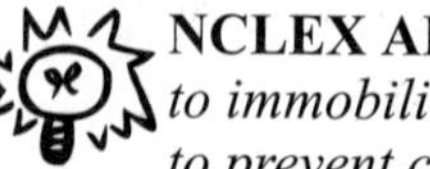
NCLEX ALERT: *Evaluate client response to immobility and response to interventions to prevent complications of immobility.*

PAIN

❑ **Pain is a complex, universal experience.**

- Pain is a sensory perceptual experience
- Pain is a totally subjective personal experience
- Pain is an early warning system; its presence triggers an awareness that something is wrong in our body (Figure 3-2).

NCLEX ALERT: *Plan measures to care for clients with anticipated or actual alteration in comfort.*

Types of pain

- Acute pain—short, predictable duration (lasting less than 6 months), immediate onset, reversible or controllable with treatment.

Example: postoperative pain which disappears as wound heals.

- Chronic pain—lasts more than 6 months, continual or persistent and recurrent.

Example: malignant (cancer) or arthritis.

- Cutaneous pain—client can identify specific area of pain which may sting or burn; may occur along a dorsal sensory nerve root.

Example: abrasions on skin, herpes zoster.

- Visceral pain—affects any of the large body cavities (abdominal viscera); characterized as diffuse, poorly localized, vague, and dull.

Example: acute pancreatitis, peptic ulcer disease, cholecystitis.

- Somatic pain—pain affecting skeletal muscle, joints, and ligaments, generally diffuse and less localized than cutaneous pain.

Example: rheumatoid arthritis, osteomyelitis.

- Referred pain—does not occur at the point of injury.

Example: myocardial ischemia felt in the left arm or shoulder; shoulder pain with cholecystitis.

Pathologic pain syndromes

- Vascular pain—associated with blood vessels; may be induced by cold.

Example: migraine headaches, peripheral vascular disease.

- Pain due to inflammation—redness, swelling, heat.

Example: peritonitis

Table 3-5: MNEMONIC TO EVALUATE PAIN

P:	Provoking or palliative factors
Q:	Quality
R:	Region
S:	Severity
T:	Timing

- Phantom pain—follows an amputation of a body part; described as throbbing, burning, stabbing, boring, vice-like, or in a cramped, twisted position.

Example: client feels "phantom sensations" in the area of the amputation, as if the part were still present.

- Malignant pain—pressure on nerve endings or interference of blood supply to area due to cancer.
- Pretended pain (malingering)—client expresses that there is pain when he actually has no pain.
- Psychogenic pain—due to emotional factors rather than physiologic dysfunction.

Assessment

***NURSING PRIORITY:** In addition to the pain and discomfort associated with a surgical procedure, it is important to assess other possible sources of discomfort, such as full bladder, occluded catheter or tube, gas accumulation, IV infiltration, or compromised circulation due to position/pressure.*

A. Subjective data collection.
   1. Determine pain location, onset, precipitating and alleviating factors.
   2. Assessment of duration, intensity, and severity of pain.
   3. Characteristics of pain (e.g., stabbing, throbbing, knife-like, crushing, cramping, suffocating, etc.).
   4. Meaning of the pain experience to the client.

B. Objective data collection.
   1. Appearance, motor behavior, facial expression.
   2. Affective behavior (e.g., crying, irritability, withdrawal, etc.).
   3. Verbal behavior (e.g., expressions of anger, fear, frustration).
   4. Increased blood pressure, pulse, and respirations.
   5. Dilated pupils, decreased urinary output, increased muscle tension, nausea, vomiting.
   6. Inspection and palpation of painful area and range of motion of involved part.
   7. See Table 3-5: Mnemonic to Evaluate Pain and Table 3-6: Assessing the Harmful Effects of Pain.

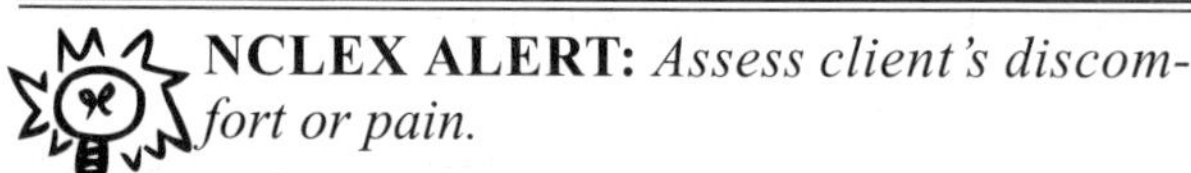

NCLEX ALERT: *Assess client's discomfort or pain.*

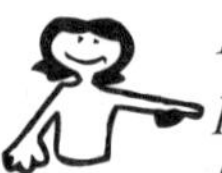

PEDIATRIC PRIORITY: *Use a variety of pain assessment strategies such as* ***QUEST.***
Q*uestion the client.*
U*se pain rating scales*
E*valuate behavior*
S*ecure parent's involvement*
T*ake into account pathology.*

Noninvasive Pain Relief Measures

Behavioral Techniques

A. Relaxation Techniques.

NURSING PRIORITY: *Low levels of anxiety or pain are easier to reduce or control than are higher levels. Consequently, pain relief measures should be utilized before pain becomes severe.*

1. Relaxed muscles result in decreased pain level.
2. Use a printed relaxation exercise which the nurse either reads or is prerecorded on a cassette tape.
3. Relaxation exercises focus on deep breathing and alternate tensing and relaxing of various body parts in a systematic manner.
4. Meditation—focuses attention away from pain.
5. Rhythmic breathing—method of relaxation and distraction by focusing on the breath.
6. Music may assist in relaxation.

NCLEX ALERT: *Provide holistic/complementary therapy (therapeutic touch, relaxation, biofeedback, etc)*

B. Guided imagery.
   1. Creative visualization—therapeutic use of images from one's imagination to focus away from pain sensation by emphasizing pleasant memories and experiences.
   2. Often combined with relaxation and biofeedback.

C. Hypnosis—produces a state of altered consciousness which is characterized by extreme responsiveness to suggestion.

D. Distraction or focusing the client's attention away from the painful sensations.
   1. When stimuli are deficient in amount in the client's environment, his threshold for sensory input tends to lower, which leads to increased pain sensation.
   2. Make environment more "normal" for client, (e.g., brief, frequent visits by nurse, bringing a snack), teaching physical exercises (pointing toes, contracting lower leg muscles).

E. Biofeedback—provides client with information about changes in bodily functions of which he is usually unaware, (e.g., blood pressure, pulse).

F. Cutaneous stimulation—alleviates pain through stimulation of skin.
   1. Use of pressure, massage, bathing, and heat or cold therapy to promote relaxation.
      a. Applied to different areas of the body.
      b. Contra lateral stimulation—when stimulating the skin near the pain site is ineffective; the side *opposite* of the painful area is stimulated for pain relief.

NCLEX ALERT: *Provide alternative measures for pain relief (TENS, imaging, massage, repositioning, etc.)*

   2. Change positions frequently and support body parts.
   3. Encourage early ambulation after surgery.
   4. Elevate swollen body parts.
   5. Check drainage tubes to insure that they are not stretched, kinked, or pulled.

G. Therapeutic touch - holistic approach using touch to realign energy fields (laying on of hands).

H. Transcutaneous electric nerve stimulation (TENS).

Table 3-6: ASSESSING THE HARMFUL EFFECTS OF PAIN

ACUTE PAIN	CHRONIC PAIN
Disturbs sleep	Fatigue
Appetite decreases	Weight gain
Fluid intake decreases	Poor concentration
Nausea and vomiting	Job loss
	Divorce
	Depression

NURSING PRIORITY: *The nurse should administer PRN pain medication to clients experiencing acute pain without fear of addicting the client to the medication.*

1. Delivers an electrical current through electrodes applied to the skin surface of the painful region or to a peripheral nerve.
2. Instruct client to adjust TENS unit intensity until it creates a pleasant sensation and relieves the pain.

Medications for Pain Relief

A. Nurse-administered PRN analgesic medications (Appendix 3-2: Analgesics).

NURSING PRIORITY: *Utilize a preventive approach in alleviating pain by giving narcotics before the pain occurs, if it can be predicted, or at least before it reaches severe intensity. This is particularly important in regards to care of the new postoperative client.*

1. Steps in administering PRN medications.
   a. Assess client to determine source, quality of pain, characteristics of pain.
   b. Analyze nursing assessment data; determine most appropriate nursing intervention.
   c. Check client's chart.
      (1) Last medication received and how administered.
      (2) The time administered.
      (3) Current physician's order.
   d. Implement appropriate pain intervention and document.
   e. Decrease stimuli in room; determine other factors influencing discomfort.
   f. At 15 and 30 minute intervals, assess client's response to pain intervention and document nursing actions.

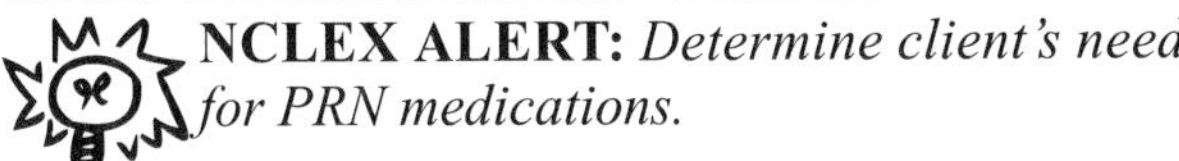

NCLEX ALERT: *Determine client's need for PRN medications.*

2. Types of medications.
   a. Narcotic analgesics are used for relieving severe pain (Appendix 3-2).

   Example: morphine, codeine, hydromorphone.

   b. Non-narcotic analgesics act at peripheral sites to reduce pain (Appendix 3-2).
   c. Potentiating drugs used to intensify the action of the narcotic agent (Appendix 3-3).

B. Patient-controlled analgesia (PCA).
   1. Client controls delivery of pain by intravenous infusion of medication via a PCA pump.
   2. Titrating the hourly dose within a preset range of mg/hour.

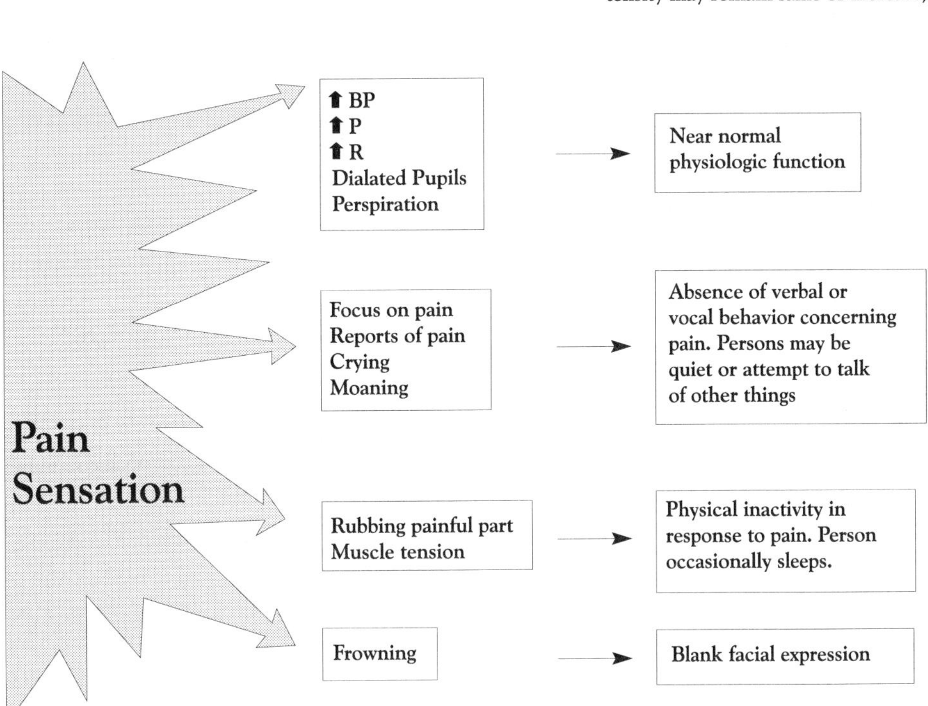

Figure 3-2: Pain

3. PCA pump procedure.
   a. Pain should be under control when PCA is initiated.
   b. Delivers a specific amount of medication as controlled by client.
   c. May be programed to deliver constant infusion with client controlling bolus infusion.
   d. A lockout time is established to prevent client from overdosing, only one dose can be administered in a set period of time, even though the client may push the button several times in succession.
   e. Important to advise family to not administer medication - theory is when client is uncomfortable he will utilize it.
   f. May obtain an override, or injection for the client who goes to sleep and awakens with severe pain unrelieved by the PCA.
   g. An example order may be: .05-1.5 mg of morphine every 5-6 minutes with a maximum of 10mg over one hour.
4. Advantages of PCA.
   a. More effective pain control.
   b. Decreased client anxiety (doesn't have to wait for medication).
   c. Increased client independence.
   d. Decreased level of sedation.
   e. Clients tend to use less narcotics.

C. Patient controlled epidural analgesia (PCEA).
1. Injection of medication via a small catheter into the epidural space of the spinal cord, common pain medications are morphine and fentanyl.
2. Relieves pain without causing sympathetic and motor nerve block.
3. May be intermittent or constant infusion.
4. To decrease hypotension episodes, make sure client is well hydrated prior to beginning of infusion.
5. Goal is to establish a comfort level and the client can perform activities necessary to his recovery (turn, cough, deep breath, eat, etc.).
6. Complications
   a. See Appendix 3-2, Narcotic Analgesics.
   b. Temporary lower extremity motor or sensory deficits - can be the result of a hematoma or infection, notify the anesthesiologist.
   c. Urinary retention - palpate supra pubic area, client may require urinary catheterization.

D. Acupuncture—insertion of thin metal needles into the body at designated points to relieve pain.

Evaluation

A. Identify client behavior response prior to the intervention and compare with response following intervention.

B. Maintain ongoing assessment and modify dosage and nursing interventions as indicated.

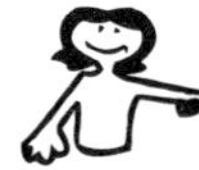

ELDERLY CARE PRIORITY: *Analgesics tend to last longer; there is increased risk for side effects and toxic effects.*

PERIOPERATIVE CARE

NCLEX ALERT: *Determine if client is prepared for a procedure or surgery.*

Preoperative care

A. Client Profile.
1. Age—elderly are more likely to have chronic health problems as well as age related factors and infants have more difficulty maintaining homeostasis than do the adult and child (Box 3-1).

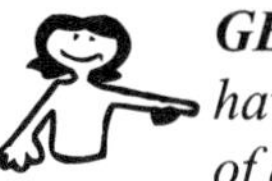

GERIATRIC PRIORITY: *Older clients have less physiologic reserve (the ability of an organ to return to normal after a disturbance in its equilibrium) than younger clients.*

2. Obesity—predisposes client to postoperative complications of infection and wound dehiscence.
3. Preoperative interview.
   a. Chronic health problems and previous surgical procedures.
   b. Past-and current drug therapy, including over-the-counter medications.
   c. History of drug allergies and dietary restrictions.
   d. Client's perception of illness and impending surgery.
   e. Discomfort or symptoms client is currently experiencing.
   f. Religious affiliation.
   g. Family or significant others.
4. Psychosocial needs—fear of the unknown is the primary cause of preoperative anxiety.

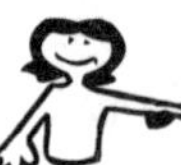

GERIATRIC PRIORITY: *The older client may require repeated explanation, clarification, and positive reassurance.*

5. Medications—may predispose client to operative complications.
   a. Anticoagulants - potentiate bleeding.
   b. Antidepressants - MAO inhibitors increase hypotensive effects of anesthetic agents.
   c. Tranquilizers - increase the risk of hypotension; may be used to enhance anesthetic agent.
   d. Thiazide diuretics - create electrolyte imbalance, particularly potassium.
   e. Steroids - prolonged use impairs the physiological response of the body to stress.
6. Check routine laboratory studies.
   a. Complete blood count; chemistry profile.
   b. Urinalysis.
   c. VDRL or FTA-ABS.
   d. Chest x-ray.
   e. Electrocardiogram (EKG) clients over 40 years old.
   f. f. Coagulation studies for clients with known problems or to establish a baseline.

B. Preoperative Teaching—goal is to decrease the client's anxiety and prevent postoperative complications.
1. Preoperative teaching content.
   a. Deep breathing and coughing exercises.
   b. Turning and extremity exercises.
   c. Pain medication policy.
   d. Adjunct equipment used for breathing - nebulizer, O_2 mask, spirometry.
   e. Explanation of NPO policy.
   f. Anti-embolism stockings, and or pneumatic compression devise to decease venous stasis.
2. Pediatric implications in preoperative teaching.
   a. Plan the teaching content around the child's developmental level and previous experiences.
   b. Use concrete terms and visual aids.
   c. Plan teaching session at a time in the child's schedule when he/she will be most conducive to learning.
   d. Use correct terms for body parts and clarify terms with which the child is unfamiliar.
   e. Introduce anxiety-provoking information last (increased anxiety may decrease comprehension).
   f. Use role-playing to either explain procedures to the child, or to allow the child to do a return demonstration.
   g. Fear of anesthesia is very common in children.
   h. Incorporate the parents in the teaching process.

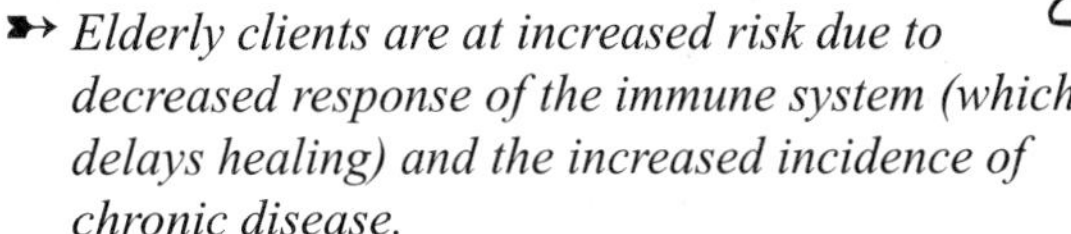

Box 3-1: Elderly Care Focus
Preoperative and Postoperative Considerations

➸ *Elderly clients are at increased risk due to decreased response of the immune system (which delays healing) and the increased incidence of chronic disease.*

- *Cardiovascular*—decreased cardiac output and peripheral circulation along with arrhythmias and increased incidence of arteriosclerosis and atherosclerosis can lead to hypotension or hypertension, hypothermia, and cardiac problems.
- *Respiratory*—decreased vital capacity, reduced oxygenation, and decreased cough reflex can lead to an increased risk of atelectasis, pneumonia, and aspiration.
- *Renal*—decreased renal excretion of wastes and renal blood flow along with increased incidence of nocturia can lead to fluid overload, dehydration, and electrolyte imbalance.
- *Musculoskeletal*—increased incidence of arthritis and osteoporosis can lead to trauma on bones and joints with positioning in the operating room, if pressure points and limbs are not padded.
- *Sensory*—decreased visual acuity and reaction time can lead to safety problems associated with falls and injuries.

➸ *The older client may require repeated explanation, clarification, and positive reassurance.*

➸ *Elderly clients often have a poor nutritional status which can directly influence healing and postoperative recovery.*

C. Physical Preparation of Client.
1. Skin preparation - purpose is to reduce bacteria on the skin (may be done in surgery or on the unit).
   a. Area of preparation is always longer and wider than area of incision.
   b. Antiseptic soap is used to cleanse area.
   c. Area may or may not be shaved.
2. Gastrointestinal preparation.
   a. Food and fluid restriction—6 to 8 hours preoperatively or NPO at midnight on the night prior to surgery..
   b. Enemas or cathartics—maybe administered the evening prior to surgery to prevent fecal contamination in the peritoneal cavity.
3. Promote sleep and rest—sleeping medication to promote rest, (i.e., barbiturate).

D. Legal Implications.
- Each surgical procedure must have the voluntary, informed, and written consent of the client or of the person legally responsible for the client.

Table 3-7: NURSING CARE OF CLIENT UNDERGOING REGIONAL ANESTHESIA

PROBLEM	NURSING INTERVENTIONS
Preparation For Procedure	1. Explain procedure. 2. Preoperative preparation and consent form signed for surgical client 3. Assess client for effectiveness as anesthesia is initiated. 4. Client will remain awake throughout procedure.
Hypotension	1. Report B/P less than 100 systolic, or any significant decrease. 2. Place client flat. 3. Administer O_2. 4. Increase IV rate if client is not prone to CHF.
Respiratory Paralysis	1. Avoid extreme Trendelenburg position before level of anesthesia is set. 2. Evaluate client's respiratory status. 3. Have ventilatory support equipment available.
Nausea And Vomiting	1. Antiemetics. 2. Anticipate nausea if client becomes hypotensive. 3. Suction, or position client to prevent aspiration.
Loss Of Bladder Tone	1. Evaluate for bladder distention.
Trauma To Extremities	1. Support extremity during movement. 2. Remove legs from stirrups simultaneously.
Headache	1. Insure adequate hydration before, during, and after procedure. 2. Maintain recumbent position 6 to 12 hrs. after procedure. 3. Administer analgesics.

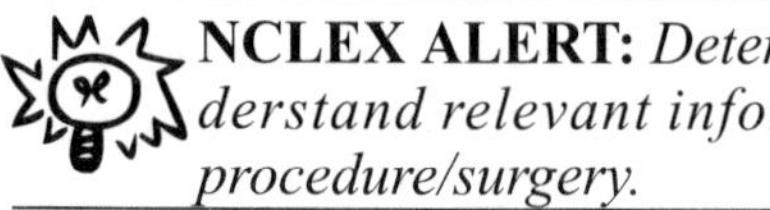

NCLEX ALERT: *Determine if client understand relevant information prior to procedure/surgery.*

1. Physician—gives the client a full explanation of the procedure, including complications, risks and alternatives.
2. Client's informed consent record (permit) must be signed by the physician, the client, and a witness (i.e., usually the staff nurse).

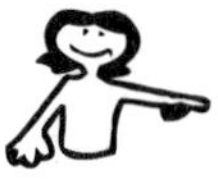

NURSING PRIORITY: *The consent record (permit) must be signed prior to the client receiving the preoperative medication.*

3. The signed consent record (permit) is part of the permanent chart record and must accompany the client to the operating room.

Day of Surgery

A. Nursing Responsibilities.
   1. Routine hygiene care.
   2. Vital signs within four hours of surgery.
   3. Remove jewelry; wedding bands maybe taped on finger.
   4. Remove fingernail polish.
   5. Dress client in patient gown.
   6. Determine if dentures and removable bridge work need to be removed prior to surgery.
   7. Continue NPO status.
   8. Check client's identification band; validate the information and see it is secure.
   9. Check skin preparation.
   10. Identify family and significant others who will be waiting for information regarding client's progress.
   11. Check the chart for completeness regarding laboratory reports, consent form, significant client observations, history and physical records.

B. Preoperative Medications (Appendix 3-3).

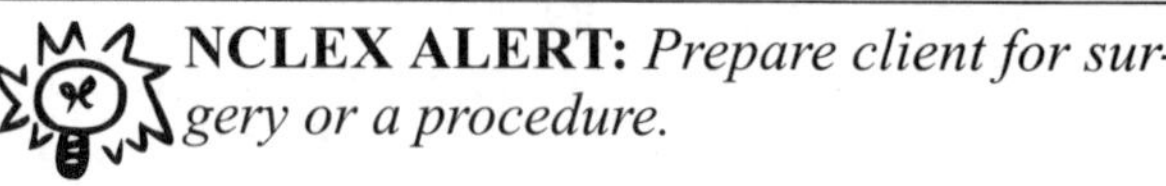

NCLEX ALERT: *Prepare client for surgery or a procedure.*

1. Purpose.
   a. Induce anesthesia rapidly and pleasantly.
   b. Reduce anxiety.
2. Nursing Responsibilities.
   a. Make sure all consent forms are signed and the client understands the procedure.
   b. Ask client to void prior to administration of medication.
   c. Obtain baseline vital signs.

d. Administer medication 45 minutes to 1 hour prior to surgery, or as ordered.
e. Raise the side rails and instruct the client not to get out of bed.
f. Remove dentures or bridges if necessary.
g. Observe for side effects of medication.
h. Allow parent to accompany child as far as possible.

Anesthesia

A. General anesthesia.

1. Intravenous anesthesia—used as an induction agent prior to the inhalation agent.
2. Inhalation anesthesia—used to progress client from stage II to stage III of anesthesia.

B. Regional anesthesia—used to anesthetize one region of the body; client remains awake and alert throughout the procedure.

1. Topical—anesthetizing medication applied to mucous membrane or skin; blocks peripheral nerve endings.
2. Local infiltration - injection of anesthetic agent, only blocks peripheral nerves around area.

Table 3-8: COMMON POSTOPERATIVE COMPLICATIONS

Complication	Signs and Symptoms	Nursing Intervention
Atelectasis	Dyspnea, decreased or absent breath sounds over affected area, asymmetrical chest expansion, hypoxia	Prevention: turn, cough and deep breath, adequate hydration, encourage ambulation. Position client on unaffected side. Maintain humidification, oxygen (see Chp. 15)
Shock	Decreasing blood pressure, weak pulse, restless, confusion, oliguria	Initiate IV access, keep NPO, maintain bedrest. Position supine with legs elevated and knees straight. Monitor ventilation and vital signs frequently. (see Chp 16)
Wound Infection	Redness, tenderness, fever, tachycardia, leukocytosis, purulent drainage.	Prevention: identify high risk clients, maintain sterile technique with dressing changes. Culture incision to determine organism. Evaluate progress and prevent spread of infection. **NCLEX ALERT:** *Assess a wound for signs of infection.*
Wound Dehiscence	Unintentional opening of the surgical incision.	Evaluate for hemorrhage, measures to prevent further pressure at incision site.
Wound Evisceration	Protrusion of a loop bowel through the surgical wound.	Cover bowel with sterile saline soaked dressing. Do not attempt to replace loop of bowel. Notify physician, client will most likely return to surgery for further exploration. **NCLEX ALERT:** *Provide emergency care for a wound disruption.*
Urinary Retention	Inability to void after surgery, bladder may be papable, voiding small amounts, dribbling.	Determine preoperative risks: medications, length of surgery, history of prostate problems. Determine amount of fluid intake and when to anticipate client to void – generally within 8hrs. Palpate suprapubic area, run tap water, provide privacy. Catheterize if necessary.
Gastric dilatation, Paralytic ileus	Nausea, vomiting, abdominal distension, decreased bowel sounds.	Prevention: geriatric clients at increased risk, encourage activity as soon as possible, maintain nasogastric tube suction, NPO, maintain IV's with hydrating solution. See Chp. 18

3. Peripheral nerve block - anesthetizes individual nerves or nerve plexuses (digital, brachial plexus). Does not block the autonomic nerve fiber; medication injected to block peripheral nerve fibers.
4. Spinal anesthesia - local anesthetics are injected into the subarachnoid space. May be used with almost any type of major procedure performed below the level of the diaphragm.
5. Epidural anesthesia - anesthetic agent is introduced into the epidural space, cerebral spinal fluid cannot be aspirated.

C. Nursing Considerations for Regional Anesthesia (spinal/epidural) (See Table 3-7).

D. Conscious sedation — the administration of an IV medication to produce sedation, analgesia, and amnesia.

1. Characteristics
   a. Client can respond to commands, maintains his protective reflexes and does not need assistance to maintain his airway.
   b. Amnesia most often occurs after the procedure.
   c. Slurred speech and nystagmus indicate the end of conscious sedation.

NCLEX ALERT: *Identify one's professional practice limitations. Primary responsibility is monitoring the client while under conscious sedation. The administration of medications to obtain the sedation level is the responsibility of the physician or an experienced RN.*

2. Nursing Implications.
   a. Obtain base line assessment prior to procedure, implications for care are the same as for a client receiving a general anesthesia.
   b. Client is assessed continuously, vital signs are recorded every 5-15 minutes.
   c. Monitor level of consciousness, client should not be unconscious, but relaxed and comfortable.
   d. Client should respond to physical and verbal stimuli, protective airway reflexes remain intact.
   e. Potential complications include loss of gag reflex, aspiration, hypoxia, hypercapnia and cardiopulmonary depression.
3. Does not require extensive post recovery time.

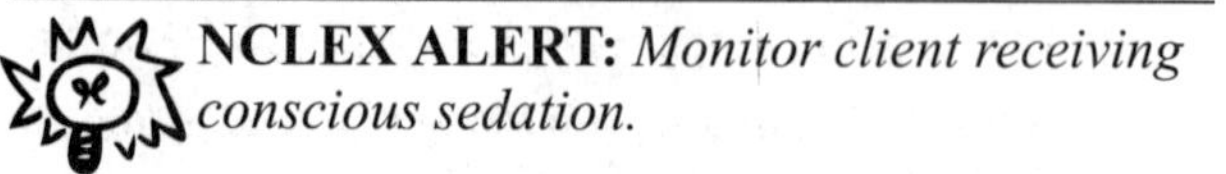

NCLEX ALERT: *Monitor client receiving conscious sedation.*

Immediate Postoperative Recovery

A. Admission of client to recovery area.

1. Position to promote patent airway, and to prevent aspiration.
2. Obtain baseline assessment.
   a. Vital signs.
   b. Status of respirations, pulse oximetry.
   c. General color.
   d. Type and amount of fluid infusing.
   e. Special equipment.
   f. Dressings.
3. Determine specifics regarding the operation from the O.R. nurse.
   a. Client's overall tolerance of surgery.
   b. Type of surgery performed.
   c. Type of anesthetic agents used.
   d. Results of procedure—was the condition corrected?
   e. Any specific complications to watch for.
   f. Status of fluid intake and urinary output.

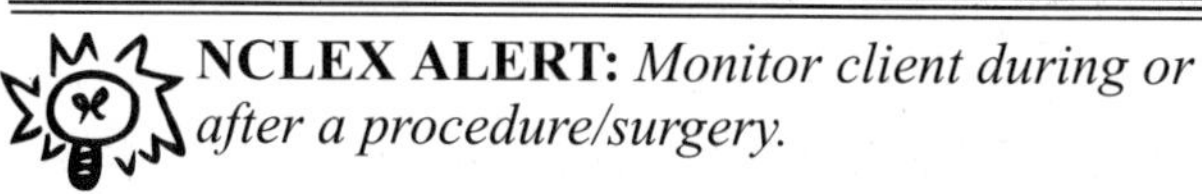

NCLEX ALERT: *Monitor client during or after a procedure/surgery.*

B. Nursing management during recovery.

✦ *Goal: to maintain respiratory function.*

NURSING PRIORITY: *The client's respiratory status is a priority concern on admission to and throughout the postoperative recovery period.*

1. Leave airway in place until pharyngeal reflex (gag reflex) has returned.
2. Position client on side (lateral Sims') or on the back with the head turned to the side to prevent aspiration.
3. Suction excess secretions and prevent aspiration.
4. Encourage coughing and deep breathing.
5. Administer humidified oxygen.
6. Auscultate breath sounds.

✦ *Goal: to maintain cardiovascular stability.*

1. Check vital signs q15 minutes until stable.
2. Report blood pressure that is continually dropping 5 to 10 mm Hg. with each reading.
3. Report increasing consistent bradycardia or tachycardia.
4. Evaluate quality of pulse and presence of dysrhythmia.

5. Evaluate adequacy of cardiac output and tissue perfusion.

✦ *Goal: to maintain adequate fluid status.*

NURSING PRIORITY: *Antidiuretic hormone (ADH) secretion is increased in the immediate postoperative period. Administer fluids with caution; it is easy to fluid overload a client.*

1. Evaluate blood loss in surgery and response to fluid replacement.
2. Maintain rate of IV infusion.
3. Measure urine output.
4. Evaluate for bladder distention.
5. Evaluate electrolyte status.
6. Evaluate hydration status.
7. Observe amount and character of drainage on dressings or drainage in collecting containers.
8. Assess amount and character of gastric drainage if nasogastric tube is in place.
9. Evaluate amount and characteristics of any emesis.

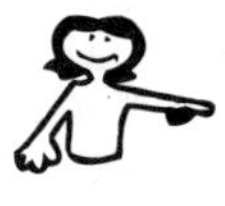

NURSING PRIORITY: *When client is vomiting, prevent aspiration by positioning on the left side and suctioning if appropriate.*

✦ *Goal: to maintain incisional areas.*

1. Evaluate amount and character of drainage from incision and drains.
2. Check and record status of Hemovac, Jackson-Pratt, or any other wound drains.

✦ *Goal: to maintain psychological equilibrium.*

1. Speak to client frequently in calm, unhurried manner.
2. Continually orient client, important to tell client that surgery is over and where he is..
3. Maintain quiet, restful atmosphere.
4. Promote comfort by maintaining proper body alignment.
5. Explain all procedures, even if client is not fully awake.
6. In the anesthetized client, sense of hearing is the last to be lost and the first to return.

✦ *Goal: client meets criteria to return to room.*

1. Vital signs stable and within normal limits.
2. Client awake and reflexes have returned.
3. Dressings intact with no evidence of excessive drainage.
4. Client can maintain a patent airway without assistance.

GENERAL POSTOPERATIVE CARE

NCLEX ALERT: *Anticipate situations with questions regarding basic postoperative nursing care, as well as questions that are for a specific surgical condition or procedure. Nursing implications for specific surgical procedures may be found under the major systems in the care of the medical surgical patient.*

✦ *Goal: to maintain cardiovascular function and tissue perfusion.*

1. Monitor vital signs, q4h.
2. Evaluate skin color and nail beds for paleness and cyanosis.
3. Monitor level of hematocrit.
4. Assess client's tolerance to increasing activity.
5. Encourage early activity and ambulation.

✦ *Goal: to maintain respiratory function.*

1. Have client turn, cough, and deep breathe q2h.
2. Use blow bottles, incentive spirometry to promote deep breathing.
3. Administer nebulizer treatment and bronchodilator
4. Maintain adequate hydration to keep mucous secretions thinned and easily mobilized.

✦ *Goal: to maintain adequate nutrition and elimination.*

1. Assess for return of bowel sounds and normal peristalsis.
2. Do not begin PO fluids until gastrointestinal function returns.
3. Assess client with a nasogastric tube for return of peristalsis.
4. Encourage fluids, unless contraindicated.
5. Assess client's tolerance of PO fluids; usually begin with clear liquids.
6. Progress diet as client's condition and appetite indicate, or as ordered.
7. Record bowel movements; normal bowel function should return on the 2nd-3rd postoperative day (providing the client is eating).
8. Assess urinary output.
   a. Client should void 8 to 10 hours after surgery.
   b. Assess urine output should be at least 30 cc/hr.
   c. Promote voiding by allowing client to stand or use bedside commode.

d. Avoid catheterization if possible.

✦ *Goal: to maintain fluid and electrolyte balance.*

1. Assess for adequate hydration.
   a. Moist mucous membranes.
   b. Adequate urine output.
   c. Good skin turgor.
2. Assess lab reports of serum electrolytes.
3. Assess character and amount of gastric drainage through the nasogastric tube.
4. Assess urine output as it correlates with fluid intake; maintain good I & O records.
5. Evaluate lab data for decreased renal function.

✦ *Goal: to promote comfort.*

1. Determine non- pharmacological pain relief measures
2. Administer analgesics.

Study Questions—Concepts of Nursing Practice

1. What is the most effective method to obtain an accurate blood pressure on a client?

① Obtain a cuff that covers the upper one-third of the client's arm.
② Position the cuff approximately 4" above the antecubital space.
③ Use a cuff that is wide enough to cover the upper two-thirds of the client's arm.
④ Identify the Korotkoff sounds, and take systolic reading at 10mm Hg after the first sound.

2. How does the school health nurse, working with sexually active teenagers, incorporate the concept of secondary prevention into practice?

① Setting up a birth-control clinic in the school health office.
② Attending health curriculum meetings to assure that contraceptive information is included in a unit on sexuality.
③ Teaching a group of parents about the problems of adolescent pregnancy.
④ Referring a pregnant adolescent for prenatal care.

3. Prior to discharge, the nurse teaches the back surgery client proper body mechanics. What client observations indicate the instruction was successful?

① Bends from the waist to lift a heavy object.
② Carries a heavy object away from his body.
③ Squats down to pick up a heavy object.
④ Leans backward when carrying a heavy object.

4. A 4-month-old client has a rectal temperature of 103.6°F. What is the best nursing action to decrease the temperature?

① Place in a cool mist croupette with compressed air.
② Sponge trunk and extremities with tepid water.
③ Encourage to take clear liquids such as apple juice.
④ Sponge with a solution containing half water and half alcohol.

5. What is the physiological principle behind the effective use of epidural anesthesia during labor?

① Both sensory and motor fibers to the uterus arise from the seventh and eighth thoracic vertebrae.
② Both sensory and motor fibers to the uterus arise from the first lumbar vertebrae.
③ Pain motor tracts from the cervix and vagina passes through the pudendal nerve and the motor fibers of the lower motor neurons before transmitting to the brain for interpretation of pain.
④ The pain of uterine contractions is carried by the eleventh and twelfth thoracic nerves, and motor fibers to the uterus arise from the seventh and eighth thoracic vertebrae.

6. To prevent complications of immobility, which activities would the nurse plan for the first postoperative day following a colon resection?

① Turn, cough and deep breathe every 30 minutes around the clock.
② Out of bed and ambulate to a bedside chair.
③ Passive range of motion three times a day.
④ It is not necessary to worry about complications of immobility on the first postoperative day.

7. What is the focus of the primary prevention strategies associated with pregnant adolescents?

① Identifying available support systems for pregnant adolescents.
② Assessing the risk status of a pregnant adolescent.
③ Advising pregnant adolescents on how to tell their parents about their pregnancy.
④ Providing adolescents with information about birth control clinics.

8. In the recovery room, the postoperative client suddenly becomes cyanotic. What is the first nursing action?

① Begin oxygen per nasal cannula.
② Call for assistance.
③ Suction the nasopharynx.
④ Insert an oral airway.

9. Where on the chest would the nurse place the stethoscope to evaluate a client's apical heart rate?

① On the right side at the midclavicular line, fourth intercostal space.
② On the left side at the midclavicular line, fifth intercostal space.
③ On the sternum, directly over the heart.
④ On the left side, mid-axillary level.

10. When the nurse admits a 2-year-old client with cerebral palsy, what is the most important information to consider in planning initial nursing care?

① Detailed description of previous hospitalizations.
② List of immunizations received.
③ Family history of illnesses.
④ General description of activities of daily living.

11. A one year old infant has ibuprofen (Advil) ordered every 6 hours. It has been 6 hours since the last dose and his parent has requested he receive his pain medication. When the nurse enters the room, the child is asleep. The parent requests the pain medication be given because the child is still restless in sleep. What is the best nursing action?

① Refuse to awaken the child.
② Wake the child and give the medication.
③ Tell the parent to call as soon as the child awakens.
④ Explain the purpose and use of pain medications to the parent.

12. What is important for the nurse to do in order to obtain a comprehensive medical history?

① Make sure the client is comfortable in their surroundings.
② Ask the most difficult questions first.
③ Ask about the family dynamics last.
④ Document events and dates in chronological order.

13. The nurse is admitting a woman who is scheduled for a total hip replacement. How is the most effective way to initiate the interview?

① Sit quietly until the client initiates the conversation.
② Start the interview with easy questions to build a rapport.
③ Try not to seem too friendly to soon.
④ Do not dwell on the diagnosis and its effect on the client.

14. A client is scheduled for surgery in the AM. Pre-operative orders have been written. What is most important to be done prior to surgery?

① Remove all jewelry or tape wedding rings.
② Verify all laboratory work is complete.
③ Inform family or next of kin.
④ Have all consent papers signed.

Answers and rationales to these questions are in the section at the end of the book entitled "Chapter Study Questions: Answers & Rationales."

Appendix 3-1:
NURSING PROCEDURE ■ POSITIONING ■

POSITIONS	PLACEMENT	USE
Fowler's	Head of bed 45-60 degree angle; hips flexed	The height may be determined by client preference, or tolerance. Frequently used for client with respiratory compromise.
Semi-Fowler's	Head of bed 30- 60 degree angle; hips flexed.	
Low Fowler's	Head of bed 15-30 degree angle; hips may or may not be flexed	
Trendelenburg	Head of bed lowered and foot raised, knee gatch straight	Thoracic percussion, vibration, and drainage procedure. Compromises respiratory function, client should not be left in position for extended time.
Modified Trendelenburg	Head of bed is flat or slightly elevated, legs are elevated about 20°, knees should be straight	Used for client in shock - promotes movement of fluids from lower extremities into circulation. Minimizes respiratory compromise.
Lateral (side-lying or Sims')	Head of bed lowered; pillows under arm and legs	For client comfort; increases uterine perfusion in pregnancy and prevents supine vena caval syndrome
Lithotomy	On back with thigh flexed against abdomen and legs supported by stirrups	Examination of female reproductive tract and rectum, cystoscopy, and surgical procedures
Prone	Head of bed flat, client on abdomen, head turned to side	To promote drainage postoperative tonsillectomy, to prevent contractures in AKA clients, imperforate anus, spina bifida
Supine	Bed in flat position, small pillow under head	Client comfort

NCLEX ALERT: *Position client to prevent complications.*

✓ **Key Points: Moving the Client Up in Bed**
- Lower the head of the bed so that it is flat or as low as the client can tolerate.
- Place one arm under the client's shoulders and the other arm under the client's thighs.
- Instruct the client to bend legs, put feet flat on bed, and push.
- Do not pull client up with pressure or pulling in the axillary area.

✓ **Key Points: Dangling at the Bedside**
- Raise the head of the bed until the client is sitting upright.
- Place one arm around shoulders and grasp knees with the other arm.
- In one motion, swing client's legs over bedside to sitting position.
- Assist client to remain in position to determine and or prevent orthostatic hypotension.

✓ **Key Points: Moving from Bed to Chair**
- Move client to the side of the bed closest to the edge where the client will be getting up.
- Raise head of bed to assist client in pivoting to the side of the bed.
- Move client to edge of bed and place feet flat on floor.
- Have client reach across chair and grasp arm.
- Stabilize client by positioning your foot at the outside edge of client's foot.
- Pivot client into chair using leg muscles instead of back muscles.
- Pull client back and up in chair for better posture.

✓ **Key Points: Logrolling the Client**
- Used for neck and back injury or surgical client.
- Maintain proper alignment on head and back areas while turning.
- Before moving patient, place a pillow between knees.
- Move client in one coordinated movement.

Appendix 3-1:
NURSING PROCEDURE ■ POSITIONING ■

NCLEX ALERT: *Maintain correct body alignment*

Clinical Tips for Problem Solving

If client is unable to assist with movement, then —

- Use a turn sheet to provide more support for client.
- Obtain additional assistance to help in moving the client.

If client is unable to maintain any type of position without assistance, then —

- Use trochanter roll made from bath blankets to align the client's hips to prevent external rotation.
- Use foam bolsters to maintain side-lying positions.
- Use folded towels, blankets, or small pillows, position client's hands and arms to prevent dependent edema.

If skin begins to break down, then —

- Keep client off affected area until healed.
- Change client's position every two hours.
- Check with physician for therapeutic mattress or medications for decubitus care.

Appendix 3-2:
ANALGESICS

MEDICATIONS	SIDE EFFECTS	NURSING IMPLICATIONS

❖ GENERAL NURSING IMPLICATIONS ❖

— Assess pain parameters, blood pressure, pulse, and respiratory status before and periodically after administration.

— Administer before pain is severe for better analgesic effect.

— Elderly or debilitated clients may require decreased dosage.

NARCOTIC ANALGESICS: Bind to opiate receptors in the central nervous system (CNS), altering the perception of and emotional response to pain. Controlled substances (Schedule II).

Strong Opiod Analgesics

MEDICATIONS	SIDE EFFECTS	NURSING IMPLICATIONS
Morphine sulfate (MS):PO, SQ, IM, IV Meperidine (**Demerol**): PO, SQ, IM Fentanyl Citrate (**Fentanyl, Sublimaze**): IM, IV, PO, transdermal	Respiratory depression Orthostatic hypotension Sedation, dizziness, dizziness, lightheadedness, dysphoria Constipation Tolerance, physical and psychological dependence	1. Morphine and meperidine are commonly used for PCA. 2. Demerol - use with caution in children and elderly clients due to increased toxicity and seizures. 3. Use with caution in clients who are respiratory compromised. 4. *Pediatric implication:* Medication calculated according to age and weight. 5. Increased toxicity in clients with hypothyroidism, renal, and liver conditions. 6. Requires documentation as indicated by Controlled Substance Act. 7. Instruct patient to change position slowly to minimize orthostatic hypotension.

Moderate to Strong Opiod Analgesics

MEDICATIONS	SIDE EFFECTS	NURSING IMPLICATIONS
Codeine: PO, SQ Hydromorphone (**Dilaudid**): PO, SQ, IM, IV, suppository Oxycodone (**Percodan, Percocet, Tylox**): PO Hydrocodone (**Vicodin**) PO Propoxyphene (**Darvon, Darvocet**): PO	Sedation, euphoria, respiratory depression, constipation, urinary retention, cough suppression	1. Usually administered by mouth 2. Codeine is extremely effective cough suppressant 3. Physical dependence is minimal 4. Warn patient to avoid activities requiring alertness until effects of drug are known.

Moderate Opiods

MEDICATIONS	SIDE EFFECTS	NURSING IMPLICATIONS
Butorphanol (**Stadol**) IM, IV, nasal spray, Nalbuphine (**Nubain**):SQ, IV, IM Pentazocine (**Talwin, Talwin Nx**): PO, SQ, IM, IV		

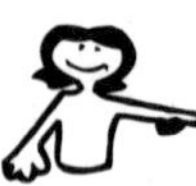

NURSING PRIORITY: *Concurrent administration with non-narcotic analgesics may enhance pain relief because they act at different sites.*

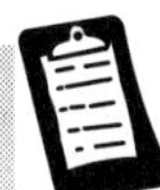

Appendix 3-2: ANALGESICS

MEDICATIONS	SIDE EFFECTS	NURSING IMPLICATIONS
NON-NARCOTIC ANALGESICS: Act peripherally to prevent the formation of prostaglandins in inflamed tissue, inhibiting the stimulation of pain receptors. Also, inhibit prostaglandin synthesis in the CNS and stimulate peripheral vasodilation to cause antipyresis.		
Acetaminophen (**Tylenol, Datril, Tempra**): PO Aspirin (**ASA**, Acetylsalicylic Acid): PO Ibuprofen (**Motrin, Nuprin, Advil**): PO Naproxen (**Naprosyn**); Naproxen sodium (**Anaprox, Aleve**): PO Piroxicam (**Feldene**): PO Sulindac (**Clinoril**): PO	GI pain and upset, nausea, vomiting, diarrhea, heartburn Dizziness, headache, Tinnitus (aspirin)	1. Nonsteroidal anti-inflammatory agents may prolong bleeding time and increase the effects of oral anticoagulants. 2. Chronic use of acetaminophen with other nonsteroidal anti-inflammatory agents may increase the chance of renal and liver damage. 3. ***Uses:*** **Mild to moderate pain**: acetaminophen, aspirin, ibuprofen, naproxen. **Fever:** acetaminophen, aspirin, ibuprofen **Inflammation:** aspirin, naproxen **Arthritis:** aspirin, ibuprofen, naproxen, piroxicam, sulindac **Dysmenorrhea:** ibuprofen, naproxen

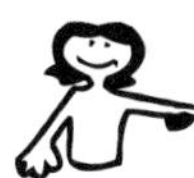

NURSING PRIORITY: *Advise patient that CDC warns against giving aspirin to children or adolescents with influenza.*

MEDICATIONS	SIDE EFFECTS	NURSING IMPLICATIONS
NARCOTIC ANTAGONISTS: Competitively block the effects of narcotics, without producing analgesic effects.		
Naloxone (**Narcan**)	Hypotension, hypertension, dysrhythmias	1. Assess respiratory status, blood pressure, pulse and level of consciousness until narcotic wears off. Repeat doses may be necessary if effect of narcotic outlasts the effect of the narcotic antagonist. 2. Remember that narcotic antagonists reverse analgesia along with respiratory depression. Titrate dose accordingly and monitor pain level. 3. ***Uses:*** Used to reverse CNS and respiratory depression in narcotic overdose. 4. ***Contraindications and precautions:*** Use with caution in narcotic-dependent patients; may cause severe withdrawal symptoms.

Appendix 3-3: PREOPERATIVE MEDICATIONS

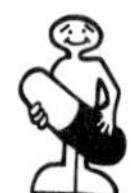

CLASSIFICATION	SIDE EFFECTS	NURSING IMPLICATIONS
SEDATIVES: Decrease anxiety prior to or during surgery.		
Amobarbital (**Amytal**): PO Pentobarbital (**Nembutal**): PO, rectal Secobarbital (**Seconal**): PO, IV, IM, rectal. Lorazepam **(Ativan)**: PO, IM, IV.	May produce paradoxical effects in elderly. Confusion and dizziness.	1. Decrease stimuli in the room after administration. 2. Offer emotional support to the anxious client. 3. **Ativan** has decreased incidence of paradoxical response.
Midazolam hydrochloride (**Versed**) IM	Decreased respirations, pain at IM or IV site. Nausea , vomiting	
TRANQUILIZERS: Decrease anxiety prior to surgery.		
Diazepam (**Valium**): PO Droperidol (**Inapsine**): PO Lorazepam **(Ativan)**: PO	Hypotension. May cause dizziness, clumsiness, or confusion.	1. Decrease stimuli in room after administration. 2. Offer emotional support to anxious client.
ANTIHISTAMINES: Potentiates effect of preoperative narcotic, decreases postoperative nausea, and has sedative effects.		
Promethazine hydrochloride (**Phenergan**): PO, IM Hydroxyzine hydrochloride **(Vistaril, Atarax)**: PO, IM	Blurred vision, hypotension, flushed skin	1. May be administered with Demerol as preoperative medication. 2. **Vistaril** must be given deep IM (preferably Z track) to prevent tissue irritation.
NARCOTIC ANALGESICS - see Appendix 3-2		
ANTICHOLINERGIC: Reduces oral, bronchial, gastrointestinal secretions; decreases gastrointestinal motility; bronchodilates; decreases incidence of laryngospasm.		
Atropine: PO, IM, IV Scopolamine: PO, IM Glycopyrrolate (**Robinul**): PO, IM, IV	Flushed face Dilated pupils Increased cardiac rate Urinary retention	1. Children and elderly are at increased risk for side effects. 2. Advise clients regarding atropine flush. 3. Administer with caution to the glaucoma, MI, and CHF client. 4. Postural hypotension may result if client ambulates after parenteral administration. 5. Monitor for urinary retention and decreased bowel sounds.

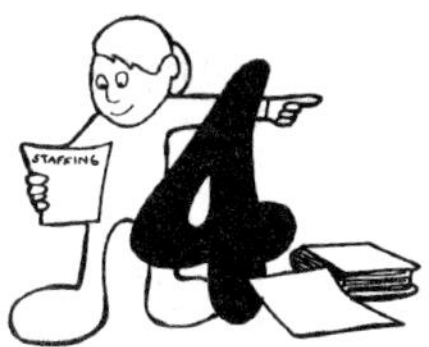

CONTROL FUNCTIONS AND MANAGEMENT

LEGAL ASPECTS

Nursing Practice Regulations

A. Common Elements of Nurse Practice Acts.
1. Definition of practice.
2. Establishment and authorization of regulatory agency.
3. Methods of licensure.
   a. Examination—successfully complete National Council Licensure Examination for Registered Nurses (NCLEX-RN™).
   b. Endorsement—applying for a license in a state or jurisdiction when already licensed in another state.
   c. Requirements for foreign graduates.
      (1) Complete requirements for NCLEX-RN.
      (2) Individual states may require completion of the Commission on Graduates of Foreign Nursing Schools (CGFNS) test *prior* to NCLEX-RN.
4. Penalties for failure to conform to requirements of the act.
   a. Failure to obtain license.
   b. Failure to practice according to standards.
   c. Grounds for disciplinary action.

B. How to protect your license (Table 4-1).

C. Related Statutes.
1. Reporting Acts—regulate what events must be reported to authorities; vary from state to state.
   a. Child Abuse.
   b. Gunshot wounds.
   c. Communicable diseases.
   d. Ophthalmia neonatorum.
   e. Phenylketonuria.
   f. Criminal acts.
2. Good Samaritan Laws—enacted by individual states.
   a. Purpose: to encourage health care providers to assist at accidents and emergencies.
   b. Elements of Good Samaritan Statutes (Table 4-2).

Table 4-1: PROTECT YOUR LICENSE

- ✦ Do not let anyone else borrow it.
- ✦ Do not let anyone copy it unless you write "copy" across it. In some states it is illegal to copy your license.
- ✦ If you lose it, report it immediately and take the necessary steps to obtain a duplicate.
- ✦ Be sure that the Board of Nursing knows whenever you change your address, whether you move across the street or across the nation.
- ✦ Practice nursing according to the scope and standards of practice in your state.
- ✦ Know your state law so you will not do anything which could cause you to be disciplined by the removal of your license.

Reprinted with permission from: Stark, S. "Legal Issues," in Zerwekh, J. and Claborn, J. *Nursing Today: Transition & Trends*, 3rd ed., Philadelphia: W.B. Saunders, 2000, p.391.

Liability for Actions

A. Individual Liability—every person is liable for his or her own conduct. Liability may be shared by another person or group (i.e., the doctor, another nurse, or the hospital), but it cannot be removed by the statements or actions of another.

B. Vicarious Liability—shares but does not lessen individual liability.
1. Respondent Superior—employer can be held liable for actions of employee.
2. Supervisory Negligence—supervisors can share liability if:
   a. Assignments are not within nurse's capabilities.
   b. Assignments are not appropriate for educational level of nurse.
   c. Assignments are not within legal limitations of practice.
   d. Supervision provided the activities of assigned nurse must meet actual limits and abilities of that individual.
3. Physician may share liability in either of the above cases, but *cannot* alter an individual nurse's personal liability by a statement of *agreement to assume liability.*

Criminal Law

A. Wrongs against society as a whole.

B. Punishment, usually prison term or fine.

C. Examples.
1. Violation of Practice Act.
2. Murder.
3. Manslaughter.
4. False imprisonment.
5. Narcotics violations.
6. Assault and battery.

Civil Law

A. Wrongs against private individuals or groups.

Table 4-2: GOOD SAMARITAN STATUTES

- ✦ Care must be provided in good faith.
- ✦ Care must be gratuitous; no compensation is made for the care rendered.
- ✦ A higher standard of care may be required of health care workers due to their higher level of expertise.
- ✦ Nurses will be expected to provide care at the level of an ordinary nurse in a similar circumstance.
- ✦ Does not cover a person who is soliciting business or representing an agency.
- ✦ Does not cover the care rendered in an emergency room situation.
- ✦ Care provided should not be willfully or wantonly negligent.

Reprinted with permission from: Stark,, S. "Legal Issues," in Zerwekh, J. and Claborn, J. *Nursing Today: Transition & Trends,* 3rd ed., Philadelphia: W.B. Saunders, 2000, p. 394.

B. Compensation for victim.

C. Torts—intentional or unintentional civil wrong.

1. Negligence—unintentional harm to another which occurs through failure to act in a reasonable and prudent manner.
2. Malpractice—professional practice which injures someone through failure to meet the proper standard of care.
   a. Elements of malpractice suit.
      (1) A professional must owe a duty: nurse-client relationship established.
      (a) Assignment to specific nursing team or client.
      (b) Nursing care given to patient regardless of formal assignment.
      (c) Emergency or need for immediate care by any client.
      (2) A professional must breach the duty by doing something wrong or not doing something needed.
      (3) Harm must occur to client.
      (4) Direct cause and effect relationship between the breach and the harm.
      (5) Foreseeability—a professional could reasonably expect injury to occur as a result of the breach of duty.
3. Invasion of Privacy—Protection of constitutional right to be free from undesired publicity and exposure to public view.

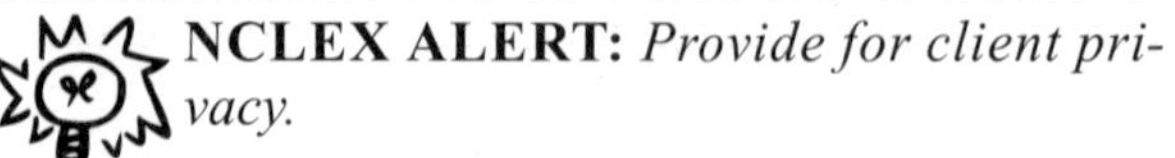

NCLEX ALERT: *Provide for client privacy.*

   a. Proper covering of physical body.
   b. Medical records.
      (1) Records should be released only with written client consent.
      (2) Release for medical "need to know" limited to caregivers only.
   c. Belongings must be protected and may not be searched without specific authorization. A client's list of belongings should be explained to and signed by the client.
   d. Confidentiality.
      (1) Conversations confidential; in some states protected by specific statute.
      (2) Photographs and viewing of procedures require consent of client.
      (3) Control of visitor access to client and client information.
   e. Reporting laws are an exception.
      (1) Communicable diseases.
      (2) Gunshot and knife wounds.
      (3) Child abuse.
      (4) Others defined by state statute.
   f. Rights may be waived by the client but never by medical personnel.
4. Defamation—written or oral communication to a third, or more, persons concerning matters which may injure an individual's reputation.
   a. Client.
   b. Staff and co-workers.
   c. Defenses to defamation action.
      (1) Truth.
      (2) Privilege—disclosure required by a duty to report to an authorized person; report to supervisor concerning poor practice of another nurse.

NCLEX ALERT: *Report a health care provider's unsafe practice (e.g., improper care, using drugs, etc.).*

5. False Imprisonment—unlawfully restraining personal liberty; unlawful detention.
   a. Actual—use of physical force to prevent departure of client; inappropriate use of restraints.
   b. Implied—use of words, threats, or gestures to restrain client.
      (1) Refusing to allow client to leave hospital until bill is paid.

(2) Refusing to release newborn infant until bill is paid.

(3) Refusing to allow client to leave without signing AMA form.

c. Exceptions—depend on state laws.

(1) Refusing to allow departure of individual with communicable disease.

(2) Refusing to allow departure of incompetent or mentally ill client if imminent threat of serious injury to self or other.

6. Assault and Battery—non consensual touching.

a. Valid consent.

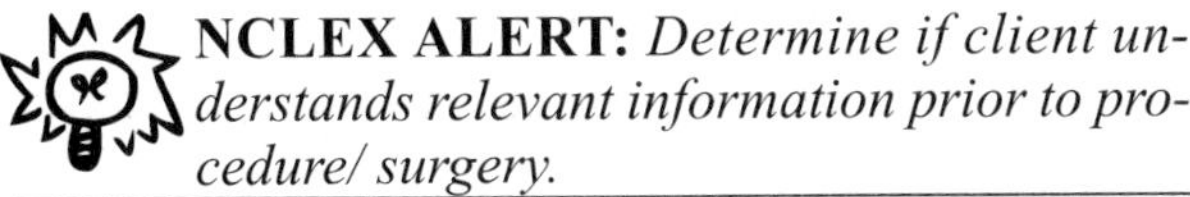

NCLEX ALERT: *Determine if client understands relevant information prior to procedure/ surgery.*

(1) Timely—some states or institutions have specific time restrictions on when consents are signed.

(2) Written—for all invasive procedures.

(3) Witnessed signature—do not witness unless you know client has all information needed to make informed decision.

(4) Procedure specified in terms the client can understand.

(5) Client understanding of significant risks of procedure.

(6) Client understanding of alternatives to procedure.

(7) Signed while client is free from mind-altering drugs or conditions.

b. Withdrawal of consent.

(1) Can be written or verbal.

(2) Can occur anytime prior to the procedure.

c. Exceptions.

(1) Life-threatening emergencies.

d. Minors—up to age 18.

(1) Parental signature generally required for consent.

(2) Some states or case laws alter this requirement for certain procedures.

(a) Birth control.

(b) Pregnancy.

(c) Sexually transmitted disease.

(d) Drug and alcohol dependency.

(e) Emancipated minor—definition may vary but usually is a minor who is self-supporting and living away from home.

e. Mentally incapacitated individual—consent required of legal guardian or, for temporary incapacities, person specifically authorized for medical consent.

Special Legal Principles

A. Standard of Care—the legal concept of a fictional, reasonable, prudent individual of the same education and profession against which another professional's performance is judged.

1. Established by considering:

a. Curriculum in schools of nursing.

b. Actual practice of nurses using "expert witnesses."

c. Statement of nursing standards.

(1) Practice Acts, and rules and regulations.

(2) Joint commissions.

(3) Professional organizations.

d. Policy and procedures manuals.

e. Prior court decisions.

2. Need not meet maximum level of performance.

3. Used to determine when a breach of duty has occurred.

B. Statute of Limitations—length of time during which a negligence suit may be filed.

1. Varies from state to state.

2. Is usually longer for minors—frequently does not begin until minor reaches 18.

3. Can be used as a defense if lawsuit not filed within time limitation.

C. Contributory Negligence—the client or some other person contributed to the injury; may be used as a defense in a lawsuit.

1. Requires competent client who is aware of risks.

2. Will deny recovery if proven.

D. Assumption of the Risk—client understands risks of event and agrees to accept them.

E. Elements of Informed Consent.

NCLEX ALERT: *Determine if client understands relevant information prior to procedure or surgery.*

1. The client must know the procedure.

2. The client must know the risks.

3. The client must know the alternatives.

Table 4-3: GUIDELINES FOR DEFENSIVE CHARTING

✦ All entries should be accurate.

✦ Make corrections appropriately and according to agency or hospital policies. Do not obliterate any information that is in the chart.

✦ If there is information that should have been charted and was not, the nurse should make a "late entry" noting the time the charting actually occurred and the specific time the charting reflects. *Example:* 10/13/99. 10:00am late entry, charting to reflect 10/12/99.

✦ All identified client problems, nursing actions taken, and the client responses should be noted. Do not describe a client problem and leave it without including nursing actions taken and the client response.

✦ Be as objective as possible in charting. Rather then charting the client tolerated the procedure well, chart the specific parameters checked to determine that conclusion. *Example:* "ambulated, tolerated well" would be more effective if charted "ambulated complete length of hall, no shortness of breath noted, pulse rate at 98, respirations at 22."

✦ Each page of the chart should contain the current date and time. Frequently, chart forms are stamped ahead of time. Each time you enter information on a new page, make sure it reflects the current time of charting.

✦ Follow through with who saw the client and what measures were initiated. Particularly note when the doctors visited; if you had to call a doctor for a problem, record the doctor's response. If orders were received, be sure they are signed according to policy. This is especially important, if you had to make several calls to the doctor.

✦ Make sure your notes are legible and clearly reflect the information you intended. It is a good idea to read over your nurse's notes from the previous day to see if they still make sense and accurately portray the status of the client. If the notes do not make sense to you the next day, imagine how difficult it would be to decipher the information at a later date.

Adapted with permission from: Stark, S. "Legal Issues," in Zerwekh, J. and Claborn, J. *Nursing Today: Transition & Trends*, 3rd. ed. W.B. Saunders, 2000, p.406.

F. Comparative Negligence—damage is apportioned between all responsible parties, including the client.

G. Ownership of Medical Records.

1. General rule is client owns information in file, agency owns actual file.
    a. Reasonable cost for copying.
    b. Reasonable limitations regarding viewing.
2. Some states have laws specifically controlling ownership of medical records.

H. Res Ipsa Loquitor—the thing speaks for itself.

1. Used when client injury occurs and it is difficult or impossible to prove how the injury occurred or who was responsible.
2. Allows jury to infer that defendant was negligent without expert testimony.
3. Required elements.
    a. Injury of type that would not occur unless someone was negligent.
    b. Cause of the injury under exclusive control of defendant.
    c. Client did not contribute to own injury.

Important Protective Procedures

A. Documentation—written record of events surrounding client's hospital stay.

1. Protects client by promoting good communication among health care providers.
2. Provides evidence in court of care given.
    a. Courts will not assume care is given unless it is recorded.
    b. Demonstrates meeting of standard of care.
    c. Demonstrates decision-making of nurse.

B. How to document (Table 4-3: Guidelines for Defensive Charting).

1. Be sure notes conform to the format required by the agency.
2. Use the format correctly.
    a. Complete all portions of format (i.e., SOAP or SOAPIE notes).
    b. Use opinions only in assessment portion of charting, never in areas requiring factual data.
    c. Complete an honest record of events.
        (1) Exclude reference to "incident report" filed.
        (2) Do not alter record at any time.
        (3) Record all events, even unusual events, factually.
        (4) Give all appropriate information about each note (i.e., IV site, location, color, temperature, size [swelling, etc.], dressing, and condition).
        (5) Explain omissions in care.
    d. Time, date, and sign all entries.
    e. Do not skip lines; do not leave any blank spaces for other people to chart.
    f. Correct errors properly.
        (1) Draw a straight line through error; date, initial.
        (2) Add omitted information by an "addendum" or "late entry" - give date and time of original note as well as date and time of addendum.

g. Use meaningful, specific language. Do not use words you do not understand, or unaccepted abbreviations.

NCLEX ALERT: *Document/report treatment errors or accidents.*

C. Know Your Limits.

1. Physical-Emotional—be aware of fatigue and confusion, and compensate for them.

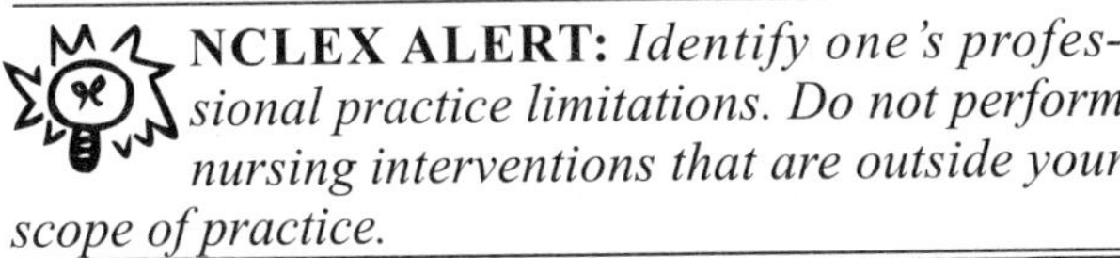

NCLEX ALERT: *Identify one's professional practice limitations. Do not perform nursing interventions that are outside your scope of practice.*

2. Practice competency—do not perform procedures without adequate preparation, knowledge and experience. Request supervision if unsure of your skills.
3. Never allow anyone to talk you into doing something you are not sure of by letting them agree to take the liability or telling you it is simple.

D. Continuing Education.

1. Mandatory in some states.
2. Important to keep knowledge and skills current.

Responsibility for Professional Practice

1. In order to maintain the standards of nursing care and to protect the client, the nurse should report anyone in the health care setting that engages in illegal, unethical or incompetent practice.

NCLEX ALERT: *Report a health care provider's unsafe practice.*

2. Examples of unethical care include:
   a. Medication errors that are made and not reported/corrected.
   b. Physical and verbal client abuse.
   c. Providing care while under the influence of alcohol or drugs.
   d. Breech of client confidentiality.
   e. Jeopardizing a client's well being by withholding or treatment.
3. The nurse should follow the line of authority within the institution for reporting the incident.
4. The American Nurses Association's Code for Nurses, the American Hospital Association's A Patient's Bill of Rights, and the individual state nurse practice acts provide the guidelines for safe, ethical nursing practice.

NCLEX ALERT: *Educate staff regarding client's rights.*

Specific Situations of Risk

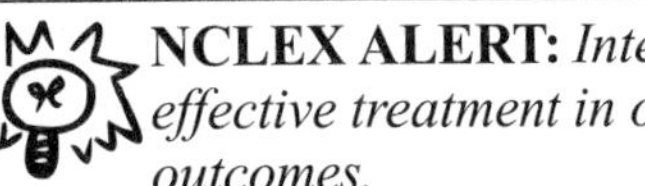

NCLEX ALERT: *Intervene to provide more effective treatment in order to improve client outcomes.*

A. Common areas of nursing liability.

1. Mistaken client identity.
2. Medication errors.
3. Failure to adequately and accurately assess client's condition.
4. Failure to take action and document changes in client's condition.
5. Failure to adequately supervise client resulting in client injury.
6. Failure to remove foreign objects from client during or after surgical procedures.
7. Illegible handwriting on client's chart and records.
8. Improper delegation of nursing responsibilities.
9. Correct interpretation and implementation of physician's orders.
10. Floating to a client care area where the nurse does not feel qualified to provide competent care.

B. Physical Injury.

1. Inappropriate siderail usage.
2. Inadequate attention during ambulation.
3. Obstacles or dangers on floor or in path.
4. Improper transportation.
   a. Inadequate locks on doors and equipment.
   b. Inadequate and inappropriate use of restraints.
5. Client burns.

C. Medication Errors.

1. Use five rights to protect client.
2. Know dosage, significant side effects, contraindications and interactions of all drugs given.
3. Never give drugs without complete order with name, route, dose, frequency.
4. Challenge orders when necessary.

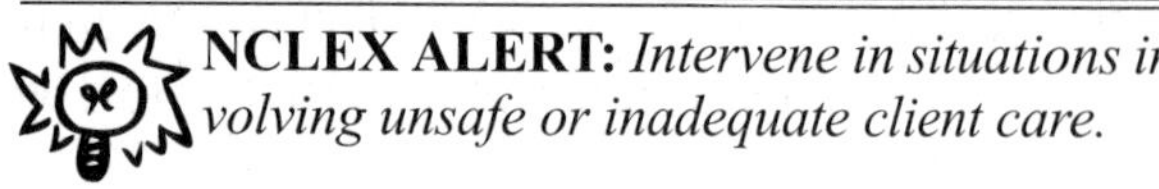
NCLEX ALERT: *Intervene in situations involving unsafe or inadequate client care.*

D. Telephone and Other Verbal Orders.
   1. Use telephone orders in emergency only, following policy of institutions involved.
   2. Do not take verbal orders with physician present in any situation which is not an extreme emergency.
   3. Verify all orders at the time they are received, and again, should any questions arise.
   4. Obtain needed signature promptly.

E. Changes in client's condition.

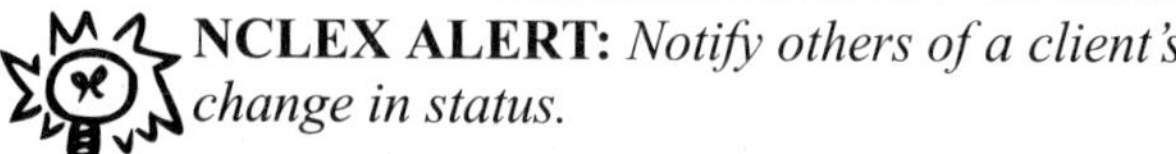
NCLEX ALERT: *Notify others of a client's change in status.*

   1. Notify appropriate individuals.
   2. Challenge failure to provide appropriate care.
   3. Failure to obtain needed medical assistance.

F. Restraints.
   1. Should be adequate and appropriate for the purpose.
   2. Requires a physician's order to utilize a restraint on a client.
   3. In an emergency situation, restraints may be used without a doctor's order for a very limited period of time.
   4. Safe nursing practice includes:
      a. Check restrained client q30 minutes and provide for physiological needs.
      b. Remove restraints and provide ROM q2h.
      c. Documentation—time of each check and neurovascular status of client's extremities.
      d. Remove restraints as soon as possible.
      e. Tie restraints to the bed frame, not to the side rails.

NCLEX ALERT: *Identify appropriate use of restraints or safety devices.*

G. Shift Report - purpose is to inform the oncoming nurse of the immediate needs and progress of the client. The oncoming nurse is responsible for the nursing care required on their shift.
   1. Do not read everything on the care plan or Kardex.
   2. The oncoming nurse is responsible for the nursing care required on their shift.
      a. Status of IV's, and amount of fluid to count.
      b. Any abnormal conditions (vital signs, pain, special treatments).
      c. Status of client with regard to their diagnosis. Examples: cardiac client-presence of absence of chest pain and dysrhythmias; surgical client -voiding, incision status; orthopedic client - circulation distal to cast or traction.

NCLEX ALERT: *Give a change of shift report.*

H. Internal disasters - fire
   1. Immediately return to your unit if a fire code is called.
   2. If clients on your unit are not in immediate danger, close all of the doors to the client rooms.
   3. If you need to evacuate your unit because of immediate danger, evacuate clients in this order:
      a. Ambulatory clients first because they can move the quickest.
      a. Remove clients in wheelchairs or walkers next.
      b. Last to remove are the clients who are bedridden.
   4. Know the types of fire extinguishers:
      Class A - water or solution for paper or linens.
      Class B - foam extinguisher for grease, chemical or electric fires.
      Class C -multipurpose for paper , linens, or electrical fires.
   5. Acronym - RACE
      R- Rescue
      A- Alert
      C- Confine
      E- Evacuate

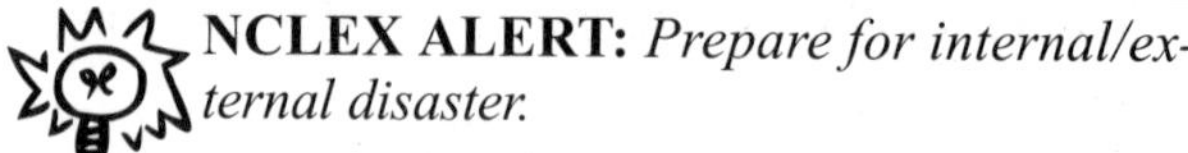
NCLEX ALERT: *Prepare for internal/external disaster.*

I. Advance medical directives - an inquiry regarding a client's advance directives or desire to prepare one is required for clients receiving Medicare funds and entering the hospital or an extended care facility.
   1. Living Will—a written document describing the client's wishes and special instructions regarding life support measures in the event the client is incapacitated.
   2. Durable power of attorney for healthcare—identifies the person whose takes the responsibility to ensure that previously agreed health care directives as

well as a living will are carried out according to the client's direction.

NCLEX ALERT: *Inform client of his/her rights (e.g., advanced directives, confidentiality, etc.).*

ETHICAL CONCERNS

Death and Dying Issues

A. Euthanasia—implies painless actions to end the life of individuals suffering from incurable or terminal diseases.
   1. What are the concerns regarding the *quality* of life and suffering versus *quantity* of life?
   2. Do clients have the choice and the "right to die"?
   3. What are the implications of passive euthanasia (withdrawal of life support) versus voluntary euthanasia (dying individual wants to control the time of death)?

B. No CODE (DNR Order).
   1. Physician's order must be written.
   2. Family members in agreement with "No CODE."
   3. Frequently in agreement with client's advanced medical directive.
   4. "Slow CODE," "No Heroics," "No Ventilation," "Pull the Plug," are legal issues that are not clearly defined.

MANAGEMENT CONCEPTS

Patterns of Health Care Delivery

A. Functional nursing.
   1. Series of tasks performed by several people.
   2. Fragmented, impersonal nursing care.

B. Team nursing.
   1. Groups of clients assigned to a team leader (usually an RN).
   2. Team leader coordinates care for a group of clients.
   3. Team conference—assess client needs and revise plan of nursing care.

C. Primary nursing.
   1. RN plans and directs care of client for a 24-hour period.
   2. Associate nurse takes over responsibility care when primary nurse is "off duty."
   3. Brought RN back to client's bedside.

D. Case managed care.
   1. Based on previously identified client outcomes to be achieved within a specific time frame.
   2. RN "manages" a caseload of clients for which he/she is responsible from preadmission to postdischarge.
   3. Ideally, case manager is at an advanced level of nursing practice.

Making Client Care Assignments and Delegating Duties

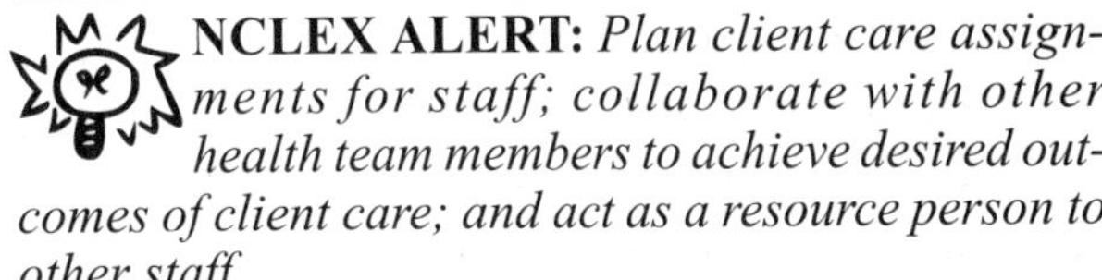

NCLEX ALERT: *Plan client care assignments for staff; collaborate with other health team members to achieve desired outcomes of client care; and act as a resource person to other staff.*

A. Guidelines for making assignments (Tables 4-4 and 4-5).

B. Assign a nursing task to an appropriately qualified person.
   a. Client care assistant (nurse's aide, unlicensed assistive personnel, certified nursing assistant)—bed making, bathing, feeding, ambulating, general activities of daily living. Activities that have very specific guidelines.

NCLEX ALERT: *Supervise delivery of care by assistive personnel.*

   b. Licensed practical/vocational nurse (LPN/LVN) —nursing procedures (i.e., suctioning, catheterization) requiring knowledge of sterile technique, medication administration, implements basic nursing process after RN has evaluated client and determined plan of care..
   c. Registered nurse (RN)— develops nursing care plan, implements teaching plans, and plans for client discharge.

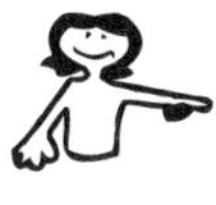

NURSING PRIORITY: *Discharge planning, initial client assessment, and planning for education are the responsibility of the RN.*

(1) Performs the initial assessment on admission and after surgery or treatment.

(2) Analyzes assessment data and determines appropriate nursing diagnoses and nursing actions.

(3) Assign most ill or unstable client to RN.

(4) Responsible for making decisions regarding client care.

Table 4-4: DELEGATION TERMS

- ✦ **Delegation:** ". . .entrusting the performance of selected nursing tasks to competent persons in selected situations. The nurse retains the accountability for the total nursing care of the individuals." (NCSBN, 1990).
- ✦ **Supervision:** "Provision of guidance by a qualified nurse for the accomplishment of a nursing task or activity with *initial direction* of the task or activity and *periodic inspection* of the actual act of accomplishing the task or activity." (NCSBN, 1990).
- ✦ **Accountability:** "Being answerable for what one has done, and standing behind that decision and/or action." (Hansten & Washburn, 1994).

C. Considerations for assigning client rooms

1. Clients needing frequent nursing assessment or intervention should be assigned a room near the nurse's station.
2. Group client assignments geographically together to assist in the work organization schedule of the nurse.
3. Consider the client diagnosis in planning assignments of care and client room assignments.
   a. Consider the immunosuppressed clients needs - do not put them at increased risk for opportunistic infections.
   b. HIV + client should not share room with a client with an upper respiratory infection, client with wound infection should not share room with a client with an open lesion due to poor circulation.
   c. Be aware of clients that will require some level of isolation and a private room. For example children with rotavirus, respiratory syncytial virus; clients with methicillin resistant staphylococcus (MRS).
   d. When a group of clients are assigned to one nurse, consider the opportunity for cross infections. For example, a client who is immunosuppressed and a client with MRS should not be assigned to the same nurse.
4. Nurse Practice Acts of each state may dictate the specific activities of the LPN and RN.

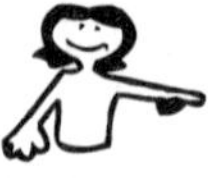

NURSING PRIORITY: *Client safety is a priority concern when planning assignments.*

D. Prioritizing client care assignments.

1. Identify the most ill or unstable client on your assignment and care for that client first.
2. Physiological needs are a priority - education and communication needs can wait until physiological needs are met. Of the physiological needs airway, breathing and circulation (ABC's) are priority.

Table 4-5: FOUR RIGHTS OF DELEGATION

- ✦ ***Right Task***—Can the task be delegated?
- ✦ ***Right Person***—Who is the competent person for the selected situation or task?
- ✦ ***Right Communication***—How do I get the person selected for the task to understand what I want?
- ✦ ***Right Feedback***—How do I give feedback during my "periodic inspection?" (Hansten & Washburn, 1994).
- ✦ ***Right Education***—Does the person have the right type of education to perform the procedure or care for the client?

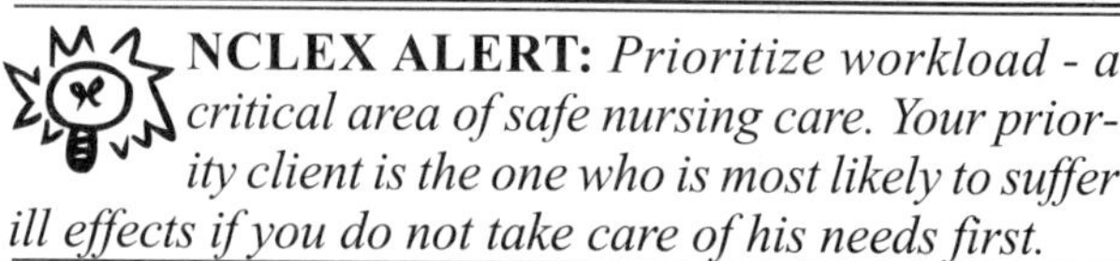

NCLEX ALERT: *Prioritize workload - a critical area of safe nursing care. Your priority client is the one who is most likely to suffer ill effects if you do not take care of his needs first.*

Quality Management

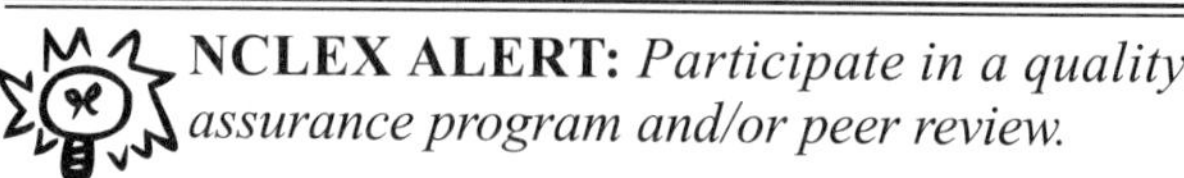

NCLEX ALERT: *Participate in a quality assurance program and/or peer review.*

A. Continuous quality improvement (CQI)—to constantly and continuously look for opportunities to improve client care.

1. Results from CQI audits are utilized to identify problem areas and to improve client care.
2. CQI—evaluates all aspects of nursing care (i.e., nutrition services, radiology, etc.).
3. Usually monitored by the quality assurance department of the hospital.

B. Quality assurance process.

1. Setting standards.
   a. Use of general standards of care, (i.e., ANA's **Standards of Nursing Practice**) along with each institution's and each client care unit's standards.
   b. *Example of a standard:* Every client will have a written nursing care plan.
2. Determining criteria to meet standards.
   a. Provides a measurable indicator to evaluate performance.
   b. *Example:* Nursing care plan is to be developed and written by a registered nurse within 10 hours of admission.
3. Evaluating performance or how well the criteria has been met.
   a. Usual method is reviewing documented records (chart).
   b. *Example:* Checking the chart to see if care plan is in place within the 10 hour time period.

4. Making plans for change.
   a. Because no performance standards can be perfectly met all the time, methods and plans to correct deficits need to be identified (nursing audit).
   b. *Example:* Determine how much deviation from the standard is acceptable before changes are made—15 out of 20 clients admitted have a care plan recorded within 10 hours of admission.
5. Follow-up on how effective changes were.
   a. Checking to see if changes were made.
   b. *Example:* After first audit of charts and suggested changes are made, a second audit of 20 charts determines whether an improvement in getting the care plan on the chart in 10 hours occurred.

C. Methods of monitoring nursing care.
1. Nursing audit—examining the client's records either retrospectively (after discharge) or concurrently (while client is receiving care).
2. Peer review—practicing nurses evaluating peer performance based on standards and criteria.
3. Utilization review—mandated by JCAHO to determine appropriate allocation of resources.
4. Patient satisfaction—questionnaire to clients as to satisfaction regarding the care they received.⌘

Study Questions—Control Functions and Management

1. The nurses enters data on a chart and discovers she has written on the wrong chart. How is this error best corrected?

① White out the wrong information and write over it.
② Recopy the page with the error so chart will be neat.
③ Draw a straight line through the error, initial, and date.
④ Obliterate the error so it will not be confusing.

2. Most states have reporting laws which require health care workers to report certain situations and behavior to authorities. Which is not usually a reportable matter?

① Child abuse.
② Communicable disease.
③ Gunshot wounds.
④ Attempted suicide.

3. What is the best nursing action when the client gives information which is pertinent to care?

① Share this information with everyone in the unit.
② Share this information with those needing to know for planning care.
③ Write the information in the chart only.
④ Share this information only with other nurses on the unit.

4. What client response would the nurse identify as an indication that the client understands the informed consent document?

① The client states that the physician has explained the procedure to him.
② The nurse finds the informed consent form already signed.
③ The client can give a return verbal explanation of the informed consent document.
④ The client states that his wife read it and said it was okay.

5. While caring for an 8 year old child with a broken wrist the nurse notices red, raised streaks on the child's back. The child's father enters the room and the child becomes quiet and distant, leaning away from the father as he approaches the child. What is the best nursing action?

① Chart that the child was probably beaten by the father.
② Notify the supervisor to report possible child abuse.
③ Disregard suspicions and care for the immediate needs of the child.
④ Not worry about the incident as there is no actual proof of abuse to the child.

6. What is the nurse's best approach to avoid claims of negligence?

① A strong and binding contract for services.
② Adhere to all hospital policies.
③ Competent practice of nursing.
④ Keeping a current license.

7. Which judgment error would be considered most damaging?

① Making illegal changes in the chart.
② Arguing with the plaintiff over the case.
③ Withholding information from your attorney.

④ Being argumentative while on the witness stand.

8. A nurse is transcribing orders for a client and finds a new order for aspirin. The nurse knows that the client has a long history of GI bleeding. What action should the nurse take?

① Withhold the medication and charts why it was not given.
② Ask the client if she is allergic to aspirin.
③ Call the physician and question the order in light of the history.
④ Give the medication.

9. The physician asks the nurse to give a client a medication that the nurse knows the client is allergic to. When the nurse tries to point this out to the physician, the physician threatens to tell the nurse's supervisor. What is the best response?

① Tell the physician to give the medication himself.
② Walk away and ignore him.
③ Agree to give the medication but not initial the dose.
④ Offer a meeting between the the nurse, supervisor, and physician.

10. What is a key component in a quality assurance program?

① Patient satisfaction questionnaire.
② Determine criteria to meet standards.
③ Case management for continuity of care.
④ An acuity system for client classification.

Answers and rationales to these questions are in the section at the end of the book entitled "Chapter Study Questions: Answers & Rationales."

GENERAL CONCEPTS OF PHARMACOLOGY

❑ **No medication has a single action; all medications have the potential to alter more than one body function.**

NURSING PRIORITY: *Many medications have several actions that are desirable. Carefully evaluate the questions as to what is the desired response of the medication for the specific client situation. Example: Atropine—preoperative to decrease secretions; in cardiac client it is used to treat bradycardia.*

1. Desired action—the desired, predictable response for which the medication is administered.
2. Side effects (drug reaction)—the undesirable, or unwanted response; frequently predictable.
3. Unpredictable response—the unusual response to a medication.
   a. Idiosyncratic reaction—an individual, unexpected response to a medication.
   b. Allergic reaction—does not occur with the initial dose of medication; occurs with subsequent doses because it requires that the immune system respond with the production of antibodies in order to trigger the allergic reaction.

A. The Drug Amendments of 1962 made it mandatory that each medication have one official name.
   1. Generic name (nonproprietary)—the official designated name which the medication is listed under in official publications.
   2. Chemical name—designates the specific chemical composition of the medication.
   3. Trade (proprietary name, brand)—the name designated and registered by a specific manufacturer.

NCLEX ALERT: *Typically, the medications on the exam will be identified with both the generic and trade name, (i.e., diazepam [Valium]).*

B. Factors influencing dosage—response relationships.
   1. Age—the young infant and the elderly are generally more sensitive to medications.
   2. Medication history—the prior administration of medications may greatly affect the client's response.
      a. Tolerance—medications administered repeatedly begin to produce progressively decreased effects.
      b. Cumulative effects—more medication is being administered than is being removed.
      c. Medication interactions—the effects of one medication may be increased, decreased or eliminated by the prior administration of another medication.
   3. Presence of disease process, specifically kidney and liver problems.
   4. Method of administration.
   5. Adequate cardiac output.
   6. Emotional factors—clients are more likely to respond to a medication in a positive manner if they have confidence in their physician and anticipate the therapeutic effects.

Drug Interactions

A. Pharmacokinetic Interaction

❑ **Drug interaction can be defined as an altered, or modified, action or effect of a drug as a result of interaction with one or more drugs. It is not to be confused with adverse drug reaction or drug incompatibility.**

1. Drug interaction can change the absorption, distribution, metabolism, or excretion of one or both drugs. Letters **ADME** are often used to represent these processes (see Table 5-1: Pharmacokinetic Interactions of Drugs).
   a. **A**bsorption—drugs can block, decrease, or increase absorption. Does this by increase or decrease gastric emptying time, changing gastric pH, or by forming drug complexes.
   b. **D**istribution—altered distribution occurs when two drugs that bind to the same plasma proteins are taken.
   c. **M**etabolism—a drug may affect the metabolism of another drug by stimulating or inhibiting enzymes secreted from the liver.
   d. **E**xcretion—a change in urine pH, cardiac output can effect the excretion of a drug.
2. Adverse drug reaction—undesirable drug effect ranging from mild untoward effects to severe responses, including hypersensitivity reaction and anaphylaxis.

3. Drug incompatibility—a chemical or physical reaction that occurs among two or more drugs *in vitro* (outside the body).

B. Pharmacodynamic Interactions

1. Additive effect—get twice the effect.

Example: Desirable additive effect occurs when giving a diuretic and a beta blocker for hypertension or giving two analgesics, aspirin and codeine, for increased pain relief. Undesirable additive effect can occur from two vasodilators (**Apresoline**) and nitroglycerin for angina can lead to severe ↓ BP.

1. Synergistic or potentiation effect—greater than twice the effect.

*Example: Desirable synergistic effect is when **Demerol** and **Phenergan** are combined causing **Phenergan** to potentiate the effect of **Demerol**. Undesirable synergistic effect occurs when alcohol and a sedative-hypnotic such as **Valium** are combined increasing CNS depression.*

2. Antagonistic effect—the effect of either or both drugs is decreased.

*Example: When you give an adrenergic beta blocker (**Inderal**) with an adrenergic beta stimulant (**Isuprel**), the action of each drug is canceled.*

A. Drug—food interactions.

1. Food can bind with drugs and delay drug absorption.

Table 5-1: PHARMACOKINETIC INTERACTIONS OF DRUGS

DRUG	EFFECT
ABSORPTION	
Laxatives	Speeds gastric emptying time. Increases gastric motility. Decreases drug absorption.
Narcotics Anticholinergics	Slows gastric emptying time. Decreases gastric motility. Increases drug absorption or decreases absorption depending on where the drug is delayed (gastric vs. intestinal).
Aspirin	Decreases gastric pH. Increases drug absorption.
Antacids	Increases gastric pH. Slows absorption of acid drugs.
Antacids and tetracycline	Forms drug complexes. Blocks drug absorption.
DISTRIBUTION	
Anticoagulant and anti-inflammatory (sulindac)	Competes for protein-binding sites. Increases free drug (i.e., anticoagulant)
METABOLISM	
Barbiturates	Promotes induction of liver enzymes. Increases drug metabolism. Decreases drug plasma concentration of the second drug.
Antiulcer (cimetidine)	Inhibits liver enzymes release. Decreases drug metabolism of **Valium, Dilantin,** morphine, etc. Increases drug plasma concentration of the second drug.
EXCRETION	
Any drug that decreases cardiac output or decreases renal blood flow.	Decreases drug excretion. Increases drug plasma concentration.
Antiarrhythmic (quinidine)	Decreases renal excretion of second drug,, (e.g., digoxin). Increases digoxin concentration.
Antigout (probenecid)	Decreases excretion of penicillin by competing for tubular reabsorption. Increases penicillin concentration.
Antacid (sodium bicarbonate)	Changes urine pH to alkaline. Promotes excretion of weak acid drug
Aspirin, ammonium chloride	Changes urine pH to acid. Promotes excretion of weak base drugs

Example: Tetracyclines bind with dairy products→ ↓ in plasma tetracycline.

2. Food increases the absorption of nitrofurantoin (**Macrodantin**)—anti-infective, metoprolol (**Lopressor**)—beta blocker, and lovastatin (**Mevacor**)—anti-lipemic.
3. MAO inhibitors (**Marplan**)—antidepressants when taken with tyramine-rich foods, (i.e., cheese, wine, organ meats, beer, yogurt) may lead to a hypertensive crisis.

B. Drug—laboratory interactions.

1. Abnormal plasma or serum electrolytes can affect drugs.

Example: Digitalis toxicity can occur when a client's serum potassium and magnesium are decreased serum calcium increased.

Table 5-2: PEDIATRIC PHARMACOLOGY AND NURSING IMPLICATIONS

PHYSIOLOGIC CONSIDERATIONS	BODY EFFECTS & POSSIBLE DRUG RESPONSES
ABSORPTION	
Neonates (< 1 month old) Infants (1 month - 1 year): alkaline gastric juices immature liver and kidneys → ↓ metabolism and extretion	Reduced gastric acid production; gastric pH is higher than in adults. Drugs, such as penicillin, that are absorbed poorly in a low gastric pH are absorbed faster in the higher pH. Smaller drug dose may be required. Slow gastric emptying time due to a slow or irregular peristalsis may slow drug absorption. Drugs given orally usually take longer to reach peak plasma levels. Adults and older children have a faster absorption rate. Elimination by the liver is reduced, thus a smaller drug dose is required. Topical drugs may be absorbed faster than in adults because infants have a proportionally greater body surface area. In addition, their skin is thin and drugs pass through more readily. The increased systemic absorption could result in adverse effects.
DISTRIBUTION PHASE	
Overall immaturity of organs affects drug action→ drug dosage needs to be adjusted. Infants and children have lower blood pressure. The liver and brain are proportionally larger and receive more blood flow; the kidneys receive less. Infant's body composition is 65% to 75% water; premature infant's is 85% water.	Water-soluble drugs are diluted in the large volume of their body fluid. Due to drug dilution from the large volume of water, a larger drug dose is needed to achieve the desired plasma drug level. Since infants have decreased plasma protein-binding sites, lower doses are needed. With fewer available binding sites, there is more free drug. Drug doses should be decreased with most antibiotics, including cephalosporins and sulfonamides; as well as with phenobarbital and theophylline. All drugs should be checked for recommended pediatric dose range. The blood-brain barrier is not completely developed in the infant, so more drug passes into the cerebral cells.
METABOLISM	
Rapidly developing tissues of infants and small children makes them more sensitive.	The half-life of drug may be more prolonged than it would be in an older child or adult; therefore, drug accumulation can occur.
↓ Activity of liver enzymes due to the immaturity of the infant liver.	Drug half-life in the older child can be shorter due to the increased metabolic rate. Higher doses for the older child might be needed to offset the increased metabolic rate.
EXCRETION	
Drug elimination via the kidneys is ↓ until after the first year of life. Blood flow volume through the kidneys is less than in adults, and the glomerular filtration rate is approximately 30% to 40% of the adult rate. ↓ Ability to concentrate urine.	A decrease in drug excretion leads to a longer half-life of the drug and possible drug toxicity. Many of the antibiotics and analgesics are slowly excreted. Renal excretion of the drug is the net effect of glomerular filtration, active tubular secretion, and passive tubular reabsorption. In the presence of renal disease, a child may be unable to excrete a drug, leading to drug accumulation and possible toxicity.

Table 5-3: GERIATRIC PHARMACOLOGY AND NURSING IMPLICATIONS

PHYSIOLOGIC CONSIDERATIONS	BODY EFFECTS & POSSIBLE DRUG RESPONSES
ABSORPTION	
GI: ↑ pH (alkaline) gastric secretions ↓ Peristalsis with delayed intestinal emptying time	↓ Gastric acidity alters absorption of weak acid drugs, such as aspirin. ↓ In gastrointestinal motility rate (peristalsis) may delay onset of action
Cardiac: ↓ Cardiac output ↓ Blood flow	↓ Blood flow to the gastrointestinal tract (40-50% less) is due to a ↓ in cardiac output. Because of the reduction of blood flow, absorption is slowed but not decreased.
DISTRIBUTION	
↓ Body water and fluids ↑ Fat to water ratio ↓ Serum protein and albumin	Water-soluble drugs are more concentrated. Fat-soluble drugs are likely to accumulate. There are fewer protein-binding sites, resulting in more free drug. Drugs with a high affinity for protein compete for protein-binding sites with other drugs. Drug interactions result due to a lack of protein sites and an increase in free drugs.
METABOLISM	
Liver: ↓ Enzyme function ↓ Blood flow ↓ Total liver function	↓ Liver function causes a reduction in drug metabolism. With a reduction in metabolic rate, the half-life of drugs increases, and drug accumulation can result. Metabolism of a drug inactivates the drug and prepares it for elimination via the kidneys. Drug toxicity might occur when the half-life is prolonged.
EXCRETION	
Renal: ↓ Blood flow by 40-50% ↓ Functioning nephrons (kidney cells) ↓ Glomerular filtration rate by 40-50%	With a decrease in renal function, there is a decrease in drug excretion, and drug accumulation results. Drug toxicity should be assessed continually while the client is on the drug.

NURSING PRIORITY: The ***peak drug level*** *is the highest plasma concentration of a drug at a specific time. The* ***trough level*** *is the lowest plasma concentrations of a drug and measures the rate at which the drug is eliminated. Trough levels are drawn a few minutes before the drug is given, regardless whether it is oral or IV. These levels are drawn on drugs that have a narrow therapeutic index and are considered toxic, (i.e., aminoglycosides and other antibiotics).*

Drug Therapy Considerations Across the Lifespan.

1. Pediatric implications (Table 5-2).
2. Geriatric implications (Table 5-3).

MEDICATION ADMINISTRATION

NURSING PRIORITY: The nurse's responsibility in administering medication is influenced by three primary factors: nursing guidelines for safe medication administration, pharmacological implications of the medication, and the legal aspects of medication administration.

Nursing Responsibilities in Medication Administration

A. Administer according to the "5 Rights."
   1. Right medication.
   2. Right dosage.
   3. Right route of administration.

4. Right time.
5. Right client.
6. *Sixth right*—right charting (documentation).

NCLEX ALERT: *Administer medications according to the "5 rights" of medication administration.*

B. A nurse should administer only those medications which she has prepared.

C. Be familiar with medication.
1. General purpose the client is receiving the medication.
2. Common side effects.
3. Average dose or range of safe dosage.
4. Any specific safety precautions prior to administration (digitalis—check apical pulse; heparin—check clotting times).

D. Document medication against physician's orders according to institution policy.

E. Evaluate client's overall condition and assess for changes which may indicate the medication is contraindicated (e.g., morphine would be contraindicated in a client developing increased intracranial

F. Evaluate compatibility with other medications the client is receiving.

G. Use appropriate aseptic technique in preparing and administering medication.

H. Do not leave medications at the client's bedside without a doctor's order to do so.

I. If client is to administer his own medication, review with him correct administration, (i.e., eyedrops).

NCLEX ALERT: *Evaluate client's use of medications (prescription and over the counter medications).*

LEGAL IMPLICATIONS

Nurse's Legal Responsibilities in Administration of Medication

A. The nurse administers a medication only by order of a licensed physician and according to provisions of the specific institution.

B. The nurse should not automatically carry out an order if the dosage is outside the normal range or if the route of administration is not appropriate; she should consult the physician.

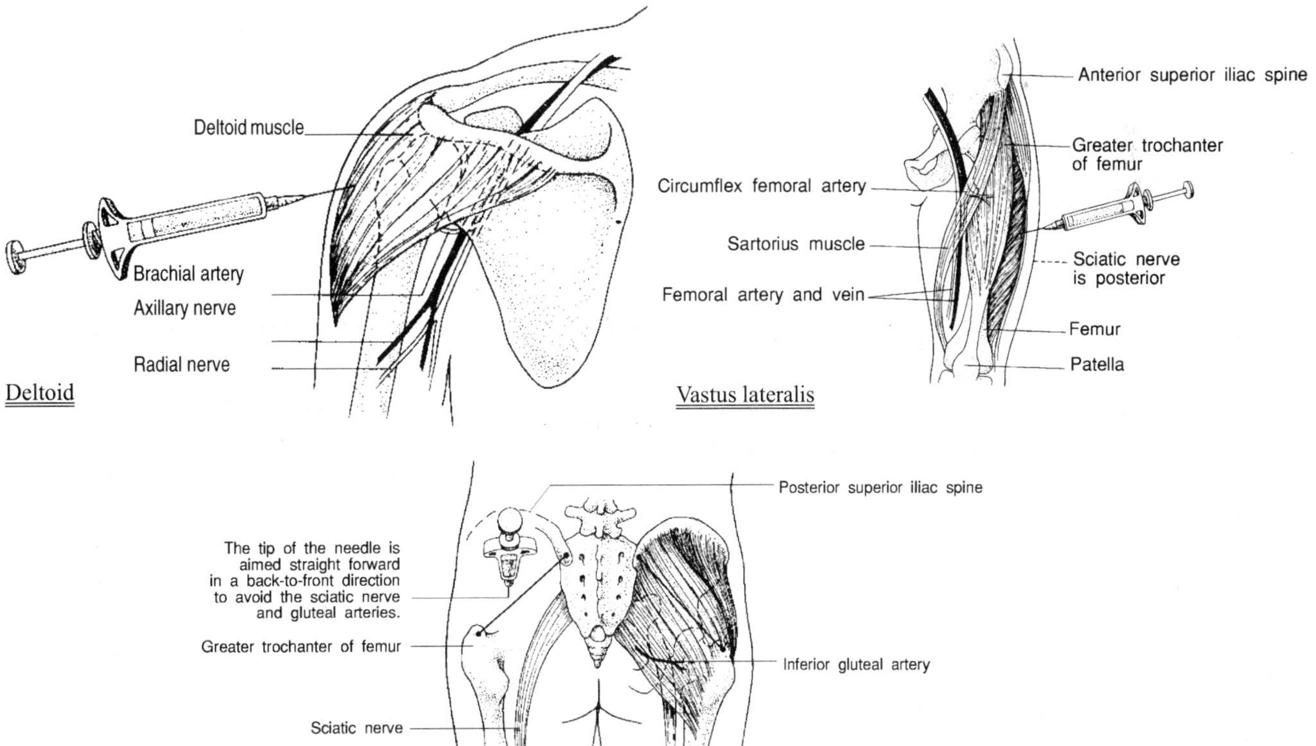

Figure 5-1:
INTRAMUSCULAR INJECTION SITES

Table 5-4: INTRAVENOUS MEDICATION ADMINISTRATION

METHOD	INJECTION RATE	NURSING IMPLICATIONS
Push or bolus	0.1 to 10 cc injected over 30 seconds to 5 minutes depending on medication	1. Drug is not diluted and is injected directly into the client's venous system. 2. Access may be direct injection into the vein or through an existing IV infusion. 3. Use access port closest to the client. 4. Has a rapid effect on the CNS and cardiopulmonary systems.
Intermittent infusion or piggyback (IVPB)	Medication is diluted in 25-100 cc and infused over 15 to 60 minutes. Concentrated medications require higher dilution and longer infusion time.	1. Drug is diluted to decrease toxicity and hypertonicity of the solution. 2. Method of choice for multiple daily doses.
Constant and variable-rate infusion	0.2 to 1,000 cc per hour	1. Method for medications which need to be highly diluted (chemotherapeutic drugs). 2. Provides for continuous medication infusion.

NCLEX ALERT: *Pay particular attention to medications that have specific nursing implications. Questions may be based on when you would contact the physician regarding the appropriateness of a medication order.*

C. The nurse is legally responsible for the medication she administers, even when the medication is administered according to a physician's order.

D. The nurse is responsible for evaluating the client prior to and after the administration of a PRN medication.

E. The nurse must administer the medication according to the nursing responsibilities previously discussed.

F. The medication should be charted as soon as possible after administration.

G. When taking verbal orders on the phone, carefully repeat all the orders to verify they are correct.

H. Medication errors:
1. If an error is found in a physician's drug order, it is the nurse's responsibility to question the order.
2. Always report medication errors to the physician immediately.
3. It is the nurse's responsibility to carefully assess the client for effects of the erroneous medication.
4. Medication errors should be documented in an incident report and on the client's chart.

Methods of Medication Administration

(Note: This section on medications should not be used as a procedure guideline. The purpose is to note specific characteristics of each method. All medications are administered according to previously discussed nursing responsibilities in medication administration).

NCLEX ALERT: *Administer oral, intramuscular, intravenous, and subcutaneous medications; insert a suppository; and determine need for administration of PRN medications.*

A. Oral medication.
1. Assess level of consciousness and ability to follow directions.
2. Evaluate swallow reflex.

B. Topical medications.
1. Skin application—evaluate condition of skin in area medication is to be applied; if appropriate, rotate sites to prevent irritation.
2. Sublingual—allow medication to dissolve under the tongue; client should not chew or swallow.
3. Nasal—position client to allow nose drops or spray to enter nares directly without contaminating the eyes.
4. Eyes—medication must be specifically indicated for ophthalmic use.
   a. Instill one or two drops in the middle of the lower conjunctival sac.
   b. Do not allow tip of applicator to come in contact with the eye.
   c. Do not drop medication directly on the cornea.
   d. Direct client to close their eyes gently to distribute the medication.
   e. Make sure you administer the correct medication in the correct eye.
5. Ears—medication is instilled into the auditory canal.

a. Position client with affected ear upward.

b. Children under three—pull pinna down and backward.

c. Older children, adults—pull pinna up and backward.

d. Administer solution at room temperature.

e. Keep client in the same position for appropriate time to prevent medication from coming out.

6. Suppositories

(1) Rectal—absorption from rectal mucosa is slower and less predictable than in systemic medications.

(2) Frequently given for nausea and vomiting.

(3) May be preferred route for infant.

(4) Insert blunt end advanced first through the rectal sphincter, especially if client is having difficulty retaining the suppository when the tapered end is inserted first.

a. Vaginal—absorption across vaginal mucous membranes.

(1) Should maintain supine position after insertion.

(2) Should not douche unless advised by physician.

C. Transdermal medication—medication is stored in a patch or is measured on a dose-determined applicator that is placed on the skin and absorption occurs through the skin.

1. Provides more consistent blood levels and avoids GI problems.

2. Patch sites should be rotated and areas cleansed after use.

3. Patch should not be applied over inflamed areas.

4. Do not allow transdermal medications to come in contact with your skin, as absorption of medication can occur in the nurse.

5. Patch needs to come in contact with skin (excessive body hair may need to be removed).

D. Inhalation medication—medication is in an aerosol form and is inhaled and absorbed throughout the respiratory tract (See chapter 15).

1. Position in semi-Fowler's.

2. Check instructions for inhaler use and make sure client understands.

E. Parenteral medications—the administration of medications by some method of injection.

1. Intradermal injection—administered just below the skin surface.

a. Use syringe with appropriate calibrations since amount is very small in volume (.01 to .10 cc).

b. Use small gauge (26) needle, $\frac{3}{8}$ to $\frac{1}{2}$ inch long.

c. Select area where skin is thin (inner surface of forearm, middle of back).

d. Insert needle bevel edge up at 15 ° angle.

e. Frequently used for tuberculin testing, local anesthetic, allergy testing.

2. Subcutaneous injection—medication injected into fatty tissue, just below the dermis.

a. Medication should be small in volume (0.5 to 1.5 cc), and nonirritating.

b. Areas on outer surface of upper arm, anterior surface of the thigh, or the abdomen are frequent sites.

c. Use 25 or 26 gauge needle, $\frac{1}{2}$ to 1 inch long, and insert at 45° angle.

3. Intramuscular injection—injection of medication into the muscle.

a. The amount of medication is usually 0.5 to 3.0 cc.

b. Appropriate sites (Figure 5-1).

(1) Deltoid and dorsal gluteal.

(2) Ventrogluteal and vastus lateralis .

c. Use 1-1$\frac{1}{2}$ inch needle; gauge of needle depends on viscosity of medication; insert needle at 90° angle.

d. Aspirate when needle is in place; if no blood returns, administer medication.

e. Z-track technique is utilized to prevent medication from leaking back through the needle track and irritation or staining subcutaneous tissue.

(1) After medication is drawn up, change the needle.

(2) Pull skin over to one side at the injection site.

(3) Inject medication into taut skin at site selected.

(4) Remove the needle and release the skin. As the stretched skin returns to its original position, the needle track is sealed.

(5) The preferable site is the dorsogluteal area.

f. Intramuscular injections in children.

(1) Vastus lateralis is common site in infants.

(2) Dorsogluteal area is generally not used unless child is walking.

(3) Needle is inserted about 1 inch.

4. Intravenous administration—injection of medication into the blood (Table 5-4).

a. Administration of large volumes of liquid by infusion.

b. Administration of irritating medications by piggyback method.

(1) Dilute medication according to directions, usually 50-150 cc D_5W.

(2) Assess patency of primary infusion.

(3) Connect medication and adjust flow rate for the time designated, usually 30 to 45 minutes.

(4) Administration of medications through piggyback intravenous method enhances the action of the medication.

c. Administration of specific medication in present IV infusion by *IV push* method.

(1) Carefully carry out the nursing responsibilities discussed previously.

(2) Inject the medication slowly and observe the client's response.

(3) Be aware of the institution's policy regarding guidelines for IV push medications.

Forms of Medication Preparations

A. Solids.

1. Capsule—medication is placed in cylindrical gelatin container.
2. Pills, tablets—medication is pressed into solid form of various shapes and colors.
   a. Enteric coated—prevents medication from being released in stomach; dissolves in intestine. Do not crush enteric coated tablets.
   b. Lozenge—flavored tablet that is held in the mouth for slow release of medication.
3. Suppositories—generally keep in cool area; will melt at body temperature; may produce local or systemic effect.
   a. Rectal.
   b. Vaginal.
   c. Urethral.
4. Ointments—used for external application.
5. Powders—finely ground medications which are stable only in dry form; frequently mixed with solution prior to administration.

B. Solutions.

1. Spirits—alcohol solutions of volatile substances (camphor spirits).
2. Syrups—medication prepared in an aqueous sugar solution.
3. Elixirs—solutions containing alcohol, sugar and water; may or may not have medicine ingredients.
4. Suspensions—finely ground particles of medication dispersed in a liquid; shake all suspensions well before preparing dose (antacids).
5. Emulsions—medication is dispersed in an oil or fat solution; shake all emulsions well before preparing dose.
6. Liniments, lotions—medication is dispersed in a mixture of oil, soap, alcohol, water; used for external application.

Calculation of Medication Dosages

Frequently, medications are not ordered by the physician in the amounts supplied by the pharmacy. In these situations, it is necessary for the nurse to calculate the correct dosage. Another important area of calculation is in the administration of intravenous solutions. It is essential that the nurse have a good working knowledge of the fundamental principles of mathematics in order to calculate medications correctly.

- **Equivalent Conversions—medication dosages used in a mathematical formula must be in the same system of measurement**

Convert grains to milligrams: multiply by 60 (60 mg = 1 gr).

$$\frac{1}{2}\, gr = ?\, mg$$

$$\frac{1}{2}\, gr\ x\ \frac{60}{1} = 30\, mg$$

Convert milligrams to grains: divide number of milligrams by 60.

$$30\, mg = ?\, gr$$

$$30\ div\ by\ 60 = \frac{1}{2}\, gr$$

Convert grams to milligrams: multiply by 1,000.

$$5\, gm = 5{,}000\, mg$$

Convert milligrams to grams: divide by 1,000.

$$500\, mg = .5\, gm$$

- **Oral medication calculations**

$$Dose\ \frac{desired}{Dose}\ on\ hand = amount\ \ to\ \ give$$

Example: *Order reads to give* ***KEFLEX*** *500 mg. Dose on hand is 250 mg capsules.*

$$\frac{500}{250} = 2\ capsules$$

$$Dose\ \frac{desired}{Dose}\ on\ hand\ x\ quantity = amount\ to\ give$$

Example: *Order reads to give ampicillin 350 mg. Dose on hand is 250 mg. in 5 cc.*

$$\frac{350}{250}\, x\, 5 = X$$

$$350 \; div \; by \; 250 = 1.4$$

$$1.4 \; x \; 5cc = 7cc$$

The problem can also be set up in algebraic proportion:

$$\frac{350mg}{X} = \frac{250mg}{5cc}$$

$$250X = 1{,}750$$

$$X = 7cc$$

Parenteral medication calculations

$$Dose \frac{desired}{Dose} \; on \; hand \; x \; qty \; of \; solution = amt \; to \; give$$

Example: *Order reads 75 mg of* ***DEMEROL****. On hand is 100 mg in 1 cc.*

$$\frac{75mg}{100mg} \; x \; 1cc = X$$

$$75 \; div \; by \; 100 = .75$$

$$.75 \; x \; 1cc = .75cc \; or \; \frac{3}{4} \; cc$$

Set up in algebraic proportion, the equation reads:

$$\frac{75mg}{x} = \frac{100mg}{1cc}$$

$$100X = 75$$

$$X = .75cc \; or \; \frac{3}{4} \; cc$$

Example: *Order reads to give ⅙ gr Morphine sulfate. On hand is 15 mg in 2 cc.*

$$\frac{1}{6} gr = ? \; mg$$

$$\frac{1}{6} \; x \; \frac{60}{1} = 10mg$$

$$\frac{10mg}{15mg} \; x \; 2cc = amount \; to \; give$$

$$10 \; div \; by \; 15 = .67cc$$

$$.67 \; x \; 2cc = 1.3cc$$

Intravenous medication calculation

To determine how long an infusion will run, divide the total number of cc to infuse by the hourly infusion rate.

$$Amount \; to \frac{infuse}{Hourly} \; rate = Number \; of \; hours$$

Example: *Order reads 1,000 cc at 125 cc per hour. How long will it take the 1,000 cc to infuse?*

$$\frac{1000}{125} = X$$

$$1000 \; div \; by \; 125 = 8 \; hours$$

To determine how many cc per hour an infusion will run, divide the total number of cc to infuse by the infusion time.

$$Amount \; to \frac{infuse}{Total} \; infusion \; time = cc \; per \; hour$$

Example: *Order reads 1,000 cc to run every 8 hours. How many cc per hour?*

$$1000cc \; div \; by \; 8 \; hours = 125cc \; per \; hour$$

Calculating drop factors—check the intravenous equipment to determine how many drops are delivered in 1 cc. For example purposes, a drop factor of 10 gtt per 1 cc is used. The following are two formulas to calculate this factor.

$$Total \frac{cc}{Times} \; in \; min = cc \; per \min \; x \; drop \; factor \; = gtt \; per \min$$

Example: *1,000 cc is ordered to infuse in 8 hours. Set drop factor is 10 gtt per cc.*

$$\frac{1000cc}{480min} = 2.08 \; cc \; per \; minute$$

$$2.08 \; x \; 10 = 20.8 \; or \; 21 \; gtt \,/\, \min$$

Example: *500 cc is ordered to infuse in 2 hours. Set calibration is 10 gtt per cc.*

$$\frac{500cc}{120min} = 4.16 \; x \; 10 = 41.6 \; or \; 42 \; gtt \,/\, \min$$

Determine the number of cc per hour and divide by 60 (60 minutes in 1 hour). This equals the number of cc (ml) per minute. Multiply by set calibration of number of gtts per cc.

$$Number \; of \; cc \; per \frac{hour}{60} = cc \; per \min$$

$$cc \; per \; minute \; x \; set \; calibrations = \backslash \; gtt \,/\, \min$$

Example: *500 cc is ordered to infuse in 2 hours. Set calibration is 10 gtt per cc. (250 cc/hr to infuse).*

$$\frac{250cc}{60} = 4.16cc \; per \min$$

$$4.16cc \; x \; 10 = 41.6 \; or \; 42 \; gtt \,/\, \min$$

Note: There may be a 2 to 4 gtt difference when using different formulas.

Study Questions—Pharmacology

1. The nurse is preparing to administer an intramuscular injection to a infant who is 8 months old. Which muscle would be the most appropriate injection site?

① Biceps.
② Dorsogluteal.
③ Vastus lateralis.
④ Ventrogluteal.

2. The doctor has indicated that ampicillin and gentamicin are to be given piggyback in the same hour, every 6 hours (12-6-12-6). How would the nurse administer these drugs?

① Both drugs together IV push.
② Each drug separately, flushing between drugs.
③ Retrograde both drugs into the tubing.
④ One drug every four hours and one every six hours.

3. The physician orders an IV piggyback of Cefotan 1 gm in 100 cc D_5W to run over 30 minutes. The drip factor for the tubing is 10 gtt/cc. How many drops per minute would you run the IV?

① 33 gtt/min.
② 25 gtt/min.
③ 12 gtt/min.
④ 50 gtt/min.

4. What should the nurse take into consideration when giving medication to an elderly client?

① Multiple simultaneous drugs can be dangerous.
② The elderly client metabolizes and excretes the drugs differently from younger and more active clients.
③ Medication affects the elderly client during the early hours of the morning.
④ Medication has an effect on the respiratory system of the elderly.

5. What is the first step the nurse should do to ensure that the right medication is being given to a client?

① Check the client's ID band.
② Read the information insert for directions as to correct administration.
③ Check the order with the medication administration sheet.
④ Check the expiration date on the medication.

6. The nurse pours a dose of medication, then finds that the client no longer needs the dose. What is the most appropriate nursing action?

① Record the dose as taken to keep the count correct.
② Charge for the dose because the dose must be paid for.
③ Record the medication as "not taken" and waste the poured dose.
④ Pour the medication back into the container.

7. Which preparation of a drug absorbs more rapidly?

① Ointment applied to the skin.
② Liquid medicine given orally.
③ Oral gelatin capsules.
④ Enteric-coated tablets.

8. Medications taken orally must undergo a change after contact with body fluids in order to be used by the body. What is this process?

① concentration.
② elimination.
③ transference.
④ absorption.

9. The nurse is verifying whether or not to give a medication to a client. What should she check first?

① Client's name.
② Expiration date of the drug.
③ Route of delivery.
④ Chart to see if the drug was ordered.

10. A client is to get Demerol 75 mg IM for pain. While drawing up the medication, the nurse draws up an extra 0.3cc of air in the syringe. What is the rationale for this action?

① Seal the injection site with an air bubble.
② Give the site enough space in case the client is a bleeder.
③ Clear the drug from the needle and seal the site.
④ Decrease the possibility of infection at the site.

Answers and rationales to these questions are in the section at the end of the book entitled "Chapter Study Questions: Answers & Rationales."

Appendix 5-1: CONVERSIONS

■ Celsius to Fahrenheit

Fahrenheit reading $= \frac{9}{5}$ *x Celsius reading + 32*

Example: Celsius is 50°

Fahrenheit $= \frac{9}{5}$ x 50 + 32

90 + 32 = 122° *Fahrenheit*

■ Pounds and grams

1 lb = 454 grams

To convert pounds to grams, multiply the number of pounds by 454.

7.5 + 454 = 3,405 gm.

To convert grams to pounds, divide the number of grams by 454.

Example: An infant weighs 3,405 gm.

$\frac{3,405}{454}$ = 7.5 lb. Or 7 lb. 8 oz.

■ Kilograms and pounds

1 kilogram = 2.2 lbs.

To convert kilograms to pounds, multiply the number of kilograms by 2.2

10 kg x 2.2 lb. = 22 lb.

To convert pounds to kilograms divide the number of pounds by 2.2

$\frac{44}{2.2}$ = 20 kg.

■ Grains and milligrams

1 grain = 60 milligrams

To convert grains to milligrams, multiply the number of grains by 60.

$\frac{1}{8}$ gr = ? mg

$\frac{1}{8}$ 60 = 7.5 mg

To convert milligrams to grains, divide the number of milligrams by 60.

7.5 mg = ? gr

7.5 ÷ 60 = .125

$\frac{125}{1000} = \frac{1}{8}$

Appendix 5-2: ABBREVIATIONS AND SYMBOLS

aa . . . . of each
ac . . . . before meals
ad lih. . . . . as desired
bid . . . . twice daily
c̄ . . . . with
Ca . . . . calcium
CBC . . . . complete blood count
C1 . . . . chlorine
dr . . . . dram
et . . . . and
ext. . . . . extract
fl or fld . . . . fluid
GI . . . . gastrointestinal
gm. . . . . gram
gr . . . . grain
gt/gtt . . . . drop/drops
H20. . . . . water
H202 . . . . hydrogen peroxide
HS . . . . bedtime (hour of sleep)
in . . . . inch
K. . . . . potassium
L . . . . liter
1b or # . . . . pound
liq. . . . . liquid
lytes . . . . electrolytes
m. . . . . minim
ml . . . . milliliter
Mg . . . . magnesium

N. . . . . nitrogen
Na . . . . sodium
NPO . . . . nothing by mouth
od . . . . every day
OD . . . . right eye
OOB. . . . . out of bed
OS . . . . left eye
os . . . . mouth
OU . . . . both eyes
oz. . . . . ounce
pc . . . . after meals
po. . . . . by mouth
prn . . . . as needed
q . . . . every
qid . . . . four times a day
qod . . . . every other day
qs . . . . as much as required
qt . . . . quart
q2h. . . . . every 2 hours
g3h. . . . . every 3 hours
s̄ . . . . without
ss. . . . . one half
stat . . . . immediately
tab . . . . tablet
tbs . . . . tablespoon
tid . . . . three times a day
tsp. . . . . teaspoon
WBC . . . . white blood count; white blood cell

❑ ***Homeostasis*, for the purposes of this chapter, is defined as the mechanism for maintaining a steady state in the body.**

FLUID AND ELECTROLYTES

Physiology

A. Basic concepts of body fluid.
  1. Water is a primary body fluid. It is used to transport nutrients as well as to remove waste products.
    a. Infant—70 to 80% of body weight is water.
    b. Adult—50 to 60% of body weight is water.
    c. Elderly Adult—45 to 55% of body weight is water.
  2. Electrolytes—electrically charged particles.
    a. Anion—carries a negative charge.
    b. Cation—carries a positive charge.
    c. Electrolytes found in intracellular fluid and in extracellular fluid are essentially the same; however, the concentrations differ.
  3. Intracellular fluid—provides the cell with internal fluid necessary for cellular function.
    a. Approximately 40% to 50% of total body fluid.
    b. Electrolytes.
      (1) Potassium (primary).
      (2) Magnesium.
      (3) Phosphate.
  4. Extracellular fluids (ECF)—transport system for cellular waste, oxygen, electrolytes and nutrients, assists to regulate body temperature, lubricates and cushions joints.
    a. Approximately 30% to 40% of total body water.
    b. An infant maintains a larger percentage of extracellular fluids than does an older child or adult.
    c. Vascular—circulating plasma volume.
    d. Interstitial—fluid surrounding tissue cells.
    e. Electrolytes.
      (1) Sodium (primary).
      (2) Chloride.
      (3) Calcium.

B. Dynamic transport of fluid and electrolytes.
  1. Passive transport—movement of body fluids caused by the concentration and the molecular weight of the fluid.
    a. Diffusion—movement of molecules from an area of high concentration to an area of low concentration.
    b. Osmosis—movement of water through a semipermeable membrane from an area of low electrolyte concentration to an area of high concentration; *osmotic pressure* is term used to describe osmosis (water goes where the salt is.)
    c. Filtration—the movement of water and electrolytes through a semipermeable membrane from an area of high pressure to an area of low pressure; *hydrostatic pressure* is term used to describe the force of filtration.
  2. Active transport—movement of substances from an area of low concentration to an area of high concentration with the expenditure of energy.
  3. Oncotic pressure—the osmotic pressure created by plasma proteins.
  4. Hydrostatic pressure—the pressure created by the volume in the vascular bed.
  5. Filtration occurs in the arterial end of the capillaries because the hydrostatic pressure is higher than the oncotic pressure. Fluid then moves out of the vascular bed into the tissue.
  6. At the venous end of the capillaries, the oncotic pressure is greater and the fluid moves back into the vascular volume.
  7. Osmolarity refers to the concentration of the dissolved particles in a solution; osmolarity controls the movement of fluid in each of the compartments.
    a. Hyper-osmolar—increased concentration of particles or solutes in a solution; fluid will move into this space to dilute the concentration.
    b. Hypo-osmolar—decreased concentration of particles, more water and less solutes; fluid will move out of this space to increase the concentration of solutes.
    c. Iso-osmolar (isotonic)—normal distribution of solutes and water in body fluid.

C. Fluid shifts.
  1. Plasma to interstitial fluid shift.
    a. Edema—accumulation of fluid in interstitial spaces.
      (1) Increase in hydrostatic pressure, as in a client with fluid overload (congestive heart failure).
      (2) Decrease in oncotic pressure, as in a client with excessive protein loss (renal disease).

(3) Break in the integrity of vessel walls, as in a client experiencing burns and trauma.

b. Hypovolemia may occur as a result of excessive fluid shift into the interstitial spaces, resulting in circulatory collapse (burn clients.)

2. Interstitial to plasma fluid shift—movement of edema back into the circulatory, volume as in client with mobilization of burn edema, or in the excessive administration of hypertonic solution causing the interstitial water to be returned to the plasma; client may demonstrate symptoms of circulatory overload.

3. Fluid spacing— third spacing occurs in tissue injury from an increase in capillary permeability and from an increase in vascular fluid volume.

(1) Ascites.

(2) Burn edema.

(3) Sequestration of fluid in the bowel.

D. Homeostatic mechanisms.

1. Endocrine system.

a. Hypothalamus secretes antidiuretic hormone (ADH) which regulates the water reabsorption by the kidneys.

b. Adrenal cortex secretes aldosterone, which promotes sodium retention and potassium excretion, thereby causing an increase in plasma volume.

2. Lymphatic system—assists to return excessive protein and fluid that escapes into the tissue back to the plasma volume.

3. Cardiovascular system maintains blood pressure to insure adequate renal perfusion.

4. Kidney maintains fluid volume and concentration of urine via the glomeruli filtration rate.

Fluid Imbalances (ECF)

A. Fluid deficit—extracellular fluid volume deficit (dehydration, ECFVD); hypovolemia results from vascular fluid volume loss.

1. Sensible fluid loss-fluid loss of which an individual is aware, such as urine.

2. Insensible fluid loss—fluid loss of which an individual is not aware (approximately 1,000 cc of fluid is lost every 24 hours through the skin and lungs in a normal adult.)

3. Causes of fluid deficit (all result from loss of both water and sodium).

a. Decreased fluid intake.

b. Failure to absorb or reabsorb water, as in diarrhea and intestinal disorders.

c. Loss of fluid through the gastrointestinal tract, as in vomiting, nasogastric suctioning.

d. Excessive renal excretion due to renal disease and inappropriate ADH secretion.

e. Iatrogenic loss due to overuse of diuretics or inadequate replacement of fluid loss.

f. Excessive fluid loss through skin and lungs due to febrile state.

g. Impaired integrity of the skin as in burns, wounds, and hemorrhage.

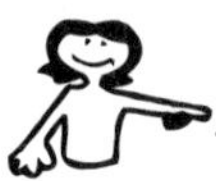

NURSING PRIORITY: *Sodium is the major electrolyte that affects fluid balance. "Where goes the sodium, so goes the water."*

4. Clinical manifestations.

a. Thirst, longitudinal tongue furrows.

b. Dry skin and dry mucous membranes.

c. Poor skin turgor (assess skin on the abdomen or the inner thigh in children, skin turgor is a poor indicator on elderly clients.)

d. Weight loss.

e. Oliguria.

f. Decreased blood pressure.

g. Decreased central venous pressure.

h. Postural hypotension.

i. Mottled skin color changes in infants and children.

j. Weakness, confusion, speech difficulty in elderly.

5. Laboratory findings.

a. Increased specific gravity.

b. Increased blood urea nitrogen (BUN >25mg/dL) without increase in creatinine.

c. Increased hematocrit (the normal ratio of hematocrit to hemoglobin is three to one). *For example:* 12 grams hemoglobin to 36 percent hematocrit.

d. Hyperglycemia (> 120mg/dL).

NCLEX ALERT: *Monitor client's hydration status (I&O, edema, signs and symptoms of dehydration.).*

B. Extracellular fluid volume excess (circulatory overload, ECFVE)—the retention of sodium and water in the intravascular and interstitial spaces.

1. Causes of fluid excess.

a. Excessive oral fluid intake.

b. Failure to excrete fluids, as in renal disease and cardiac failure.

c. Iatrogenic—fluid increase due to excessive infusion of hypotonic fluids.
d. Excess intake of sodium.
2. Clinical manifestations.
a. Pitting edema, sacral edema.
b. Pulmonary edema (dyspnea).
c. Bounding pulse, bradycardia.
d. Weight gain.
e. Lethargy.
f. Variable urine volume.
g. Changes in level of consciousness
h. Increased central venous pressure.
i. Jugular vein distention (JVD).
j. Increased blood pressure.
3. Laboratory findings—depends on the area of the body the shift occurs.
a. Decreased specific gravity of urine (<1.010).
b. Decreased hematocrit.
c. Decreased serum sodium.

C. Extracellular fluid volume shift (third spacing)—shift in the location of the extracellular fluid between the intravascular and interstitial spaces.
1. Causes of fluid shift.
a. Vascular to interstitial space shift due to tissue damage such as blisters, sprains.
b. Large fluid shifts occur in severe injuries, burns, intestinal perforations and obstruction, and lymphatic obstruction.
2. Clinical manifestations.
a. Decreased circulating volume, resulting in symptoms of hypovolemia.
b. Localized symptoms when the fluid is obstructing an organ, as in the intestinal tract.

D. Nursing management of client with fluid imbalances.
1. Assessment.
a. Evaluate client's history and predisposing factors contributing to the problem.
b. Assess for direction of fluid problem: fluid excess or deficit.
c. Evaluate appropriate lab data.
d. Evaluate client's ability to tolerate and correct the problem.
e. Elderly clients are more likely to develop ECFVE due to chronic diseases (renal, cardiac).
2. Nursing intervention.
a. Maintain accurate intake and output records.
b. Obtain accurate daily weight.

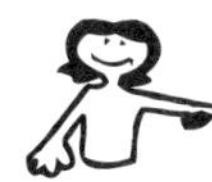

NURSING PRIORITY: Daily weight is the most reliable indicator of fluid loss or gain in all clients, regardless of age.

c. Evaluate for presence of edema.
d. Maintain IV replacement fluids at prescribed flow rate.
e. Monitor central venous pressure.
f. Monitor vital signs. (Blood pressure is not a reliable indicator of problems of fluid balance in young children).
g. Maintain good skin care to prevent breakdown.
h. Assess lab data for changes in the problem.
i. Carefully monitor elderly, cardiac and pediatric clients for tolerance of fluid replacement.
3. See Appendices on Electrolyte Imbalances and Replacement (Appendices 6-1 through 6-6).

INTRAVENOUS FLUID REPLACEMENT THERAPY

Isotonic solutions

1. Solutions contain water and either a carbohydrate (dextrose) or sodium chloride.
2. May be used to dilute medications or to keep the vein open.

Hypotonic Solution

1. Solutions contain water, carbohydrates for calorie needs, and basic electrolytes.
2. Types of solutions.
a. .45% or ½ strength normal saline
b. D_5W.
c. Combination of ½ normal saline and D_5W.

Hypertonic Solutions

1. 3% NaCl or 5% NaCl both are hypertonic and only used to treat situations of hyponatremia.
2. Administered slowly, can cause intravascular volume overload, carefully monitor serum sodium.

Nutritional Solutions

1. Contain very high percentage of dextrose.
2. Contain mixture of essential and non-essential amino acids.
3. Concentrated solutions are used in total parenteral nutrition and must be administered via a central line.
4. Types of nutritional solutions.
a. 10% Dextrose solution.

b. Protein solutions (Aminosyn, Freamine).

c. Fat emulsions.

Volume Expanders

1. Solutions are used when there has been a massive loss of plasma volume (burns and hemorrhage).
2. Because the solution increases the circulating volume, fluid volume overload may occur.
3. Produces rapid expansion of plasma volume; gradually reverses over 12 hours and is generally cleared within 24 hours.
4. Solutions used for volume expansion.
   a. Dextran 40 (Rheomacrodex)
   b. Dextran 70 (Macrodex).
   c. Plasma and human serum albumin prepared from whole blood.

Nursing Implications in Administration of Intravenous Fluid

Selection of the IV site

NCLEX ALERT: *Starting IV therapy (catheter or needle), maintenance of the site, and fluid infusion are common responsibilities of the RN.*

1. Veins in the lower extremities and veins that are sclerosed or irritated from previous use should be avoided.
2. Avoid areas of flexion, especially the antecubital area.
3. Adults and older children—distal veins of the upper extremities should be used first. Subsequent venipuncture should be proximal or higher than the previous site.
4. Infants—scalp veins are frequently used because of easy access, less movement in the area, and it is easier to stabilize the insertion site.

Key Points for Venipuncture

1. Select the smallest gauge catheter or needle to deliver the infusion. Large gauge catheters are used for administration of blood and large amounts of fluid.
2. Needles are frequently used for short term infusions (less than 8 hours); catheters are used for continuous infusion.
3. Site selection
   a. Begin with the cephalic or basilic vein of the hand.
   b. Avoid areas over joints, this decreases the stability of the site.
   c. Select a site in a distal vein of the hand or the forearm; if this is unsuccessful, or if infiltration occurs, the infusion can be resited in an area above the original site.
   d. Veins in the lower extremities are to be avoided.
4. Apply the tourniquet and insert the needle with the bevel up at a 15° to 30° angle.
5. After the needle has advanced into the vein and there is good blood return, release the tourniquet.
6. Wear gloves during insertion of the needle and as long as there is possibility of skin contact with the client's blood.
7. Appropriately secure the infusion device.
   a. Cover the insertion site; do not place tape directly over the insertion site.
   b. Label the site with time, date, catheter/needle size, and initials of nurse.
   c. Do not encircle the arm with tape; this can restrict circulation to the extremity.

NCLEX ALERT: *Manage care of a client with a peripheral IV.*

Key Points for Intravenous Infusions

1. Factors influencing rate fluid administration.
   a. Type of fluid.
   b. Age of client.
   c. Cardiac and renal status.
   d. Size of the vein and gauge of catheter/needle.
   e. Client's response to fluids.
2. The rate of flow should be carefully calculated (Chapter 5).
3. Label the infusion container.
   a. Time container was hung.
   b. Rate of infusion.
   c. Any medications that were added.
   d. Frequently the bags of fluid are numbered in consecutive order of administration.
4. Maintain accurate intake and output records.
5. Average maintenance fluid rate is 3,000 cc over 24 hours.
6. Solutions that are cloudy or contain precipitant should not be used.
7. Heparin lock.
   a. Utilized for intermittent access.
   b. May be flushed with a heparin or saline flush solution (100u per 1cc) at regular intervals.

c. Site may be converted to fluid infusion if necessary.

8. IV infusion sites are changed on a regular basis, preferably prior to inflammation, irritation, or fluid extravasation occurring at the site. Common time frame is for the site to be changed every 72 hours.

9. Pediatric Considerations.

a. Children are very susceptible to rapid fluid shifts, with resultant cerebral edema. IV solutions of normal saline or percentages of normal saline are frequently used to decrease the possibility of an untoward fluid shift.

b. Volume chambers holding no more that a 2-hour supply of fluid, or controlled infusion devices should be used on children to prevent the inadvertent rapid infusion of too much fluid.

c. Always make sure infants and young children are voiding prior to beginning IV infusion of fluids containing added potassium.

Factors Affecting Flow of IV Fluids

1. Rate of flow is directly proportional to height of solution.
2. Rate of flow is directly proportional to diameter of tubing and gauge of needle or cannula.
3. Rate of flow is inversely proportional to length of tubing. Excessive tubing will decrease the flow rate.
4. Rate of flow is inversely proportional to the viscosity of the solution; the more viscous the fluid, the slower the rate of flow.

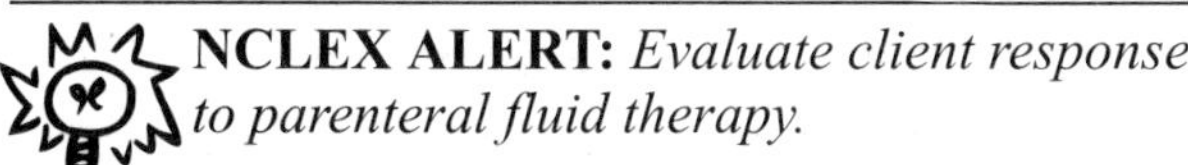

NCLEX ALERT: *Evaluate client response to parenteral fluid therapy.*

Indications for Use of Infusion Control Devices

1. To deliver a medication that requires a precise rate of administration (dopamine, pitressin, aminophylline).
2. To deliver fluids that would precipitate adverse effects if administered too rapidly (hyperalimentation).
3. To deliver fluids in controlled amounts to a client very sensitive to volume administered (infants, children under 10 years old, clients with pulmonary edema).

Complications of Intravenous Therapy

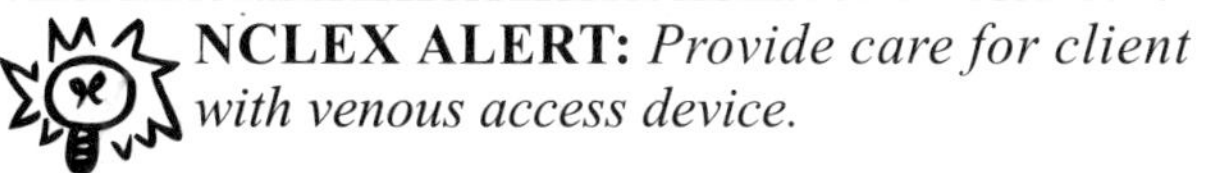

NCLEX ALERT: *Provide care for client with venous access device.*

Infiltration

1. Common causes—dislodging of the needle by client movement or obstruction of fluid flow.
2. Signs and symptoms—edema, *blanching of skin*, discomfort at site, fluid which is flowing slowly or has stopped; *cooler skin temperature.*
3. Preventive nursing management— use the smallest gauge of catheter possible; use an armboard to stabilize catheter, especially in restless, confused clients, or those with catheters placed in the antecubital fossa area; check frequently for coolness of skin around site; avoid looping tubing below bed level; check IV flow rate at least every 2 hours.
4. Nursing interventions—discontinue IV solution and remove catheter; apply cold compress if within first 30 minutes of infiltration, then apply warm moist heat to increase fluid absorption (if not contraindicated); if infiltrated solution contains an irritating medication (chemotherapy, vasoconstritive fluids), call the physician for orders to counteract effects of medication in the subcutaneous tissue.

Phlebitis

1. Common causes—overuse of a vein, irritating infusion solutions or medications, catheter in vein for too long a period of time, or use of large gauge catheters.
2. Signs and symptoms—tenderness, pain along the course of the vein, edema, *redness at insertion site*, red streak along course of vein, extremity with IV *feels warmer* than other extremity.
3. Preventive nursing management—change IV site every 72 hours, use large veins to administer irritating solutions, stabilize cannula, dilute medications adequately and infuse at prescribed rates, choose the smallest gauge catheter possible to administer solutions.
4. Nursing interventions—apply warm compresses to stimulate circulation and promote absorption.

Air Embolism

1. Common causes—air enters system from improper use of IV pumps; during irrigation of a plugged catheter in violation of hospital policy; injecting air into IV tubing when giving medication through injection site; not removing air from IV tubing. Central lines are higher risk, as negative thoracic pressure can pull atmospheric air into line when tubing is changed.
2. Signs and symptoms—hypotension, cyanosis, tachycardia, increased venous pressure, and loss of consciousness.

3. Preventive nursing management—remove all air from administration sets when changing tubing, do not irrigate catheters, assess IV pumps for correct infusion rate. When changing central line tubing, place client supine and have him hold his breath during the actual line change.
4. Nursing interventions—immediately turn client on left side and place in Trendelenburg position (air will rise to the feet or right ventricle), thus decreasing the risk of the air entering the pulmonary circulation.

ACID-BASE BALANCE

Basic Concepts of Acid-Base Balance

A. Terms used to describe acid-base balance.
   1. pH—the chemical abbreviation for negative logarithm of hydrogen ion concentration.
   2. CO_2—carbon dioxide.
   3. $PaCO_2$—pressure of dissolved carbon dioxide gas in the blood.
   4. O_2—oxygen.
   5. PaO_2—pressure of dissolved oxygen gas in the blood.
   6. HCO_3^- —bicarbonate.
   7. mmHg—millimeters of mercury.
   8. H+—hydrogen ion concentration.

B. Normal blood gas values.
   1. pH 7.4 (7.35-7.45).
   2. PaO_2—80 to 100 mmHg.
   3. $PaCO_2$—35 to 45 mmHg.
   4. HCO_3^-—22 to 28 mEq/L.

C. The hydrogen ion (H+) concentration determines the acidity or alkalinity of a solution; the higher the H+concentration the more acid the solution.

D. Acid-base ratio is determined by sampling arterial blood. This provides a reliable index of overall body function.

E. The body maintains a normal or neutral state of acid-base balance. The stable concentration of H+ balance is reflected in arterial blood with a relatively constant pH of 7.35 to 7.45.

F. It is necessary for the pH to remain relatively constant for the various enzyme systems of all body organs to function correctly.

G. O_2 saturation levels reflected in blood gas readings do not have a direct effect on the acid-base balance.

H. A state of acid-base decompensation exists when the acid-base levels are either below 7.35 or above 7.45.

I. Compensation—the system not primarily affected is responsible for returning the pH to a more normal level.

J. Correction—the problem in the system primarily affected is corrected, thereby returning the pH to a more normal level.

K. $PaCO_2$ imbalance—the origin or primary system is respiratory, or is compensating for a metabolic problem.

L. HCO_3^- imbalance—the origin or primary system is metabolic, or it is compensating for a respiratory problem.

M. The major clinical manifestations of an acid-base imbalance are indicative of CNS involvement. The severity of the symptoms will depend on the length of time the imbalance exists, as well as the severity of the deviation.
   1. Acidosis (metabolic or respiratory): Symptoms are indicative of depression of CNS; this is not uncommon.
   2. Alkalosis (metabolic or respiratory): Symptoms are indicative of increased stimulation of the CNS; death is a rare occurrence.

N. The normal ratio of HCO_3^- to $PaCO_2$ is 20 to 1. If this ratio is present the pH is normal.

Regulation of Acid-Base Balance

A. Buffer system—the most rapid-acting of the regulatory systems. The buffer system is activated when there is an excess acid or base present.
   1. A buffer is a chemical that helps maintain a normal pH.
   2. The buffer system chemicals are paired. The primary buffer chemicals are sodium bicarbonate and carbonic acid. The buffers are capable of absorbing or releasing hydrogen ions as indicated.
   3. The body buffers an acid more effectively than it neutralizes a base.
   4. An effective buffer system depends on normal-functioning respiratory and renal systems.

B. Respiratory system—the second most rapid response in the regulation of acid-base balance. Carbonic acid is transported to the lungs, where it is converted to carbon dioxide and water, then excreted.
   1. The amount of carbon dioxide in the blood is directly related to the carbonic acid concentrations.
   2. Increased respirations will decrease carbon dioxide levels, thus decreasing the carbonic acid concentration and resulting in decreased H+ and an increase in the pH.
   3. Decreased respirations will cause retention of carbon dioxide, increasing the carbonic acid concentrations and resulting in increased H+ concentration, and a decrease in the pH.
   4. With excessive acid formation, the respiratory center in the medulla is stimulated, which results in an in-

crease in the depth and rate of respirations. This causes a decrease in the carbon dioxide levels and returns the pH to a more normal point.

5. With excessive base formation, the respiratory rate slows in order to promote retention of carbon dioxide and decrease the alkalotic state. Carbon dioxide is considered an acid substance because it combines with water to form carbonic acid. The $PaCO_2$ levels are influenced only by respiratory causes.

C. Renal system—the slowest, but most effective, mechanism of acid-base regulation.
   1. The kidneys reabsorb sodium (Na), and produce and conserve sodium bicarbonate ($NaHCO_3^-$).
   2. In acidosis the H+ is increased, therefore the H+ is excreted before the potassium (K+) ion, thereby precipitating hyperkalemia. When the acidosis is corrected, the potassium will move back into the cell.
   3. In alkalosis the H+ is decreased; there is an augmented renal excretion of the K+ ion, thereby precipitating hypokalemia.

Alterations in Acid-Base Balance

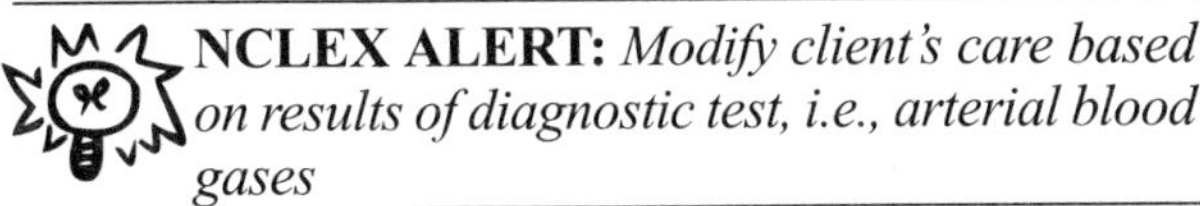

NCLEX ALERT: *Modify client's care based on results of diagnostic test, i.e., arterial blood gases*

A. **Respiratory acidosis**—characterized by excessive retention of carbon dioxide due to hypoventilation; therefore, there is increased carbonic acid concentration, producing an increase in hydrogen ions and a decrease in the pH (decreases below 7.35).
   1. Causes.
      a. Depression of the respiratory center.
         (1) Head injuries.
         (2) Oversedation with sedatives and/or narcotics.
         (3) Infection of CNS.
      b. Conditions affecting pulmonary function.
         (1) Obstructive pulmonary diseases.
         (2) Pneumonia.
         (3) Cystic fibrosis.
         (4) Atelectasis.
         (5) Occlusion of respiratory passages.
      c. Conditions which interfere with chest wall excursion.
         (1) Thoracic trauma.
         (2) Diseases affecting innervation of thoracic muscle (Guillain-Barré, myasthenia gravis, polio).
   2. Clinical manifestations.
      a. Dyspnea on exertion.
      b. Rapid, shallow respirations (hypoventilation).
      c. Disorientation, decreased level of consciousness.
      d. Tachycardia, dysrhythmias.
      e. Muscle weakness.
   3. Blood gas values.
      a. pH decreases below 7.35.
      b. $PaCO_2$ increases above 45.
      c. HCO_3- remains normal.
   4. Compensation/Correction.
      a. Compensation—renal system will compensate by retaining bicarbonate and excreting increased amounts of hydrogen ions.
      b. Correction—vigorous pulmonary hygiene to improve ventilation and decrease $PaCO_2$ levels, or mechanical ventilation in states of decreased respiratory drive.
   5. Nursing management.
      a. Use preventive management.
         (1) Have client turn, cough and deep breathe every two hours postoperatively.
         (2) Use narcotics judiciously in the immediate post-op period.
         (3) Maintain adequate hydration.
      b. Use semi-Fowler's position to facilitate breathing.
      c. Thoroughly assess client's pulmonary function.
      d. Try postural drainage and percussion, followed by suction, to remove excessive pulmonary secretions.
      e. Anticipate need for mechanical ventilation if client does not respond to pulmonary hygiene.
      f. Anticipate use of bronchodilator either systemically (aminophylline) or aerosol (Albuterol).
      g. Administer O_2 with caution, as it may precipitate CO_2 narcosis.
      h. Evaluate for hyperkalemia.
      i. Support renal system to promote adequate compensation.

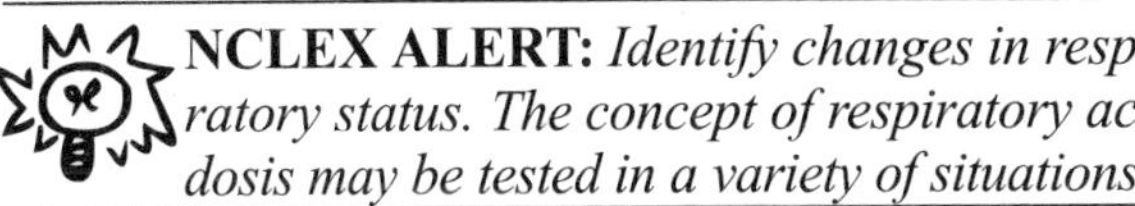

NCLEX ALERT: *Identify changes in respiratory status. The concept of respiratory acidosis may be tested in a variety of situations.*

B. **Respiratory alkalosis**—characterized by a low $PaCO_2$ due to hyperventilation. An excessive amount of CO_2 is exhaled, resulting in a decrease of H+ and an increase in pH (above 7.45).
   1. Causes of respiratory alkalosis.
      a. Primary stimulation of CNS.

(1) Emotional origin (hysteria, fear, apprehension).

(2) CNS infection (encephalitis).

(3) Salicylate poisoning.

b. Reflex stimulation of CNS.

(1) Hypoxia-stimulates hyperventilation.

(2) Fever.

(3) Cardiac conditions.

c. Mechanical ventilation resulting, in "overbreathing."

d. Thickened alveolar-capillary membrane - CHF, pneumonia, pulmonary emboli.

2. Clinical manifestations.

a. Deep, rapid breathing (hyperventilation).

b. CNS stimulation resulting in confusion, syncope, seizures.

c. Hypokalemia.

d. Muscle twitching and weakness.

e. Tingling of extremities.

3. Blood gas values.

a. pH increases above 7.45.

b. $PaCO_2$ decreases below 35.

c. HCO_3^- remains normal.

4. Compensation/Correction.

a. Compensation—renal system will compensate by increasing bicarbonate excretion and retaining hydrogen ions, therefore returning pH to a more normal level.

b. Correction—prevents loss of carbon dioxide from respiratory systems.

5. Nursing Management.

a. Identify and eliminate (if possible) causative factor.

b. Evaluate need for sedation.

c. Use rebreathing mask to increase CO_2 levels.

d. Remain with client to decrease anxiety levels.

C. **Metabolic alkalosis**—characterized by an increase in the bicarbonate levels in the serum leading to a decrease in the H+ and an increase in the pH (increase above 7.45).

1. Causes (either an increase in serum HCO_3^- or a decrease in serum H+ concentration).

a. Diuretic therapy—loss of H+, Cl^-, K+ precipitates an increase in the bicarbonate level in the serum.

b. Excessive loss of H+ ions.

(1) Prolonged nasogastric suctioning without adequate electrolyte replacement.

(2) Excessive vomiting, resulting in loss of hydrochloric acid and K+.

c. Prolonged steroid therapy—loss of H+, Cl^-, and K+ ions leading to an increased retention of bicarbonate by the kidneys.

2. Clinical manifestations.

a. Nausea, vomiting, diarrhea.

b. Increased irritability, disorientation.

c. Restlessness, muscle twitching.

d. Hypokalemia.

e. Shallow, slow respirations (hypovolemia).

f. Dysrhythmias.

3. Blood gas values.

a. pH increases above 7.45.

b. $PaCO_2$ normal.

c. HCO_3^- increases above 26.

4. Compensation/Correction.

a. Compensation—respiratory system will compensate by retaining carbon dioxide (hypoventilation) in order to compensate for the alkalosis.

b. Correction—replacement of electrolytes and fluids lost due to excessive renal excretion or due to excessive gastric loss of acid.

5. Nursing management.

a. Preventive.

(1) Provide foods high in potassium and chloride for client on diuretics.

(2) Administer potassium supplement to clients on long-term diuretics.

(3) Administer IV solution with replacement electrolytes.

b. Maintain accurate intake and output records.

c. Evaluate the lab values for a decrease in serum potassium levels.

d. **Diamox** maybe used to increase excretion of bicarbonate.

D. **Metabolic Acidosis**—characterized by a decrease in bicarbonate level in the serum, leading to an increase in H+ and a decrease in the pH (decreases below 7.35).

1. Causes (deficit of a base or an increase in acid).

a. Incomplete oxidation of fatty acids.

(1) Diabetic acidosis.

(2) Starvation.

(3) Salicylate poisoning.

b. Abnormal loss of alkaline substances.

(1) Deep, prolonged vomiting may cause excessive loss of base products.

(2) Severe diarrhea and loss of pancreatic secretions.

c. Renal insufficiency—kidney loses its ability to compensate for acid overload, thus H+ ions are not excreted, nor is HCO_3^- retained in normal amounts.

d. Salicylate poisoning due to accumulation of ketone bodies produced as a result of the increased metabolic rate.

2. Clinical manifestations.
   a. Disorientation.
   b. Deep, rapid respirations (Kussmaul).
   c. Increased lethargy.
   d. Dysrhythmias.
   e. Hyerkalemia.
3. Blood gas values.
   a. pH decreases below 7.35.
   b. PCO_2 remains normal.
   c. HCO_3^- decreases below 22.
4. Compensation/Correction.
   a. Compensation—respiratory system compensates by increasing rate and depth of respirations in order to blow off CO_2 and increase the pH.
   b. Correction—identify the underlying problem and promote optimal function.
5. Nursing management.
   a. Assist in identification of underlying problem.
   b. Administer sodium bicarbonate IV to neutralize acid and return pH to normal.
   c. Evaluate diabetic for ketoacidosis and administer insulin accordingly.
   d. Assess renal function and hydration status.
   e. Maintain accurate intake and output records.
   f. Evaluate lab values for hyperkalemia.
   g. Support respiratory systems in order to promote compensation.

INFLAMMATION

❑ **Inflammation is the tissue response to localized injury or trauma. It is an expected response to tissue injury.**

Basic Concepts of Inflammation

A. Three major categories.
1. Simple acute.
   a. Occurs rapidly.
   b. Neutrophils (WBC) are usually the predominant cell.
   c. Non specific, occurs with every injury.
   d. Essential for normal tissue repair.
2. Immunologically mediated, delayed hypersensitivity.
   a. Typical inflammatory response.
   b. Directly caused by an antigen-sensitized lymphocyte reaction.
   c. Involves a longer time to develop.
   Example: tuberculin skin testing, subacute bacterial endocarditis (SBE), and organ transplant rejection.
3. Chronic.
   a. Characterized by pain, redness, and swelling.
   b. Does not subside in two weeks but has a damaging course that lasts for weeks, months, or even years.
   c. Predominant cell types are lymphocytes, plasma cells, and macrophages.
   Example: rheumatoid arthritis, tuberculosis, chronic glomerulonephritis.

B. Inflammatory response.
1. Vascular response.
   a. Initial local vasoconstriction due to tissue injury.
   b. Release of histamine, kinin, and prostaglandin leads to local vasodilatation.
   c. Hyperemia and increased capillary permeability lead to changes in osmotic pressure and a leakage of fluid (exudate).
2. Systemic response.
   a. Fever.
   b. Leukocytosis (shift to the left, with increased numbers of neutrophils in circulation).
   c. Weight loss.
3. Increased pulse and respiration.
   a. Increase sedimentation rate.

C. Cardinal signs of inflammation (see Table 6-1).
1. Local response.
   a. Redness.
   b. Heat.
   c. Pain.
   d. Swelling.
   e. Loss of function.

D. Healing process.
1. Regeneration—replacement of lost cells and tissues with cells of the same type.
   a. Rapid regeneration of cells from skin, mucous membrane, gastrointestinal, urinary, and reproductive tracts occurs.
   b. Central nervous system cells (neurons) and cardiac muscle cells do not regenerate. Healing occurs by repair with scar tissue.

Table 6-1: CARDINAL SIGNS OF INFLAMMATION

CLINICAL SYMPTOM	PATHOPHYSIOLOGY
Redness	Hyperemia from vasodilation.
Heat	Increased metabolism at site and local vasodilation.
Pain	Pressure from fluid exudate on adjacent nerve endings, which leads to nerve stimulation; change in local pH.
Edema	Fluid shift and accumulation in interstitial spaces.
Loss of function	Decreased movement due to swelling and pain

2. Replacement—healing in a more complex process by replacement of lost cells with connective tissue; leads to scar formation.
   a. Primary intention healing.
      (1) Healing takes place with wound margins neatly approximated.
      (2) *Example:* a surgical incision.
   b. Secondary intention healing.
      (1) Wound edges are wide and irregular and may not be approximated; large amounts of exudate may be present.
      (2) Increased amount of granulation tissue; healing takes place upward and from the edges inward.
      (3) *Example:* pressure ulcers.

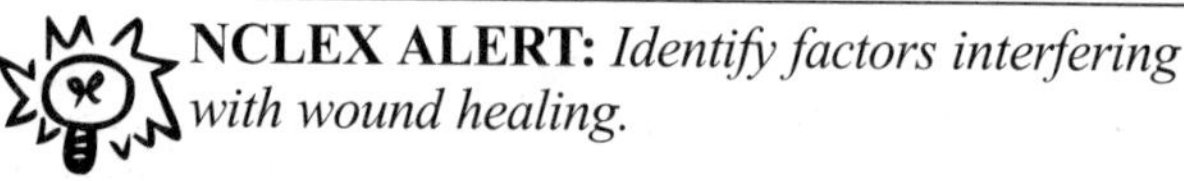

NCLEX ALERT: *Identify factors interfering with wound healing.*

E. Factors delaying the healing process.
   1. Nutritional deficiency, specifically protein and vitamin C.
   2. Decreased blood supply (edema or peripheral vascular disease, etc.).
   3. Antiinflammatory drugs (i.e., corticosteroid).
   4. Infection.
   5. Advanced age.
   6. Obesity.

INFECTION

❑ **Infection is the process by which an organism (pathogen, pathogenic agent) invades the host and establishes a parasitic relationship.**

Box Text 6-1: Elderly Care Focus
Infections

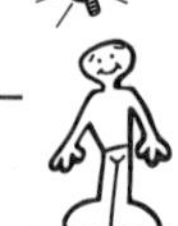

- May be manifested by changes in behavior - confusion, disorientation.
- May not exhibit fever or pain.
- Closely monitor client response to antibiotics , especially with regard to renal function.
- Maintain adequate hydration.
- Monitor GI function; diarrhea is common with antibiotics.

Chain of Transmission

A. Pathogens.
   1. Incubation period—the period of time from exposure to the pathogen until symptoms of infection occur in the host.
   2. A person can be asymptomatic and still transmit a pathogen that will produce an infection in someone else.
   3. Toxigenicity refers to the destructive potential of the toxin that is released by the pathogen.
   4. Types of pathogens.
      a. Viruses.
      b. Bacteria—gram-negative and gram-positive.
      c. Fungi.
      d. Chlamydia.
      e. Protozoa.
      f. Mycoplasma.

B. Reservoir.
   1. Environment within which the organism can live and multiply; is provided by some organic substance, human or animal.
   2. A carrier provides an environment for the pathogen to grow and multiply, but shows no symptoms of the infection.

C. Exit port.
   1. How the infection leaves the host.
   2. Common ports of exit include feces and body fluids.
   3. Understanding port of exit is necessary to prevent transmission of pathogen.

D. Route of transmission.
   1. Method by which the pathogen moves to another host.
   2. Direct transmission is immediate transfer from one host to another, as in sexually transmitted diseases, or inhalation of contaminated droplets from respiratory infections.
   3. Indirect transmission occurs via an intermediate carrier (mosquitoes, contaminated water, contaminated food).

E. Port of entry into susceptible host.

1. May enter the host via inhalation, ingestion, through the mucous membranes, or percutaneously.
2. Biological and personal characteristics of the new host will determine the lines of defense the host will have against the invading pathogen.

F. Control of transmission.
1. Transmission of a contagious disease can be broken by interfering with any link of the transmission chain.
2. Treatment is aimed at breaking the transmission chain at the most vulnerable and cost-effective point.
   a. Barrier precautions—gloves, gowns, condoms.
   b. Proper handling of food and water supplies.
   c. Avoidance of high-risk behavior—unsafe sex, IV drug use.
   d. Good handwashing technique and good personal hygiene.
3. Important to consider chain of transmission in order to protect health care workers (See Table 7-2: Immunizations for Health Care Workers).
4. Host susceptibility can be greatly reduced through immunizations.

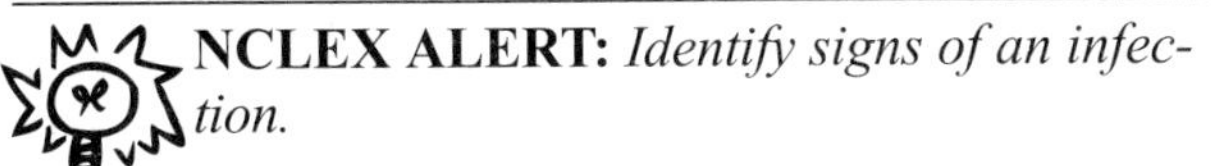
NCLEX ALERT: *Identify signs of an infection.*

Nursing Intervention

✦ *Goal: to promote healing*
1. Increase fluid intake.
2. Diet high in protein, carbohydrates and vitamins, specifically vitamins A, C, and B complex.
3. Immobilize an injured extremity with a cast, splint, or bandage.
4. Administer antipyretic medications (See Appendix 6-8).

✦ *Goal: to decrease pain.*
1. Cold packs after initial trauma may assist to decrease swelling and pain.
2. Heat may be used later to promote healing and to localize the inflammatory agents.
3. Elevate the injured area to decrease edema and promote venous return.

✦ *Goal: to prevent infection.*
1. Handwashing is the single most effective mechanism for preventing spread of infection.
2. Monitor vital signs—increase in pulse, respiration, and temperature occurring four to five days postoperative may indicate infectious process.
3. Check for *staphylococcus* and *pseudomonas* (produce purulent-draining wounds).

Table 6-2:
SIGNS OF INFECTION

✦ **Generalized:**
Fever, localized inflammattion, joint pain, fatigue, increased WBCs.

✦ **Gastrointestinal:**
Diarrhea, nausea and vomiting.

✦ **Respiratory:**
Purulent sputum, sore throat, chest pain, congestion.

✦ **Urinary tract:**
Urgency and frequency, hematuria, purulent discharge, dysuria, flank pain.

4. Maintain aseptic technique in dressing changes and in wound irrigations.
5. Maintain standard precautions.(Appendix 6-9).
6. Administer antibiotic medications. (Appendix 6-10).

✦ *Goal: to prevent complications.*
1. Determine presence of leukopenia or impaired circulation if the client is receiving steroids or drugs that depress bone marrow, or has been exposed to a communicable disease; these all impair the inflammatory response.
2. Protect healing wounds from injury such as pulling or stretching.
3. Identify clients with compromised immune response; are at high risk for opportunistic infection.

METHICILLIN RESISTANT STAPHYLOCOCCUS AUREUS (MSRA)

❑ **A strain of bacteria that has developed a resistance to common antibiotics.**

A. Bacteria is commonly carried in nasal passages. It is not harmful to healthy person, but will cause infection in susceptible host.

B. Clients who have received multiple antibiotics and who have had multiple hospitilizations are at increased risk.

Treatment

Cultures then antibiotics sensitive to bacteria.

Nursing Intervention

✦ *Goal: Decrease spread of infection*
1. Routine cultures of health care workers.
2. Identification of clients at increased risk.
3. Add contact isolation barrier to the standard precautions:
   - Private room
   - Gown and gloves

- Masks are not necessary unless the client has lower respiratory infection.
- Teach family importance of gloves and gowns.

4. Notify nurse epidemiologist when client is diagnosed with MSRA
5. Handwashing is critical, even after removal of gloves.

Study Questions—Homeostasis

1. The nurse identifies which set of blood gas values as consistent with a diagnosis of respiratory acidosis in a client?

① pH 7.0; PCO_2 42.
② pH 7.46; PCO_2 38.
③ pH 7.35; PCO_2 44.
④ pH 7.32; PCO_2 48.

2. A client is experiencing difficulty with edema and fluid overload. What nursing intervention would be the most accurate in evaluating the client's fluid balance?

① Measure the intake and output.
② Check for thirst and tissue turgor.
③ Evaluate changes in daily weight.
④ Evaluate vital signs every 3 hours.

3. Postoperative orders are D5 1\2 NS with 40 mEq/L of KCL. The liter of Lactated Ringers has not completely infused. What will the nurse do?

① Finish the current liter of fluid.
② Ask the client if he needs to void.
③ Hang the ordered IV.
④ Assess the IV site.

4. A child has been exposed to high levels of lead. What is important for the nurse to check when conducting an assessment?

① Decreased appetite and hyperirritability.
② Increased attention span and drowsiness.
③ History of high hemoglobin and hematocrit.
④ History of jaundice and bruising.

5. What information is important to teach a client who is on steroid therapy?

① Record daily weights to determine weight gain.
② Increase dose of medication as needed.
③ Do not discontinue medication abruptly.
④ Increase fluid intake.

6. What medication would increase the client's risk of infection?

① Beta blockers.
② Steroids.
③ Aspirin.
④ Calcium channel blockers.

7. What organ system regulates the electrolyte balance in the body?

① Kidneys.
② Heart.
③ Parathyroid.
④ Liver.

8. On a nursing assessment, the nurses finds the client's skin to be flushed and dry. The nurse should continue an assessment for what problem?

① Sodium imbalance.
② Altered renal function.
③ Fluid deficit.
④ Hypovolemia.

9. Which problem can result when the client has a fever?

① Fluid loss.
② Hyponatremia.
③ Hypokalemia.
④ Fluid overload.

10. A elderly client has an order for continuous fluid replacement at 75cc per hour. The nurse is preparing to start the IV. Where should she begin and what is the equipment of choice?

① A 22 gauge butterfly, right arm anticubital area.
② An 18 gauge, 3 inch IV cannula (intracath), inserted in the left hand.
③ An 18 gauge, 1 inch IV cannula (intracath), in the anticubital area of left arm.
④ A 22 gauge, 1 inch intercath, top of the left hand.

11. A client returns from surgery. He is NPO and has a nasogastric tube in place. His IV is ordered to run at 125 cc per hour. What type of fluid will most likely be used in this client?

① D_5W.
② Ringer's Lactate.
③ 0.9% sodium chloride.
④ $D_{10}W$.

Answers and rationales to these questions are in the section at the end of the book entitled "Chapter Study Questions: Answers & Rationales."

Appendix 6-1: ELECTROLYTE IMBALANCES: POTASSIUM

CAUSES	SYMPTOMS	NURSING IMPLICATIONS
NORMAL SERUM LEVELS (POTASSIUM): 3.5 - 5.0 mEq/L		
HYPOKALEMIA: Serum K+ below 3.5 mEq/L		
Decreased intake of K^+ GI loss: vomiting diarrhea fistulas nasogastric suction without replacement Excessive renal excretion: diuretics increasing aldosterone Alkalosis Steroid therapy (Administration of insulin and glucose moves K^+ into cell)	Muscle weakness and cramps Hyporeflexia Confusion, drowsiness, fatigue Tachycardia EKG changes: flat T wave, S-T depression, U waves, PVCs Postural hypotension GI: anorexia, vomiting, diarrhea	1. Identify source of depletion. 2. Monitor K^+ levels. 3. Encourage foods high in K^+. 4. Replace K^+ (oral and IV). 5. Maintain accurate intake and output records. 6. Evaluate for digitalis toxicity (lowered K^+ potentiates digitalis). 7. Evaluate for alkalosis. 8. Provide client education regarding diuretics. 9. Administer potassium supplements.
HYPERKALEMIA: Serum K above 5.0 mEq/L		
Decreased urinary excretion renal failure decreased aldosterone decreased secretion Massive tissue injury: burns trauma Excessive administration of IV K+ Acidosis	Drowsy Muscle weakness to flaccid paralysis Hyperreflexia EKG changes: peaked T waves prolonged P-R widened QRS dysrhythmias: tachycardia bradycardia complete block cardiac arrest Oliguria, anuria	1. Identify origin of increase. 2. Monitor K^+ levels. 3. Administer diuretics, if renal function adequate. 4. Administer hypertonic glucose and insulin to initiate K^+ transfer into cell. 5. Utilize exchange resins: (**Kayexalate**). 6. Administer sodium bicarbonate if client is acidotic. 7. Be prepared for a cardiac emergency. 8. Maintain accurate intake and output records.

Appendix 6-2: MEDICATIONS TO CORRECT POTASSIUM IMBALANCE

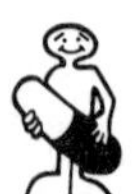

MEDICATIONS	ACTION	NURSING IMPLICATIONS
POTASSIUM SUPPLEMENTS		
ORAL: Potassium chloride (KCl) Potassium triplex Potassium citrate Potassium gluconate (**Kaon**) **IV:** Potassium chloride Potassium acetate	Principle intracellular action and essential for many physiological processes. Used in treatment and prevention of hypokalemia.	1. Oral preparations generally have unpleasant taste; administer with full glass of water or juice. 2. Potassium is irritating to gastric mucosa. 3. Pediatric implications: make sure child/infant is urinating adequately before beginning supplement. 4. Parenteral K^+ *must* be diluted and administered by IV drip. **Do not give K^+** by IM or IV push. 5. IV K^+ solutions are irritating to the vein. If pain occurs, either slow infusion rate or dilute in larger volume of fluid. 6. Administer with caution to cardiac clients and those on digitalis preparations.
EXCHANGE RESIN		
Sodium polystyreal sulfonate (**Kayexalate**): PO or rectal retention enema	In the intestine the hydrogen ion is exchanged for the potassium; this binds excess potassium and removes it from the serum. Medication is not absorbed systemically.	1. Laxatives are given to facilitate excretion of the resin. 2. Cleansing enema must precede the **Kayexalate** retention enema. 3. Carefully evaluate the client with CHF and/or hypertension. 4. Monitor serum electrolytes. 5. Use with caution in clients requiring sodium restriction.

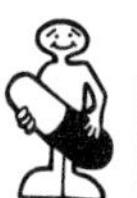

Appendix 6-3: ELECTROLYTE IMBALANCES: SODIUM

CAUSES	SYMPTOMS	NURSING IMPLICATIONS
NORMAL SERUM LEVELS (SODIUM) 135 - 145 mEq/L		
HYPOVOLEMIC HYPONATREMIA: Serum Na^+ decrease 135 mEq/L		
Inadequate Na^+ intake Decreased renal excretion: diuretics adrenal insufficiency increased ADH Edema Excessive administration of D_5W Fresh water near-drowning Cystic fibrosis Excessive sweating Gastrointestinal losses Diabetic acidosis Massive tissue injury: burns trauma	*Solution deficit (sodium loss):* CNS problems: decreased level of consciousness seizures Weak, restless Oliguria Abdominal cramps Postural hypotension Increased hematocrit Flushed skin *Dilutional hyponatremia (water excess):* CNS problems: confusion headache seizures Muscle twitching Increased urine	1. Decreased hematocrit. Identify source of depletion. 2. Maintain accurate intake and output records, and daily weight (best measurement of fluid status). 3. Irrigate nasogastric tubes with normal saline. 4. Administer 0.9% NaCl IV (normal saline) if client has sodium deficit. 5. Restrict fluid intake if client has fluid excess. 6. Elderly and infants at higher risk because of variations in total body water. 7. Occurs in clients who are NPO, on diuretics, perspiring, vomiting, having diarrhea; burns, or excessive administration of D5W. 8. Occurs in renal disease, Addison's disease, and diabetic acidosis. 9. Carefully monitor clients receiving D5W.
HYPERNATREMIA: Serum Na^+ above 145 mEq/L (sodium retention or water loss)		
Decreased fluid intake Excessive salt intake Increased renal retention: renal disease Cushing's syndrome (adrenal hyperfunction) decreased ADH Salt water near-drowning	*Fluid excess (sodium retention):* Pitting edema Weight gain Lethargic Decreased CVP Decreased hematocrit *Fluid deficit: (hemoconcentration of Na^+*, water loss) Concentrated urine Dry mucous membranes Flushed skin Tachycardia Increased temperature	1. Identify origin of increase. 2. Maintain accurate intake and output records, and daily weight. 3. Administer D_5W IV if fluid is normal or there is a deficit. 4. Administer diuretics to remove excess Na^+. 5. Restrict fluid intake if client has fluid excess. 6. Assess skin condition. 7. Assess for pitting edema. 8. Assess for CHF.

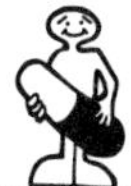

Appendix 6-4: MEDICATIONS TO CORRECT SODIUM IMBALANCE

MEDICATION	ACTION	NURSING IMPLICATIONS
SODIUM SUPPLEMENTS		
Sodium chloride (NaCl, table salt) Saline solutions: 0.9% and 0.45% saline solution for infusion	Necessary ion in maintaining osmotic pressure in intravascular and extracellular fluids. Necessary component for acid-base buffer system.	1. Administer with caution in clients with CHF, renal problems, edema, or hypertension. 2. Maintain daily weights, I & O to evaluate fluid retention. 3. Evaluate serum Na^+ levels.

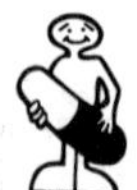

Appendix 6-5: ELECTROLYTE IMBALANCES: CALCIUM

CAUSES	SYMPTOMS	NURSING IMPLICATIONS
NORMAL SERUM LEVELS (Calcium): 9 - 11 mg % or 4 - 5 mEq/L		
HYPOCALCEMIA: Serum Ca^{++} below 8.6 mg % of below 4 mEq/L %, or 3.5 mEq/L -infants		
Acute pancreatitis Steatorrhea Dietary lack of Ca^{++} and vitamin D Renal failure Hypoparathyroid Excessive transfusion of citrated blood Metabolic alkalosis Overuse of antacids and laxatives	Tetany: + Chvostek's sign + Trousseau's sign Neuromuscular irritability Numbness and tingling in extremities Seizures Abdominal cramping and distention Hyperreflexia Dysrhythmias	1. Identify origin of deficiency. 2. Keep Ca^{++} replacement medications easily accessible for post-operative thyroid and parathyroid clients. 3. Assess for tetany. 4. Evaluate adequacy of Ca^{++} intake in infants. 5. Reduce environmental stimuli in both adults and infants. 6. Institute seizure precautions. 7. Provide client education regarding Ca^{++} intake.
Infants: ***Early onset*** - decreased activity of parathyroid; infants of diabetic mothers; premature infants; exchange transfusion ***Late onset*** - decreased dietary intake	***Early onset in infant***: edema, apnea, intermittent cyanosis, vomiting, abdominal distention ***Late onset in infant:*** Increasing CNS excitability	
HYPERCALCEMIA: Serum Ca^{++} above 10.5 mg% above 5 mEq/L		
Metastatic malignancy Hyperparathyroidism Thiazide diuretics Prolonged immobilization	Anorexia Nausea, constipation CNS depression Decreasing muscle tone Renal calculi Pathological fractures Dysrhythmias	1. Identify origin of increase. 2. Administer diuretics to facilitate removal of serum Ca^{++}. 3. Increase client's fluid intake 3,000 to 4,000 cc daily to decrease calculi formation. 4. Decrease Ca^{++} intake. 5. Encourage client mobility. 6. Provide client education regarding supplemental vitamins. 7. Handle client carefully to prevent pathological fractures. 8. Assess client on digitalis for symptoms of toxicity

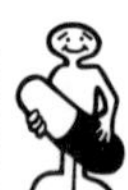

Appendix 6-6: MEDICATIONS TO CORRECT CALCIUM IMBALANCE

MEDICATION	ACTION	NURSING IMPLICATIONS
CALCIUM SUPPLEMENTS		
Calcium lactate, PO Calcium gluconate **(Kalcinate)** IV, PO Calcium carbonate, PO (Loop diuretics are used to enhance excretion of calcium.)	Primary component of bones and teeth Activator for coagulation enzyme factors Necessary for cardiac muscle function IV infusion for treatment of hypocalcemic tetany Adjunctive therapy to prevent hypocalcemia during exchange transfusion.	1. May be given in conjunction with vitamin D to enhance absorption. 2. PO supplements utilized best if given 1½ hours before meals. 3. Prevent IV infiltration, as Ca^{++} solutions cause tissue hypoxia and sloughing. 4. Do not add Ca^{++} preparations to solutions containing carbonates or phosphates. 5. Use with caution for client receiving digitalis. 6. Monitor infusion rate carefully; sudden increase in serum Ca^{++} level may precipitate severe cardiac dysrhythmias.

Appendix 6-7: ANTI-INFLAMMATORY MEDICATIONS

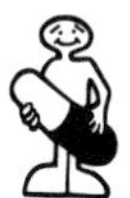

❖ GENERAL NURSING IMPLICATIONS ❖

— Give oral medications with or after meals.
— IV injection should be over at least 1 minute.
— Following long-term therapy, withdrawal from steroids should be gradual.
— Increased amounts of adrenocorticosteroids may be required during stress periods such as surgery.
— Assess for complications associated with prolonged usage (infections, psychological changes, fluid retention).

MEDICATION	SIDE EFFECTS	NURSING IMPLICATIONS
ADRENOCORTICAL STEROIDS: ***Anti-inflammatory action:*** *Inhibit release of proteolytic enzymes during inflammation, decreases the number of lymphocytes, used as an immunosuppressant for delaying organ rejection* ***Cardiovascular:*** *Potentiate vasoconstriction effects of norepinephrine; elevated blood pressure.* ***Carbohydrate, fat protein metabolism****: produce hyperglycemia, glycosuria; facilitate breakdown of protein in muscle, and promote mobilization of fatty acids from adipose tissue.* ***Stress effect:*** *During stress (sympathoadrenal response) a release of corticosteroids occurs.*		
Cortisone acetate (**Cortisone**): PO, IM, topical ophthalmic ointment Hydrocortisone: (**Cortef**):IM, PO Dexamethasone (**Decadron**): PO, topical, IM or ophthalmic Prednisone (**Deltasone, Meticorten**): PO Methylprednisolone (**Medrol**): PO, IM, IV	Increased susceptibility to infections GI upset, gastric irritation Osteoporosis Psychological disturbances (depression, euphoria) Hypocalcemia Hyperglycemia Hypertension (caused by sodium and water retention) Cushing's syndrome: moon face, buffalo hump, distended abdomen, thin arms and legs, excessive hair growth	1. Administer medication before 9 a.m. to decrease adrenal cortical suppression. 2. Encourage daily dose with breakfast. 3. Monitor for psychological changes. 4. Decrease salt intake in diet; encourage high protein and potassium diet. 5. Weigh daily. 6. Topical steroids usually do not provoke physical evidence of absorption unless applied to large areas or over prolonged periods. ***Teaching:*** Take medication with food. Diet should include adequate K^+ intake and decreased Na^+ intake. Do not stop taking the medication without a doctor's order. Avoid immunizations if on long-term therapy. Report to health care provider: stress situations, sore throat, fever, or other signs of infection, or a weight gain of 5 lb or more in a week.

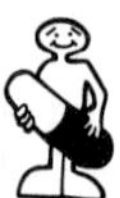

Appendix 6-8: NON-STEROID ANTI-INFLAMMATORY (NSAID) MEDICATIONS

MEDICATIONS	SIDE EFFECTS	NURSING IMPLICATIONS
❖ GENERAL NURSING IMPLICATIONS ❖ — Give with a full glass of water, either with food or just after eating. — Drink increased water during the day (total of 2,000-3,000 ml daily). — Store in child-proof containers and out of reach of small children. — Do not exceed recommended doses.		
NSAIDs: Inhibit prostaglandin synthesis.		
Acetaminophen: **(Tylenol, Datril, Tempra)**: PO, rectal	Minimal gastric irritation; does not affect prothrombin time. Hepatotoxic in large doses: vomiting, anorexia, diaphoresis, weakness, RUQ tenderness, jaundice; fever, ↑liver function studies.	1. Assess for toxicity by observing for symptoms of CNS stimulation. 2. If used concomitantly with anticoagulants, dosage may need to be reduced to avoid hemorrhage. 3. Available in flavored liquid and tablets for children. 4. ***Uses***: analgesic for relief of headache, joint pain; reduces fever.
Acetylsalicylic acid: **(Aspirin, ASA)**: PO	***Salicylism:*** skin reactions, redness, rashes, ringing in the ears, GI upset, hyperventilation, sweating and thirst. ***Long-term usage:*** erosive gastritis with bleeding.	1. Interacts with oral anticoagulants and may significantly increase the prothrombin time. 2. If available, administer as enteric-coated or buffered tablets. 3. Be aware that aspirin is the most common agent responsible for accidental poisoning in small children. 4. Do not give aspirin to children unless under the specific direction and supervision of a physician;associated with Reye's syndrome in children.. 5. Observe clients who are on anticoagulant therapy and also diabetic clients who may have symptoms of hypoglycemia, salicylate potentiates antidiabetic oral drugs. 6. ***Uses:*** pain, fever, inflammatory conditions such as arthritis, gout.
Ibuprofen **(Advil, Motrin)**: PO	Dyspepsia (heartburn, nausea, epigastric distress) Dizziness Rash, dermatitis	1. May increase effects of anticoagulants. 2. Do not crush enteric-coated form. 3. Do not exceed 3.2 gm/day. 4. Avoid taking it concurrently with aspirin. 5. ***Uses:*** arthritis, fever, pain, muscle cramps.
Naproxen **(Naprosyn)**: PO	Headache Dyspepsia Dizziness, drowsiness Peripheral fluid retention.	1. May increase effects of anticoagulants. 2. Avoid tasks requiring alertness until response to drug is established. 3. ***Uses:*** arthritis, primary dysmenorrhea, pain.
Indomethacin: **(Indocin)**: PO	GI upset Nephrotoxicity Lightheadedness Fatigue	1.Caution client against performing hazardous task requiring mental alertness or physical coordination. 2. Assess renal function in clients on long-term therapy. 3. ***Uses:*** rheumatoid arthritis, osteoarthritis; relieves pain and swelling in acute gouty arthritis.
Celecoxib **(Celebrex)**: PO	GI upset Headache	1. Should not be used in clients with history of asthma. 2. Should not be used by clients who have a history of allergy to apsirin. 3. **Uses:** osteoand rheumatoid arthritis, dysmenorrhea.

Appendix 6-9: INFECTION CONTROL PROCEDURES

GENERAL INFORMATION:

- Many clients with disease-specific isolation precautions now require only standard precautions.
- The specific substances covered by standard precautions include blood and all other body fluids, body secretions, and body excretions, except sweat, even if blood is not visible.
- Transmission-based precautions are followed, in addition to standard precautions, whenever a client is known or suspected to be infected with contagious pathogens.

STANDARD PRECAUTIONS:

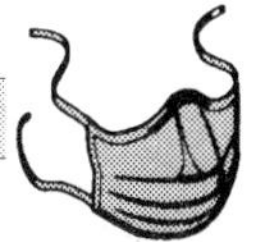

1. Wash your hands immediately if they become contaminated with blood or body fluids; also wash your hands before and after client care and after removing gloves.
2. Wear gloves if you will or could come in contact with any body fluid, or contaminated surfaces or objects.
3. Change your gloves between tasks and procedures on the same client.
4. Wear a gown, eye protection (goggles, glasses), or face shield, and a mask during procedures likely to generate droplets of blood or body fluids.
5. Carefully handle used client care equipment soiled with body fluids.
6. Ensure that hospital procedures for routine care, cleaning and disinfection of environmental surfaces, beds, bedrails, and bedside equipment are followed.
7. Handle contaminated linens in a manner that prevents contamination and transfer of microorganisms.
8. Handle used needles or other sharp implements carefully. Do not bend, break, reinsert them into their original sheaths, or handle them unnecessarily. Discard them intact immediately after use into an impervious disposal box.
9. Place clients who cannot maintain appropriate hygiene or who contaminate the environment in a private room.
10. If you have an exudative lesion, avoid all direct client contact until the condition has resolved.

IN ADDITION TO STANDARD PRECAUTIONS:

AIRBORNE TRANSMISSION-BASED PRECAUTIONS:

1. Place the client in a private room that has monitored negative air pressure in relation to surrounding areas.
2. Wear respiratory protection (masks or face shields) when entering the room.
3. Limit client transport and client movement out of the room.
4. Clients with measles, varicella, tuberculosis

DROPLET TRANSMISSION-BASED PRECAUTIONS:

1. Place the client in a private room.
2. Wear a mask when working within 3 feet of the client.
3. Keep visitors 3 feet from the infected client.
4. Limit movement of the client from the room. If the client must leave the room, have him wear a surgical mask, if possible.
5. Clients with invasive neisseria meningitis, mycoplasma pneumonia, streptococcal group A infections, pertussis.

CONTACT TRANSMISSION-BASED PRECAUTIONS:

1. Place the client in a private room.
2. Wear gloves whenever you enter the room. Always change gloves after contact with infected material. Remove gloves before leaving the client*s room and wash your hands.
3. Wear a gown when entering the client's room if your clothing will have extensive contact with the client, environmental surfaces, or if the client has diarrhea or is incontinent. Remove the gown before leaving the client's room.
4. Limit movement of the client from the room.
5. Avoid sharing any client care equipment.
6. Clients with diseases easily transmitted by direct contact- gastrointestinal, respiratory, skin, or wound infections

Appendix 6-10: ANTIBIOTIC MEDICATIONS

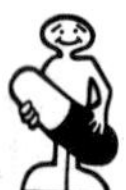

MEDICATIONS	SIDE EFFECTS	NURSING IMPLICATIONS

❖ GENERAL NURSING IMPLICATIONS ❖

— Cultures should always be taken prior to the administration of the first dose.
— Teach the client to finish the entire prescribed course of medication even though he may feel well.
— Schedule at evenly spaced intervals around the clock.
— Give most oral antibiotic drugs on an empty stomach (1 hour before or 2 hours after meals).
— Take drugs with a full glass of water.
— Observe for hypersensitivity:
  anaphylaxis—hypotension, respiratory distress, urticaria, angioedema, vomiting, diarrhea.
  serum sickness—fever, vasculitis, generalized lymphadenopathy, edema of joints, bronchospasm.
— Observe for superinfection:
  stomatitis—sore mouth, white patches on oral mucosa, black furry tongue
  diarrhea
  monilial vaginitis—rash in perineal area, itching, vaginal discharge
  new localized signs and symptoms—redness, heat, edema, pain, drainage, cough
  recurrence of systemic signs and symptoms—fever, malaise

PENICILLIN: Bactericidal; interferes with the formation of the bacterial cell wall.

MEDICATIONS	SIDE EFFECTS	NURSING IMPLICATIONS
Penicillin G (**Bicillin**): PO, IM Penicillin V (**PenVee K, V-cillin K**): PO Amoxicillin (**Amoxil**): PO with clavulanate — (**Augmentin**): PO Ampicillin (**Omnipen, Polycillin**): PO, IM, IV Cloxacillin (**Tegopen**): PO Ticarcillin (**Ticar**): IM, IV	Parenteral injection is more hazardous than oral administration. Diarrhea, especially in children. Allergic reactions: skin rashes, joint pain, dermatitis, kidney damage. Anaphylactic reaction (hypersensitivity): decreased B/P, increased pulse, respiratory distress, diaphoresis.	1. Observe for allergic reactions and have emergency equipment available. 2. Amoxicillin can be scheduled without regard to meals. 3. Observe client for 30 minutes after IM or IV administration for symptoms of allergic reactions. 4. Clients with beta hemolytic strep infections should be on penicillin for a minimum of 10 days to prevent development of rheumatic fever or glomerulonephritis. 5. May reduce the effectiveness of oral contraceptives. 6. Discard liquid forms of penicillin after 7 days at room temperature and 14 days when refrigerated. 7. For IV administration, generally dilute reconstituted penicillin in 50 to 100 ml of 5% dextrose or 0.9% sodium chloride injection and infuse over 30 to 60 minutes. 8. ***Uses:*** pneumonia, meningitis, gonorrhea, otitis media, urinary tract infections, syphilis, and as prophylaxis for clients with rheumatic fever.

AMINOGLYCOSIDE: ***Bactericidal:*** interferes with formation of bacterial cell wall.

MEDICATIONS	SIDE EFFECTS	NURSING IMPLICATIONS
Gentamycin (**Garamycin**): IM, IV Amikacin (**Amikin**): IM, IV Kanamycin sulfate (**Kantrex**): PO, IM, IV Neomycin sulfate (**Mycifradin sulfate**): PO, IM, topical, ophthalmic	Toxicity: Ototoxicity—hearing loss is irreversible. Nephrotoxicity— albuminuria, casts, oliguria. Skin rash, headache, hypotension, pain, and tenderness at injection site.	1. Assess peak and trough levels to determine toxic levels. 2. Neurotoxicity may be increased if given soon after surgery. 3. Assess for ototoxicity (change in hearing, ringing in the ears, dizziness, or unsteady gait) and nephrotoxicity (monitor BUN and creatinine). 4 . Are generally not used for long-term therapy. 5. Drink 2000-3000 ml. of fluid daily. 6. ***Uses:*** broad spectrum; primarily used for gram- negative sepsis and serious gram-negative infections including, *E. coli*, *Klebsiella*, *proteus*, and *staphylococcus*; infections of the urinary tract, and neonatal meningitis.

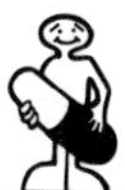

Appendix 6-10:
ANTIBIOTIC MEDICATIONS

MEDICATIONS	SIDE EFFECTS	NURSING IMPLICATIONS
CEPHALOSPORINS: ***Bacteriostatic:*** broad-spectrum, interfere with the formation of the bacterial cell wall.		
1st generation—Cefadroxil (**Duricef, Ultracef**):PO Cephalexin (**Keflex**): PO Cephalothin sodium (**Keflin**): IM, IV Cefazolin (**Kefzol**, **Ancef**): IM, IV 2nd generation— Cefuroxime (**Ceftin**): PO, IM, IV Loracarbef (**Lorabid**): PO Cefoxitin (**Mefoxin**): IM, IV 3rd generation—Cefixime (**Suprax**): PO Ceftriaxone (**Rocephin**): IM, IV	Hypersensitivity. Superinfection. GI upset, neutropenia (decreased WBC), pain at injection site, renal damage seizures.	1. Give oral cephalosporins with food or milk. 2. Administer IM medications deep into the muscle. 3. Use with caution in clients known to be allergic to penicillin. 4. Ceftriaxone (**Rocephin**) is only drug approved for once-daily dosing.
TETRACYCLINES: ***Bacteriostatic:*** *broad-spectrum; interfere with protein synthesis of infectious organism and thus diminishes its growth and reproduction.*		
Tetracycline (**Achromycin**): PO, IV, IM Doxycycline (**Vibramycin**): PO, IV Demeclocyline (**Declomycin**): PO Minocycline (**Minocin**): PO, IV	Loose stools, diarrhea, sore throat, photosensitivity. Deformity in teeth in children up to eight years old and in newborns whose mothers have received the drug.	1. Administer on empty stomach; withhold antacids, dairy foods, and foods high in calcium at least 2 hours after PO administration. Do not administer with milk. 2. Can give doxycycline and minocycline with food. 3. Do not give at the same time with iron preparations. Give them as far apart as possible (i.e., 2-3 hours). 4. Advise client to avoid direct or artificial sunlight. 5. Prevent or treat pruritus ani, which occurs as a side effect, by cleansing the anal region several times each day and after each BM. 6. Observe for development of superinfections 7. ***Uses:*** *with other antimicrobials for PID and STDs,. severe respiratory tract and urinary tract infections, septicemia, osteomyelitis.*
SULFONAMIDES: ***Bacteriostatic:*** *interfere with the utilization of para-aminobenzoic acid (PABA, required by bacteria for growth); halt multiplications of bacteria but do not kill fully formed microorganisms.*		
Sulfamethoxazole (**Gantanol**): PO Sulfisoxazole (**Gantrisin**): PO Sulfamethoxazole-trimethoprim (**SMZ-TMP, Bactrim, Septra**): PO, IV	Blood dyscrasia, renal dysfunction (crystalluria, hematuria, oliguria); skin and mucous membrane lesions, dizziness, headache, fatigue. Rash (Stevens-Johnson syndrome). May reduce the synthesis of vitamin K, leading to hemorrhage.	1. Encourage adequate fluid intake to prevent crystalluria. 2. Assess for side effects. 3. **Azulifidine**: urine may turn orange-yellow. 4. Be aware that long-acting sulfonamides are potentially more dangerous than short-acting preparations and should only be used cautiously. 5. **Uses:** treatment of acute and chronic cystitis, ulcerative colitis, lymphogranuloma venereum, toxoplasmosis, and chancroid.

Appendix 6-10: ANTIBIOTIC MEDICATIONS

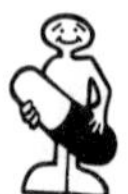

MEDICATIONS	SIDE EFFECTS	NURSING IMPLICATIONS
MACROLIDES: ***Bacteriostatic and bacteriocidal:*** inhibit microbial protein synthesis.		
Erythromycin base (**Ilosone, E-Mycin**): PO, IV, Azithromycin (**Zithromax**): PO Clarithromycin (**Biaxin**): PO	Nausea, vomiting, abdominal distress, diarrhea. Hepatotoxic: abnormal liver function studies, jaundice, fever.	1. Do not administer with or immediately prior to fruit juice or other acid drinks. 2. **Ilosone**: observe for jaundice, usually after 10 - 14 days of therapy. Also, do not store **Ilosone** suspension longer than two weeks at room temperature. 3. Uses: suppression of intestinal bacteria before colonscopy or bowel surgery, and as a substitute for penicillin.
QUINOLONES: *Bacteriostatic and bacteriocidal: broad-spectrum; inhibit microbial protein synthesis.*		
Ciprofloxacin (**Cipro**): PO Ofloxacin (**Floxin**): PO, IV	Nausea, vomiting, abdominal distress, diarrhea. Crystalluria. Hepatotoxic: abnormal liver function studies, jaundice, fever.	1. Give IV infusions over 60 minutes, and stop primary infusion if using a piggyback setup. 2. Not used in pediatric clients due to potential damage to cartilage and joints. 3. Increase fluid intake and avoid calcium-containing antacids, to prevent crystalluria. 4. ***Uses:*** suppression of intestinal bacteria before colonscopy or bowel surgery, and as a substitute for penicillin.
OTHER ANTIBIOTICS:		
Chloramphenicol sodium: (**Chloromycetin**): PO, IV	Blood dyscrasia (aplastic anemia), irreversible bone marrow depression. GI upset; in neonates, may cause the gray syndrome: ashen gray color, vomiting, loose green stools, vasomotor collapse.	1. Broad-spectrum, bacteriostatic. ***Uses:*** for typhoid fever and other serious systemic infections,(e.g., meningococcal meningitis). Not to be used for minor infections. 2. Observe for bone marrow depression, (e.g. weakness, sore throat, bruising). 3. Monitor CBC, platelets, serum iron, reticulocyte counts (q 3 days). 4. Assess for optic and peripheral neuritis, which is an indication for immediate discontinuance of the drug. 5. Observe premature and newborn infants for gray syndrome. 6. Observe for GI side effects, neurotoxic reactions, and jaundice.
Astreonam (**Azactam**): IM, IV	Diarrhea, rash, blood dyscrasias, elevated liver enzymes.	1. Classified as a beta-lactam; is effective against gram-negative bacterial infections. 2. ***Uses***: for UTIs, lower respiratory tract infections, and gynecologic/abdominal infections.
Vancomycin (**Vancocin**): PO, IV	Ototoxicity, nephrotoxicity.	1. Acts by inhibiting cell wall synthesis; very powerful drug. 2. ***Uses:*** in severe penicillin-resistant staphylococcal infection. 3. Peak and trough levels are monitored.
Metronidazole (**Flagyl**): PO, IV, Intravaginally	Anorexia, nausea, vomiting, dry mouth with a metallic taste. Abdominal cramps, and uterine pain (if given intravaginally). Superinfection.	1. ***Uses:*** to treat anaerobic infections (e.g., intra-abdominal, gynecologic, bone, and joint). 2. Urine may turn dark red-brown. 3. Avoid alcohol and alcohol-containing elixirs.

PHYSIOLOGY OF THE IMMUNE SYSTEM

A. The lymphoid system is composed of organs and cells that participate in the immune response.
   1. Primary lymphoid organs.
      a. Thymus.
         (1) Production of T-cells.
         (2) Hormones that affect T-cell differentiation.
      b. Bone Marrow.
         (1) Antigen processing.
         (2) Cell-mediated and humoral immunity.
         (3) Recognition and removal of old cells.
   2. Secondary lymphoid organs.
      a. Lymph nodes—filter out foreign material and circulate the lymphocytes.
      b. Spleen—produces lymphocytes and plasma cells, filters the blood.
      c. Mucosal-associated lymphoid tissue (MALT)—the G.I. tract, the bronchi, and the skin all contain associated lymphoid tissue.
      d. Tonsils—trap and remove invading organisms.

B. Body recognizes foreign proteins, *antigens*, which elicit a response from the immune system—the production of antibodies- which attack and destroy the invading antigens.

Immunological Responses

A. B-cell—Humoral or antibody-mediated response.
   1. B-lymphocytes (macrophages) identify and destroy foreign antigens.
   2. Some of the B-lymphocytes remain small and inactive; these cells become the memory cells. On a second exposure to the antigen, the memory cells initiate a rapid antibody response.
   3. After antigenic stimulation, the B-lymphocytes differentiate into plasma cells, which excrete large amounts of immunoglobulin.
      a. IgM—provides the initial antibody response.
      b. IgG—main serum antibody, important to the resistance of infection; the longest acting immunoglobulin; crosses placenta and provides natural passive immunity in the newborn.
      c. IgA—plays an important role against infection in respiratory passages; provides antiviral antibodies.
      d. IgE—is associated with immediate hypersensitivity reactions, anaphylactic, and atopic reactions; assists in the defense of parasitic infections.
   4. The complement response—the immune response without cell participation. The complement proteins activate one or more of the following responses.
      a. Phagocytosis— pathogenic organisms are covered with opsonin; this allows the phagocyte to recognize the foreign protein and ingest it.
      b. Inflammatory reaction—stimulation of the inflammatory cells, or chemotaxis, which results in the migration of neutrophils and macrophages to area of antigen concentration.
      c. Cytotoxic function—the protein of the complement system digests the cell membranes causing, the cell to rupture.
      d. If the complement response is not controlled, host cells may be destroyed. When the immune complexes activate complement in the walls of small vessel, tissue injury, and inflammation occur.

B. Cell-mediated response, T-cell (lymphocyte).
   1. Stem cells originate in the bone marrow and travel to the thymus, where they mature into functional T-cells.
   2. A cell-mediated reaction occurs when the antigen binds with a sensitized T-cell.
   3. Provides cellular immunity, delayed hypersensitivity reactions.
   4. Recognizes tumor cells and inhibits tumor growth.
   5. Rejects organ transplants.
   6. Produces autoimmune disorders.
   7. Inflammatory response is a nonspecific immune response. This involves the movement of the phagocyte into the affected area to restore homeostasis.

C. Properties of the immunologic response.
   1. Specificity—the formation of a specific antibody for each antigen. Antibodies produced against one bacteria will not protect the body from other bacteria.
   2. Memory—the ability to remember the specific antigen and make the appropriate antibody. Once the body responds to a particular antigen, memory cells are produced. This produces a stronger immune response the next time the body comes in contact with the same antigen.

Table 7-1: ACQUIRED IMMUNITY

TYPE	CHARACTERISTICS	EXAMPLES
Active: antibodies synthesized by body in response to antigen stimulation.	***Natural:*** contact with an antigen through exposure; develops slowly, often lifetime protection.	Recovery from childhood diseases (e.g., chicken pox, measles, mumps).
	Artificial: immunization with an antigen develops slowly; may provide protection for several years but "boosters" may be required.	Immunization with live or attenuated vaccines (Sabin, measles). Toxoid immunization (tetanus toxoid, diphtheria toxoid).
Passive: antibodies produced in one individual and transferred to another.	***Natural:*** immunity from placenta and colostrum transferred from mother to child; provides immediate temporary protection.	Maternal immunoglobin in the neonate.
	Artificial: injection of serum from immune human or animal; short-lived but immediate immunity.	Gamma globulin; injection of animal hyperimmune serum (diphtheria antitoxin, tetanus antitoxin).

3. Self-recognition—the ability of the body to recognize its own proteins and differentiate them from foreign protein. This allows foreign protein to be attacked without injury to the body's own cells.

D. Types of specific immunity.

1. Natural immunity—no prior contact with an antigen; may be related to genetic tendency or species-specific.
2. Acquired immunity—develops either actively or passively (See Table 7-1).

Factors Affecting the Immune Response

1. **Age**--infant's immune system is not fully developed; in the, elderly the immune response is hypoactive.
2. **Metabolism**—thyroid and adrenal hormone deficiencies decrease the immune response; steroids inhibit phagocytosis and inflammatory response.
3. **Emotional stress**—may precipitate a decrease in cell-mediated immunity or lymphocyte production.
4. **Hormonal influences**—females have a greater incidence of autoimmune diseases than males.
5. **Environment and lifestyle**—unsanitary living conditions and exposure to pathogens increase susceptibility to infections.
6. **Nutrition**—poor nutrition can decrease the overall immune response.

NURSING PRIORITY: *Clients that have a compromised immune system should not participate in any immunization program until they have checked with their doctor.*

DISORDERS OF THE IMMUNE SYSTEM

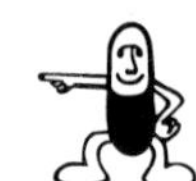

Hypersensitivity

A. Type I (immediate, IgE; antibodies involved).

1. Person sensitized by prior exposure to a particular antigen.
2. When same antigen reappears, it interacts with the IgE, which initiates mast cell degranulation; this activates the release of chemical mediators, primarily histamine.
3. Histamine—major chemical mediator.
   a. Spasm of bronchial muscles.
   b. Capillary vasodilation.
   c. Increased capillary permeability.
   d. Decreased blood pressure.
   e. Increased nasal stuffiness and bronchial secretions.
   f. Peak effect in 1-2 minutes lasts for about 10 minutes.
4. Conditions associated with Type I.
   a. Anaphylaxis (most severe).
   b. Atopic reactions (most common).
      (1) Allergic rhinitis.
      (2) Urticaria.
      (3) Bronchial asthma.

B. Type II (cytotoxic; IgG and IgM antibodies involved).

1. Complement system is activated, causing cytotoxic effects against the body's own cells.

2. The normal process of phagocytosis begins to damage normal body tissue.
3. Conditions associated with Type II.
   a. Hemolytic disease of the newborn.
   b. Myasthenia gravis.
   c. Transfusion reactions.
   d. Acute graft rejection.

C. Type III (immune complex, IgG and IgM antibodies involved).
1. Circulating immune complexes (antibody/antigen complex) are deposited in the body tissue.
2. When the immune complex is deposited in the body tissue, the complement factors may be activated. This causes local tissue inflammation and cell wall damage.
3. Categories of immune complex formation.
   a. Persistent infections (streptococcal infections) combined with a poor antibody response may lead to the formation of immune complex that eventually deposits in an affected organ.
      (1) Endocarditis.
      (2) Acute glomerulonephritis.
      (3) Serum sickness (injection with foreign serum).
   b. The body produces antibodies that attack the body's own cells (autoantibodies).
      (1) Rheumatoid arthritis.
      (2) Systemic lupus erythematous.
   c. Repeated inhalation of allergens causes immune complex formation to be deposited in the lungs and on other body surfaces.

D. Type IV (cell-mediated, delayed hypersensitivity)
1. The T-cells are sensitized to an antigen from a previous exposure.
2. The sensitized T-cells initiate the inflammatory response, leading to cellular damage and damage to the surrounding tissue.
3. Conditions associated with Type IV.
   a. Tuberculosis, skin testing.
   b. Contact dermatitis.
   c. Graft vs host rejection (skin) .
   d. Transplant rejection.

Anaphylactic Reaction

❑ **An antigen-antibody response that precipitates the release of vasoactive substances (histamine), causing profound vasodilation and increased capillary permeability.**

A. Anaphylactoid reaction does not involve allergen/antibody interaction; it is triggered by non-protein substances (IV radiographic dye).

B. The initial exposure occurs during the sensitization phase; immune antibodies are formed. The next exposure to the antigen may bring on the second phase of the response—the mediator or histamine release and activation of the complement response.

Assessment

1. Risk Factors.
   a. History of exposure to allergen.
      (1) Amount of allergen.
      (2) Absorption of ingested allergen.
      (3) Predisposition to hypersensitivity.
      (4) Antibody levels from previous exposure.
2. Clinical Manifestations
   a. Hypotension to vascular collapse.
   b. Urticaria, diffuse erythema, periorbital edema.
   c. Hoarseness, wheezing.
   d. Bronchospasm, progressing to respiratory failure.
   e. Vomiting.
   f. Generalized burning and/or itching.
   g. Sense of impending doom.

NCLEX ALERT: *Manage a medical emergency. Anaphylaxis is an immediate response, progression of symptoms is very rapid, emergency treatment must be initiated immediately if condition is suspected. Death from an anaphylactic reaction is most often due to broncho constriction.*

Diagnostics (According to symptoms and exposure to allergen)

Treatment

1. Maintain patent airway.
2. Epinephrine (dosage and route of administration depend on the client's condition).
3. Benadryl, IM or IV.
4. Oxygen.
5. IV fluids (Ringer's lactate or 5% Dextrose).
6. Continuous cardiac monitoring.
7. Corticosteroid to reduce inflammatory response.

Nursing Intervention

✦ *Goal: to assess clients for predisposition to hypersensitivity reactions.*

1. Evaluate client history regarding reactions to:
   a. Medications—especially penicillin
   b. Foods—seafoods, eggs.
   c. Insect bites.
   d. Vaccines—especially egg-cultured types.
   e. Blood products, transfusion reaction.
   f. Diagnostic agents—iodine-base contrast media.
2. If hypersensitivity is suspected, a localized skin test may be done prior to the administration of substance.
3. Prevention is the priority.

✦ *Goal: to maintain adequate ventilation.*

1. Comfortable position, preferably in bed.
2. High oxygen concentrations.
3. Anticipate utilization of airway adjuncts (oral airways, endotracheal intubation).
4. Administration of medications to reverse bronchospasm. (aminophylline, corticosteroid, epinephrine).

✦ *Goal: to restore adequate circulation.*

1. IV fluids to correct loss of fluid to third-space shifts and vasodilation.
2. Carefully titrate fluid replacement with vital signs.

***NURSING PRIORITY:** Monitor the client carefully; as fluid begins to shift back into the vascular compartment, it is very easy to fluid overload the client.*

3. Vasopressor may be utilized to increase blood pressure if fluid replacement is not effective.
4. Client may be placed in supine position with the feet and legs elevated provided this does not compromise ventilation.

✦ *Goal: client teaching to prevent recurrence.*

1. Once causative agent is identified, instruct client accordingly.
2. Depending on causative agent, client may be candidate for desensitization.
3. Advise client to wear identification tag or bracelet.

Autoimmune

A. A critical aspect of the immune response is the ability of the body to recognize normal tissue and to not invade or destroy it.

B. When the immune system can no longer recognize the normal tissue and begins to destroy healthy tissue, an auto immune response has occurred.

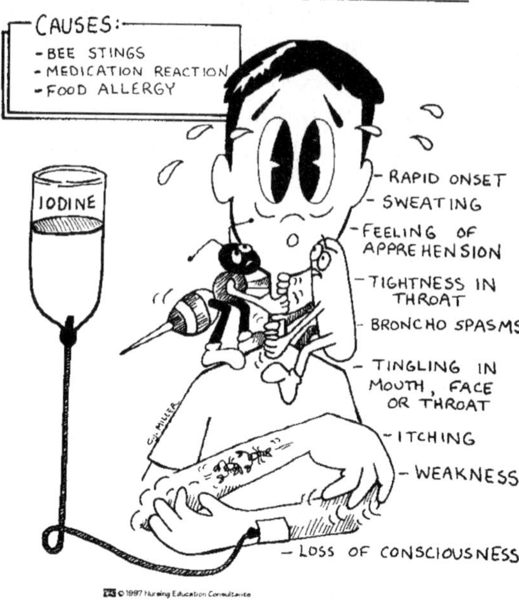

Figure 7-1: Anaphylactic Reaction
Zerwekh, J. & Claborn, J. (1997). *Memory Notebook of Nursing*, Vol. 2, Dallas, TX: Nursing Education Consultants, Inc.

C. Some autoimmune responses are very tissue specific and invade only that specific tissue, while another response may be body wide affect. Hormone factors play an unclear role; higher incidence of autoimmune disease in women than in men.

D. Autoimmune response and disease occurrence.

1. The direct action of the auto antibody on the cell surface. This causes destruction of the cell (cytotoxic); may activate the complement system.
2. Small immune complexes are formed and are deposited in the capillaries, in the joints, or in the renal structures. Tissue damage occurs due to activation of the complement system response.
3. Activation of sensitized T-cells; these cells release lymphokines, which in turn cause tissue damage.

E. Autoimmune response may be systemic or organ-specific.

1. Systemic diseases.
   a. Systemic lupus erythematosus (SLE).
   b. Rheumatoid arthritis.
2. Organ-specific diseases.
   a. Myasthenia gravis.
   b. Hyperthyroid (Graves' Disease).
   c. Addison's Disease.
   d. Insulin dependent diabetes.

Systemic Lupus Erythematosus (SLE)

❑ **An autoimmune disorder that affects multiple organs. There is a diffuse production of autoantibodies that can attack and cause damage to body organs and tissue.**

A. Tissue injury in SLE results from the attack of the autoantibodies and the deposition of the immune complex throughout the body.

B. The course of the disease varies greatly in the severity of symptoms; there are exacerbations and remissions.

Assessment

A. Risk factors.

a. More common in women, 20 to 50 years old.

b. Familial tendencies.

c. Higher incidence among non-whites.

d. May be drug-induced.

1. Clinical manifestations.

a. Initially may be nonspecific—weight loss, fatigue and fever.

b. Skin rash—characteristic "butterfly" rash over face. Erythematous rash on areas of the body exposed to sunlight.

c. Arthritis—does not cause bone erosion or joint deformity, generally affects the peripheral joints.

d. Renal system involvement.

e. Cardiovascular system.

(1) Raynaud's phenomenon.

(2) Pericarditis, may progress to endocarditis.

(3) Vascular inflammation of the small vessels. Most common sites affected are the small vessels of the fingers and the GI tract.

f. Neurologic disorders—seizures and or psychoses.

g. Hematologic disorders.

h. Emotional lability.

i. Severe depression.

j. Respiratory system—dyspnea, pleural inflammation.

k. Gastrointestinal system—general GI discomforts; inflammation may progress to involve the pancreas or the liver.

Diagnostics

1. Since symptoms vary greatly from one individual to another diagnosing the condition can be very difficult.
2. Presence of LE cells (antibodies) in the serum.
3. Antinuclear antibodies (ANA) are present and/or increased.
4. Presence of immune antibodies.
5. General bone marrow suppression—decreased red blood cells, white blood cells and platelets.
6. Increased gamma globulin levels due to increased antibodies.

Treatment

(There is no known cure.)

1. Nonsteroidal anti-inflammatory medications
2. Corticosteroids are drugs of choice in exacerbations.
3. Plasmapheresis—the mechanical removal of the toxins from the blood. May provide temporary relief during acute episodes.
4. Supportive therapy, depending on the involved organs.

Nursing Intervention

✦ *Goal: to prevent exacerbations.*

1. Maintain good nutritional status.
2. Avoid exposure to infections.
3. Teach client regarding skin problems and observation for complications.
4. Teach client personal hygiene to prevent urinary tract infections.
5. Make sure client understands how to take medications.
6. Review signs and symptoms of infection, and the importance of contacting the doctor should they occur.
7. Avoid exposure to sunlight; use a heavy sun screen when exposure is unavoidable.
8. Contact physician before participating in any immunization procedures.

✦ *Goal: to maintain adequate tissue perfusion.*

1. Assess for indications of impaired peripheral perfusion.
2. Prevent injury to extremities.
3. Assess for indications of cardiac involvement.
4. Decrease activity level if client exhibits symptoms of cardiac involvement.
5. Carefully evaluate fluid status with regard to cardiac status and weight gain.

✦ *Goal: to maintain good renal function.*

1. Monitor for peripheral edema, hypertension, hematuria, decreased output.
2. Maintain on bed rest if renal involvement is severe.
3. Monitor BUN and creatinine levels.
4. Careful evaluation for urinary tract infections.

✦ *Goal: to assist client to maintain psychological equilibrium.*

1. Observe for behavioral changes that may indicate CNS involvement.
2. Encourage client to participate in support groups and to seek counseling to deal with stress.
3. Encourage positive coping mechanisms.

Acquired Immunodeficiency Syndrome (AIDS)

❑ **A condition resulting from severe impairment of the immune system's ability to respond to invading pathogens. AIDS ultimately affects all body systems.**

A. Occurs as a result of being infected with the human immunodeficiency virus (HIV).

B. After exposure to the virus, the client may develop symptoms within 6 to 12 weeks; however, symptoms may not develop for 6 months.

C. Once a client is infected, current studies indicate he will probably harbor the virus for the rest of his life.

D. The infections that occur in the AIDS clients are called *opportunistic* because they take advantage of the suppressed immune system.

1. These infections tend to resist conventional treatment.
2. The type of infection and its extent varies with each client, depending on the extent of immunosuppression.
3. Single opportunistic infections are rare, most often client has multiple infections.

Transmission of HIV

A. Blood transmission.

1. Sharing of contaminated needles, or accidental needle sticks from an infected person account for the highest numbers of infections due to contaminated blood.
2. HIV+ females are a source of transmission of HIV to their children through perinatal transmission, regardless of vaginal or cesarean delivery.
3. Exposure to an infected client's blood via open wounds or mucous membranes.

B. Sexual transmission.

1. Homosexual males.
2. Heterosexual; either partner can infect the other.
3. Anal sex is considered to be a high-risk sexual activity.
4. Any sexual activity that involves direct contact with vaginal secretions and semen may transmit HIV.

C. HIV dies quickly outside the body because it needs living tissue and moisture to survive.

D. HIV *may not* be transmitted by:

1. Hugging, kissing, holding hands, or other nonsexual contact.
2. Inanimate objects (money, doorknobs, bathtubs, toilet seats, etc.).
3. Dishes, silverware, or food handled by an infected person.
4. Animals or insects.

Table 7-2: CDC RECOMMENDATIONS FOR IMMUNIZATION OF HEALTH CARE WORKERS

DISEASE	RECOMMENDATION
Hepatitis B	Three-dose series of HB vaccine for pre-exposure protection
Polio	Primary series of oral polio virus vaccine in childhood is sufficient
Tetanus/diphtheria	Booster dose of Td every 10 years after primary series of diphtheria and tetanus toxoids; tetanus toxoid may be repeated in 5 years if a dirty wound is sustained
Measles	College entrants and health care workers who do not have evidence of immunity to measles (physician-diagnosed measles or laboratory evidence of immunity) should have documentation of two doses of measles vaccine received on or after their first birthday; vaccine can be given as MMR*
Mumps	A single dose of live mumps vaccine received on or after the first birthday is sufficient; vaccine can be given as MMR*
Rubella	A single dose of live attenuated rubella vaccine received on or after the first birthday is sufficient; vaccine can be given as MMR*

*There is no evidence suggesting an increased risk from live measles, mumps, or rubella (MMR) vaccination to persons already immunize to these diseases as a result of previous vaccination or natural disease.

Source: Center for Disease Control. *Update on Adult Immunization. Immunization Practices Advisory Committee*, (1991).

Prevention of Transmission in Health Care Setting

A. Maintain standard (universal) precautions (Appendix 6-10).

B. Consider all blood and body fluids from all clients to be contaminated.

C. Avoid contaminating outside of container when collecting specimens.

D. Do not recap needles and syringes.

E. Cleanse work surface areas with appropriate germicide (household bleach in concentrations of 1:100 to 1:10 is effective).

F. Clean up spills of blood and body fluid immediately. Remove as much of the body fluid as possible, then wash the area with a germicide solution.

G. Follow CDC recommendations for immunization of health care workers (Table 7-2).

NCLEX ALERT: *It is essential that you know the modes of transmission of HIV, activities that do not transmit the virus, and the nursing care to protect yourself, your AIDS client, and other clients you are caring for.*

Clinical Manifestations

1. Most people are not diagnosed at time of infection because they do not seek medical care when symptoms occur, or health care providers do not take an adequate history.
2. Category A
   a. Asymptomatic HIV+ infection.
   b. Persistent lymphadenopathy.
   c. Acute primary HIV infection with accompanying symptoms.
      (1) Diarrhea.
      (2) Nausea and vomiting.
      (3) Decreased energy.
   d. May remain in category A for extended period of time.
3. Category B
   a. Symptomatic conditions attributed to the HIV infection or defect in immunity.
   b. Examples of conditions complicated by the HIV infection.
      (1) Bacterial infections (endocarditis, meningitis, pneumonia, sepsis).
      (2) Candidiasis for more than 1 month.
      (3) Fever or diarrhea lasting more than 1 month.
      (4) Hairy leukoplakia, oral.
      (5) Herpes zoster - two distinct episodes.
      (6) Pulmonary tuberculosis.
4. Category C - Conditions that are strongly associated with severe immunodeficiency and cause serious morbidity and mortality.
5. HIV related Kaposi's sarcoma.
   a. Begins with a "patch" that looks like a bruise, later will turn dark violet or black.
   b. Is not related to the CD4+ cell counts, and may occur early in the disease.
   c. Invades body organs, extremities, skin and torso.
   d. May become very painful.

Opportunistic Infections

1. *Pneumocystis carinii* pneumonia (PCP) The most common of the opportunistic infections. Typical symptoms of upper respiratory infection.

Tuberculosis.

1. Fungal infections - histoplasmosis, coccidioidomy- cosis.

Diagnostics

1. CD4+ cell count - (receptor cell on the T4 helper cell) - dramatic decrease in cell count after primary infection (T4, T4 helper, CD4+ are synonymous).
2. Enzyme immunoassay (EIA) testing - after the primary invasion there is an increase in the viral load and decrease in CD4+ count, at this time the client begins to develop antibodies to the HIV. The EIA detects these antibodies.
3. If the EIA test is positive, then the Western blot test is done to confirm the HIV positive results.
4. Multiple serum diagnostics are utilized to determine other criteria for an immunosuppressed condition.
   a. CBC—anemia, leukocytopenia.
   b. Immunoglobulin levels of IgG and IgA are usually increased.
   c. Platelet count decreased.
   d. Serum protein and albumin are decreased.
   e. Liver function tests (LFTs) are elevated.

Treatment

1. Medications - antiretroviral medications. (appendix 7-2) Therapy may be started at the time of the initial infection to decrease the damage to the immune system.
2. Other medications are utilized to treat the opportunistic infections, according to area of involvement.

3. Chemotherapeutic drugs may be used to treat Kaposi's sarcoma.

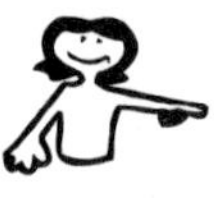

NURSING PRIORITY: Frequently the treatment for the AIDS client causes problems in other areas: the high dose antibiotics may increase the level of leukopenia, the chemotherapy medications will further decrease the bone marrow functions. The AIDS client on chemotherapy is going to be even further immunosuppressed.

Nursing Intervention

✦ *Goal: client and public education regarding transmission of disease.*

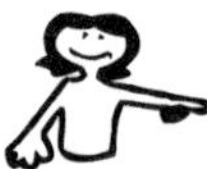

NURSING PRIORITY: Public and client teaching regarding the transmission of the HIV is vital in the control of this disease.

1. Safe sex.
   a. Maintain monogamous relationships.
   b. Sex with female or male prostitutes is a high-risk activity.
   c. Avoid all sexual activities that cause cuts or tears in the vagina, on the penis, or in the rectum.
   d. Males should wear a condom for all sexual activity if multiple partners are involved.
   e. If the HIV status of a sexual partner is not known, a condom should always be used during intercourse.
   f. Anyone who has been involved in any high-risk sexual activities, or has injected IV recreational drugs, should have a blood test to determine presence of the HIV.

Self-Care

1. Maintain personal hygiene; wash hands frequently.
2. Do not share personal items such as toothbrushes, razors, and enema equipment.
3. Do not get pregnant.
4. In a health care setting, always advise of HIV positive status.
5. Do not receive a live-virus vaccine (can be fatal in immunosuppressed clients).
6. Kitchen and bathroom facilities may be shared, provided normal sanitary practices are observed.
7. Clean up spills of body fluids or waste immediately with a solution of 1 part bleach to 10 parts water. A bleach solution should be used to disinfect kitchen and bathroom floors, showers, sinks, and toilet bowls.
8. Towels and washcloths should not be shared without laundering.
9. Sanitary napkins, tampons, and any bloody dressing should be wrapped in a plastic bag and placed in a trash container.
10. Needles should not be recapped. Dispose of them in an impenetrable sealed container.
11. Clients with AIDS do not have to remove pets. Have someone else change litter boxes and birdcages, when possible; if this is not feasible, use gloves.
12. Do not donate blood or plasma, body organs, or semen.

✦ *Goal: to maintain ventilation (with pulmonary involvement).*

1. Client frequently on limited activities or bedrest.
2. Supplemental oxygen.
3. Avoid contact with upper respiratory infections.
4. Adequate fluid intake, humidifier.
5. Frequent assessments for pulmonary changes and hypoxemia.
6. Coughing and deep breathing exercises.
7. Carefully evaluate respiratory function if narcotic analgesics are used.
8. Carefully assess activity tolerance.

✦ *Goal: to assist client to minimize the effects of neurologic changes.*

1. Frequent assessment of neurologic status.
2. Assess for visual changes.
3. If client is confused, provide care directed to reorientation.
4. Provide a safe and supportive environment, according to the neurological deficits.

✦ *Goal: to assist client to maintain psychosocial equilibrium.*

1. Encourage client to express his feelings and concerns.
2. Do not be judgmental regarding client's lifestyle.
3. Maintain frequent contact with the client.
4. Encourage client to maintain as much independence as possible.
5. Assist client to take advantage of services available—social worker, financial aid, support groups.
6. Client should be advised as to patient rights.

Pediatric AIDS

❑ **Majority of children with AIDS were infected in the perinatal period. There are minimal cases related to blood transfusions or medications used by hemophiliacs.**

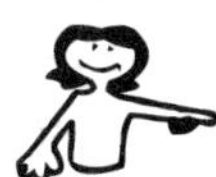

NURSING PRIORITY: HIV+ mothers should not breast-feed their infants.

Assessment

1. Risk factors.
   a. Pediatric infection from transfused blood is virtually non existent.
   b. Sexual activity is the major cause of HIV in adolescents.
   c. Infants born to mothers who are HIV+ account for a large majority of HIV infection in children.
2. Clinical manifestations.
   a. Infants who become symptomatic prior to their first birthday have a poor long-term prognosis.
   b. HIV+ infants usually develop symptoms by 18-24 months of age.
   c. Children rarely develop Kaposi's sarcoma.
   d. Failure to thrive and failure to meet developmental mile stones is common.
   e. Chronic or recurrent diarrhea
   f. Malabsorption syndrome, failure to gain weight.
   g. Hepatosplenomegaly, lymphadenopathy.
   h. Oral thrush (candidiasis).
   i. Opportunistic infections.
3. Diagnostics.
   a. Enzyme-linked immunosorbent assay (ELISA).
   b. Maternal antibodies may persist for 18 months.
4. Treatment—essentially same as for adult.

Nursing Intervention Specific to Children

✦ *Goal: to maintain homeostasis.*

1. Infants and children should receive the standard immunizations against childhood diseases with the exception of varicella (chickenpox) and OPV. Inactivated oral polio (IPV) is encouraged.
2. Nutritional support.
3. Educate adolescents regarding safe sex.
4. Generally, high-risk HIV infants are not circumcised.

Home Care

1. Teach the parents how to care for the child.
   a. How to administer medications.
   b. Symptoms of infections.
   c. Proper handling of diapers.
   d. Avoid contact with blood or body fluids.
2. Teach parents how to prevent transmission of disease.
3. Course of disease in infants and children is very unpredictable.

Organ Transplantation

❑ **Transplant has become the treatment of choice for clients with end-stage disease of the kidney, liver, heart, and lung, etc.**

Assessment

A. Types of rejection.
1. Hyperacute.
   a. Onset within 48 hours.
   b. General malaise, high fever.
   c. Must remove organ to stop rejection.
2. Acute.
   a. Occurs within 3 months to 2 years.
   b. Cell-mediated response, recipient becomes sensitized to the donor antigens.
   c. Symptoms relate to transplanted organ system affected; may be treated with immunosuppressant medications.
3. Chronic.
   a. Occurs months to years after transplant.
   b. May be asymptomatic or display symptoms directly related to failure of transplanted organ.
   c. Treatment usually not successful.

Treatment

Immunosuppressive medications (Appendix 7-1) are given in combination therapy. Often they are started prior to the transplant.

Nursing Intervention for Immunocompromised Clients

✦ *Goal: to monitor for and/or prevent opportunistic infections.*

1. The type, location, and severity of the infection depend on the disease progress and the client's immunosuppressive state.
2. Antimicrobial medications are given in high doses for an extended period. Medications may cause neutropenia.
3. Observe for *pneumocystis carinii* pneumonia (PCP) and other opportunistic infections (i.e., tuberculosis, fungal infections).
4. Protect client from iatrogenic infections.
5. Observe for neurological infections, specifically meningitis.
6. Observe hospitalized client and/or teach client symptoms of opportunistic infections.

a. Persistent unexplained fever, night sweats.
b. White spots in the mouth.
c. Persistent diarrhea and weight loss.

7. Teach client how to prevent infection.
   a. Careful hand washing.
   b. Do not use unpasteurized dairy products.
   c. Cook all vegetables, meats, and fruit before eating; this eliminates sources of microorganisms.
   d. Avoid contact with animal waste or bird cages, this decreases further contact with microorganisms.

✦ *Goal: to maintain adequate nutritional intake.*
1. Teach client regarding nutrition and caloric intake.
2. Encourage high-calorie snacks through out the day.
3. Encourage client to eat several small meals throughout the day.
4. May need to include dietary supplements such as Ensure or Isocal.
5. Assess client for lactose intolerance.
6. Avoid foods or beverages that may cause oral, esophageal, or gastric irritation.
7. Tube feedings or parenteral nutrition may be necessary.

✦ *Goal: to maintain fluid and electrolyte status.*
1. Evaluate weight gain and loss.
2. Observe for chronic diarrhea.
3. Encourage fluids that assist to maintain electrolyte balance.
4. Maintain IV fluids as appropriate.

✦ *Goal: to prevent decubiti formation and excoriation of the skin.*
1. Wash perineal and anal area, allow to dry thoroughly.
2. Observe bony prominence for adequacy of circulation and development of decubiti.
3. Do not put any lotions on reddened areas or open lesions.
4. Teach client importance of frequent change in position.

✦ *Goal: to assist client to maintain psychological equilibrium.*
1. Encourage client to express feelings and concerns.
2. Encourage client to maintain as much independence as possible.
3. Assist client to take advantage of community services available.
4. Advise client of patient rights and consent for treatment.⌘

Study Questions—Immune System

1. To evaluate the progress of the client's systemic lupus erythematous (SLE), the nurse evaluates which diagnostic findings?

① Increased serum complement fixation correlates with reduction of "butterfly" rash.
② The severity of the SLE correlates with the level of the LE (cell) formation.
③ Overall bone marrow proliferation correlates with symptoms of inflammation.
④ Absence of ANA antibodies correlate with a diminishing immune process.

2. A 15-month-old child is immunosuppressed. Which immunizations will not be given to the child?

① DPT, Hepatitis B.
② *Hemophilus influenza B.*
③ Polio and Varicella.
④ MMR and DPT.

3. The nurse understands that signs/symptoms in a client experiencing itching, erythema, and raised lesions are characteristic of which type hypersensitivity?

① Anaphylactic.
② Delayed type.
③ Immune complex.
④ Cytotoxic.

4. Which medications may be included in the medical treatment plan of care for a client with severe systemic lupus erythematosus (SLE)?

① Chlordiazepoxide (**Librium**).
② Ampicillin (**Amoxil**).
③ Acyclovir (**Zovirax**).
④ Methotrexate (**Mexate**).

5. What is an allergic reaction that can quickly deteriorates into shock and death?

① Anaphylaxis.
② Contact dermatitis.
③ Serum sickness.
④ Hay fever.

6. When a person's immune system reacts against itself, this self-tissue destruction is called?

① Anaphylaxis.
② Macrocytosis.
③ Phagocytosis.
④ Autoimmunity.

7. What is the condition when a client's body is unable to defend itself from an invading microorganism?

① Immunodeficiency.
② Anaphylaxis.
③ Phagocytosis.
④ Autoimmunity.

8. What type of immunity occurs when a client receives a vaccination?

① Autoimmunity.
② Natural active immunity.
③ Acquired passive immunity.
④ Acquired active immunity.

9. A client is exposed to an antigen through illness or vaccination. What is developed in the client's body due to this exposure?

① Macrophage.
② Eosinophil.
③ Erythrocytes.
④ Antibodies.

10. A natural chemical defense found in the body which works as a part of the body's immune system is found in:

① The liver.
② Pancreatic enzymes.
③ Gastric secretions.
④ The mucosa of the large bowel.

11. A client is worried he may have been exposed to AIDS. What will the nurse explain to this client?

① Symptoms of AIDS develop immediately in sexually active individuals.
② Clients may remain asymptomatic for an indefinite period of time, even their entire lifetime.
③ Symptoms of AIDS are immediately seen when the client tests HIV positive.
④ After exposure to the virus, symptoms may develop within 6-12 weeks or as long as 6 months.

12. The nurse is caring for a client who is categorized as HIV+, Category A. What would the nurse anticipate finding on the nursing assessment?

① Fatigue, weight loss, night sweats.
② Confusion, disorientation, loss of coordination.
③ Dyspnea, tachycardia on exertion, fever.
④ Red, raised lesions on neck and face, fever.

Answers and rationales to these questions are in the section at the end of the book entitled "Chapter Study Questions: Answers & Rationales."

Appendix 7-1: IMMUNOSUPPRESSIVE MEDICATIONS

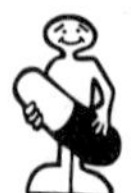

MEDICATIONS	ACTION	SIDE EFFECTS	NURSING IMPLICATIONS

❖ GENERAL NURSING IMPLICATIONS ❖

— Avoid exposure to infection; wash hands frequently.
— Wear protective clothing; use sunscreen.
— Report any sore throat, fever, or other signs of infection to health care provider.
— Take medication at the same time each day to maintain consistent blood levels.
— No vaccines or immunity-conferring agents while client is immunosuppressed.
— Depending on level of immunosuppression, client may need protective isolation.

IMMUNOPSUPPRESIVE MEDICATIONS: Inhibit the immunological response.

MEDICATIONS	ACTION	SIDE EFFECTS	NURSING IMPLICATIONS
Azathioprine (**Imuran**): PO or IV	Inhibits RNA and DNA protein synthesis. Suppresses T-cell (cell-mediated) Leukopenia, bone marrow depression, pancreatitis, liver dysfunction, immunosuppression. Used to suppress kidney transplant rejection.	Dose-and duration-dependent. Bone marrow suppression: leukopenia, thrombocytopenia, anemia. Nausea, vomiting, anorexia. Alopecia, rash.	1. Interacts with allopurinol, causing an increase in **Imuran** toxicity. 2. Avoid use in pregnancy. 3. Take with food or milk to decrease GI upset. 4. Should not be given to client with active infection. 5. Follow up CBCs at least monthly while on medication. 6. Closely monitor client for development of infections.
Cyclosporine (**Sandimmune**): PO, IV Methotrexate (**Mexate**) Cyclophosphamide (**Cytoxan**)	Inhibits T-lymphocyte proliferation and function. See Appendix 8-1. See Appendix 8-1.	Dose-and-duration dependent. Infections, nephrotoxicity, hypertension, hirsutism, gum hyperplasia, tremors.	1. Monitor renal function as nephrotoxicity occurs frequently. 2. Avoid use in pregnancy. 3. Use the pipette supplied by manufacturer to measure dose, mix with 4-8oz. of water, milk, or juice. 4. Evaluate blood pressure and report elevations (especially occurs with heart transplants). 5. Monitor liver function studies. 6. Good oral hygiene to reduce gum problems. 7. Teach client that he should not stop taking the medication or change dosage without physician's order. 8. Serum blood levels are monitored at regular intervals. 9. Hirsutism that occurs is reversible.
Anti-lymphocyte globulin **(ALG)** Murine monoclonal anti-lymphocyte therapy **(OKT3)**	Antibody which blocks function of T-cell by reacting with T_3 antigen	Fever, chills, hypotension, bronchospasm, Aseptic meningitis **(OKT3)**	1. Over 50% of clients experience a fever. 2. Have epinephrine and supportive emergency care available, as allergic reaction can occur at any time during therapy.
Methylprednisolone sodium **(SoluMedrol)**	See Appendix 6-8		

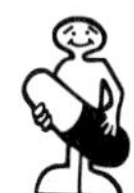

Appendix 7-2:
ANTIVIRALS MEDICATIONS

MEDICATIONS	SIDE EFFECTS	NURSING IMPLICATIONS

❖ GENERAL NURSING IMPLICATIONS ❖

— Medications may be used in combination to obtain better therapeutic results.
— Avoid exposure to infection; wash hands frequently.
— Report any sore throat, fever, or other signs of infection to health care provider.
— No vaccines or immunity-conferring agents while client is immunosuppressed.
— Depending on level of immunosuppression, client may need protective isolation.
— Most of the medications are to be avoided during pregnancy.
— Medications do not cure AIDS or reduce the risk of transmission of HIV.

ANTIVIRAL MEDICATIONS: Inhibit viral DNA or RNA replication in the virus, preventing replication and leading to viral death.

MEDICATIONS	SIDE EFFECTS	NURSING IMPLICATIONS
Nucleoside Reverse Transcriptase Inhibitors (NRTIs)		
Zidovudine (**AZT, Retrovir**): PO Stavudine (**d4T, Zerit**): PO Didanosine (**ddl, Videx**): PO Zalcitabine (**ddC, Hivid**): PO	Anemia, severe headache, nausea, insomnia	1. Monitor CBC. 2. Take zidovudine q4h around the clock. 3. Take zalcitabine q8h around the clock. 4. Didanosine take on an empty stomach. Chew tablets thoroughly or crush and disperse in 3 oz of water. Do not mix with fruit juice. 5. Take stavudine q12h. 6. Closely monitor client for development of infections.
Protease Inhibitors (PIs)		
Indinavir (**Crixivan**): PO	Nephrolithiasis, GI upset, abdominal pain, headache	1. Monitor renal function as occurs. 2. Take one hour before or after low-fat meals.
Nelfinavir (**Viracept**): PO	Diarrhea, nausea, flatulence	
Non-Nucleoside Reverse Transcriptase Inhibitors (NNRTIs)		
Nevirapine (**Viramune**): PO	Possible severe rash (Steven-Johnson syndrome), hepatotoxic, fever, nausea	1. Monitor liver function studies.
Delavirdine (**Rescriptor**): PO	Rash, GI upset	
Nucleoside Analogs		
Acyclovir (**Zovirax**): PO, IV, topical Famciclovir (**Famvir**): PO Valacyclovir (**Valtrex**): PO	Nausea, vomiting, headache, CNS disturbance (especially in elderly)	1. Needs to be administered within 24 hours of herpes zoster outbreaks.

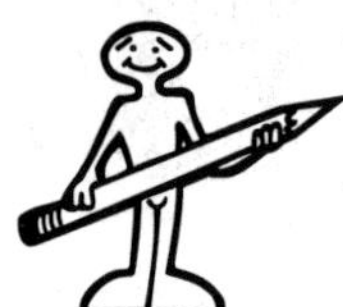

Notes

ABNORMAL CELL GROWTH 8

CHARACTERISTICS OF CANCER

❑ **Cancer must be regarded as a group of disease entities with different causes, manifestations, treatment, and prognoses. The basic disease process begins when normal cells undergo change and begin to proliferate in an abnormal manner.**

Major Dysfunction in the Cell

A. Cellular proliferation—cancer cells divide in an indiscriminate, unregulated manner.

B. Loss of contact inhibition. Cells have no regard for cellular boundaries; normal cells respect boundaries and do not invade adjacent areas or organs.

C. Tumors (neoplasm).

1. Benign—encapsulated neoplasm that remains localized in the tissue of origin.
   a. Exerts pressure on surrounding organs.
   b. Will decrease blood supply to the normal tissue.
2. Malignant—nonencapsulated neoplasm that invades surrounding tissue. Depends on the stage of the neoplasm as to whether or not metastasis (or spread to distant body parts) has occurred. Four primary mechanisms by which the neoplasm spreads.
   a. Vascular system—cancer cells penetrate vessels and circulate until trapped. The cancer cells may penetrate the vessel wall and invade adjacent organs and tissues.
   b. Lymphatic system—cancer cells penetrate the lymphatic system and are distributed along lymphatic channels.
   c. Implantation—cancer cells implant into a body organ. Certain cells have an affinity for particular organs and body areas.
   d. Seeding—a primary tumor sloughs off tumor cells into a body cavity, such as the peritoneal cavity.
3. Common sites for metastasis—brain, liver, lungs, spinal cord, and bone.

Etiology

A. Viruses—incorporate into the genetic structure of the cell.

B. Physical agents—exposure to sunlight, radiation, chronic irritation or inflammation, and tobacco use.

C. Chemical agents—produce toxic effects by altering DNA structure in body sites distant from chemical exposure (e.g., dyes, asbestos, tars, smoke, etc.); most often affects liver, lungs, and kidneys.

D. Genetic and familial factors—DNA damage occurs in cells where chromosomal patterns are abnormal (e.g., Wilms' tumor, acute leukemias, etc.).

E. Dietary factors—risk of cancer increases with long-term ingestion of fats and oils from animal sources; alcoholic beverages; salt-cured, smoked meats; and nitrate containing foods.

F. Hormonal agents—tumor growth promoted by disturbances in hormonal balance of the body's own (endogenous) hormones or administration of exogenous hormones (i.e., diethylstilbestrol (DES), prolonged estrogen replacement, oral contraceptives).

Prevention

A. **Ten steps of cancer prevention.**

1. Increase intake of fresh vegetables (especially those of the cabbage family).
2. Increase fiber intake—reduces risk of breast, prostate, and colon cancer.
3. Increase intake of vitamin A—reduces risk of larynx, esophageal, and lung cancer.
4. Increase intake of foods rich in Vitamin C—may protect against stomach and esophageal cancer.
5. Keep weight in normal range—obesity associated with cancer of uterus, gall bladder, breast, and colon.
6. Reduce amount of intake of dietary fat—increased risk of breast, colon, and prostate cancer.
7. Reduce intake of salt-cured, smoked, and nitrate-cured foods—linked to stomach and esophageal cancer.
8. No cigarette smoking—increased risk of lung cancer.
9. Reduce alcohol intake—increased risk of liver cancer.
10. Avoid overexposure to sunlight—risk of skin cancer.

B. Secondary prevention.

1. PAP test—for sexually active women, and/or women over age 18, it is recommended that the test be done annually.
2. Digital rectal examination—men and women annually after age 40.
3. Proctosigmoidoscopy— after age 50, should be done every 3 to 5 years in both men and women.
4. Check for occult blood in stool—done after age 50 on an annual basis.
5. Mammography—Baseline between ages 35-40, then again 40-49, then yearly after age 50.

6. Breast self-examination—conducted monthly (Chapter 22).
7. Pelvic examinations—every 3 years from age 20-40, yearly after age 40.
8. Testicular self examination—monthly from age 20-40. (Chapter 22)

C. Cancer's early warning signs (Table 8-1).

Classification of Malignant Tumors

A. Cellular origin.
1. Carcinoma—originates in epithelial tissue (skin and lining of body tissue).
2. Adenocarcinoma—originates in glandular tissue (breast, prostate).
3. Sarcoma—originates in connective and supporting tissue (bone, nerves).
4. Embryonal—originates in embryonic tissue.
5. Lymphomas—originate in the lymphatic system.
6. Leukemias—originate in blood-forming organs.

B. TNM Classification (staging) (Table 8-2).

Table 8-1: CANCER'S EARLY WARNING SIGNS

ADULTS
C Change in bowel or bladder habits.
A A lesion or sore that does not heal.
U Unusual bleeding or discharge.
T Thickening or lump in the breast.
I Indigestion or difficulty swallowing.
O Obvious changes in wart or mole.
N Nagging cough or persistent hoarseness.
(Note that the first letter of each sign spells "**CAUTION**").

CHILDREN
1. Marked changes in bowel and bladder; nausea and vomiting for no apparent cause.
2. Generally run-down condition; increased susceptibility to infection.
3. Spontaneous bleeding episode (epistaxis); failure to stop bleeding in normal time period.
4. Swellings, lumps or masses anywhere in the child's body.
5. Persistent crying or pain for which there is no apparent cause.
6. Any change in size of mole or birthmark.
7. Unexpected stumbling or lack of coordination in the child.

Source: American Cancer Society, *Cancer Facts and Figures*, (New York: American Cancer Society, 1992).

TREATMENT OF CANCER

Diagnostics

A. Common cancer diagnostic studies.
1. X-ray examination.
2. Computerized axial tomography (CAT).
3. Cytology studies.
4. Radioisotope scans.
5. Magnetic resonance imaging (MRI).
6. Mammography.
7. Lymphangiography.
8. Position emission tomography (PET).
9. Ultrasound.
10. Tumor markers (Table 8-3).
11. Colposcopic exam of cervix.

B. Biopsy.
1. Needle—tissues obtained by aspiration, or with a large bore needle; a sample is removed.
2. Incisional—tumor mass may be too large for removal; this may be done for staging the disease level.
3. Excisional—involves removal of the entire tumor.
4. Endoscope biopsy—direct biopsy through an endoscopy of the area (gastrointestinal, respiratory, genitourinary tracts).

Goals of Cancer Therapy

A. Cure—client will be disease-free and live to normal life expectancy.

B. Control—client's cancer is not cured but controlled by therapy over long periods of time.

C. Palliative—maintain as high a quality of life for the client when cure and control are not possible.

D. Prophylaxis—provide treatment when no tumor is detectable but when client is known to be at risk for tumor development, spread, or recurrence.

Modalities of Cancer Treatment

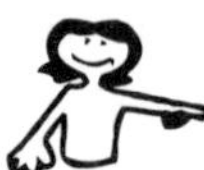

NURSING PRIORITY: *Therapy generally involves utilizing two or more modalities of treatment.*

A. Surgery.
1. Diagnostic surgery—obtains tissue samples for diagnostic purposes and determine methods of treatment.
2. Staging surgery—determines the extent of the cancer, presence, and location of metastatic lesions.
3. Curative surgery—removal of cancers that are localized to the area of origin; extent of resection determined by the type of tumor.
4. Palliative surgery—does not impair the growth or spread of the cancer, but improves the client's quality of life. May be done to relieve pain, decrease obstruction, relieve pressure, and to prevent hemorrhage.
5. Reconstructive surgery—restoration of the client's form, function, and appearance after radical surgery for cancer.

Table 8-2: TNM STAGING CLASSIFICATION

T - Tumor size.
N - Degree of involvement of lymph nodes.
M - Absence or presence of metastasis.

T - Primary tumor
T_0 - no evidence of tumor.
T_{1s} - carcinoma in situ.
T_1-T_4 - ascending degrees of increase in tumor size and involvement.

N - Regional lymph nodes
N_0 - no clinical evidence of regional node involvement.
N_x - regional lymph nodes cannot be evaluated clinically.
N_1-N_3 - ascending degrees of nodal involvement.

M - Metastasis
M_0 - no evidence of distant metastasis.
Mx - distant metastasis cannot be assessed.
M_1 - ascending degrees of metastatic involvement, including lymph nodes.

Example: T_{1s}, N_x, M_0 - cancer in situ; unable to clinically assess distant lymph nodes; there is no evidence of metastasis.

Source: American Joint Committee on Cancer, *Manual for Staging Cancer.* Chicago: Author.

6. Preventive surgery—for clients who are in a high-risk category, certain surgical procedures may prevent the future development of cancer.

B. Chemotherapy—overall goal of chemotherapy is to destroy the cancer cells without excessively damaging the normal cells.

NURSING PRIORITY: *The therapeutic ratio is the guiding principle of chemotherapy. The aim is to administer an antineoplastic agent dose large enough to eradicate cancer cells, but small enough to limit adverse effects to safe and tolerable levels.*

1. Medications highly toxic and attack healthy cells as well as the cancer cells.
2. Combination chemotherapy more effective than single dose therapy.
3. Adjuvant therapy—after the initial therapy (surgical or radiation) medications are used to eliminate any remaining cancer cells.
4. Myelosuppressive effects peak in 7 to 14 days after the chemotherapy, white blood cell and platelet count are at the lowest levels.

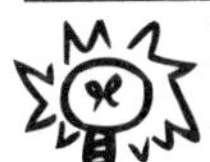

NCLEX ALERT: *Follow procedures for handling bio-hazardous materials (e.g. chemotherapeutic agents, radiation sources, etc.)*

5. Vascular access methods of administration.
   a. Peripherally inserted central catheters (PICC's) external access central lines.
   b. Implanted venous infusion access—catheters are tunneled from exit site to the venous insertion site (Port-A-Cath, Hickman catheter, Groshong catheter).
   c. Ommaya reservoir—catheter placed into the cerebrospinal fluid for infusion.

C. Nursing implications in chemotherapy.
1. Assess client for symptoms of bone marrow depression (increased bruising and bleeding, sore throat, fever).
2. Prevent exposure of client to people with communicable diseases.

NURSING PRIORITY: *Safety guidelines for administration: Avoid any accidental spillage; wear latex gloves when handling drugs; use Luer-Lok fittings on all IV tubing; dispose of all equipment used to administer antineoplastic agents according to policies and procedures governing toxic and chemical waste disposal (leak-proof and puncture-proof containers).*

3. Prior to therapy, establish a baseline regarding I & O, bowel habits, oral hygiene, psychological status, and family relationships.
4. Inform client of side effects and nursing measures to reduce resulting discomfort.
5. Monitor I & O; maintain adequate hydration to prevent urinary complications.

Table 8-3: TUMOR MARKERS

TUMOR MARKER	CANCERS IN WHICH MARKER MAY BE FOUND
Carcinoembryonic antigen (CEA)	Colon-rectal (values >5ng/ml) Breast Lung
Alpha-fetoprotein (AFP)	Testicular (nonseminomatous) Liver Lung Pancreatic
Prostatic acid phosphatase (PAP)	Metastatic prostate
Prostate-specific antigen (PSA)	Primary and metastatic prostate
Cancer antigen (CA) 125	Ovarian
Pancreatic oncofetal antigen	Pancreatic
Calcitonin	Medullary cancer of the thyroid

6. Inform client that alopecia, if it occurs, is usually transient.

7. Check for possible drug interactions with chemotherapeutic agents.

D. Radiation therapy—radiation destroys the cell's ability to reproduce by damaging the cellular DNA. Cells that are rapidly reproducing are vulnerable to the effects of radiation. Normal healthy cells recover more effectively from the damage caused by radiation.

1. Types of radiation therapy.

a. External beam therapy (teletherapy): radiation source is outside the body. The radiation source is directed toward the area of the tumor and draining lymphatics.

(1) Decreases the incidence of skin surface damage.

(2) Client should not wash off the markers for the radiation sites.

NURSING PRIORITY: *Clients who receive radiation therapy should not be bathed with soap over the radiation site, avoid use of lotions and powders.*

b. Implant therapy (brachytherapy, closed therapy, sealed source therapy)—the sealed source of radiation is implanted directly into the tumor or into a body cavity around a tumor.

(1) Delivers a large amount of radiation to a small area of the body. May be used to treat uterine and cervical cancer.

(2) A hollow applicator may be inserted surgically and the radioactive source inserted in a treatment area and removed when the client returns to the room. This decreases risk of accidental exposure due to displacement.

c. Unsealed source (radio pharmaceutical or isotope)—radioisotopes may be given IV, or into a body cavity, or orally. Body fluids become contaminated.

2. Adverse effects of radiation therapy.

NURSING PRIORITY: *Adverse effects are related to radiation dose delivered within a specified time, method of delivery, and client's overall health status.*

a. Skin reactions.

(1) Skin erythema.

(2) Dry desquamation of the skin in the treatment field.

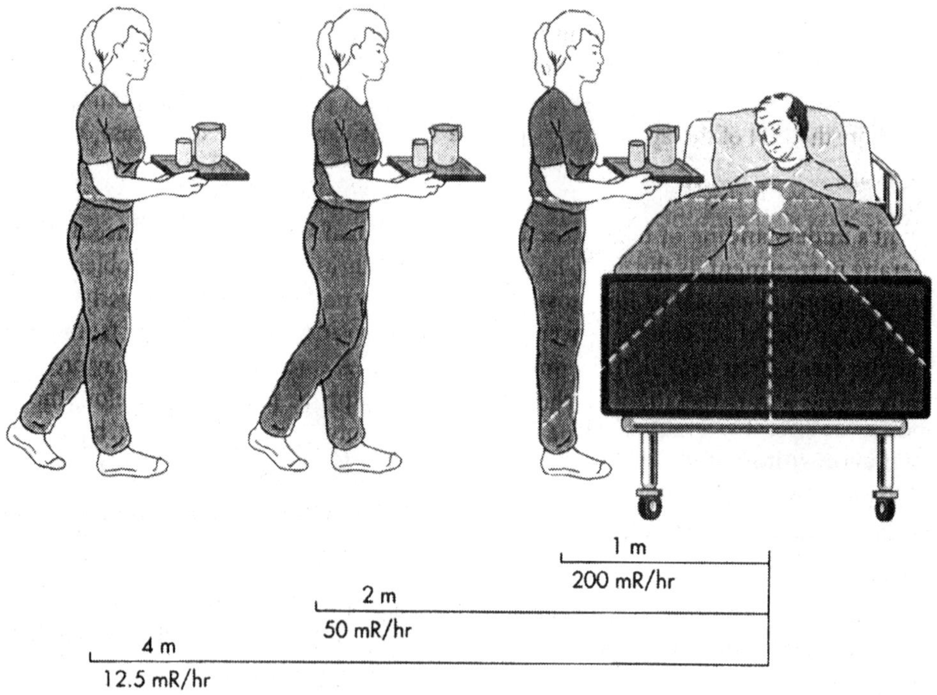

Figure 8-1: Radiation Safety
The nurse nearest the source of radioactivity (the client) is more exposed. At two feet, exposure is 15 times that at eight feet.
Reprinted with permission: Phipps, WJ, Sands, JK,& Marek, JF (1999). *Medical Surgical Nursing: Concepts & Clinical Practice*, 6th ed. Philadelphia: Mosby, p. 291.

(3) Wet desquamation particularly in areas of skin folds (breast, perineum, axilla); skin may be blistered.

(4) Loss of hair on the skin in the treatment field.

(5) Skin pigmentation and discoloration.

b. Gastrointestinal disturbances

3. Safety precautions to prevent excessive exposure (Figure 8-1).

a. Time—client care should be coordinated to provide for client needs, but limit the nurse's exposure time.

b. Distance—the greater the distance from the source the less the exposure. Except when giving direct care, attempt to maintain distance of six feet from the source of radiation.

c. Shielding—in practice lead shielding is difficult to work with, generally not necessary if time and distance principles are observed.

NCLEX ALERT: *Follow protocol when handling bio-hazardous materials (e.g., radiation therapy, chemotherapeutic agents). Time, Distance, and Shielding are critical concepts in caring for a client with a radiation implant.*

4. Nursing implications for a client with an internal radiation source (sealed source).

a. Private room and bath.

b. A lead container and tongs should be present in the client's room.

c. If implant becomes dislodged, it should be picked up with the forceps and returned to the lead container. Notify radiation therapist or officer immediately.

d. Observe time, distance, and shield precautions.

e. Examples include uterine implants, testicular implants, implants used in head and neck tumors.

f. Inform all people coming in contact with the client of the specific precautions necessary.

g. Utilize badges or radiation monitors for care givers having direct client contact.

h. Know where the radiation source is.

i. Client's excretions are not radioactive because radioisotopes are not in the circulation.

j. List on the chart.

(1) Type of radiation.

(2) Time inserted.

(3) Anticipated removal time.

(4) Specific precautions for the type radiation utilized.

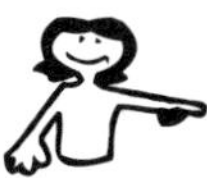

NURSING PRIORITY: *Check linens, bedpans, and other items for signs of a dislodged implant.*

5. Nursing implications for the client receiving systemic radiation therapy.

a. Systemically administered radionuclides (radioisotopes) may cause radioactive body secretions.

b. Keep linens and trash in room until they have been checked for radioactivity by radiation therapy department.

E. Immunotherapy—based on the theory that certain substances stimulate the immune response and/or attack the tumor cells directly.

F. Pediatrics—long-term effects of treatment on the child.

1. Impaired growth and development, especially from radiation to growth centers of the bone during early childhood and adolescence.

2. Damage to the central nervous system.

3. Gonadal aberrations, including reproductive, hormonal, genetic, and teratogenic effects.

4. Disturbances to other organs, including pneumonitis, pericarditis, pleurisy, hypothyroidism, and cystitis.

Nursing Intervention

✦ *Goal: to maintain client at optimum psychosocial level.*

1. Encourage verbalization.

2. Assist client to understand disease process and therapeutic regime.

3. Include family in the care.

4. Assist client to cope with changes in body image due to alopecia.

a. Inform client if hair loss is anticipated, alopecia is most often temporary and regrowth may begin before chemotherapy ends.

b. Encourage to select and wear a wig or turban.

c. Instruct client with regards to hair care.

(1) Use mild protein-based shampoo and cream conditioner to help prevent hair dryness.

(2) Advise client to shampoo only every 3 to 5 days.

(3) Teach client to pat, *not rub*, hair dry after shampooing to avoid excessive handling of brittle hair.

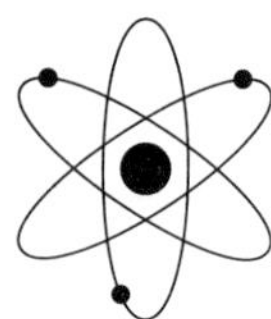

Table 8-4: RADIATION SAFETY PRECAUTIONS

- Private room and bath.
- Plan care so minimal time is spent in the room.
- When prolonged care is required, wear a lead shield or apron.
- Wear a monitoring device to measure exposure.
- Mark on the room and in the Kardex that pregnant women, infants, and young children should not come in contact with the client during treatment.
- Check all linens and materials removed from the bed for presence of foreign bodies that could be a source of radioactivity.
- Keep long-handled forceps and lead container in the room of a client with an implant in place.
- Do not wash off marks placed on client's body for purpose of identifying area for external radiation.

(4) Encourage client to avoid excessive brushing to prevent tearing or unnecessary manipulation of hair.

(5) Suggest client sleep on a satin pillowcase to decrease hair tangles and friction.

(6) Encourage client to discontinue use of electric hair dryers, hot rollers or crimpers, hair clips, sprays, dyes, or permanents to prevent further hair damage.

d. Prevent or minimize hair loss by inducing scalp hypothermia.

5. Assess client's support systems.
6. Recognize client's emotional outbursts and anger as part of his coping process.
7. Encourage measures to maintain ego.
   a. Allow him to participate in his own care and make decisions.
   b. Maintain active listening.
   c. Encourage personal lifestyle (clothing, makeup, hobbies, etc.).

✦ *Goal: to maintain nutrition.*

1. Diet—appropriate to age level.
   a. Increase calories, increase protein.
   b. Supplemental vitamins.
   c. Small frequent feedings.
   d. Increase fluid intake.
   e. Between-meal supplements.
2. Hyperalimentation (See Chapter 18).
3. Prevent and/or decrease complications associated with nutrition.
   a. Anorexia.
   b. Nausea and vomiting.
   c. Stomatitis.
      (1) Meticulous oral hygiene (brushing with a nonabrasive dentifrice (such as baking soda or saline) and flossing after each meal and at bedtime.
      (2) Observe oral mucosa daily.
      (3) Provide nonirritating foods.
      (4) Keep mucous membranes moist; encourage fluid intake to prevent dehydration.

✦ *Goal: to maintain normal elimination pattern.*

1. Provide adequate fluids and fiber in diet to prevent constipation.
2. Prevent and/or decrease complications of diarrhea.
   a. Antidiarrheal medications.
   b. Low residue, high protein, bland diet.
   c. Evaluate lab reports for electrolyte values.
   d. Evaluate fluid status.
   e. Prevent anal excoriation.
      (1) Thorough cleansing of rectal area with mild soap and water.
      (2) Avoid irritation of the rectal area.
      (3) Use ointments and sprays to decrease discomfort and promote healing.
3. Fresh fruits and vegetables should be eaten only after cooked, peeled or washed thoroughly.
4. Prevent urinary tract infections, primarily cystitis.
   a. Maintain adequate fluid intake (3000 cc per day).
   b. Administer ascorbic acid to promote urine acidity.
   c. Frequent assessment for symptoms of cystitis (See Chapter 23).
   d. Avoid bladder catheterization if possible.
   e. Encourage frequent voiding.
5. Assess for the development of vesicovaginal or rectovaginal fistulas.
6. Minimize embarrassment of incontinence and provide appropriate hygiene measures.

✦ *Goal: to prevent and/or decrease infectious process.*

1. Careful assessment of temperature elevations.
2. Administer antibiotics.

Table 8-5: NURSING IMPLICATIONS AND CHEMOTHERAPY

PROBLEM	NURSING IMPLICATIONS
Bone marrow depression: Increased bleeding, anemia, decreased resistance to infection (leukopenia)	1. Observe for bleeding tendency (bruising, hematuria, bleeding gums, etc.). 2. Report any unexplained temperature elevation. 3. No active vaccinations while on medication. 4. Report any unusual fatigue. 5. Decrease invasive procedures, minimize injections.
Pulmonary toxicity	1. Monitor for non-productive cough, fever, dyspnea, and tachypnea. 2. Most cases are cumulative dose-related and may be fatal.
Hyperuricemia (increased serum levels of uric acid)	1. Encourage fluid intake up to 3,000 cc daily if allowed. 2. Assess for flank and abdominal pain. 3. Assess for swelling of the lower extremities and joint pain. 4. May be treated with allopurinol.
Alopecia	1. Encourage client to obtain a wig after beginning of symptoms. 2. Ice packs to the scalp may reduce hair loss. 3. A scalp tourniquet during medication infusion may also reduce hair loss. 4. Avoid sunlight to exposed scalp.
Stomatitis (mucositis)	1. Good oral hygiene. a. Frequent mouth rinse to keep mucous membranes moist. b. Brush teeth with a small, soft toothbrush. c. Remove dentures to prevent further irritation. 2. Avoid alcohol, spicy or hot foods; mechanical soft, bland diet ordered.
GI: Anorexia, nausea and vomiting, diarrhea, and constipation	1. Assist client to maintain good nutrition. a. Discuss with client and dietitian food preferences. b. Correlate meals with antiemetic medications. c. Treat stomatitis with anesthetic mouthwashes to decrease discomfort while eating. 2. Evaluate client for fluid and electrolyte imbalances. 3. Evaluate skin around anal area in the client with diarrhea, prevent excoriation. 4. Identify clients prone to constipation and maintain high fluid and high fiber intake. 5. Observe for occurrence of a paralytic ileus. 6. May need to withhold food and fluid 4 to 6 hours before treatment. 7. Small feedings and high fluid intake.
Tissue irritation, necrosis, ulceration	1. Monitor site during infusion. Only one venipuncture on a vein to avoid leakage. 2. If multiple drugs administered, flush between each. 3. Extra precaution should be taken to prevent extravasation (infusion of chemotherapy medication into subcutaneous tissue), tape securely, aspirate for blood return, observe for continuous flow of IV.

NCLEX ALERT: *Observe client for side effects of a chemo-therapeutic agent. If extravasation occurs:*

(a) stop the infusion -remove any remaining drug in the tubing or needle and aspirate the infiltrated area.
(b) ***do not*** *remove the needle.*
(c) contact physician and consult hospital policy and precautions of specific medication.
(d) antidote medication may be instilled directly into the infiltrated area.
(e) ice may be applied to site and extremity elevated for the first 24-48 hrs. after extravasation.

3. Meticulous personal hygiene.
4. Child should be isolated from communicable diseases, especially chicken pox. Evaluate optimum time for child to return to school.
5. Frequent assessment for potential infectious processes.
6. Explain how skin reactions following radiation therapy may not develop for 10-14 days, and may not subside until 2-4 weeks following treatment.

✦ *Goal: to prevent and/or decrease hematological complications (See Chapter 14).*

1. Evaluate for decreasing platelets and thrombocytopenia.

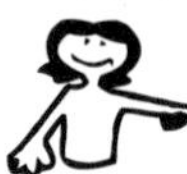

NURSING PRIORITY: *Institute bleeding precautions if platelet count is less than 50,000/mm3.*

2. Administer platelets and whole blood transfusions as indicated.
3. Evaluate areas of potential bleeding.
   a. Nosebleed (epistaxis).
   b. Urinary tract (hematuria).
   c. Stool (melena).
   d. Mucous membranes.

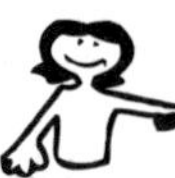

NURSING PRIORITY: *Advise client to use electric razor and a soft-bristle toothbrush.*

4. Anemia.
   a. Maintain adequate rest; encourage client to pace activities to avoid fatigue.
   b. Maintain adequate oxygenation.
   c. Assess for problems with erythropoiesis.
   d. Evaluate respiratory and cardiac systems for mechanisms of compensation.
   e. Encourage a diet high in protein, vitamins, and iron.

✦ *Goal: to maintain activity level.*

1. Encourage daily activities within limitations of disease process.
2. Assist client to evaluate activity patterns and encourage periods of rest.
3. Avoid fatigue.

✦ *Goal: to relieve pain (See Chapter 3).*

1. Evaluate client's and family's response to pain.
2. Evaluate characteristics of pain.
3. Promote general comfort.
4. Administer medications for pain relief.

✦ *Goal: to recognize complications specific to radiation and chemotherapy.*

1. Alopecia.
2. Hemorrhagic problems.
3. Gastrointestinal distress.
4. Bone marrow depression (myelosuppression).
   a. Thrombocytopenia.
   b. Anemia.
   c. Neutropenia.
5. Skin reactions.
6. Decreased immune response.

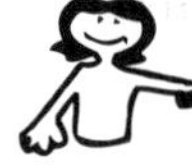

NURSING PRIORITY: *It is important for the nurse to be able to differentiate between toxic effects of medication and radiation therapy and the progression of disease process.*

Self-Care

1. Limit number of people having direct contact with the client.
2. Good oral hygiene - no flossing, soft toothbrush, avoid irritating foods.
3. Client should avoid coming in direct contact with animal excreta (cat litter boxes, bird cages, etc.).
4. Teach client to take his temperature daily and report temperature over 100°F (38°C).
5. Use antipyretics cautiously- tend to mask infection.
6. Peak of neutropenia occurs within 7 to 14 days after the administration of the chemotherapy.
7. Teach and manage radiation induced skin reactions.
   a. Moisturize skin 3-4x/day with Eucerin or Lubriderm.
   b. Gentle cleansing with normal saline; gently patted or air- dried; expose areas to air for 10-15min t.i.d., if moist desquamation occurs.
   c. Avoid use of perfumes, deodorants, and talcs.
   d. Wear loose-fitting cotton clothing.
   e. If dry desquamation, apply topical steroids, cornstarch, or Benadryl.

Study Questions—Abnormal Cell Growth

1. In the treatment of the leukemic client, what is the main goal of chemotherapy?

① Prevent all future relapses.
② Assist the client into remission.
③ Decrease intervals between exacerbations.
④ Increase the positive effects of radiation.

2. In evaluating a client's reaction to external radiation, what is a common nursing observation three weeks after beginning therapy?

① A sudden weight loss.
② Abnormal skin pigmentation.
③ Vertigo when sitting up quickly.
④ Urinary retention and infection.

3. What are the nursing interventions regarding the care of a client with a vaginal radium implant?

① Clamp and drain the Foley at intervals.
② Provide a high residue diet.
③ Place the client in a semiprivate room.
④ Raise the head of the bed no more than 20 degrees.

4. What is an important aspect of client teaching regarding external radiation therapy?

① Remain isolated after treatments.
② Fast prior to the treatment.
③ Schedule treatments monthly.
④ Leave skin markings between treatments.

5. A client is receiving chemotherapy with several antineoplastic agents. Which nursing observation is considered a side effect of chemotherapy?

① Slow slurred speech.
② Increased leukocytes on CBC.
③ Gingivitis and oral ulcers.
④ Sinus dysrhythmias with bradycardia.

6. The nurse would identify which diagnostic test as a confirmation of a diagnosis for cervical cancer?

① A computerized tomography (CT) scan.
② Elevated HCG level.
③ Colposcopic examination.
④ Uterine scan.

7. The nurse is evaluating a central line before administering the client's chemotherapy. What it important for the nurse to check?

① Systemic sepsis.
② Date of the last dressing change.
③ Inflammation and irritation at insertion site.
④ Type of fluid infusing into line.

8. The nurse explains to a young adult female client that the most common area for finding cancer in women is the:

① Ovaries.
② Fallopian tubes.
③ Cervix.
④ Urinary bladder.

9. The nurse is giving discharge planning to a cancer client on doxorubicin (Adriamycin). What is important to tell the client?

① Report symptoms of hematuria.
② Increase oral fluids.
③ Avoid folic acid intake.
④ Report symptoms of dyspnea.

10. A client is receiving busulfan (Myleran). The nurse would notify the physician with which assessment finding?

① Nonproductive, dry cough.
② WBC 7000, Hb 13gm, Hct 38%.
③ Nausea and vomiting.
④ Low serum uric acid.

Answers and rationales to these questions are in the section at the end of the book entitled "Chapter Study Questions: Answers & Rationales."

Appendix 8-1: ANTINEOPLASTIC AGENTS

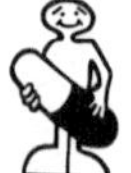

MEDICATIONS	SIDE EFFECTS	NURSING IMPLICATIONS

❖ GENERAL NURSING IMPLICATIONS ❖
— Observe for therapeutic effects (increased appetite and sense of well-being, improved mobility, and decreased pain).
— Observe for adverse effects (See Table 8-5).
— Dosage is usually based on client's body weight.
— Monitor laboratory values for bone marrow suppression.
— Avoid contact with skin when preparing medications by wearing disposable gloves, protective eyewear, and barrier protective clothing. Wear a mask when handling powder forms of drug. Prepare drug on disposable tray or towel, so that it may be discarded.

NCLEX ALERT: *Follow procedures for handling bio-hazardous materials,(e.g., chemotherapeutic agents).*

ALKYLATING AGENTS: Bind to various cell constituents causing a cytotoxic effect; imitate the action of radiation, as their effect is similar to ionizing radiation (radiomimetic); cell cycle nonspecific.

MEDICATIONS	SIDE EFFECTS	NURSING IMPLICATIONS
Busulfan **(Myleran)** Chlorambucil **(Leukeran)** Cisplatin **(Platinol)** Cyclophosphamide **(Cytoxan, Neosar)** Mechlorethamine [nitrogen mustard] **(Mustargen)**	Alopecia (cyclophosphamide) Gonadal suppression (busulfan, mechlorethamine) Hyperuricemia (cisplatin) Ototoxicity, tinnitus, hypomagnesemia, hypokalemia, hypocalcemia, nephrotoxicity (cisplatin) Hemorrhagic cystitis, hematuria (cyclophosphamide) Pulmonary toxicity (busulfan, chlorambucil, cyclophosphamide)	1. Frequently assess patient taking cisplatin for dizziness, tinnitus, hearing loss, loss of coordination, and numbness or tingling of extremities; may be irreversible. 2. Encourage increased fluid intake with clients on **Cytoxan** and cisplatin. If hemorrhagic cystitis occurs with **Cytoxan**, medication is discontinued. 3. Pulmonary toxicity with **Myleran** may lead to pulmonary fibrosis. 4. Allopurinol for uric acid excretion. *See Table 8-5: for nursing implications and side effects of chemotherapy.*

ANTI METABOLITES: Take the place of normal proteins required for DNA synthesis; cell cycle specific.

MEDICATIONS	SIDE EFFECTS	NURSING IMPLICATIONS
Cytarabine **(ARA-C)** Cytosine arabinoside **(Cytosar-U)** Fluorouracil **(5-FU, Adrucil) (Efudex, Fluoroplex)** Mercaptopurine **(6-MP, Purinethol)** Methotrexate sodium **(Folex, Mexate)**	Alopecia (cytarabine, fluorouracil, methotrexate) Stomatitis (cytarabine, fluorouracil, methotrexate) Hyperuricemia (cytarbine, mercaptopurine, methotrexate) Diarrhea, phototoxicity (fluorouracil) Hepatotoxicity (cytarabine, mercaptopurine, methotrexate)	1. Assess patients taking fluorouracil for stomatitis and diarrhea. These symptoms may necessitate discontinuation. 2. Ensure that the patient taking high doses of **5 FU** or methotrexate receives folinic acid or citrovrum factor (Leucovorin rescue) to prevent toxicity. 3. Teaching: tell client taking fluorouracil or methotrexate to use sun screen and wear protective clothing to prevent photosensitivity reactions. 4. Methotrexate: (a.) Client shouldn't take supplemental folic acid. (b.) Assess for glycosuria. (c.) Assess client for GI bleeding and gastric ulceration. (d.) Contraindicated in first trimester of pregnancy (abortifacient). (e.) Avoid alcohol intake.

Appendix 8-1:
ANTINEOPLASTIC AGENTS

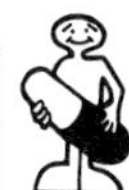

MEDICATIONS	SIDE EFFECTS	NURSING IMPLICATIONS
ANTITUMOR ANTIBIOTICS: Interfere with DNA synthesis; cell cycle nonspecific (except for bleomycin).		
Dactinomycin **(Actinomycin-D, Cosmegen)** Daunorubicin **(Cerubidine)** Doxorubicin **(Adriamycin)** Bleomycin **(Blenoxane)**	Alopecia, stomatitis, phlebitis at IV site, gonadal suppression, hyperuricemia Congestive heart failure, dysrhythmia (daunorubicin) Cardiomyopathy, EKG changes (doxorubicin) Pulmonary toxicity, fever, hyperpigmentation (bleomycin)	1. Monitor vital signs frequently during administration. 2. Assess patient taking daunorubicin for congestive heart failure (dyspnea, rales, peripheral edema, weight gain). 3. Assess patient taking doxorubicin for myocardial toxicity (CHF - dyspnea, dysrhythmia, hypotension, weight gain).
HORMONAL AGENTS: Cause immunosuppression and block normal hormones in tumors that are sensitive.		
Diethylstilbestrol **(DES)** Megestrol **(Megace)** Tamoxifen **(Nolvadex)** Testosterone **(Andro, Depo-Testosterone, Testex)** Prednisone **(Deltasone)**	Edema, hypercalcemia (diethylstilbestrol, tamoxifen, testosterone) Impotence, gynecomastia in males (diethylstilbestrol, testosterone)	1. Teaching: clients taking tamoxifen may have severe bone pain, which may indicate drug effectiveness and will resolve over timed. Pain may be controlled with analgesics. 2. Diethylstilbestrol and testosterone may alter the effects of oral anticoagulants, oral hypoglycemic agents, and insulin. 3. Tamoxifen decreases the effectiveness of concurrently administered estrogen.
PLANT ALKALOIDS: Vinca alkaloids prevent mitosis by antagonizing hormone-stimulated processes necessary for cell proliferation rather than causing a cytotoxic reaction; cell cycle specific.		
Vinblastine **(Velban)** Vincristine **(Oncovin)**	Peripheral neuropathy (vincristine) Hyperuricemia Stomatitis, anorexia, constipation Phlebitis at IV site Alopecia	1. Prevent gastric problems of constipation with high fiber diet, adequate hydration, stool softeners. 2. Minimize hair loss by applying cold compresses to scalp prior to administration of medication. 3. Older adults are especially sensitive to the neurotoxic effects of vincristine. 4. Allopurinol for the hyperuricemia.
INTERFERONS: Interfere with the replication of various viruses, affect cell motility and proliferation.		
α2(A) Interferon **(Roferon-A)**	Fever, chills Nephrotoxicity Fatigue, malaise, anorexia Elevation of liver enzymes	1. Monitor vital signs. 2. Monitor liver function studies. 3. Teach client to avoid individuals who have received live immunizations and to avoid receiving an immunization while on the drug.

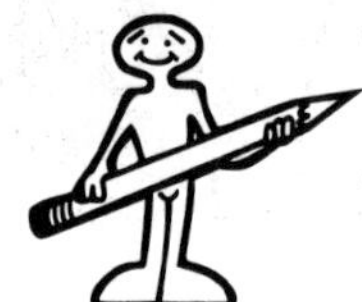

Notes

PSYCHIATRIC NURSING CONCEPTS

SELF-CONCEPT

- *Self-concept*—all beliefs, convictions and ideas that constitute an individual's knowledge of himself and influence his relationships with others.
- *Self-esteem*—an individual's personal judgment of his own worth obtained by analyzing how well his behavior conforms to his self-ideal.
- *Self-ideal*—an individual's perception of how he should behave based on certain personal standards.

NURSING PRIORITY: *A healthy self concept, (i.e., a positive self-esteem) is essential to psychologic well being; it is universal, (i.e., something everyone wants and needs).*

Assessment

A. Factors affecting self-esteem.
1. Parental rejection in early childhood experiences.
2. Lack of recognition and appreciation by parents as child grows older.
3. Overpossessiveness, overpermissiveness, and control by one or both parents.
4. Unrealistic self-ideals or goals.

GERIATRIC PRIORITY: *The use of wheelchairs, canes, walkers, hearing aids, or any combination of these will impact the self-esteem of the elderly client.*

B. Behaviors associated with low self-esteem.
1. Self-derision and criticism—describes himself as stupid, no good, a born loser.
2. Self-diminution—minimizes one's ability.
3. Guilt and worrying.
4. Postponing decisions and denying pleasure.
5. Disturbed interpersonal relationships.
6. Self-destructiveness and boredom.
7. Polarizing view of life.

NCLEX ALERT: *Promoting a positive self- concept is basic to all psychotherapeutic interventions. Look for options that focus on this concept; acknowledging the client as a person is an example.*

Nursing Intervention

A. Expand self-awareness.
1. Promote an open, trusting relationship.
2. Work and expand on whatever ego strength the client possesses.
3. Maximize the client's participation in the therapeutic relationship.

B. Self-exploration.
1. Encourage the client to accept his own feelings and thoughts.
2. Assist the client to clarify his concept of self and relationship with others through appropriate self-disclosure.
3. Explore with client maladaptive thinking patterns such as:
   a. Catastrophizing—thinking that the worst will happen.
   b. Minimizing and maximizing—tendency to minimize the positive and maximize the negative.
   c. Black-and-white thinking—tendency to look at situations in extremes, no middle ground.
   d. Overgeneralization—if something happens once, it will happen again.
   e. Self-reference—tendency to believe that people are particularly aware of their mistakes.
   f. Filtering—selectively pulling out certain details out of context while neglecting to look at more positive facts.
4. Communicate empathically, not sympathetically, and encourage client that he has the power to change himself.

C. Self-evaluation.
1. Encourage client to define and identify problem.
2. Identify irrational beliefs such as:
   a. "I must be loved by everyone."
   b. "I must be competent and not make mistakes."
   c. "My whole life is a disaster if it doesn't turn out exactly as planned."
3. Identify areas of strength by exploring areas such as hobbies, skills, work, school, character traits, personal abilities, etc.

PEDIATRIC PRIORITY: *If parents assist children to accomplish goals that are important to them, children begin to develop a sense of personal competence and independence.*

4. Explore client's adaptive and maladaptive coping responses.
   a. Determine "pay-offs" for maintaining self-defeating behaviors such as:
      (1) Procrastination.
      (2) Avoiding risks and commitments.
      (3) Retreating from the present situation.
      (4) Not having to accept responsibility for one's action.
   b. Identify the disadvantages of the maladaptive coping responses.

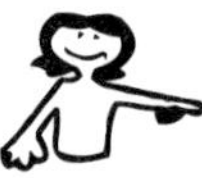

NURSING PRIORITY: *An individual's functional level of overall self-esteem may change markedly from day to day and moment to moment.*

D. Realistic planning.
   1. Assist client to identify alternative solutions.
   2. Encourage creative visualization to enhance self-esteem through goal setting.
   3. Assist client to set realistic goals by encouraging him to participate in new experiences.

E. Commitment to action.
   1. Providing an opportunity for client to experience success is essential.
   2. Reinforce strengths, abilities, and skills.

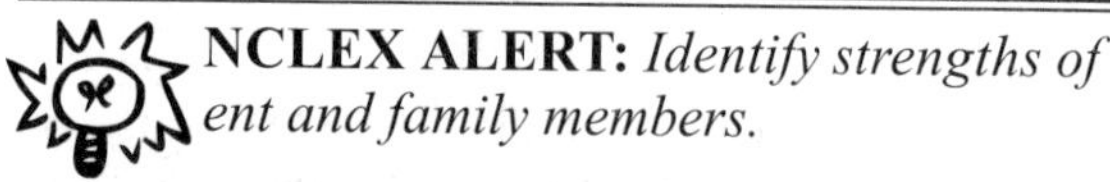

NCLEX ALERT: *Identify strengths of client and family members.*

BODY IMAGE

Evaluation of Body Image Alteration

A. Types of body image disturbances.
   1. Changes in body size, shape, and appearance (rapid weight gain or loss, plastic surgery, pregnancy).
   2. Pathological processes causing changes in structure or function of one's body (arthritis, Parkinson's disease, cancer, heart disease).
   3. Failure of a body part to function properly (paraplegia or stroke).
   4. Physical changes associated with normal growth and development (puberty, aging process).
   5. Threatening medical or nursing procedures (catheterization, radiation therapy, organ transplants).

B. Principles.
   1. Body characteristics that have been present from birth or acquired early in life seem to have less emotional significance than those arising later.
   2. Bodyimage changes, handicaps, or changes in body function that occur abruptly are far more traumatic than ones that develop gradually.
   3. The location of a disease or injury greatly affects the emotional response to it; internal diseases are generally less threatening than external diseases (trauma, disfigurement).
   4. Changes in genitals or breasts are perceived as a great threat and reawaken fears about sexuality and virility.

Alterations of Body Image: Four Phases

A. Impact phase.
   1. Shows behaviors of despair, discouragement, and passive acceptance.
   2. Often projects guilt onto others.
   3. Senses failure in own body.
   4. Anger and hostility often turned inward.

B. Retreat phase.
   1. Becomes aware of the injury, illness, loss, or disfigurement.
   2. Child and older adult retreat into regressive behavior.
   3. Adolescent and adult retreat into denial.

C. Acknowledgment phase.
   1. A period of mourning the loss.
   2. Acknowledges loss regardless of the degree involved; no longer can hide or retreat from situation.
   3. Begins to focus on strengths rather than losses.

D. Reconstruction phase.
   1. Adapts to changes in body image.
   2. Encouraged to try new approaches to life.

Specific Situations of Altered Body Image and Nursing Intervention

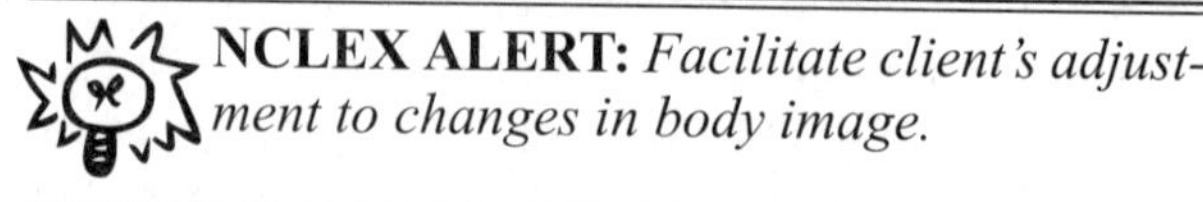

NCLEX ALERT: *Facilitate client's adjustment to changes in body image.*

Obesity

Assessment

A. Body weight exceeds 20% above the normal range for age, sex, and height.

B. Feeding behavior is gauged according to external environmental cues (i.e., availability of food, odors, stress) rather than hunger (increased G.I. motility).

C. Increased incidence of diabetes, cardiovascular disease, and poor healing; skin fold thickness greater than 0.2 inches measured with skin fold calipers.

D. Often has symptoms of depression, fatigue, dyspnea, tachycardia, and hypertension.

Intervention

A. Encourage behavior modification programs.

B. Promote activities and interests not related to food or eating.

C. Identify client's need to eat and relate the need to preceding events or situations.

D. Decrease guilt and anxiety related to being obese.

E. Provide long-range nutritional counseling.

F. Encourage an exercise program.

G. Assess for complications (hypertension, cardiovascular disease).

Stroke (CVA)

Assessment

A. Change of body function due to loss of bowel and bladder control, speech, and cognitive skills.

B. Disordered orientations in relationship to body and position sense in space; body image boundaries disrupted.

Intervention

A. Decrease frustration related to speech problems by encouraging speech effort, speaking slowly, and clarifying statements.

B. Promote reintegration of altered body image due to paralyzed body part by tactile stimulation and verbal reminders of the existing body part.

Amputation

Assessment

A. Feelings of loss; lowered self-esteem; guilt; helplessness.

B. Depression, passivity, and increased emotional vulnerability.

C. Phantom limb pain in most clients—increased experience if amputation occurs after four years of age, and almost universal experience after age eight.

D. Phantom limb pain stronger in upper limbs and lasts longer than in lower limbs.

Intervention

A. Anticipatory guidance and therapeutic preparation of a client who is to undergo amputation.

B. Discussion of phantom limb phenomenon and exploration of client's fears regarding amputation.

C. Assist family to work through their feelings and to accept client as a whole person.

D. Acknowledge phantom limb pain; reassure client that this is a normal process.

Pregnancy

Assessment

A. Produces marked changes in a woman's body, resulting in major alterations in body configuration within a short period of time.

B. Second trimester—becomes aware that her body is widening and requires more body space.

C. Third trimester—very much aware of increased size; may feel ambivalent about the changes in her body.

D. Perceives her body as vulnerable, yet as a protective container for the unborn.

E. Mate experiences changed body image and sympathetic symptoms during woman's pregnancy.

Intervention

A. Explanation and reassurance of the normal physiologic changes that are occurring.

B. Provide discussions of alterations in body image for both mates.

C. Encourage verbalization of feelings relating to changed body image.

Cancer

Assessment

A. Cancer clients may suffer many changes in body image.

B. Removal of sex organs (breasts, uterus) has a significant impact on client's sexuality.

C. Disfiguring head and neck surgery has devastating impact to body image, since the face is one of the primary means by which people communicate.

D. Symptoms of depersonalization, loss of self-esteem, and depression may occur.

Intervention

A. Provide anticipatory guidance to help client cope with crisis of changed body image.

B. Set long-term goals to help cancer client adjust to physiological and psychological changes occurring.

Enterostomal surgery

Assessment

A. Client often shocked at initial sight of ostomy.

B. May experience lowered self-esteem, fear of fecal spillage, alteration in sexual functioning, feelings of disfigurement and rejection.

Intervention

A. Preoperative explanation by use of drawings, models, or pictures of how stoma will appear.

B. Reassurance that reddish appearance of stoma and large size will diminish in time.

C. Encourage discussion and recognize importance of client taking with a "successful ostomate."

HUMAN SEXUALITY

Key Nursing Concepts

A. Growth and development.

1. Observable differences in male and female behavior are seen as early as infancy.
2. Core gender identity develops in the normal child about three or four years of age.
3. Sexual problems seen in childhood are as follows: sexual misconception, gender identity disturbances, and home settings which cause sexual confusion.
4. Rapid biologic changes seen in adolescence result in anxiety about maturation.
5. The adolescent is faced with the following: establishing his or her identity; accepting a changed body image; coping with new energy; and resolving reappearing Oedipal conflict.
6. Sexual problems seen in adolescents include: guilty feelings regarding masturbation, integrating transient homosexual experiences into heterosexual relationship; resolving conflicts related to pre-marital intercourse; and obtaining sex-related health services (i.e., birth control).
7. The young adult faces the task of establishing a pattern of heterosexual intimacy.
8. The middle-aged adult faces the task of adjusting to physiologic changes in sexual function and the responsibilities of parenting.
9. Sexual activity and interest may persist into old age, provided the individual is healthy and has an interesting partner.

B. Principles.

1. Human sexuality is best understood when approached holistically (i.e., from the physiological, psychological, sociological, and cultural perspectives).
2. The process of hospitalization alters one's concept of self as a sexual being.
3. Sexual role identity may be altered during the illness process.
4. Cultural variables influence one's expression of sexuality.
5. Hospitalized patients may act out sexually to test the response of others to their sexuality, or to gain control of a situation, or to attract attention.
6. Sexual problem treatment is short-termed and behavior-oriented; the goal is to decrease fear of performance and to facilitate communication.
7. Nursing plays a key role in sex-health education; nurses need to be aware of their own personal attitudes toward sex to respond helpfully to clients.

Changes in Sexuality

A. Effect of illness and injury on sexuality.

1. Depression episodes often precipitate a decrease in libido.
2. Sexual preoccupations and overtones may be experienced by the psychotic client.
3. Certain medications contribute to sexual dysfunction, failure to reach orgasm in women, and impotence or failure to ejaculate in men (e.g., reserpine, phenothiazine, and estrogen use in men decrease libido, while androgen use in females increases libido).
4. Clients with spinal cord injuries may lose sexual functioning because of full or partial paralysis.
5. Trauma and disfigurement may precipitate an alteration in sexuality and leave the client with no time to prepare for the loss.

B. Effect of the aging process on sexuality.

1. Physiological changes in the woman relate to decreasing estrogen supply: decrease in vaginal lubrication, shrinkage in size and elasticity of vaginal canal, and decrease in breast size.
2. Physiological changes in the man include a decrease in testosterone, decrease in spermatogenesis, a longer length of time to achieve erection along with a decrease in the firmness of erection.
3. Prolonged abstinence from sexual activity can lead to disuse syndrome in which the physiological changes are experienced to a greater degree.

CONCEPT OF LOSS

NCLEX ALERT: *Identify coping mechanisms of client and family, assist client to adjust to role changes (e.g., puberty, retirement, death), provide emotional support to the client or family, and assess client's response to illness.*

A. Definition.

1. Includes both biological and physiological aspects; loss of function.
2. Components of loss include death, dying, grief, and mourning.
   a. Death: represents finality, the end of one's biological being.
   b. Dying: the social process of organizing activities that prepare for death; provides others, as well as the client, a way to prepare for the future.
   c. Grief: the sequence of subjective states that follow loss and accompany mourning.
   d. Mourning: the psychological processes that are aroused by the loss of a loved object or person.
   e. Disenfranchised grief: loss which is not or cannot be openly expressed and acknowledged by others. **Examples**: Miscarriage, birth of a disabled child, death of an ex-spouse, loss of hair during chemotherapy, death of a pet.

Assessment

A. Characteristic stages.
1. Death and dying (Kübler-Ross, 1969).
   a. Denial and isolation.
   b. Anger.
   c. Bargaining.
   d. Depression.
   e. Acceptance.
2. Grief.
   a. Shock and disbelief.
   b. Developing awareness.
   c. Restitution or resolution of the loss.

B. Clinical Signs.
1. Impending death.
   a. Loss of muscle tone.
      (1) Bowel/bladder incontinence.
      (2) Difficulty speaking, swallowing, loss of gag reflex.
      (3) Decreased GI motility (e.g., flatus, abdominal distention, retention of feces).
   b. Slowing of the circulation.
      (1) Mottling and cyanosis of extremities.
      (2) Cool skin (first in feet, later the hands, ears and nose).
   c. Changes in vital signs.
      (1) Decreased pulse (weaker) and blood pressure.
      (2) Rapid, shallow, irregular, or abnormally slow respirations; mouth breathing.
   d. Sensory impairment.
      (1) Blurred vision.
      (2) Impaired senses of taste and smell.

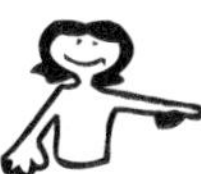

NURSING PRIORITY: *Hearing is thought to be the last sense lost.*

2. Imminent death.
   a. Dilated, fixed pupils.
   b. Inability to move; loss of reflexes.
   c. Faster, weaker pulse; lowered blood pressure.
   d. Cheyne-Stokes respirations.
   e. Noisy breathing, often referred to as the *death rattle*, due to collection of mucus in the pharynx.
3. *Clinical* death.
   a. Total lack of response to external stimuli.
   b. No muscular movement, especially breathing.
   c. No reflexes.
   d. Flat encephalogram.

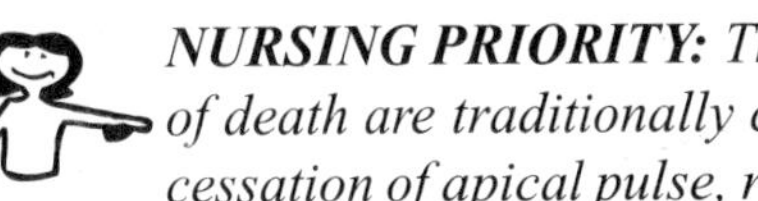

NURSING PRIORITY: *The clinical signs of death are traditionally considered to be cessation of apical pulse, respirations, and blood pressure. However, with the advent of advanced life support systems, identifying death is more difficult.*

Coping and Reactions to Death Throughout the Life Cycle

1. ***Infant—toddler (ages 1-3).***
   a. Reactions to death and dying.
      (1) No specific concept of death—think only in terms of living.
      (2) React more to pain and discomfort of illness and immobilization; separation anxiety; intrusive procedures; change in ritualistic routine.
   b. Nursing intervention.
      (1) Assist parents to deal with their feelings.
      (2) Encourage parents' participation in child's care.
      (3) Promote decreased separation anxiety.

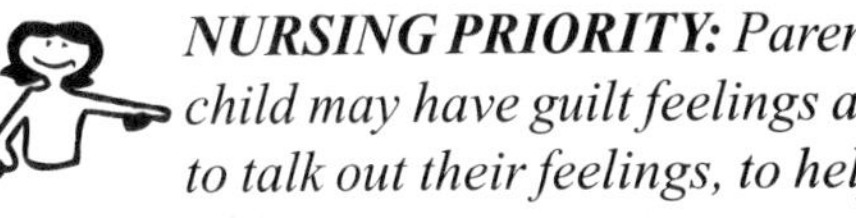

NURSING PRIORITY: *Parents of a dying child may have guilt feelings and may need to talk out their feelings, to help each other and the child.*

2. ***Preschooler (ages 3-5).***
   a. Reactions to death and dying.

(1) Death is viewed as a departure, a kind of sleep.

(2) No real understanding of the universality and inevitability of death.

(3) Life and death can change places with one another.

(4) Death is viewed as gradual or temporary; the person is still alive but under a different set of conditions.

(5) Often views illness and death as a punishment for his thoughts or actions.

(6) If a pet dies, may request a "funeral" or "burial" or some type of ceremony to symbolize their loss.

b. Nursing Intervention.

(1) Utilize play for expression of thoughts and feelings regarding death and dying.

(2) Provide a clear explanation of what death is; death is final and not sleep.

(3) Permit a choice of attending a funeral; if child decides to attend, explain what will take place.

PEDIATRIC PRIORITY: *A young child's fear of death is often aloneness, being away from the parents. It is important for parents to interact with the nurse in the child's presence so that the nurse can be identified as a trustworthy substitute caretaker.*

3. ***School age (ages 5-12).***

a. Reactions to death and dying.

(1) Death is personified; fantasies of a separate person or distinct personality (e.g., skeleton-man, devil, ghost, or death-man).

(2) Often, fantasies about the unknown are very frightening.

(3) Fear of mutilation and punishment is often associated with death; anxiety is released by nightmares and superstitions.

b. Nursing Intervention.

(1) Respond to questions regarding funerals, burials, and postdeath services.

(2) Accept regressive or protest behavior.

(3) Encourage verbalization of feelings and emotional reactions.

4. ***Adolescent (ages 12-18).***

a. Reactions to death and dying.

(1) Has a mature understanding of death.

(2) Concerned more with the here and now (i.e., the present).

(3) May have strong emotions about death (anger, frustration, despair); silent, withdrawn.

(4) Often worries about physical changes in relationship to terminal illness.

(5) May ask very difficult, open questions regarding death.

b. Nursing Intervention.

(1) Support maturational crises relating to identity.

(2) Encourage verbalization of feelings.

(3) Promote peer and parental emotional support.

(4) Respect need for privacy and personal expressions of anger, sadness or fear.

(5) Model appropriate grieving behavior.

5. ***Adult.***

a. Concerned about death as a disruption in lifestyle and its effect on significant others.

b. Associates loss as unmet goals, constricting future plans, and threat to emotional integrity.

6. ***Older adult.***

a. Aware of death as inevitable; life is over.

b. Emphasis on religious belief for comfort; a time of reflection, rest, and peace.

CULTURAL DIVERSITY

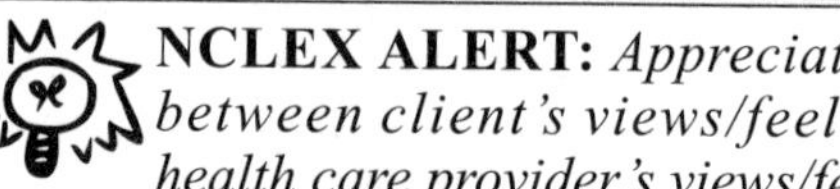

NCLEX ALERT: *Appreciate differences between client's views/feelings and the health care provider's views/feelings.*

Special Considerations

1. Cultures vary widely in their traditions.
2. In the United States each particular ethnic group has its own cultural system and specific way of behavior and evaluating illness and wellness.

NURSING PRIORITY: *Certain psychopathologies change diagnostic category entirely in different cultures. Misinterpretation and misunderstanding of clients' presenting symptoms can lead to problems in the nurse-client relationship, (e.g., notion of possession [good] of the Holy Ghost among the American Pentecostal groups might be viewed as expression of symptoms of a mental disorder).*

3. *Culture shock* occurs whenever a person leaves a familiar country, region, lifestyle or occupation and enters a radically different environment.

Examples: *Entering the hospital; moving to a new neighborhood.*

Assessment of Cultural Aspects

1. Communication styles.
   a. Does the client speak English fluently? If not, what language is preferred?
   b. Is an interpreter needed?

NURSING PRIORITY: *If an interpreter is needed, it is preferable to avoid using family members. Also, it is helpful to learn key words from interpreter, to assist the nurse in implementing care.*

2. Ethnic or religious group.
   a. What particular group does client identify with?
   b. How closely does the client adhere to the traditional beliefs of the group?
3. Nutrition.
   a. Are there certain ethnic or religious preferences among foods selected or prepared?
   b. Are there foods to be encouraged when a person is ill?
4. Family relationships.
   a. Is the family matriarchal or patriarchal?
   b. What role in the family does the client hold?
5. Health beliefs.
   a. Does the client rely on folk medicine practices?
   b. Has the client been recently treated by a curandero, Voodoo doctor, medicine man, or Chinese herbalist?

NURSING PRIORITY: *Strong evidence suggests that factors such as genetics, environment, diet, and cultural beliefs are responsible for ethnic variations in psychotropic drug use (e.g., poor metabolism of certain psychotropic drugs because of genetic factors has been found responsible for drug effects in Asians, blacks, and native Americans).*

PSYCHOSOCIAL ASSESSMENT

❑ **Complete assessment includes descriptions of the intellectual functions, behavioral reactions, emotional reactions, dynamic issues of the client relative to adaptive functioning, and response to present situations.**

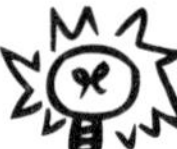

NCLEX ALERT: *Assess client's reponse to illness, identify coping mechanisms of client and family, and assess a family's emotional reaction to client's illness.*

Psychiatric History

❑ **Purpose: to obtain data from multiple sources, (e.g., client, family, friends, police, mental health personnel), in order to identify patterns of functioning that are healthy as well as patterns that create problems in the client's everyday life.**

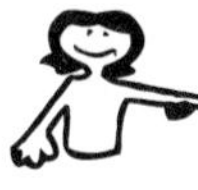

GERIATRIC PRIORITY: *Allow ample time to gather psychosocial data from elderly clients, as they are often starved for someone to listen to them.*

A. General history of client.
   1. Obtain general demographic information—address, age, religious affiliation, occupation, insurance company, etc.
   2. Pertinent personal history such as birth, growth and development, illness, and marital history.
   3. Previous mental health hospitalizations or treatment.

B. Components of psychiatric history.
   1. Chief Complaint—main reason client is seeking psychiatric help.
      a. Use client's own words as to why he/she is hospitalized or seeking help.
      b. Check for recent difficulties or alterations in relationships, level of functioning, behavior, perceptions, or cognitive abilities.
   2. Presenting symptoms—onset and development of symptoms or problems.
      a. Check for increased feelings of depression, anxiety, hopelessness, suspiciousness, confusion, fear.
      b. Assess for changes in bowel habits, insomnia, lethargy, weight loss or gain, anorexia, palpitations, pruritus, headaches.
   3. Family history
      a. Have any family members sought psychiatric treatment?
      b. Who was important to client in childhood? Adolescence?
      c. Was there physical or sexual abuse?
      d. Did parents drink or use drugs?
   4. Personality profile
      a. Assess client's interests, feelings, mood, and usual leisure or hobby activities.

b. How does client cope with stress?

c. Inquire about sexual patterns—sexually active? sexual orientation? sexual difficulties?

d. Have client describe social relationships—Friends, Who is important to client? What is a usual day like?

Mental Status Examination

❑ **The mental status examination differs from the psychiatric history in that it is used to identify an individual's *present* mental status.**

NCLEX ALERT: *Identify changes in client's mental status.*

Aspects of the Examination

NURSING PRIORITY: *Assess level of consciousness, vision, and hearing first (e.g., alert, lethargic, stuporous, or comatose) and ability of the client to comprehend the interview.*

A. General appearance, attitude, and behavior.

1. Descriptors: posture, gait, activity, facial expression, mannerisms.
2. Disturbances include deviations of activity, distortions in mobility (waxy flexibility or dyskinesia), uncooperativeness, changes in personal hygiene.

B. Characteristics of talk and stream of thought.

1. Descriptors: emphasis on form, rather than content of client's verbal communication; loudness, flow, speed, quality, logic, level of coherence.
2. Disturbances include the following patterns:

a. Mutism—no verbal response.

b. Circumstantiality—cumbersome detail in client's communication.

c. Perseveration—pattern of repeating same words or movements.

d. Flight of ideas—rapid, loosely connected thoughts.

e. Blocking—sudden silence, often associated with intrusion of delusional thoughts or hallucinations.

f. Echolalia—repeating of the last word heard.

g. Neologism—coining of new words.

h. Verbigeration—repeating words, sentences, or phrases several times.

i. Pressured speech—an increase in the quantity of speech, usually becoming loud, rushed, and emphatic.

C. Emotional state.

1. Descriptors: client's report of subjective feelings (mood or affect) and examiner's observation of client's pervasive or dominant emotional state.
2. Disturbances include deviations such as elation, depression, apathy, incongruence, disassociation.

D. Content of thought.

1. Descriptors: What is central theme? How does client view himself (self-concept)? Is suicidal or homicidal ideation present? If so, what is potential lethality?
2. Disturbances include: special preoccupations and experiences such as hallucinations, delusions, illusions, depersonalization, obsessions or compulsions, phobias, fantasies, and daydreams.

E. Sensorium and intellect.

1. Determines degree of client's awareness and level of intellectual functioning, general ability to grasp information and calculate; abstract thinking; memory (recall of remote past experiences or recent past experiences, retention and recall of immediate impressions; reasoning and judgment).
2. Disturbances of orientation in terms of time, place, person, and self; memory, retention, attention, information, and judgment are assessed through use of standardized tests and questions.

NURSING PRIORITY: *It is often helpful to start the mental status examination off with determining the sensorium and intellect, since the validity and reliability of obtaining data require the client to be reasonably oriented.*

F. Insight evaluation.

1. Determines whether the client can understand and appreciate the nature of their condition and the need for treatment.

STRESS AND ADAPTATION

❑ ***Stress*** **is a state produced by a change in the environment that is perceived as challenging, threatening, or damaging to the individual's equilibrium.**

❑ ***Adaptation*** **is a constant, ongoing process that occurs along the time continuum, beginning with birth and ending with death.**

Stressors

1. Physiologic stressors.

a. Chemical agents—drugs, poisons, alcohol.

Table 9-1: SELYE'S GENERAL ADAPTATION SYNDROME

Stage I —	**Alarm Reaction**
Mobilization of the body's defensive forces (anti-inflammatory) and activation of the "fight - flight" mechanism.	
Stage II — Stage of Resistance	
Optimal adaptation to stress within a person's capabilities.	
Stage III — Stage of Exhaustion	
Loss of the ability to resist stress because of depletion of body resources; failure to adapt leads to death.	

b. Physical agents—heat, cold, radiation, electrical shock, trauma.

c. Infectious agents—viruses, bacteria, fungi.

d. Faulty immune mechanisms.

e. Genetic disorders.

f. Nutritional imbalance.

g. Hypoxia.

2. Psychosocial stressors.
   a. Accidents and the survivors (airplane crash, hurricane, and earthquake survivors.
   b. Death of a close friend, neighbor being robbed and beaten.
   c. Horrors of history: Auschwitz, Hiroshima, Chernobyl.
   d. Fear of aggression, mutilation, and destruction.
   e. Events of history brought into our living room.
   f. Life crises—situational, developmental, role.
   g. Inherent conflicts in all social relations.
3. Environmental stressors.
   a. Noise pollution.
   b. Temperature pollution.
   c. Air and chemical pollution.

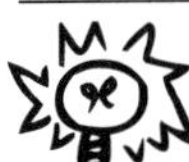

NCLEX ALERT: *Implement measures to reduce environmental stressors.*

Stress Response

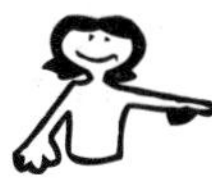

NURSING PRIORITY: *Understanding of the stress response is basic to many nursing interventions.*

1. Sympathetic-Adrenal Medullary Response (Table 9-2: Selye's General Adaptation Syndrome): **"Fight or Flight."**
   - Increased pulse, blood glucose, and coagulability of blood; pupils dilated; mental activity enhanced; cold, clammy skin; respirations rapid, and shallow.
2. Pituitary-Adrenal Cortical Response.
   - Increased production of ACTH, mineralocorticoids (aldosterone), and release of glucagon.
   - The sympathetic-adrenal medullary response occurs within seconds.
   - The pituitary-adrenal cortical response (also, called Selyean response, after Hans Selye) includes the fight - flight response and takes minutes to hours to produce a desired effect.

Stress Reduction Methods

1. Proper nutrition.
2. Regular exercise, physical activity, and recreation.
3. Meditation, breathing exercises, creative imagery.
4. Communication, time management.
5. Biofeedback, rolfing (massage of deep connective tissue to achieve realignment of body structure), therapeutic touch, bioenergetics (decrease muscle tension by releasing feelings through physical exertion and verbal techniques).
6. Relaxation response (Benson, 1975).
   a. Quiet environment.
   b. Passive attitude.
   c. Comfortable position.
   d. A mental device or object, such as a word, sound, or phrase to occupy the mind and keep out thoughts.
7. Group process and social support.
8. Thought stopping, self-hypnosis, refuting irrational self-talk.

CONCEPT OF ANXIETY

❑ **An emotion, a subjective experience; a feeling state that is experienced as vague uneasiness, tension, or apprehension; occurs when the ego is threatened; provoked by the unknown; precedes all new experiences.**

A. Assessment (Table 9-2).

B. Nursing Management (Table 9-3).

NCLEX ALERT: *Plan measures to help a client cope with anxiety. Anxiety is often tested in situations regarding the medical-surgical client.*

Table 9-2: ASSESSMENT OF ANXIETY

PHYSIOLOGICAL	PSYCHOLOGICAL
SYMPATHETIC RESPONSES	***BEHAVIORAL RESPONSES***
Tachycardia	Restlessness
Elevated blood pressure	Agitation
Increased perspiration	Tremors (fine to gross shaking of the body)
Dilated pupils	Startle reaction
Hyperventilation with difficulty breathing	Rapid speech
Cold, clammy skin	Lack of coordination
Dry mouth	Withdrawal
Constipation	
PARASYMPATHETIC RESPONSES	***COGNITIVE RESPONSES***
Urinary frequency	Impaired attention
Diarrhea	Poor concentration
	Forgetfulness
	Blocking of thought
	Decreased perceptual field
	Decreased productivity
	Confusion
RELATED RESPONSES	***AFFECTIVE RESPONSES***
Headaches	Tension
Nausea or vomiting	Jittery feeling
Sleep disturbances	Worried
Muscular Tension	Apprehension,, nervousness
	Irritability
	Dread
	Fear
	Panic
	Fear of impending doom

COPING/ DEFENSE/ EGO/ MENTAL MECHANISMS

❑ **Specific defense processes used by individuals to relieve or decrease anxieties caused by uncomfortable situations that threaten self-esteem.**

A. Related principles.

1. The primary functions are to decrease emotional conflicts, provide relief from stress, protect from feelings of inadequacy and worthlessness, prevent awareness of anxiety, and maintain an individual's self-esteem.
2. Everyone uses defense mechanisms to a certain extent. If used to an extreme degree they distort reality, interfere with interpersonal relationships, limit one's ability to work productively, and may lead to pathological symptomatology.

B. Common defense mechanisms (Appendix 9-1).

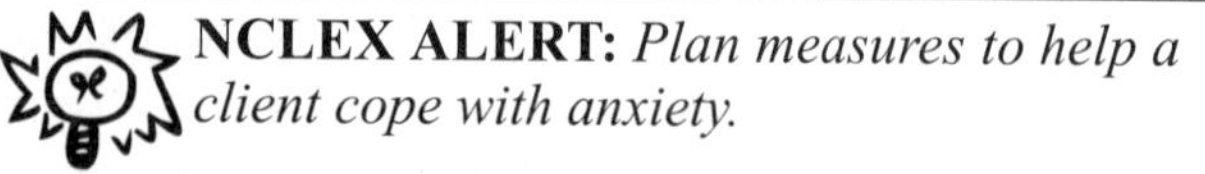
NCLEX ALERT: *Plan measures to help a client cope with anxiety.*

C. Nursing management.

1. Accept coping mechanisms.
2. Discuss alternative coping mechanisms and problem-solving situations.
3. Assist the client in learning new or alternative coping patterns for a healthier adaptation.
4. Utilize techniques to decrease anxiety.

THERAPEUTIC NURSING PROCESS

❑ **Therapeutic interpersonal relationship is the interaction between two persons: the *nurse* promotes goal-directed activities that help to alleviate the discomfort of the *client* by promoting growth and satisfying interpersonal relationships.**

Characteristics

- Goal-directed.
- Empathetic understanding.
- Honest, open communication.
- Concreteness; avoids vagueness and ambiguity.
- Acceptance; nonjudgmental attitude.
- Involves nurse's understanding of self, and personal motives and needs.

Interview Process

- To establish rapport with the client.
- To obtain pertinent client data.
- To initiate client assessment.
- To make practical arrangements for treatment.

Phases

1. Initial phase—goal is to *build trust.*
   a. Explore the client's perceptions, thoughts, feelings and actions.
   b. Identify problem.
   c. Assess levels of anxiety of self and client.
   d. Mutually define specific goals to pursue.
2. Working phase—goal is *to establish objectives* or working agreement (a contract).
   a. Encourage client participation.
   b. Focus on problem-solving techniques; choose between alternate courses of action and practice skills.
   c. Explore thoughts, feelings, and emotions.
   d. Develop constructive coping mechanisms.
   e. Increase independence and self-responsibility.
3. Termination phase—goal is *to evaluate goals* set forth and terminate relationship.

Table 9-3: NURSING MANAGEMENT OF ANXIETY

LEVEL OF ANXIETY	ASSESSMENT	GOAL	NURSING MANAGEMENT
MILD	Increased alertness, motivation, and attentiveness.	To assist client to tolerate some anxiety.	1. Help client identify and describe feelings. 2. Help client develop the capacity to tolerate mild anxiety and use it consciously and constructively.
MODERATE	Perception narrowed, selective inattention, physical discomforts.	To reduce anxiety; LTG: directed toward helping client understand cause of anxiety and new ways of controlling.	1. Provide outlet for tension such as walking, crying, working at simple, concrete tasks.
SEVERE	Behavior becomes automatic; connections between details are not seen; senses are drastically reduced.	To assist in channeling anxiety.	1. Recognize own level of anxiety. 2. Link client's behavior with feelings. 3. Protect defenses and coping mechanisms. 4. Identify and modify anxiety-provoking situations.
PANIC	Overwhelmed; inability to function or communicate; possible bodily harm to self and others; loss of rational thought.	To be supportive and protective.	1. Provide nonstimulating, structured environment. 2. Avoid touching. 3. Stay with client. 4. Medicate client with tranquilizers if necessary.

a. Plan for termination early in formation of relationship (in initial phase).

b. Discuss client's feelings about termination.

c. Evaluate client's progress and goal attainment.

***NURSING PRIORITY:** To effectively interview, be sure to start with a broad, empathetic statement; explore normal behaviors before discussing maladaptive behaviors; phrase inquiries or questions sensitively to decrease client's anxiety; ask client to clarify vague statements; focus on pressing problems when client begins to ramble; interrupt nonstop talkers as tactfully as possible; express empathy toward client while he is expressing feelings.*

Communication Theory

❑ **Definition-"All those processes by which people influence one another" (Ruesch, 1968).**

1. Levels of communication.

   a. Verbal communication-occurs through the medium of words, spoken or written.

   b. Nonverbal communication-includes everything that does not involve the spoken or written word; involves the five senses.

      (1) Vocal cues-tone of voice, quality of voice, nervous coughing and sounds of hesitation.

      (2) Action cues-body movement, posture, facial expressions, gestures and mannerisms.

      (3) Object cues-dress, appearance to convey a certain "look" or message.

      (4) Space-distance between two people; intimate, personal, public space.

      (5) Touch-universal and basic to all nurse-client relationships; response to it is influenced by the setting, cultural background, type of relationship, sex of communicators, and expectations.

2. Therapeutic nurse-client communication techniques.

   a. Planning and Goals.

      (1) Demonstrate active listening; face-to-face contact.

      (2) Demonstrate unconditional positive regard, interest, congruence, respect.

      (3) Develop trusting relationship; accept client's behavior and display nonjudgmental, objective attitude.

      (4) Be supportive, honest, and authentic.

      (5) Focus on emotional needs and emotionally charged area.

      (6) Focus on here and now behavior and expression of feelings.

      (7) Attempt to understand another point of view.

Table 9-4: THERAPEUTIC COMMUNICATION

RESPONSE	EXAMPLE
1. Exploring	"What seems to be the problem?" "Tell me more about..."
2. Reflecting	"I am really mad at my mother for grounding me." "You sound angry."
3. Focusing	"Give an example of what you mean." "Let's look at this more closely."
4. Clarifying	"I'm not sure that I understand what you're saying." "Do you mean...?"
5. Using general leads	"Go on..." "Talk more about..."
6. Broad opening leads	"Where would you like to begin?" "Talk more about..."
7. Validating	"Did I understand you to say...?"
8. Informing	"The time is..." "My name is..."
9. Accepting	"Yes." "Okay." Nodding "Uh hmm."
10. Sharing observations	"You appear anxious. I noticed that you haven't been coming to lunch with the group."
11. Presenting reality	"I do not hear a noise or see the lights blinking." "I am not Cleopatra; I am your nurse."
12. Summarizing	"During the past hour..."
13. Using silence	Nurse remains silent.

(8) Develop an awareness of the client's likes and dislikes.

(9) Encourage expression of both positive and negative feelings.

(10) Use broad openings and ask open-ended questions; avoid questions that can be answered by yes or no.

(11) Use reflections of feelings, attitudes and words.

(12) Explore alternatives rather than answers or solutions.

(13) Focus feedback on *what* is said rather than *why* it is said.

(14) Paraphrase to assist in clarifying client statement.

(15) Promote sharing of feelings, information, and ideas rather than giving advice.

b. Examples of therapeutic communication responses (Table 9-4).

c. Examples of nontherapeutic communication responses (Table 9-5).

NCLEX ALERT: *Listen to client's concerns and use therapeutic interventions to increase client's understanding of his/her behavior.*

INTERVENTION MODALITIES

Crisis Intervention

❑ **A crisis is a self-limiting situation in which usual problem-solving or decision-making methods are not adequate.**

1. A crisis offers opportunities for growth and renewal.
2. Crisis intervention strategy views people as capable of personal growth and able to control their own lives.
3. Types of crisis intervention strategies:
   a. Individual crisis counseling.
   b. Crisis groups.
   c. Telephone counseling.
4. Crisis intervention requires support, protection, and enhancement of the client's self-image.

Table 9-5: NONTHERAPEUTIC COMMUNICATION

RESPONSE	EXAMPLE
1. False reassurance	"Don't worry, you will be better in a few weeks." "Don't worry, I had an operation just like it; it was a snap."
2. Giving advice	"What you should do is..." "If I were you, I would do..."
3. Rejecting	"I don't like it when you..." "Please, don't ever talk about..."
4. Belittling	"Everybody feels that way." "Why, you shouldn't feel that way."
5. Probing	"Tell me more about your relationship with other men."
6. Overloading	"Hi, I am JoAnn, your student nurse. How old are you? What brought you to the hospital? How many children do you have? Do you want to fill out your menu right now?"
7. Underloading	Not giving enough information so that the meaning is clear; withholding information.
8. Clichés	"Gee, the weather is beautiful outside."

Group Therapy

❑ **A structured or semi-structured process in which individuals (7 -12 members ideal size) are interrelated and interdependent and who may share common purposes and norms.**

1. Emphasis on clear communication to promote effective interaction.
2. Disturbed perceptions can be corrected through consensual validation.
3. Socially ineffective behaviors can be modified through peer pressure.
4. See Table 10-3: Group Modalities for Elderly Clients.

NCLEX ALERT: *Participate in a group session for clients with psychosocial disorders.*

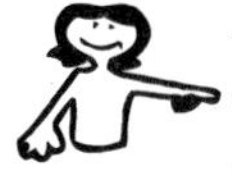

NURSING PRIORITY: Reality testing ability in the client is an important consideration in the selection of group members. A person who is psychotic would not be a good selection as a group member.

Family Therapy

NCLEX ALERT: *Provide emotional support to family, assess dynamics of family interactions, assess family's understanding of illness and emotional reaction, and help family adjust to role changes.*

❑ **A treatment modality designed to bring about a change in communication and interactive patterns between and among family members.**

1. A family can be viewed as a system that is dynamic. A change or movement in any part of the family system affects all other parts of the system.
2. Family seeks to maintain a balance or "homeostasis" among various forces that operate within and upon it.
3. Emotional symptoms or problems of an individual are an expression of the emotional symptoms or problems in the family.
4. Therapeutic approaches involve helping the family members look at themselves in the here-and-now and recognize the influence of past models on their behavior and expectations.

Milieu

NCLEX ALERT: *Maintain a therapeutic milieu/environment.*

❑ **A scientifically, planned, purposeful manipulation in the environment aimed at causing changes in the behavior and personality of the client.**

1. Nurse is viewed as a facilitator and a helper to clients rather than a therapist.
2. The *therapeutic community* is a very special kind of milieu therapy in which the total social structure of the treatment unit is involved as part of the helping process.
3. Emphasis is placed on open communication, both within and between staff and client groups.

Mind-Body-Spirit Therapies

❑ **Alternative therapies different from traditional Western medicine; often influenced by traditional Chinese medicine, which focuses on maintaining**

unity with nature and balancing our energy systems.

1. Acupuncture —movement of energy through meridians of the body to restore energy balance.
2. Imagery—change reality by creating a different mental picture.
3. Therapeutic touch —manipulate and direct client's energy through the use of the practitioner's hands and direct energy from the practitioner to the client to enhance healing.
4. Massage—through touch unblocks energy flow and connects client with practitioner.
5. Relaxation—imagery and progressive tensing and relaxing muscle groups throughout the body.
6. Bioenergetics—removes blockages to promote the flow of bio-energy or Ch'i.
7. Transcendental meditation—quiet meditation, focusing on getting beyond the self and becoming one with the universal energy source.
8. Others—exercise, nutrition, prayer, religious practices.

Somatic Therapies

1. Restraints.
   a. Must consider client's civil liberties.
   b. Mechanical restraints include camisoles, wrist and ankle restraints, sheet restraints, and cold wet sheet packs.

NURSING PRIORITY: It is important to have a physician's order for applying restraints and to provide for clients' biologic needs, (e.g., hygiene, elimination, nutrition, and method of communication).

2. Seclusion.
   a. Confinement to a room that may be locked. Often, the room is without a mattress or linens and the client is in a hospital nightgown.
   b. There is limited opportunity for communication.

NCLEX ALERT: *Legal requirements for the care of the secluded client vary from state to state and specifics are usually not tested on the NCLEX-RN.*

Psychosurgery

❑ **Surgical interruption of selected neural pathways that govern transmission of emotion between the frontal lobes of the cerebral cortex and the thalamus.**

1. Recent resurgence of interest in psychosurgery as knowledge of neuroanatomy and "mapping" the cerebral cortex has become more sophisticated.
2. Area of moral and ethical debate, especially since nerve tissue once damaged cannot regenerate.

Electroconvulsive Therapy (ECT) *(See Chapter 10)*

Other Therapies

1. Psychodrama—the use of structured and directed dramatization of client's emotional problems and experiences.
2. Activities therapy—a number of vital programs come under this, such as music therapy, occupational therapy, art therapy, recreational therapy, ROPES, dance or movement therapy, etc.

COMMON BEHAVIORAL PATTERNS

NCLEX ALERT: *Identify inappropriate behavior, utilize client behavior modification techniques, and use therapeutic interventions to increase client understanding of his/her behavior.*

Interpersonal Withdrawal

❑ **Behavior characterized by avoidance of interpersonal contact and a sense of unreality.**

1. Physical withdrawal—client sits or stands apart from others; may hide, assume a catatonic posture, or (in extreme form) attempt suicide.
2. Verbal withdrawal—avoidance through silence or (in extreme form) mutism; silence may indicate resistance, a pensive moment, or the indication that nothing more is to be said.

Nursing Intervention

1. Avoid punishment of client.
2. Decrease isolation.
3. Invite the client to speak.
4. State the amount of time you are willing to stay with the client whether he/she chooses to speak or not.
5. Change the context of the contact (for example, go for a walk together).
6. Encourage the client to share responsibility for the continuance of the relationship.

Regression

❑ **A selective, defensive operation in which the individual resorts to earlier, childish, or less complex patterns of behavior which once brought the client attention or pleasure.**

Nursing Intervention

1. Avoid fostering dependency and childlike attitudes.
2. Be patient and understanding.
3. Confront client directly about his/her plan.
4. Compliment client when he/she does something unusually well or assumes more responsibility.
5. Promote problem solving, reality orientation, and involvement in social activities.
6. Avoid punishment following periods of regression; instead, explore the meaning of the regressive behavior.

Anger

❑ **An unconscious process used in order to obtain relief from anxiety that is produced by a sense of danger; it involves a sense of powerlessness.**

- Fear of expressing anger is related to fear of rejection.

Nursing Intervention

1. Have client acknowledge or name feelings.
2. Explore source of personal fear or perceived threat (e.g., illness, disability, disfigurement or emotional crisis).
3. Encourage verbalization of anxiety.
4. Explore appropriate external expression of feelings.
5. Avoid arguing with client.
6. Acting out behavior is often an indirect expression of anger; it attracts attention and often represents the feelings the person is experiencing.

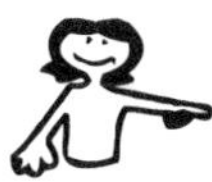

NURSING PRIORITY: *Nontherapeutic responses to a client's anger are defensiveness, retaliation, condescension, and avoidance.*

Hostility/Aggressiveness

❑ **An antagonistic feeling; the client wishes to hurt or humiliate others; the result may be a feeling of inadequacy or self-rejection due to a loss of self-esteem.**

Nursing Intervention

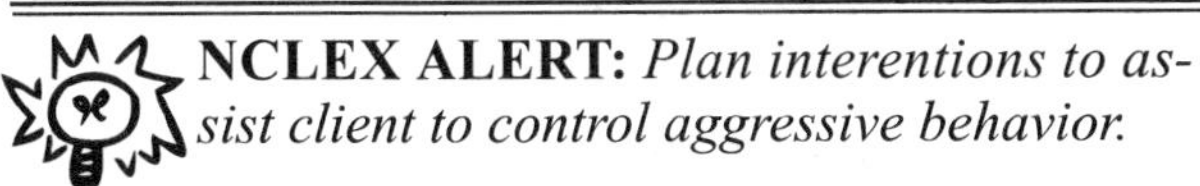

NCLEX ALERT: *Plan interentions to assist client to control aggressive behavior.*

1. Prevent aggressive contact by early recognition of increased anxiety.
2. Maintain client contact rather than avoid it.
3. Encourage verbalization of feelings associated with a threat of frustration (helplessness, inadequacy, anger).
4. Reduce environmental stimuli.
5. Avoid reinforcement behavior (i.e., joking, laughing, teasing, competitive games).
6. Encourage an alternative expression of aggression such as use of Bataccas (cylindrical clubs of a soft, padded material), pillows, or foam balls so that injury is avoided.
7. Use distraction, or remove the client from the immediate environment to re-establish self-control.
8. Set limits on unacceptable behavior.
9. Protect other clients.

NURSING PRIORITY: *When two clients are arguing, engage the dominant client first by using distraction or removing the client from the setting to allow time for de-escalation and processing of the situation.*

Violence

❑ **Behavior that is physically assaultive and risks injury to the self, others, and environment.**

Nursing Intervention

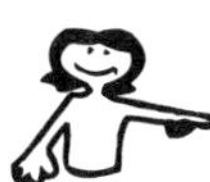

NURSING PRIORITY: *Immediate intervention should focus on control and safety, followed by discussion to alleviate guilt and identify alternative behaviors to help prevent future episodes of violence.*

1. Establish eye contact.
   a. Conveys attention and concern.
   b. Elicits more information.
   c. Ask the person to look at you.

GERIATRIC PRIORITY: *Expect some elderly clients to have vision problems; they may not know who you are.*

2. Avoid asking, "Why?"; instead ask, "What's bothering you?"
   a. *Why* questions are threatening and decrease self-esteem.
   b. Open-ended questions identify the problem, convey concern, and produce more information.

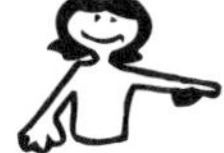

GERIATRIC PRIORITY: *Hearing problems occur with the elderly; don't shout or talk rapidly.*

3. Speak to client softly, slowly, and with assurance.
4. Give directions clearly and concisely. Tell the patient what you want him or her to do.
5. Encourage client to verbalize feelings.
   a. Give the person an outlet for the physical tension, "Walk with me — tell me what happened."
   b. Keep the conversation slow. Pace yourself. "Wait, I can't follow that. Tell me what you said."
   c. Listen more than talk.
   d. Let the person walk, move, or pound, and vent the tension before you talk.
6. Position yourself near the door.
   a. Don't block the door.
   b. Don't box the patient into a corner.
7. Self-protection and protection of other clients is a primary concern.
   a. Never see a potentially violent client alone; call security or other personnel.
   b. Keep a comfortable distance from client; don't intrude on his or her personal space.
      (1) With mild or moderate anxiety in the patient — sit near, about 2 feet away.
      (2) With severe or panic anxiety — stay 4 to 6 feet back (or farther).
   c. Be prepared to move quickly; violent clients act fast and unpredictably.
   d. Ascertain that client has no weapons before approaching.
   e. Be supportive and intervene to increase client's self-esteem.
   f. Be honest — tell the person you are concerned that he or she is out of control, but you are not going to let anyone get hurt.
   g. Stay with the person, but don't touch until you've asked permission and it has been given to you.
8. When client is in control, review and process the situation in order to alleviate client's guilt and to discuss alternatives should client become anxious or angry in the future.

Manipulation/Acting Out

❑ **A type of controlling behavior in which an individual uses others to meet his/her own needs or to achieve specific goals; often disguises underlying feelings of inadequacy, inferiority, and unworthiness; an attempt to protect against failure or frustration and to gain power over another.**

Nursing Intervention

1. Be consistent and firm in the expectations of behavior.
2. Allow some freedom within set limits.
3. Consistent enforcement of set limits.
4. Be alert to client's attempt to intimidate; allow verbal anger.
5. Avoid involvement and intellectualization.
6. Watch carefully for client's use of manipulative patterns; be alert to the many guises in which it may be manifested.
7. Keep staff united, firm, and consistent.
8. Encourage open communication about real needs and feelings.
9. Maintain a sense of authority.
10. Do not accept gifts, favors, flattery or other guises of manipulation.

Dependence

❑ **A behavior pattern characterized by adopting a helpless, powerless stance; a reliance on other people to meet a basic need.**

Nursing Intervention

1. Assess client's abilities and capacities.
2. Set firm and consistent limits on behavior.
3. Provide only help needed.
4. Encourage problem-solving and decision-making skills; emphasize accountability.
5. Avoid making decisions or assuming responsibility for client's ability to make decisions.
6. Maintain an attitude of firmness and confidence in client's ability to make decisions.
7. Discourage reliance beyond actual needs.
8. Give positive reinforcements for development of independent growth-facilitating behavior.
9. Encourage successful participation in social relationships.

Shame

❑ **The inner sense of being completely diminished or insufficient as a person (e.g., feeling less than).**

Nursing Intervention

1. Assist client to begin to *externalize* rather than internalize feelings of shame.
2. Encourage client to share feelings honestly with individuals they feel "safe" with.
3. Involve clients in "debriefing," which is writing and talking about past shame experiences.
4. Encourage client to make positive self-affirmations and involve themselves in creative visualization activities to improve self-concept.

Detachment

❑ **The behavioral process characterized by aloofness, superficiality, denial, and intellectualization in interpersonal contact.**

Nursing Intervention

1. Establish awareness of the process of detachment.
2. Explore fears and fantasies inhibiting emotional expression.
3. Encourage verbalization from global generalities to specific personal comments.
4. Provide clarification of client's unclear responses.
5. Emphasize awareness and exploration of feelings.

ABUSE

❑ **Abuse is difficult to define, as the term has been politicized and is not clinical or scientific.**

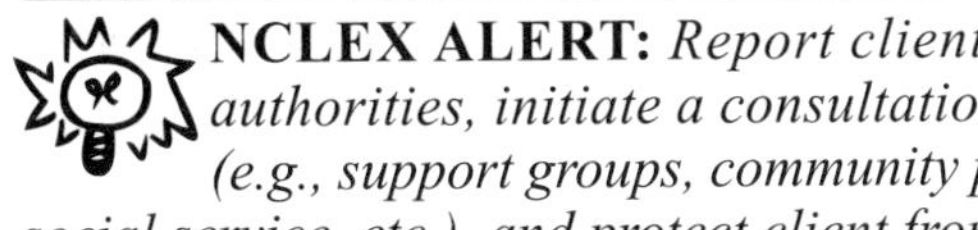

NCLEX ALERT: *Report client abuse to authorities, initiate a consultation/referral (e.g., support groups, community programs, social service, etc.), and protect client from injury.*

Types of Abuse

A. ***Physical abuse***—non-accidental, intentional injury inflicted on another person.

B. ***Physical neglect***—willing deprivation of essential care needed to sustain basic human needs and to promote growth and development.

C. ***Emotional abuse***—use of threats, verbal insults, or other acts of degradation that are intended to be injurious or damaging to another's self-esteem.

D. ***Emotional neglect***—absence of a warm, interpersonal atmosphere that is necessary for psychosocial growth, development, and the promotion of positive feelings of self-worth and self-esteem.

E. ***Sexual abuse***—lack of comprehension and consent on the part of the individual involved in sexual activities that are either exploitative or physically intimate in nature (e.g., fondling, oral or genital contact, masturbation, unclothing, etc).

F. ***Incest***—sexual activity performed between members of a family group.

Intrafamily Abuse and Violence

Patterns of dysfunctional, violent families can frequently be traced back for several generations. Adult behavior and role models for parenting are influenced by the childhood experiences within the family system.

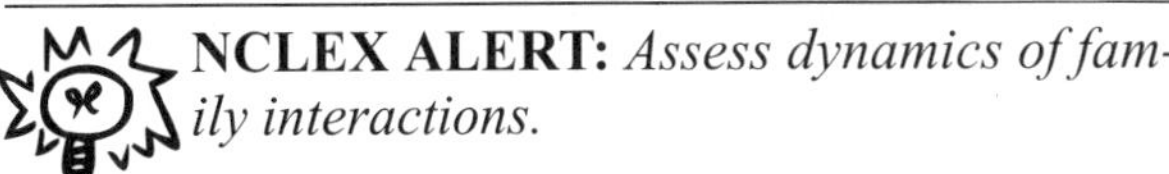

NCLEX ALERT: *Assess dynamics of family interactions.*

A. The incorporation of violence within the family teaches the children that the use of violence is appropriate. When the children grow up and form their own families, they tend to recreate the same parent-child, husband-wife relationships experienced in their original family.

B. Frequently, the abuser has inappropriate expectations of family members, who may expect perfection and may be obsessed with discipline and control.

C. Family members are confused regarding their role in the family; parents may be unable to assume an adult role in the family. Adult family members who feel inadequate in their role may use violence in an attempt to prove themselves and to maintain superiority.

D. Family is usually isolated, both physically and emotionally. The family tends to have few friends, and frequently is isolated from the extended family. Family members are ashamed of what is occurring and tend to withdraw from social contacts in fear that the family activities might become known to others.

Characteristics of Abuse

A. The person who abuses.
   1. Inability to control impulses; explosive temper; low tolerance for frustration.
   2. Possesses greater physical strength than the victim.
   3. Low self-esteem.
   4. Tends to project shortcomings and inadequacies onto others.
   5. Emotional immaturity; decreased capacity to delay satisfaction.
   6. Suspicious of everyone; fear of being exposed; tend to isolate themselves from their families.
   7. High incidence of drug and alcohol abuse.

B. Victim.
   1. Low self-esteem and depression.
   2. Experiences feelings of dependency, helplessness, or powerlessness.
   3. Client has experienced abuse as a child; there is a greater tendency to demonstrate violence in his adult relationships.
   4. Feels responsible for abuse or neglect that is inflicted upon him; may feel guilty that he is at fault—called *hostage response*.

Table 9-6: DOCUMENTATION FOR SUSPECTED ABUSE

Procedure:

1. Obtain the client's or parent's permission before photographing the victim.
2. Do not make assumptions as to whom the assailant or abuser was; chart the exact client/child's words used to describe the abuser.
3. Record information very objectively; do not record your feelings, assumptions, or opinions of the incident or how it occurred.

History:

1. Specific time, date, and location the client says the incident occurred.
2. Reported sequence of events prior to the abuse/attack.
3. Period of time between the abuse/attack and initiation of medical attention.
4. Presence of other people/children in the immediate vicinity of the abuse/attack.
5. Include verbal quotations from the client.
6. Be very specific and objective in recording observations of the client and the person who brought the client to the emergency room; observe and record the interaction of the child and the parents.

Physical Examination:

1. Be very specific in describing the location, size, shape of bruises and lacerations. If possible, photograph the client to demonstrate the extent of the injury.
2. If possible, describe the location and extent of injuries on an anatomical diagram.
3. Identify presence of other injuries.
4. Describe the victim's reaction to pain, level of pain and location of pain.

C. Common similarities between person who abuses and victim.

1. Poor self-concept and feelings of insecurity.
2. Feelings of helplessness, powerlessness, and dependence.
3. Difficulty or inability to handle anger.

Child Abuse

A. Child neglect—the failure to provide for the child the basic necessities; may be classified as physical or emotional neglect.

1. Failure to thrive—infant or child is not within the normal ranges on the growth chart.
2. Infant or child does not appear to be physically cared for. Inappropriate diapering, diaper rash, strong urine smell to the body may be seen in infants who have been neglected.
3. Evidence of malnutrition.
4. Lack of adequate supervision; child is allowed to engage in dangerous play activities, and sustains frequent injuries.
5. Language development may be delayed.
6. Withdrawal; inappropriate fearfulness.
7. Parents may be apathetic and unresponsive to the child's needs. The nurse is most often able to observe the parent-child interaction in school situations, doctor's office, or in the emergency room.

B. Physical child abuse.

1. Symptoms.
   a. Bruises and welts from being beaten with a belt, strap, stick, coat hanger, or from being slapped repeatedly in the face.
   b. Rope burns from being tied up or beaten with a rope.
   c. Human bite marks.
   d. Burns.
      (1) Burns on the buttocks from being immersed in hot water.
      (2) Pattern of burns—round, small burns from cigarettes; patterns that suggest an object was used.
      (3) Burns frequently are on the buttocks, in genital area, or on the soles of the feet.
   e. Evidence of various fractures in different stages of healing.
   f. Internal injuries from being hit repeatedly in the abdomen.
   g. Head injuries—skull, facial fractures.
2. Behavior symptoms.
   a. Withdrawal from physical contact with adults.
   b. Inappropriate response to pain or injury; failure to cry or seek comfort from parents.
   c. Infant may stiffen when held; child may stiffen when approached by adult or parent.
   d. Very little eye contact with adults.
   e. Child may try to protect abusing parent for fear of punishment if abuse is discovered.
3. Parent or caretakers.

a. Conflicting stories regarding accident or injury.
b. Explanation of accident is inconsistent with injuries sustained (fractured skull and broken leg from falling out of bed).
c. Initial complaint is not associated with child's injury (child is brought to the ER with complaints of the "flu," and there is evidence of a skull fracture).
d. Exaggerated concern or lack of concern related to level of child's injury.
e. Refusal to allow further tests or additional medical care.
f. Lack of nurturing response to injured or ill child; no cuddling, touching, or comforting child in distress.
g. Repeated visits to various medical emergency facilities.
h. Do not have realistic expectations of the child; do not understand stages of growth and development (severely spanking or beating a 1-year-old for lack of response to toilet training).

Nursing Intervention

✦ *Goal: to establish a safe environment.*

1. It is important for the nurse to be knowledgeable of the legal responsibilities in regard to state practice acts and child abuse laws (See Table 9-6: Documentation for Suspected Abuse).
2. All fifty states have a designated agency that is available on a 24-hour basis for reporting child abuse.
3. All states have mechanism for removing the child from the immediate abusive environment.

✦ *Goal: to educate the parents and help them identify assistance for long-term supportive care.*

1. Educate parents in regard to normal growth and development of children, the role of discipline, and the necessity for having realistic expectations.
2. Become familiar with available community resources such as crisis centers, crisis hotlines, parent effectiveness training groups, Parents Anonymous groups, etc.

Incest

A. Assessment.

1. Victim is usually female; perpetrator of abuse is primarily male, usually between ages 30 and 50, and often the victim's father or other member of the immediate family.
2. Incest is a symptom of severe dysfunction in an individual and within the family.
3. Perpetrators of sexual exploitation.
   a. Emotionally dependent men.

Box 3-1: Elderly Care Focus
Elder Abuse

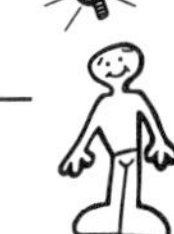

➸ *Types of elder abuse*

- Physical—willful infliction of injury.
- Neglect—withholding goods or services (such as food or attention) to the detriment of the elder's physical or mental health.
- Psychological—withholding affection or imposing social isolation.
- Exploitation—dishonest or inappropriate use of the older person's property, money, or other resources.

➸ *Neglect indicators*

- Poor hygiene, nutrition, and skin integrity.
- Contractures.
- Urine burns/excoriation.
- Pressure ulcers.
- Dehydration.

   b. Feelings of inferiority and low self-esteem.
   c. Frequently seduce their victims by being endearing and "good" to the child.
   d. Often, these men are the pillars of the community and are involved in many youth activities.
   e. Frequently, the mother is unaware of the problem. If she suspects it, she may feel guilty for having such ideas.
4. Sexually exploited child.
   a. Child may fear retaliation if anyone finds out, may fear that she will not be believed if she tells anyone.
   b. Child may feel guilty for participating in the sexual activity and afraid of disruption of the family if it is revealed.
   c. Violence rarely accompanies the incest relationship.
   d. The child may be emotionally and physically dependent on the abusing parent.

Nursing Intervention

✦ *Goal: to educate children that their bodies belong to themselves and are private.*

1. Instruct them to report any type of touching, fondling, or caressing which makes them feel uncomfortable.
2. Provide educational material to assist parents in their discussion with their children about sexual assault and inappropriate fondling.

✦ *Goal: to support the parents and the child, and help them identify assistance for long-term supportive care.*

1. Provide support and the opportunity for the child and family member to discuss their feelings.

Table 9-7: CHECKLIST OF NURSING MANAGEMENT FOR RAPE VICTIM

✓ **MEDICAL—LEGAL:** ▪ Valid written consent for examination, photographs, lab tests, release of information, and laboratory samples. ▪ Appropriate "chain of evidence" documentation — follow agency protocol. ▪ Protect legal rights.	✓ **DOCUMENT HISTORY:** ▪ Age, marital status, and parity. ▪ Menstrual and contraceptive history. ▪ Time of last coitus prior to assault. ▪ Change of clothes, bath, douche? ▪ Use of drugs or alcohol. ▪ Who, what, when, where. ▪ Penetration, ejaculation, condom, extragenital acts.
✓ **ASSIST WITH PHYSICAL EXAMINATION:** ▪ Vital signs and general appearance. ▪ Examine for extragenital trauma -mouth, breasts, neck. ▪ Examine for cuts, bruises, scratches - photograph. **Pelvic Examination**: ▪ Vulvar trauma, erythema, hymen, anal, and rectal status. ▪ Matted hair or free hairs. ▪ Vaginal examination -unlubricated speculum; foreign body, discharge, blood, lacerations; uterine size; adnexa, especially hematomas.	✓ **OBTAIN LABORATORY SAMPLES**—use appropriate *evidence collection kits* and label carefully. ▪ Saline irrigation of vagina - 2 cc and swab; acid phosphatase, blood groups antigen of semen, and precipitin test against human sperm and blood. ▪ Vaginal smears - Pap and Gram stain. ▪ Oral or rectal swabs and smears. ▪ Blood tests for serology, blood type, alcohol level. ▪ Cultures - cervix plus other areas, if indicted. ▪ Urine -pregnancy test, drugs. ▪ Hair - comb and clip; obtain fingernail scrapings; comb pubic hairs; clip client's pubic hair or any matted hairs.
✓ **IMPLEMENT MEDICAL TREATMENT:** ▪ Care for injuries and emotional trauma. ▪ Antibiotic prophylaxis for STD. ▪ Antipregnancy measures—postcoital dose of **Ovral**.	✓ **FOLLOW-UP AND REFERRAL** ▪ Recommend continued follow-up and services of rape crisis center. ▪ Repeat serology testing for gonorrhea, chlamydia, and HIVat later date.

2. Assist the family to identify community resources, and strongly encourage involvement in family counseling.

Elder Abuse

A. Types of elder abuse (See Elderly Care Focus: Box 9-1).

B. Typical victim.

1. Woman of advanced age with few social contacts.
2. At least one physical or mental impairment that limits its ability to perform ADL's.

C. Assessment of elder abuse.

1. Symptoms—contusions, abrasions, sprains, burns, bruising, human bit marks, sexual molestation, untreated but previously treated conditions, erratic hair loss from hair pulling, fractures, dislocations, head and face injuries (especially orbital fractures, black eyes, and broken teeth).
2. Behavior—clinging to the abuser, extreme guardedness in the presence of the abuser, wariness of strangers, expression of ambivalence toward family/caregivers, denial of abuse for fear of retaliation, depression, social or physical isolation.

Nursing Management

✦ *Goal: to assess for elder abuse.*

1. Use a private setting for interviewing victim and perpetrator.
2. Essential that interview be accurate, documented, and unbiased.
3. Avoid signs of disapproval that might evoke shame or anger in the older client, be nonjudgmental

✦ *Goal: to establish a safe environment.*

1. It is important for the nurse to be knowledgeable of the legal responsibilities in regard to state practice acts and reporting of abuse laws (See Table 9-6: Documentation for Suspected Abuse).
2. Client and family teaching in the areas of nutrition, general physical care, etc.

Spouse Abuse

A. Most often the spouse abused is the wife; frequently the violence is a pattern in the woman's life. The violence in the family is frequently associated with alcohol; often, there is a history of the woman's parents having a violent relationship.

B. It is not uncommon that the husband or the abuser was exposed to violent family dynamics during his childhood.

C. After the violent attack, the husband is frequently remorseful, kind and loving. He may promise that he will never do it again.

D. Women tend to stay in abuse situations. Fear retaliation, loss of home and children, and more abuse should they try to escape the situation. Abuse may increase, if they express a desire to become more independent.

Physical Assessment

1. Traumatic injury to the upper body, especially the face and the breasts.
2. Signs of fear and an expression of helplessness.
3. May avoid friends and family for fear they will find out.
4. May exhibit feelings of shame, guilt, and embarrassment that she has to seek treatment of her injuries.

Nursing Intervention

✦ *Goal: primary prevention-education of the community regarding the risks of abuse.*

✦ *Goal: secondary prevention-screening activities that occur within the community.*

✦ *Goal: teritary prevention-emergency treatment, counseling, and work that goes on in shelters.*

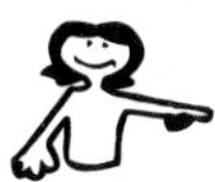

NURSING PRIORITY: *When working with an abused woman, avoid anything that sounds like blaming her for her situation.*

Rape

A. Legal definition of rape varies from state to state—forced, violent, sexual attack on an individual without his/her consent. Includes sex acts other than forced intercourse as rape; some states do not recognize rape by the husband.

B. Sexual assault is not a means of sexual gratification; it is a violent physical and emotional attack. Men attack women in an attempt to demonstrate their power and dominance; attempt to control, terrify, and degrade the woman.

C. Victims—in all age ranges; highest risk age group is 12 to 20 years old.

D. Majority of rapes are not sudden and impulsive, but they are well-planned.

E. Most women know the rapist; most rape assaults occur between people of the same race.

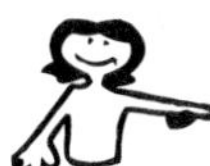

NURSING PRIORITY: *Five components essential in treating rape victim—treat and document injuries, treat and evaluate for STDs, evaluate and prevent pregnancy risk, arrange for follow-up counseling, and collect evidence according to protocols.*

Physical Assessment

1. Woman may experience a wide range of emotional responses—fear, shock, disbelief, anger, denial, guilt, embarrassment, etc. No "normal response."
2. Complete physical assessment—(Table 9-7).
3. Advise the woman to not "clean up," as the physical evidence may be destroyed, and to come immediately to the emergency room.

Nursing Intervention

✦ *Goal: to assist the client through the initial phase after the rape experience.*

1. Encourage the client to verbalize her feelings regarding the attack.
2. Assist her to set priorities and immediate needs.
3. Warm, respectful, accepting response from the nurse; protect the client from becoming overwhelmed and distressed from the initial physical examination and questioning.
4. Discuss need for follow-up care and physical examination regarding possible pregnancy and sexually transmitted disease.
5. Provide information regarding physical and emotional responses to rape.
6. Provide referral information and plan for follow-up contact within the next week.

✦ *Goal: to assist the client to work through the emotional phases that commonly occur after the initial trauma.*

1. Encourage mental health counseling the first few days after the assault.
2. Assist the client to understand and recognize the period of reorganization which frequently follows the sexual attack.
   a. Victim may experience sexual problems.
   b. May experience a strong urge to discuss the incident and feelings related to the attack.
   c. During the reorganization phase, client should have professional counseling to assist her to positively cope with the situation.⌘

Study Questions—Psychiatric Concepts

1. The mother of a 23-month-old client works in a factory at night and says if she misses any more work she will be fired. She is worried about leaving the child in the hospital at night because he is so young. What would be an appropriate nursing response?

① "He is really too young to suffer any untoward consequences."
② "It's okay to leave; just leave a favorite toy."
③ "It would be better if you could stay, but we will take good care of him."
④ "You will have a lot of expenses in the future, so you had better go to work."

2. A 9-year-old client with leukemia asks, "Will I die?" What is an initial therapeutic response based on the needs of the dying child?

① "Think about getting well instead of dying."
② "Tell me what you are thinking about dying."
③ "You need to ask your doctor."
④ "I really don't know."

3. In response to information that a 5-year-old's death is imminent, the parents express intense anger at the staff, and they are critical of the care he is receiving. What is the purpose of therapeutic intervention on the parents' behalf?

① Assure them that the doctor will be told about their concerns.
② Determine their attitude toward the child's impending death.
③ Inform them that their behavior will upset their child.
④ Allow them to express their emotions about his dying.

4. During a client care conference, there is a discussion regarding the anxiety of a 9-year-old client with leukemia. In addition to anxiety related to his death, what else might the child also experience anxiety about?

① Concerns about missing school.
② Fear of separation from his family.
③ Concerns about being dependent on staff.
④ Knowledge of the disease process.

5. An infant is scheduled for a pyloromyotomy. The mother begins to cry and says "I'm such a bad mother." What is an appropriate response by the nurse?

① "Tell me what makes you think you are a bad mother."
② "Don't cry, your baby will be fine."
③ "You are really having a bad time, aren't you?"
④ The nurse says nothing and puts her arms around the mother.

6. In order for a terminally ill client to receive quality nursing care, the head nurse needs to plan for which of the following when she assigns staff to care for the client?

① Daily change the staff nurses assigned to the client.
② Assign the same full-time staff nurses every day.
③ Use part-time nursing staff.
④ Assign a different staff nurse every other day.

7. During an intake interview on a psychiatric unit, the client makes numerous positive comments about her deceased husband, saying he was perfect. She sometimes speaks of him as if he were still alive. She told the nurse she has been depressed on and off since her husband's death three years ago. What is the client's behavior suggestive of?

① Initiating a healthy grieving process.
② Experiencing a distorted grief reaction.
③ Experiencing a delayed grief reaction.
④ Evidencing successful resolution of the grieving process.

8. Which is an appropriate initial nursing measure in caring for a female who has been raped?

① Cleanse body wounds and apply cool compresses.
② Obtain written informed consent for examination.
③ Determine if the woman has bathed or douched.
④ Obtain laboratory specimens.

9. When a child feels responsible for the physical abuse inflicted, the nurse knows the child is experiencing which of the following?

① Fear.
② Hostage response.
③ Anxiety response.
④ Guilt.

10. A nurse case worker suspects elder neglect. What assessment findings would confirm this?

① Confusion and disorientation.
② Recent hip fracture.
③ Poor nutrition and hygiene.
④ Dirty dishes in the sink.

Answers and rationales to these questions are in the section at the end of the book entitled "Chapter Study Questions: Answers & Rationales."

Appendix 9-1: UNDERSTANDING DEFENSE MECHANISMS

NAME OF DEFENSE MECHANISM	DEFINITION	EXAMPLE
Compensation	Attempting to make up for or offset deficiencies, either real or imagined by, concentrating on or developing other abilities	An unattractive girl emphasizes and cultivates intellectual abilities and is on the A honor roll at school.
Conversion	Symbolic expression of intrapsychic conflict expressed in physical symptoms	A man develops blindness after watching his friend get seriously injured in a race car accident.
Denial	Blocking out or disowning painful thoughts or feelings	An young mother with a newborn who has cleft lip tells her friends that everything is okay with her baby.
Displacement	Feelings are transferred, redirected, or discharged from the appropriate person or object to a less threatening person or object	A man gets reprimanded by his boss. Later, he yells at his wife when dinner is not ready.
Dissociation	Separating and detaching an idea, situation, or relationship from its emotional significance; helps individual put aside painful feelings and often leads to a temporary alteration of consciousness or identity	A young adolescent has amnesia surrounding a traumatic air plane crash in which she was a survivor.
Identification	Attempting to pattern or resemble the personality of an admired, idealized person	A young man chooses to become a professional football player like his father.
Introjection	Acceptance of another's values and opinions as one's own	A man who likes the country type style of living assumes the cosmopolitan.
Projection	Attributing one's own unacceptable feelings and thoughts to others	A young business woman who thinks all the women in her office want to take over her job.
Rationalization	Attempting to justify or modify unacceptable needs and feelings to the ego, in an effort to maintain self-respect and prevent guilt feelings	A man cheats on his wife and tells himself is okay because his friends cheat on their wives.
Reaction Formation	Assuming attitudes and behaviors that one consciously rejects	A man is extremely polite and courteous to his mother-in-law, whom he intensely dislikes.
Regression	Retreating to an earlier, more comfortable level of adjustment	A young preschool child begins to suck his thumb and wet the bed shortly after the birth of a sibling.
Repression	An involuntary, automatic submerging of painful, unpleasant thoughts and feelings into the *unconscious*	A woman is unable to remember a suicide attempt.
Sublimation	Diversion of unacceptable instinctual drives into personally and socially acceptable areas to help channel forbidden impulses into constructive activities	A man who has strong competitive or aggressive drives channels his energy into building a successful business.
Suppression	Intentional exclusion of forbidden ideas and anxiety producing situations from the *conscious* level; a voluntary forgetting and postponing mechanism	A young man is thinking so much about his date that it is interfering with his work. He decides to put it out of his mind till he leaves the office.
Undoing	Actually or symbolically attempting to erase a previous consciously intolerable experience or action; an attempt to repair feelings and actions that have created guilt and anxiety	A mother who has just punished her child unjustly decides to bake the child's favorite cookies.

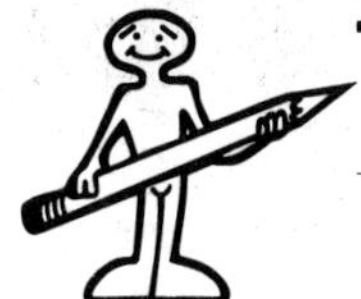

Notes

NCLEX ALERT: *Modify approaches to care in accordance with client's development stages.*

It is important to note that emotional disturbances must be evaluated within the context and framework of normal growth and development, since behavior that is acceptable at one age may be a symptom of a pathology at another age.

CHILD-RELATED DISORDERS

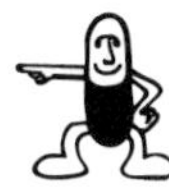

Mental Retardation

❑ **A child who is mentally retarded has an IQ of seventy or below, which is associated with deficits or impairments in adaptive behavior before the age of eighteen.**

Assessment

A. Causes.
   1. Down syndrome.
   2. Phenylketonuria (PKU).
   3. Rubella.
   4. Kernicterus (elevated bilirubin).
   5. Anoxia.
   6. Lead poisoning.
   7. Meningitis-encephalitis.
   8. Neoplasms.
   9. Tay-Sachs disease.

B. Diagnostic criteria.
   1. IQ below seventy.
   2. Deficit or impairment in adaptive behavior.
   3. Present before the age of eighteen.

C. Additional characteristics.
   1. Irritability, temper tantrums, stereotyped movements.
   2. Multiple neurological abnormalities-dysfunction with vision, hearing, or seizure activity.

Nursing Intervention

✦ *Goal: to promote optimum development within a family and community setting.*
   1. Promote feelings of self-esteem, worth, and security.
   2. Educate the parent regarding developmental age; deal with child's developmental, not chronological, age.

✦ *Goal: to promote independence by setting realistic goals.*
   1. Teach basic skills in simple terms, with steps outlined.
   2. Utilize behavior modification as a method for behavior control.
   3. Utilize the principles of *repetition, reinforcement,* and *routine* when providing information for understanding and learning.

Down Syndrome

❑ ***Down syndrome* is a common chromosomal abnormality characterized by an extra chromosome 21 (trisomy 21); incidence increases with maternal age.**

Assessment

A. Physical characteristics criteria.
   1. Head: small in size; face has flat profile, sparse hair.
   2. Eyes: inner epicanthal folds; short and sparse eyelashes.
   3. Nose: small and depressed nasal bridge (saddle nose).
   4. Ears: small and sometimes low-set.
   5. Mouth: protruding tongue; high arched palate.
   6. Neck: short and broad.
   7. Abdomen: protruding.
   8. Genitalia: small penis, cryptorchidism.
   9. Hands: short, stubby fingers; simian crease (transverse palmar crease).
   10. Muscles: hypotonic.

B. Mental characteristics.
   1. Mental retardation.
   2. Slow development.

Nursing Intervention

✦ *Goal: to promote optimal development.*
   1. Involve child and parent in early stimulation program.
   2. Promote self-care skills.
   3. Help parents identify realistic goals for child.
   4. Encourage parents to enroll child in special day care programs and education classes.
   5. Emphasize to parent that child has same needs of play, discipline, and social interaction as do other children.

Home-Care
   1. Prevent respiratory infections by teaching parents about postural drainage and percussion.

2. Encourage use of cool mist vaporizer.
3. Stress importance of changing infant's position frequently.
4. Explain to parents about feeding difficulties; encourage small, frequent feedings; feed solid food by pushing food back inside of mouth; provide foods that will form bulk to prevent constipation.
5. Discuss with parents options to home care.

✦ *Goal: to prevent Down syndrome.*

1. Encourage pregnant women at risk (over thirty-five years, family history of Down, or previous birth of a child with Down syndrome) to consider amniocentesis prior to the sixteenth week, to rule out Down syndrome.

Attention-Deficit Hyperactivity Disorder

❑ ***Attention deficit hyperactivity disorder* is a developmental disorder characterized by inappropriate inattention and impulsivity, which usually appears by age 3. Names previously used: hyperkinetic syndrome, minimal brain damage, minimal brain dysfunction, MBD.**

Assessment

A. Diagnostic criteria.
1. Inattention—child demonstrates at least three of the following:
   a. Fails to finish things he/she starts.
   b. Often doesn't seem to listen.
   c. Easily distracted.
   d. Has difficulty concentrating.
   e. Has difficulty sticking to play activity.
2. Impulsivity—child demonstrates at least three of the following:
   a. Often acts before thinking.
   b. Shifts excessively from one activity to another.
   c. Has difficulty organizing work.
   d. Needs a lot of supervision.
   e. Frequently calls out in class.
   f. Has difficulty awaiting turn in games or group activities.
3. Hyperactivity—child demonstrates at least two of the following:
   a. Runs about or climbs on things excessively.
   b. Has difficulty sitting still or fidgets excessively.
   c. Has difficulty staying seated.
   d. Moves about excessively during sleep.
   e. Is always "on the go."
4. Onset before the age of seven.
5. Duration of at least six months.

B. Additional characteristics.
1. Obstinacy.
2. Negativism.
3. Mood lability.
4. Low frustration tolerance.
5. Soft neurological signs—motor perceptual dysfunctions (e.g., poor eye-hand coordination).
6. EEG abnormalities.

Nursing Intervention

✦ *Goal: to protect the child from harm to self and others.*

1. Assist child to recognize when anger occurs and to accept feelings.
2. Teach child appropriate expression of angry feelings.
3. Redirect violent behavior with physical outlets for child's anxiety,(i.e. punching bag, jogging).
4. Confront child, withdraw attention when interactions with others are manipulative or exploitative.
5. Time-out, isolation room, and restraints when other interventions are unsuccessful.

✦ *Goal: to encourage age-appropriate, socially acceptable coping skills.*

1. If hyperactive, make environment safe for continuous large muscle movement.
2. Provide large motor activities for child to participate in.
3. Provide frequent, nutritious snacks for child to "eat on the run."

✦ *Goal: to decrease anxiety and increase self-esteem.*

1. Encourage child to seek out staff to discuss true feelings.
2. Offer support during increased anxiety; assure physical and psychological safety.

✦ *Goal: to administer prescribed drug medication.*

1. **Ritalin** may be used—usually discontinued when child enters adolescence.
2. Prolonged administration may produce a temporary suppression of normal weight gain. Child is often off medication during summer months when school is out.
3. Administer in morning (to prevent insomnia) and 30-45 minutes before meals.

Autistic Disorder

❑ **The lack of responsiveness to other people (autism), lack of involvement with others, lack of verbal communication, preoccupation with inanimate objects, and ritualistic behavior are characteristic of *infantile autism*.**

Assessment

A. Diagnostic criteria.

1. Onset before thirty months of age.
2. Lack of responsiveness and involvement with others.
3. Gross deficits in language development—speech characterized by echolalia, parrot speech, the automatic repetition of words, and pronominal reversal (the tendency to use *you* for *I*).
4. Bizarre responses to the environment.
5. *Absence* of delusions, hallucinations, and associative looseness— characteristics of childhood schizophrenia.

B. Additional characteristics.

1. Mood lability.
2. Under or over responsive to sensory stimuli.
3. Rocking or rhythmic body movements.

Nursing Intervention

✦ *Goal: to increase social awareness.*

1. Encourage a significant one-to-one relationship with an adult.
2. Promote and engage in peer interaction.
3. Develop play and self-care skills.
4. Do not force interactions. Begin with positive reinforcement for eye contact. Gradually introduce touch, smiling, hugging.

✦ *Goal: to teach verbal communication.*

1. Respond to verbalization by telling child what you do not understand.
2. Respond to nonverbal cues with verbal interpretation.
3. Observe and record context in which unclarity of spoken word occurred.
4. Use "en face" approach (face-to-face, eye-to-eye) to convey correct nonverbal expressions by example.

✦ *Goal: to decrease unacceptable behavior.*

1. Encourage child to recognize and respond to own physiological needs and urges.
2. Encourage verbalization of body needs, but do not make an issue of it.
3. Offer fluids and encourage exercise to prevent constipation.
4. Offer the bathroom at appropriate intervals throughout the day.
5. Prevent child from hurting himself or others by setting firm limits and recognizing his feelings of anger, fear, or frustration.

Separation Anxiety Disorder

❑ **Child demonstrates persistent and excessive anxiety on separation from parent or familiar surroundings.**

Assessment

A. Diagnostic criteria.

1. Unrealistic worry about harm occurring.
2. Sleep difficulties—repeated nightmares, somnambulism, and insomnia.
3. Complaints of physical symptoms on school days (e.g., stomach ache, vomiting, headache, etc.).
4. Social withdrawal, apathy, or sadness.

B. Additional characteristics.

1. Fear of the dark.
2. Excessive conformity; often demonstrates need for constant attention; may be demanding.
3. Usual age of onset is around eleven or twelve.

Nursing Intervention

✦ *Goal: to reduce the level of anxiety-provoking situations.*

1. Identify factors that produce anxiety.
2. Turn night-lights on to allay night fears.
3. Offer calm reassurance.

✦ *Goal: to differentiate between normal separation anxiety, which is seen in early childhood, and excessive anxiety, which is seen in separation anxiety disorders.*

1. To be labeled as a separation anxiety disorder, the disturbance must be of a duration of at least two weeks.
2. Children with this disorder tend to come from families that are close-knit.

Specific Disorders With Physical Symptoms

Assessment

A. Stuttering.

1. Frequent repetitions or prolongations of sounds, syllables, or words.
2. Unusual hesitations and pauses that disrupt the flow of speech.
3. Speech may be very rapid or very slow.
4. Stuttering is often absent during singing or talking to inanimate objects.

B. Functional enuresis.

1. Repeated involuntary voiding of urine during the day or night.

2. The involuntary voiding occurs after the age at which it is expected and is not due to any physical disorder.

C. Functional encopresis (fecal incontinence).
   1. Repeated voluntary or involuntary passage of feces of normal consistency in inappropriate places.
   2. Smearing feces should be differentiated from the smearing that takes place involuntarily and in the younger child (ages one or two).

Nursing Intervention

✦ *Goal: to assess and medically evaluate for any physiological cause related to stuttering, enuresis, or encopresis.*

✦ *Goal: to promote a positive self-concept by helping child overcome feelings of shame and guilt associated with disorder.*

✦ *Goal: to identify various approaches to controlling enuresis.*
   1. Administer **Tofranil**.
   2. Restrict fluids before going to bed.
   3. Encourage behavioral intervention therapies (a buzzer that wakes child when he/she starts to urinate; bladder training programs).

✦ *Goal: to identify various approaches to controlling fecal incontinence.*
   1. If retaining feces, bowel-cleaning regimen.
   2. If loose stools, needs a daily bulk laxative.
   3. If deliberate soiling, help child to express feelings through other means.
   4. Educate child about bodily signals (rectal pressure).
   5. Teach child to sit on toilet for 10-15 minutes after eating to establish regular elimination pattern.

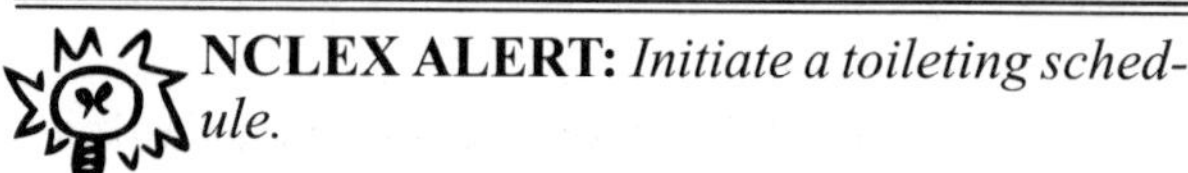

NCLEX ALERT: *Initiate a toileting schedule.*

Specific Developmental Disorders

Assessment

A. Developmental reading disorder.
   1. Impairment in the development of reading skills.
   2. Often referred to as *dyslexia*.
   3. Slow reading speed and reduced comprehension.

B. Developmental arithmetic disorder—impairment in the development of arithmetic skills.

C. Developmental language disorder.
   1. Characterized by three major types.
      a. Failure to acquire any language.
      b. Acquired language disability.
      c. Delayed language acquisition.
   2. Often the result of trauma or a neurological disorder.

Nursing Intervention

✦ *Goal: to identify specific developmental disorders in relationship to chronological age in preschool testing.*

✦ *Goal: to refer child to appropriate developmental program in school.*

Eating Disorders

❑ **This group of disorders is characterized by gross disturbances in eating behavior; it includes anorexia nervosa, bulimia, and pica.**

Assessment

A. Anorexia nervosa.
   1. Intense fear of becoming obese.
   2. Disturbance of body image.
   3. Weight loss of at least 25 percent of original body weight.
   4. No known physical illness.

B. Bulimia.
   1. Recurrent episodes of binge eating.
   2. Awareness that eating pattern is abnormal.
   3. Fear of not being able to stop eating voluntarily.
   4. Depressed mood and self-induced vomiting following the eating binges.

C. Pica.
   1. Persistent eating of nonnutritive substances for at least one month.
   2. Infants: eat paint, plaster, cloth.
   3. Older children: eat sand, bugs, rocks.
   4. Adults: eat chalk, starch, paper.

Nursing Intervention

✦ *Goal: to exhibit no signs or symptoms of malnutrition.*
   1. If client is unable or unwilling to maintain adequate oral intake, a liquid diet may be administered via nasogastric tube.
   2. Consult with dietitian; determine number of calories required to provide adequate nutrition and realistic weight gain.
   3. Explain to client details of behavior modification program.
   4. Sit with client during mealtimes for support and to observe amount ingested. A limit (usually 30 minutes) should be imposed on time allotted for meals.
   5. Observe client for at least 1 hour following meals.

6. Accompany to bathroom, if self-induced vomiting is suspected.
7. Strict documentation of intake and output.
8. Weigh client daily immediately upon arising and following first voiding, usually once or twice each week, but not more often to avoid focusing on weight. Always use same scale, if possible.
9. Do not discuss food or eating with client, once protocol has been established. Do, however, offer support and positive reinforcement for obvious improvements in eating behaviors.

✦ *Goal: to increase self-esteem as manifested by verbalizing positive aspects of self and exhibiting less preoccupation with own appearance, by discharge.*

1. Assist client to re-examine negative perceptions of self and to recognize positive attributes.
2. Offer positive reinforcement for independently-made decisions influencing client's life.
3. Offer positive reinforcement when honest feelings related to autonomy/dependence issues remain separated from maladaptive eating behaviors.
4. Help client to develop a realistic perception of body image and relationship with food.
5. Promote feelings of control within the environment through participation and independent decision-making.
6. Help client realize that perfection is unrealistic and explore this need with the client.
7. Help client claim ownership of angry feelings and recognize that expressing them is acceptable if done in an appropriate manner. Be an effective role model.

✦ *Goal: to identify eating disorder and rule out physiological etiology.*

✦ *Goal: to recognize anorexia nervosa as a life-threatening emergency—up to 15% of cases die of malnutrition and many are prone to suicide.*

ORGANIC MENTAL DISORDERS

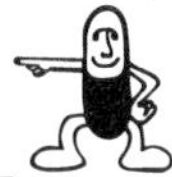

- *Organic brain syndrome* is used to refer to a constellation of psychological or behavioral signs and symptoms without reference to etiologies (e.g., delirium, dementia).
- *Organic mental disorder* designates a particular organic brain syndrome in which the etiology is known or presumed (e.g., alcohol withdrawal or delirium) (Table 10-1: Key Points—Organic Mental Syndrome).

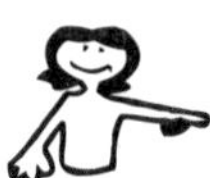

NURSING PRIORITY: The main characteristic of all these disorders is a psychological or behavioral abnormality associated with transient or permanent dysfunction of the brain. For example, metabolic disorders, substance abuse intoxications and withdrawals, and systemic illnesses tend to cause a temporary type of brain dysfunction and may be followed by complete recovery, whereas pathological processes can cause structural damage to the brain and are more likely to cause a permanent residual dysfunction or impairment.

Delirium

❑ **Delirium is a syndrome which usually develops over a short period of time. The symptom picture typically fluctuates and is often reversible and temporary.**

Assessment

A. Diagnostic criteria.
   1. A clouded state of consciousness.
   2. Memory loss for both recent and remote events; disorientation.
   3. Signs and symptoms develop over a short period of time and tend to fluctuate during the day.
   4. Confusion, hallucinations, and delusions.
   5. Sleep disturbances.
   6. Motor activity may be increased or decreased.
   7. Speech may be incoherent.
B. Additional characteristics.
   1. Emotional disturbances—anxiety, fear, depression, anger.
   2. Age at onset: common in children and after the age of sixty.
C. Etiological factors.
   1. Systemic infection—meningitis or encephalitis.
   2. Metabolic disorders—fluid/electrolyte imbalance.
      a. Hypoglycemia.
      b. Dehydration, vomiting.
   3. Hepatic or renal disease; thiamine deficiency.
   4. Drug intoxication and withdrawal.
   5. Circulatory problems associated with hypertension.
   6. Head trauma—seizure activity.

Nursing Intervention

✦ *Goal: to diminish effect of causative agent such as drugs, infectious organisms, or a circulatory-metabolic disorder.*

1. Administer medications -antipyretics, antibiotics, or sedatives.
2. Prevent further damage by assessing for possible complications.

✦ *Goal: to provide adequate nutrition.*

1. Encourage diet high in calories, protein, and vitamins, especially thiamine (B1).
2. Encourage adequate intake and output.

✦ *Goal: to prevent complications.*

1. Provide a quiet, nonstimulating environment to prevent hallucinations.
2. Assure safety needs (may fall out of bed).
3. Remove potentially harmful articles from a client's room: cigarettes, matches, lighters, sharp objects.
4. Pad side rails and headboard of client with seizure disorder.

Dementia

❑ **Dementia is a syndrome characterized by loss of intellectual abilities to such an extent that social and occupational functioning is interfered with; involves memory, judgment, abstract thought, and changes in personality. Often, the disorders are progressive and follow an irreversible course in which the damage remains permanent.**

A. Diagnostic criteria.

1. Loss of intellectual abilities that interfere with social and occupational functioning.
2. Memory impairment (JAMCO acronym for assessment).
3. Impairment in abstract thinking, judgment, and language.
4. Personality change demonstrated by exaggeration of previous personality traits.
5. Mini-Mental Status Exam show disorientation and lack of recall.

J	Judgement
A	Affect
M	Memory
C	Confusion
O	Orientation

B. Additional characteristics.

1. Anxiety or depression may be apparent.
2. Behavior may demonstrate excessive orderliness, social withdrawal, or the tendency to relate an event in excessive detail.
3. Age at onset: found predominantly in the elderly.

C. Etiological factors.

1. Neurological diseases.
   a. Huntington's chorea.
   b. Multiple sclerosis.
   c. Parkinson's disease.

Table 10-1: KEY POINTS — ORGANIC MENTAL SYNDROMES

- ✦ Clients have varying degrees of awareness of the changes that are occurring, which is emotionally painful to them.
- ✦ Often, depression is mistaken for the early onset of dementia.
- ✦ Dementia disrupts the elderly couple's final stage of family development (generativity, retirement, etc.).
- ✦ Dementia interferes with family intergenerational development where adult offspring are unable to rectify past injustices, conflicts, and disappointments with parent.
- ✦ Caregiver coping is highly stressful and can be handled in a more positive approach when there is a focus on problem-solving and education.
- ✦ Alzheimer's Disease (AD) clients have loss of: memory, intellectual functioning, orientation, affective regulation, motor coordination, and personality, with eventual loss of bowel and bladder control to the point of total incapacitation.

2. Cardiovascular disorders causing anoxia and brain damage.
   a. Cerebral arteriosclerosis.
   b. Cerebral vascular accident (CVA, stroke).
3. Central nervous system infections.
   a. Tertiary neurosyphilis.
   b. Tuberculosis and fungal meningitis.
   c. Viral encephalitis.
4. Brain trauma—chronic subdural hematoma.
5. Toxic—metabolic disturbance.
   a. Pernicious anemia.
   b. Hypothyroidism.
   c. Bromide intoxication.
   d. Wilson's disease—hepatolenticular degeneration characterized by deficient metabolism of copper.
6. Loss of brain tissue and function in presenile conditions.

***GERIATRIC PRIORITY:** The cardinal rule is: do not push too fast in getting information, assisting with activities of daily living, or insisting that the person socialize. Continued pressure and insistence on a task may result in combative behavior.*

   a. Alzheimer's disease (Table 10-2: Functional Assessment of Alzheimer's Disease).
      (1) More commonly seen in elderly geriatric clients.
      (2) Irreversible.

(3) Recent memory loss. Client can recall events and activities of 10 years ago, but not 10 minutes ago.

(4) Sundowner's syndrome—confused, disoriented behavior that becomes noticeable after the sun goes down and during the night.

(5) Wandering behavior.

(a) Restlessness and activity-seeking behavior.

(b) The "stalking of old haunts."

(6) Disorientation and inability to sustain intentions; the person forgets what she or he set out to do.

(7) Catastrophic reactions — heightened anxiety occurring during interviewing or questioning, when a person cannot answer or perform.

(8) Combative behavior.

GERIATRIC PRIORITY: *Potential situations that can lead to combative behavior are threats to self-image, new things or people in environment, illusions, pressure to remember, and direct confrontation.*

b. Pick's disease.

7. Alteration of intracranial pressure.

a. Hydrocephalus.

b. Brain tumor.

NURSING PRIORITY: *The 3 Rs—**routine, reinforcement, and repetition**—are key aspects of care, not only for the mentally retarded, but the geriatric client with dementia as well.*

Nursing Intervention

✦ *Goal: to provide a quiet, structured environment to increase consistency and promote feelings of security.*

1. Avoid dependency.
2. Establish routine for activities of daily living.
3. Meet client's physical needs.
4. Do not isolate client from others in the unit.
5. Provide handrails, walkers, and wheelchairs.
6. Do not change schedules suddenly — ***routine, reinforcement,*** and ***repetition*** are the key aspects of care.
7. Check for hazards in the environment (rugs on floor); make sure environment is well-lighted.

✦ *Goal: to promote contact with reality.*

Table 10-2: FUNCTIONAL ASSESSMENT STAGING OF ALZHEIMER'S DISEASE—FAST

Stage	Characteristics
Stage 1	—Capable of self-care.
Stage 2	—Complaint of forgetting locating of objects. —Subjective work difficulties. —Capable of self-care.
Stage 3	—Decreased ability in a demanding work setting is evident to peers. —May have difficulty in traveling to new areas. —Capable of self-care regarding activities of daily living.
Stage 4	—Decreased ability to perform complex tasks, cooking, shopping, and management of finances. —Partial self-care; needs supervision and assistance.
Stage 5	—Requires assistance selecting attire. —May need to be coaxed to bathe; fear of bathing may develop. (Elders often complain of being cold when they are exposed on the way to and from the bathing or shower area. A shower could frighten a person accustomed to tub baths and vice versa.)
Stage 6	—Decreased ability to put on clothing properly and perform personal hygiene measures. —Urinary incontinence. —Fecal incontinence. —Possible seizures. —Sundowner's syndrome.
Stage 7	—Vocabulary reduced to few words, then to just one word. —Loss of ambulatory ability, ability to sit, ability to smile, and eventually to hold uphead.

Table 10-3: GROUP MODALITIES FOR ELDERLY CLIENTS

Remotivation Therapy	Reminiscing Therapy	Psychotherapy
	Purpose of Group	
Resocialize regressed and apathetic elderly clients	Share memories Increase socialization Enhance self-esteem	Alleviation of presenting psychiatric problems Promote ability to interact with others in a group Increase ability to make decisions and function more independently
	Format	
10-15 clients in a group Meet 1-2 times per week Meetings highly structured in a classroom setting Each session has a specific topic	6-8 clients in a group Meet 1-2 times per week Topics include: holidays, travel	6-12 group members Members share problems and problem-solving with each other Group meets at regularly scheduled times
	Desired Outcomes	
Increases group members' sense of reality Encourages a more objective self-image	Assists in alleviating depression Use of process of reorganization and reintegration provides an avenue for elderly to achieve a sense of identity and positive self-concept	Decreases sense of isolation Promotes new roles and re-establishes old roles Provides group support for increasing self-esteem

NCLEX ALERT: *Orient client to reality and monitor activities of a confused client. Care of the older geriatric client is often tested, especially Alzheimer's disease.*

1. Make brief and frequent contact.
2. Give feedback.
3. Supply stimulation to motivate client to engage in activities.
4. Use concrete ideas in communication.
5. Maintain reality orientation by encouraging reminiscing (Table 10-3).

NURSING PRIORITY: *Reminiscence and life review help the client resume progression through the grief process associated with disappointing life events and increase self-esteem as successes are reviewed.*

6. Orient client frequently to reality and surroundings. Allow client to have familiar objects around him or her. Use other items, such as clock, calendar, and daily schedules.
7. Use simple explanations and face-to-face interaction. Do not shout message into client's ear.
8. Allow sufficient time for client to complete projects.
9. Reinforce reality-oriented comments and to time, place, and date.

NURSING PRIORITY: *Speaking slowly and in a face-to-face position is most effective when communicating with an elderly individual experiencing a hearing loss. Visual cues facilitate understanding. Shouting causes distortion of high-pitched sounds and in some instances creates a feeling of discomfort for the client.*

✦ *Goal: to provide diversion activities that enhance self-esteem.*

1. Provide occupational therapy, physical therapy, and recreational therapy that client enjoys.
2. Maintain a flexible schedule; keep client from becoming bored and easily distracted.
3. Recognize specific accomplishments.
4. Encourage family involvement and provide emotional support.
5. Devise methods for assisting client with memory deficit. *Examples:*
   a. Name sign and picture on door identifying client's room.
   b. Identifying sign on outside of dining room door.
   c. Large clock, with oversized numbers and hands, appropriately placed.
   d. Large calendar, indicating one day at a time, with month, day, and year identified in bold print.

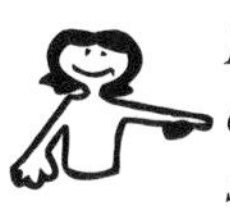

NURSING PRIORITY: The 3 Ps for clients with dementia: protecting dignity, preserving functioning, and promoting quality of life.

Anxiety Disorders

❑ **In the past, these disorders were grouped together as neuroses. Anxiety can be a predominant disturbance (panic and generalized anxiety), or anxiety is experienced as a person attempts to confront a dreaded situation (phobic disorder) or resist the obsessions and compulsions of an obsessive-compulsive disorder. In general, these are common responses to emotional problems that are very seldom treated in a psychiatric setting, since the person has neither a great defect in reality testing nor demonstrates severe antisocial behavior. Pressures of decision-making that occur in the early adult years seem to act as a precipitating event in the development of anxiety disorder (See Table 10-4: Anxiety Disorders).**

NCLEX ALERT: *Identify effects of environmental stressors on client; plan measures to deal with client's anxiety; encourage client to use problem-solving skills; teach stress reduction techniques; and provide support to client who is upset or distraught.*

Nursing Intervention

✦ *Goal: to promote techniques to reduce anxiety.*

1. Desensitization—client is exposed serially to a specific list of anxiety-provoking situations; through techniques of progressive relaxation, the client becomes desensitized to each stimulus.
2. Reciprocal inhibition—the anxiety-provoking stimulus is paired with another stimulus that is associated with an opposite feeling in order to diminish the effect of the anxiety.
3. Cognitive therapy—internal dialogue or self-talk on feelings, emotions, and behavior.
4. Regular daily exercise.
5. Other therapy—hypnosis, meditation, imagery, yoga, biofeedback training.

Somatoform Disorders

❑ **These are a group of disorders in which the person has physical symptoms suggesting a physiological etiology; however, after in-depth assessment and diagnostic testing, no organic disease or physiological abnormalities are found.**

Assessment

Types of somotoform disorders

A. Somatization disorder—recurrent, multiple complaints (from the following four areas listed below) in which medical treatment has been sought.
   1. Four pain symptoms—head, abdomen, joints, etc.
   2. Two gastrointestinal symptoms—nausea, bloating, diarrhea.
   3. One sexual symptom—sexual indifference, erectile dysfunction, abnormal menses, painful menstruation, excessive bleeding.
   4. One symptom suggesting a neurological problem—loss of sensation, blindness, double vision.

B. Conversion disorder—a loss of, or alteration in, physical functioning that suggests a physical disorder, but is related to expression of a psychological conflict or need; person appears calm while experiencing symptoms.
   1. A loss of alteration in physical function suggesting a physical disorder.
   2. Symptoms are not under voluntary control.
   3. ***La belle indifference***—an attitude toward the symptoms in which there is a lack of concern.
   4. Not a deliberate faking (malingering).
   5. "Classic conversion symptoms" usually suggest neurological disease—paralysis, aphonia, blindness, and paresthesias.

C. Pain disorder—preoccupied with pain for which there is no physical problem.
   1. Severe and prolonged pain.
   2. Pain is nonanatomical in distribution.
   3. Evidence of a stressful life situation.
   4. Complaint excessive for the observable symptoms.
   5. History of frequent visits to physician (doctor-shopping).
   6. Excessive use of analgesics without the relief of pain, along with frequent requests for surgery.

D. Hypochondriasis—distorted interpretation of existing physical signs or bodily sensations which lead the client to an unrealistic belief and a preoccupation with the fear or belief of having a serious, debilitating disease.
   1. Preoccupied with bodily functioning—focusing on heartbeat, breathing, or digestion, or on a minor aliment such as a small scratch or cough.
   2. Physical evaluation does not support the diagnosis of any physical problem.
   3. Fear or belief of having medical illness despite medical reassurance.

E. Body dysmorphic disorder—preoccupation with an imagined flaw in appearance in a normal-appearing person.

TABLE 10-4: SELECTED ANXIETY DISORDERS

Problem	Description	Nursing Intervention
Panic Disorder (with or without agoraphobia): an extreme level of anxiety.	Agoraphobia (fear of being in places or situations; crowds, traveling). May experience shortness of breath, dizziness, diaphoresis, palpitations.	**Goal: to reduce panic level anxiety feelings by reinterpreting the feelings correctly** (see Table 9-2 Panic Level of Anxiety). 1. Anticipate administration of a tricyclic antidepressant. 2. Reduce amount of caffeine in diet.
Phobia: an intense, irrational fear of a specific object, activity, or situation.	Fear of being alone or in public places. Claustrophobia (fear of close places). Acrophobia (fear of heights). Social phobia (fear of circumstances that may be humilating, e.g., speaking in public, eating in restaurants).	**Goal: to reduce phobic behavior.** 1. Do not force client to come in contact with the feared object or source of anxiety. 2. Have client focus on awareness of self. 3. Distract client's attention from phobia.
Obsessive-Compulsive Disorder: unconscious control of anxiety by the use of rituals, thoughts, obsession, or compulsions.	**Obsessions:** recurrent, persistent ideas, thoughts, or impulses that are not voluntarily produced. *Most common obsessions include thoughts of violence, contamination, and doubt.* **Compulsions:** repetitive, ritualistic behaviors that are performed in a certain fashion to relieve an unbearable amount of tension. *Most common compulsions include handwashing, counting, checking.*	**Goal: to assist in coping with the compulsive behavior.** 1. Accept rituals and avoid punishment or criticism; do not interrupt ritual, as this will increase anxiety. 2. Plan for extra time, due to slowness and client's need for perfection. 3. Prevent physical deterioration or harm, and set limits only to prevent harmful acts (such as handwashing excessively that removes the skin from the hand surface). **Goal: to encourage client to develop different ways of handling anxiety.** 1. Reduce demands on the individual. 2. Convey acceptance of client regardless of behavior. 3. Encourage alternative activity.
Post-Traumatic Stress Disorder: involves the development of characteristic symptoms following a traumatic psychological event in which the individual is unable to adapt or adjust (e.g., rape, military combat, airplane crashes, death camps, torture or abuse).	Client re-experiences the traumatic event. Client withdraws, becomes isolated and restricts emotional response. Experienes hyperalertness, insomnia, nightmares, depression and anxiety.	**Goal: to determine precipitating stress factor in client's reaction.** 1. Reduce and prevent chronic disability. 2. Encourage verbalization of the traumatic event. **Goal: to maintain personal integrity.** 1. Provide physical, social, or occupational rehabilitation. 2. Somatic therapies are used to decrease anxiety (e.g., anti-anxiety agents, etc.).
Generalized Anxiety Disorder: unrealistic or excessive anxiety and worry about life's circumstances; differs from panic disorder in that it never remits and has an early age onset.	Physical symptoms associated with disorder are restlessness, apprehension, tension, irritability, "free-floating anxiety."	**Goal: to reduce level of anxiety.** 1. Administer anti-anxiety agent. 2. Teach anxiety-reducing techniques. 3. Reduce pressure and anxiety-provoking situations around client. 4. Divert attention from symptoms.

1. Excessive concern and focus on facial defect; less commonly on other parts of the body; preoccupies and dominates client's life.
2. Social isolation and depression leading to suicidal threats and repeated hospitalizations.
3. May seek plastic surgery.

Nursing Intervention

✦ *Goal: to divert attention from preoccupation with self and symptomatology.*

1. Encourage purposeful activity that promotes interest and success.

2. Promote attitude that acknowledges personal integrity and self-worth.
3. Provide for client's physical needs as necessary.
4. Correct any misinformation and give correct information.
5. Encourage client to develop new interests and gain satisfaction from them.
6. Promote a good sense of humor.

✦ *Goal: to identify primary or secondary gain.*
1. Primary gain: symptom has symbolic meaning to client; keeps client unaware of internal conflict and anxiety.
2. Secondary gain: a gain of attention and sympathy along with reinforcement of maladjusted behavior.

✦ *Goal: to avoid secondary gains as a source of reward and reinforcement for the disorder.*
1. Focus on the individual and his/her feelings, and not on the symptoms.
2. A calm, warm, supportive approach promotes understanding and acceptance.

✦ *Goal: to avoid reinforcing the client's symptoms.*
1. Focus on feelings and not on symptoms.
2. Reduce pressure and anxiety-provoking situations around client.
3. Divert attention from symptoms.
4. Provide recreational activity.
5. Avoid pity and sympathetic approach to client's "illnesses" or "symptoms."

✦ *Goal: to be aware of personal response to the client.*
1. Recognize and understand the client's self-perception as helpless to cope.
2. Promote a nonjudgmental, understanding attitude.

✦ *Goal: to provide a supportive approach that does not focus on physical condition.*
1. Help client to understand how he/she uses illness to avoid dealing with life problems.
2. Offer empathy without sympathy.

✦ *Goal: to support alternative therapy.*
1. Behavior modification.
2. Insight-oriented psychotherapy.
3. Hypnosis.
4. Acupuncture.

Psychophysiologic Disorder

❑ **This is a physical illness that is strongly influenced by psychological factors. In previous terminology it was entitled psychosomatic disorder. It is thought that stress and anxiety arouse specific conflicts in an individual, which result in damaging effects on particular organs or organ systems that are pathophysiologically under the autonomic nervous system control. (See Figure 10-1)**

Assessment

A. Respiratory.
   1. Hyperventilation syndrome.
   2. Bronchial asthma.
B. Cardiovascular.
   1. Essential hypertension.
   2. Angina.
   3. Migraine headaches.
   4. Tachycardia.
C. Gastrointestinal.
   1. Peptic ulcer.
   2. Ulcerative colitis.
   3. Colic.
D. Integumentary.
   1. Dermatitis.
   2. Pruritus.
   3. Excessive sweating.
   4. Atopic dermatitis.
E. Musculoskeletal.
   1. Cramps.
   2. Rheumatoid arthritis.
F. Endocrine.
   1. Diabetes mellitus.
   2. Sexual dysfunctions.
   3. Hyperemesis gravidarum.
   4. Hyperthyroidism.
G. Genital/Urinary.
   1. Amenorrhea.
   2. Impotence.
   3. Secondary outbreaks of herpes genitalis Type II (HSV-2).

Nursing Intervention

Pathophysiology and nursing intervention of the above disorders are thoroughly discussed under the appropriate body system affected.

Dissociative Disorders

❑ **Involves five primary symptoms—amnesia (memory loss), derealization (objects in external environment take on a quality of unreality and estrangement), depersonalization (alteration in the perception or experience of self), identity confusion (sense of conflict, puzzlement, or uncertainty in relation to one's identity), and identity alteration (organized shift in personality that occurs without the individual's awareness).**

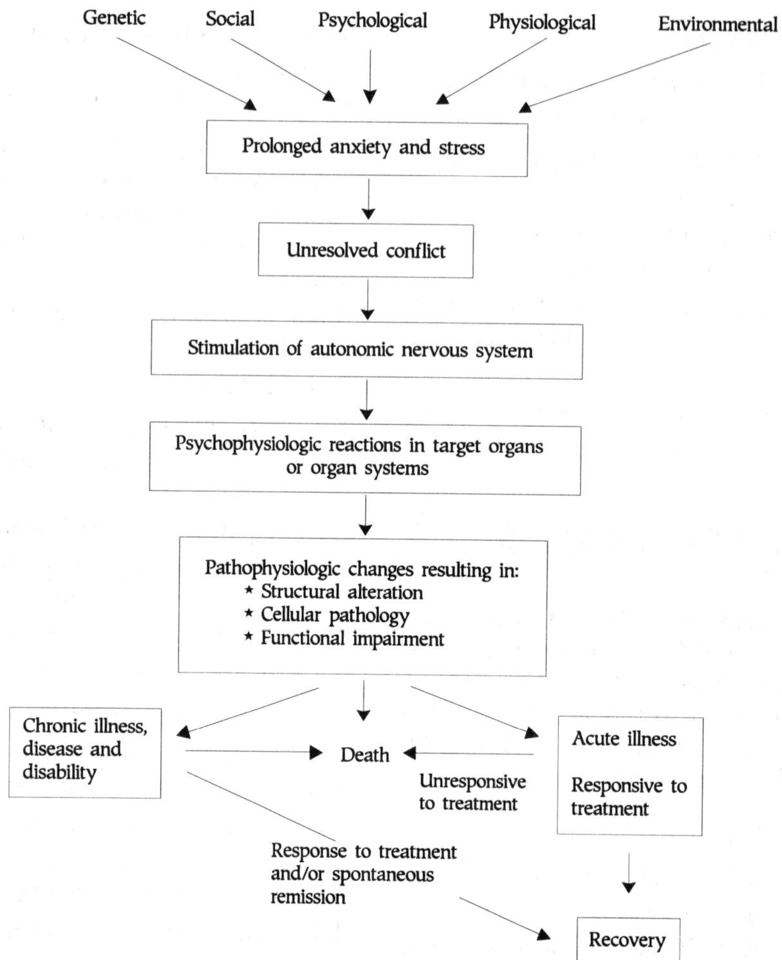

Figure 10-1: Concept of Psychopathophysiologic Disorders

Assessment

A. Dissociative amnesia.

1. A sudden inability to recall important personal information.
2. Usually begins suddenly, following severe psychosocial stress.
3. Most often observed in the adolescent and young adult female, rarely in the elderly.

B. Dissociative fugue.

1. Sudden, unexpected travel away from home with the assumption of a new identity.
2. An inability to recall one's previous identity or past.
3. No recollection of events that took place during the fugue state.

C. Dissociative identity disorder (multiple personality).

1. The existence of two or more distinct personalities, each of which determines the nature of their behavior and attitudes while uppermost in one's consciousness.
2. Transition from one personality to another is sudden and often stressful.
3. Best-known examples found in literature: Sybil and The Three Faces of Eve.

D. Depersonalization disorder.

1. An alteration in the perception of the self so that the usual sense of one's own reality is temporarily lost or changed.
2. Sensations of unreality (e.g., feelings that one's extremities have changed size).
3. Onset is rapid; disappearance is gradual.

Nursing Intervention

✦ *Goal: to assist in the ruling out that it is a physical or organic pathology which causes the dissociative disorder.*

1. Many behaviors exhibited resemble post-concussion amnesia and temporal lobe epilepsy.
2. Accurate observation and description of character, duration, and frequency of the symptoms is important.

✦ *Goal: to minimize anxiety.*

1. Redirect client's attention away from self.
2. Increase socialization activities.
3. Include family members in learning new ways to deal with client's behavior.

✦ *Goal: to provide insight into past traumatic experiences and learn new coping methods.*

1. Long-term therapy is aimed at insight into pain of past experiences and conflicts that have been repressed.
2. Encourage awareness that dissociative behaviors are reactivated by current situations that arouse emotional pain.

PERSONALITY DISORDERS

❑ **Personality disorders create disruptive lifestyles and are characterized by inflexible and maladapted behaviors. Those with personality disorders clash with society and cultural norms, and are often placed in correctional systems, mental hospitals, and child placement facilities.**

Common Characteristics

1. Problems expressed through behavior rather than as a physical symptom of stress.
2. Disruptive lifestyle is deeply ingrained and quite difficult to change; usually related to some form of abnormal behavior development of a particular pattern or trait.
3. Often comes in conflict with others.
4. Pleasure principle is dominant with inadequate superego control; has difficulty problem-solving.
5. Unable to develop meaningful relationships with others and communicate effectively.
6. Rarely acknowledges that there is a problem.

Assessment

(See Table 10-5: Personality Disorder Clusters)

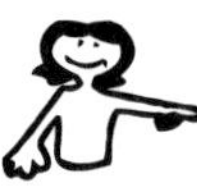

NURSING PRIORITY: *Personality disorders occur when traits become rigid and manipulative.*

Nursing Intervention

✦ *Goal: to promote communication and socialization in the paranoid personality.*

1. Decrease social isolation.
2. Verbal and nonverbal messages should be clear and consistent.
3. To decrease anxiety, plan several brief contacts rather than one prolonged contact.
4. Promote trust by following through on commitments.
5. Be open and honest to avoid misinterpretation.

✦ *Goal: to convey to the schizoid and schizotypic client the idea that you do not perceive reality the same way as he/she does but you are willing to listen, learn, and offer feedback about his/her experiences.*

✦ *Goal: to promote a positive, therapeutic, interpersonal relationship.*

1. Set realistic expectations.
2. Provide a model of mature behavior.
3. Use problem-solving technique to encourage client to make change.
4. Anticipate and deal with depression in clients who gradually develop enough insight to realize and accept responsibility for their behavior.
5. Common sources of frustration for nurses.
   a. Client's immature behavior.
   b. Poor communication skills.

✦ *Goal: to minimize manipulation and "acting out" behaviors and encourage verbal communication.*

1. Set firm, consistent limits without being punitive.
2. Be aware of how client may manipulate other staff members (e.g., playing one against the other).
3. Promote expression of feelings versus acting out.
4. Promote client's acceptance of responsibility of his/her own actions and a social responsibility to others.

NURSING PRIORITY: *Borderline clients have a tendency to cling to one staff member, if allowed, transferring their maladaptive dependency to that individual. This dependency can be avoided if client is able to establish therapeutic relationships with two or more staff members who encourage independent self-care activities.*

✦ *Goal: to assist client to manage anxiety.*

1. Anticipate client needs before they demand attention.
2. Teach client to express his/her ideas and feelings assertively.
3. Watch for signs of defensiveness, as clients are unlikely to recognize this as a mechanism of anxiety.

✦ *Goal: to set realistic limits.*

1. Break the health-attention-avoidance cycle that usually exists in relating to this type of client.
2. Support clients who are gradually making more decisions on their own.
3. Offer assistance only when needed.

Table 10-5: PERSONALITY DISORDER CLUSTERS

Cluster A	Cluster B	Cluster C
Paranoid personality: Suspicious and mistrustful of people Secretive Questions loyalty of others Jealous Overconcerned with hidden motives and special meanings Hypersensitive and alert Exaggerates Unable to relax Takes offense quickly Impaired affect Unemotional and cold No sense of humor Absence of soft, tender, sentimental feelings Distorts reality Uses projection	**Antisocial personality:** Violates rights of others Lacks responsiblity Manipulative Unable to sustain a job; frequent job changes and lengthy periods of unemployment Financial dependency Common behaviors observed— Lying, stealing, truancy Aggressive sexual behavior Sexual promiscuity Excessive drinking and drug use Criminality Vagrancy Lack of remorse	**Avoidant personality:** Fear of criticism or disapproval Hypersensitive to potential rejection View self as socially inept, personally unappealing, and inferior to others Inhibited in interpersonal relationships Reluctant to take personal risks Unwilling to get involved with people unless certain of being liked
Schizoid personality: Unable to form social relationships Cold and aloof; flat affect Indifferent to praise or criticism Has little or no desire for social involvement Appears reserved, withdrawn, and seclusive	**Borderline personality:** Unstable interpersonal relationships and moods Impulsiveness and unpredictability that may be self-damaging (e.g., spending, sex, reckless driving, drug use) Identity disturbance Recurrent suicidal behavior, gestures, or threats Self-mutilating behavior Inappropriate, intense anger; lack of anger control; shifts in mood Chronic feelings of emptiness	**Dependent personality:** Submissive; clinging behavior Fear of separation Difficulty making everyday decisions Needs others to assume responsibility Wants others to take care and nurture Feels uncomfortable or helpless when left alone Difficulty initiating projects
Schizotypal personality: Magical thinking (e.g., telepathy, superstitiousness) Ideas of reference Social isolation Recurrent illusion Oddities of thought, perception, speech, and behavior Inappropriate affect Excessive social anxiety	**Histrionic personality:** Excessive emotionality and attention-seeking Uncomfortable when not center of attention Uses physical appearance to draw attention to self Self-dramatization, theatrical, and exaggerated expression of emotion Easily suggestible **Narcissistic personality:** Grandiose self-importance Preoccupation with fantasies of success Belief that they are "special or unique" Need for excessive amount of admiration Unrealistic sense of entitlement Interpersonal exploitation Lack of empathy Arrogant and haughty	**Obsessive-compulsive personality:** Preoccupation with rules, lists, organization, schedules Perfectionistic Excessive devotion to work Overconscientious and inflexible Reluctant to delegate tasks Hoards money; frugal Rigid and stubborn in thoughts

SUBSTANCE USE DISORDERS

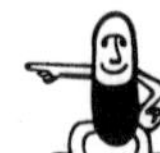

❑ ***Substance use disorders*** **are characterized by behavior changes, regular use of a substance (alcohol or drugs) which affects the central nervous system, and by withdrawal symptoms when the substance is not taken.**

❑ ***Polydrug dependence*** **involves the regular use of three or more psychoactive substances over a period of at least 6 months.**

NCLEX ALERT: *Identify signs and symptoms of substance abuse/chemical dependency.*

A. Substance abuse.
  1. A pattern of pathological use.
    a. Intoxication during the day.
    b. Inability to cut down or stop drinking.
    c. Daily need of the substance for functioning.
    d. Blackouts and medical complications from use.
  2. Impairment of social or occupational functioning.
    a. Failure to meet important obligations to friends, family, and business.
    b. Inappropriate display of erratic and impulsive behavior.
    c. Inappropriate expression of aggressive feelings.
  3. Minimum duration of at least one month of substance use.

B. Substance dependence—more severe than substance abuse; requires physiological dependence as evidenced by either tolerance or withdrawal.
  1. Tolerance.
    a. Increased amounts of the substance are required to achieve the desired effect.
    b. Markedly diminished effect with regular use of the same dose.
  2. Withdrawal—a specific syndrome of symptoms which develops when the person abruptly stops ingesting the substance.

C. Psychological dependence.
  1. Habituation—the need to take the substance.
  2. Physiological dependence not necessary.
  3. No physiological symptoms upon withdrawal.

D. Common health problems
  1. Acute problems.
    a. Poor nutritional status, loss of appetite, nausea, vomiting, and diarrhea.
    b. CNS dysfunction and irritability, seizures, tremors, motor restlessness, sensitivity to light, auditory or visual disturbances, insomnia.
    c. Susceptibility to recurrent respiratory infection.
  2. Chronic problems.
    a. Liver dysfunction, cirrhosis, pancreatitis, hypertension.
    b. Chronic brain damage and mental deterioration, poor hygiene, dermatologic changes.
    c. HIV positive.

E. Dysfunctional behavior patterns.
  1. Manipulation.

  Example: Legal difficulties, crime, physical assault, taking advantage of generosity.

  2. Impulsiveness.

  Example: Inconsistent work patterns, overdose, recklessness.

  3. Dysfunctional anger.
  4. Grandiosity.

  Example: Belief that nobody has done worse thing or has lost as much or drugged or drunk as much.

  5. Denial.
  6. Codependency—extreme emotional, social, or physical focus on another person, place, or thing.

F. Treatment modalities.
  1. Detoxification—controlled withdrawal from alcohol or drugs via a medical protocol.
  2. Drug treatment and rehabilitation—comprehensive program based on client outcomes; may include detoxification, family education, group counseling, and 12-step programs.
  3. 12-Step self-help groups—recovery built on abstinence as a daily process; requires peer support and acknowledgment that client has addiction.
  4. Drug-free residential communities—therapeutic community based on a hierarchial community structure and governance, peer support, disciplined lifestyle.
  5. Pharmacologic therapy—use of dolophine (**Methadone**) for opiate abuse to eliminate craving for drug.
  6. Psychotherapy—may be individual, group, family or a combination of all three; facilitates behavioral and lifestyle changes by dealing with personality issues and psychological conflicts.

Alcohol Dependence (Alcoholism)

❑ **A chronic pattern of pathological alcohol use is characterized by impairment in social or occupational functioning, along with tolerance or withdrawal symptoms.**

General Concepts

A. Incidence.
  1. An estimated 20 million Americans suffer from alcoholism; of those who consume alcohol, one in ten is an alcoholic.
  2. Eighty billion dollars is spent each year on alcohol-related illnesses which lead to lost wages, reduced productivity, and property damage.
  3. Chronic alcoholism shortens life span by 12 years.

B. Effects of use.
  1. ***Central nervous system depressant drug.***

2. Requires no digestion; 20 percent is absorbed unchanged from the stomach; 80 percent is absorbed from the small intestine.
3. Absorbed slowly in a full stomach.
4. Measured in the bloodstream by the blood alcohol level (BAL).
5. Can be measured within 15-20 minutes after ingestion; reaches a peak in 60 to 90 min; is completely metabolized by 12-24 hours after the last drink.
6. Decreases inhibitions and enhances mood; slows motor reactions and hence prolongs reaction time.
7. In low doses tends to increase sexual arousal, high doses decrease it.
8. Affects critical thinking, judgment, and memory.
9. Blood alcohol level of 15 percent or more is considered intoxication.

Assessment

A. Risk factors.
   1. History of alcoholism in family.
   2. History of total abstinence.
   3. Broken or disrupted home.
   4. Last or near-last child in a large family.
   5. Heavy smoking.
   6. Cultural groups: Irish, Eskimo, Scandinavian, Native American.

B. Diagnostics.
   1. Blood alcohol level (BAL).
      a. BAL determined by how much alcohol is consumed, how fast it is consumed, and body weight.
      b. The larger the person, the more alcohol he/she can tolerate.
   2. Breathalyzer.
      a. 5 to 10 percent of the alcohol is excreted through breathing.
      b. Used for monitoring the use of alcohol and to identify persons who are driving while intoxicated (DWI or DUI).
      c. Usual legal guidelines for intoxication; BAL greater than 100-150 mg percent.

C. General personality characteristics of alcoholics.
   1. Dependent behavior along with resentment of authority.
   2. Demanding, domineering, and a low tolerance for frustration.
   3. Dissatisfied with life; tendency toward self-destructive acts, including suicide.
   4. Low self-esteem and self-concept.

D. Signs and symptoms of possible alcohol abuse.
   1. Sprains, bruises, and injuries of questionable origin.
   2. Diarrhea and early morning vomiting.
   3. Chronic cough, palpitations, and infections.
   4. Frequent Monday morning illnesses; blackouts (inability to recall events or actions while intoxicated).

E. Alcohol withdrawal syndrome.
   Consuming one fifth of whiskey daily for one month is generally considered sufficient to produce alcohol withdrawal. The withdrawal syndrome develops in heavy drinkers who have increased, decreased, or interrupted the intake of alcohol.
   1. ***Alcohol withdrawal.***
      a. Anorexia, irritability, nausea, and tremulousness.
      b. Insomnia, nightmares, irritability, hyperalertness.
      c. Tachycardia, increased blood pressure, and diaphoresis.
      d. Onset within 8 hours after cessation of drinking; clears up within five to seven days.
   2. ***Delirium tremens.***
      a. Autonomic hyperactivity-tachycardia, sweating, increased blood pressure.
      b. Vivid hallucinations, delusions, confusion.
      c. Coarse, irregular tremor is almost always seen; fever may occur.
      d. Onset within twenty-four to seventy-two hours after the last ingestion of alcohol; delirium tremens usually last two to three days.
      e. Convulsions/seizures may occur ("rum fits").
      f. First episode occurs after five to fifteen years of heavy drinking.
   3. ***Alcohol hallucinosis***.
      a. Auditory hallucinations.
      b. Occurs within forty-eight hours after heavy drinking episode.
      c. Often persecutory delusions.
      d. May be potentially suicidal or homicidal.
      e. Spontaneous recovery within one week.
      f. Wernicke's encephalopathy.
         (1) An acute, *reversible* neurologic disorder.
         (2) Triad of symptoms: global confusion, ataxia, and eye movement abnormality (nystagmus).
         (3) Occurs primarily in chronic alcoholics; may develop in illnesses that interfere with thiamine (B_1) absorption (e.g., gastric cancer, malabsorption syndrome, regional enteritis).

(4) Treatment: high doses of thiamine; 100 mg IM usually reverses eye signs within two to three hours of treatment.

F. Korsakoff's Syndrome (alcohol amnesiac disorder).

1. A chronic, *irreversible* disorder, often following Wernicke's encephalopathy.
2. Triad of symptoms: memory loss, learning deficit, confabulation (filling in of memory gaps with plausible stories).

G. Other disorders associated with chronic alcoholism; esophageal varices, cirrhosis, pancreatitis, diabetes (these will be discussed in Unit 4 under the appropriate system.)

Nursing Intervention

✦ *Goal: to assess for alcoholism in client through careful questioning.*

1. Frequently used acronym suggests asking the following four questions (CAGE):
   a. Have you ever felt the need to <u>C</u>ut down on your drinking?
   b. Have you ever felt <u>A</u>nnoyed by criticism of your drinking?
   c. Have you had <u>G</u>uilty feelings about drinking?
   d. Do you ever take a morning <u>E</u>ye-opener?
2. Identify the alcoholic client in the preoperative period.
   a. Often, alcoholics are undiagnosed at the time of surgery and may go into withdrawal or DTs after the NPO period.
   b. Preoperative medication doses need to be adjusted; usually if tolerant of alcohol, clients are also tolerant of other medications, including anesthetics.
   c. Postoperative period usually takes longer for client to be fully responsive; susceptible to severe respiratory complications; has more difficulty with healing due to poor nutritional state.

✦ *Goal: to assist in the medical treatment of alcohol withdrawal.*

1. **Librium** or **Valium** for agitation (Appendix 10-1).
2. Tranquilizers (**Thorazine**) for nausea and vomiting.
3. Anticonvulsants (**Dilantin**) or magnesium sulfate given.
4. Encourage multivitamins, especially B complex and vitamin C.
5. Encourage fluids, but do not force.

✦ *Goal: to provide for the basic needs of rest, comfort, safety, and nutrition.*

1. Safety measures such as bedrest and bed rails may be necessary.
2. If client is in DTs, stay with him or her.
3. Have room adequately lit to help reduce confusion, and avoid shadows and unclear objects.
4. Monitor vital signs q 1-4 hours.
5. Encourage a high-carbohydrate, soft diet.

✦ *Goal: to recognize complications of alcohol use.*

1. Obstetric implications.
   a. Two ounces of alcohol per day may produce a BAL leading to fetal alcohol syndrome.
   b. Chronic alcoholism can lead to maternal malnutrition, especially folic acid deficiency, bone marrow suppression, infections, and liver disease.
   c. Alcohol withdrawal syndrome may occur in the intrapartal period as early as twelve to forty-eight hours after the last drink.
   d. Delirium tremens may occur in the postpartum period.
2. Neonatal implications (Fetal Alcohol Syndrome - FAS).
   a. Teratogenic effects may be seen along with growth and developmental retardation.
   b. Increased risk for anomalies of the heart, head, face and extremities.
   c. Withdrawal symptoms can occur shortly after birth; characterized by tremors, agitation, sweating, and seizure activity.
   d. Maintain seizure precautions.
3. Medical complications of alcohol abuse.
   a. Trauma-related to falls, burns, hematomas.
   b. Liver disease-cirrhosis, esophageal varices, hepatic coma.
   c. Gastrointestinal disease-gastritis, bleeding ulcers, pancreatitis.
   d. Nutritional disease-malnutrition, anemia due to iron or B_{12} deficiency, thiamine deficiency.
   e. Infections, especially pneumonia.
   f. Neurologic disease-polyneuropathy and dementia.

✦ *Goal: to assist in the long-term rehabilitation of client.*

1. Avoid sympathy, as clients tend to rationalize and use dependent, manipulative behavior to seek privileges.
2. Maintain a nonjudgmental attitude.
3. Set behavior limits in a firm but kind manner.

4. Place responsibility for sobriety on client; do not give advice or punish or reprimand client for failures.
5. Provide opportunities to decrease social isolation and encourage social groups and activities.
6. Encourage client to develop alternative coping mechanisms other than alcohol to deal with stress.
7. Refer clients and family to available community resources.
   a. Alcoholics Anonymous (AA)—a self-help group focusing on education, guidance, and the sharing of problems and experiences unique to the individual.
   b. Alanon—a self-help support group for the spouses and significant others of the alcoholic.
   c. Alateen—the support group for teenagers with an alcohol parent.
   d. Adult Children of Alcoholics (ACOA)—support group of adult child of alcoholics and dysfunctional individuals.
   e. Families Anonymous—support group for the families whose lives have been affected by the addicted client's behavior.
   f. Codependents Anonymous—support group for codependents who may be alcoholics or drug addicts, or someone who is close to an addict.
8. Promote adherence to prescribed therapeutic regimes.
   a. Disulfiram (**Antabuse**)—a drug therapy that produces intense side effects after ingestion of alcohol (severe nausea, vomiting, flushed face, hypotension, and blurred vision).
   b. Aversion therapy—a form of deterrent therapy attempting to induce alcohol rejection behavior by administering alcohol with an emetic.

Polydrug Dependence

❑ **The regular use of three or more psychoactive substances over a period of at least 6 months.**

General Concepts

A. Effects of use.
   1. Relieves anxiety.
   2. Overdose can occur.
   3. Factors affecting the degree of dependence.
      a. Physiologic and psychologic make-up of the abuser.
      b. Drug's pharmacologic action.
      c. External social and cultural factors.

B. General personality characteristics.
   1. Inability to cope with stress, frustration, or anxiety.
   2. Rebellious, immature, desire for immediate gratification.
   3. Passivity and low self-esteem and passivity.
   4. Difficulty forming warm, personal relationships.
   5. Uses defense mechanisms related to escaping—denial, rationalization, intellectualization.

Assessment

A. General assessment.
   1. Determine the pattern of drug use.
      a. Which drugs are being used by the client?
      b. How much does client use and how often?
      c. How long has client been using drugs?
      d. What combination of drugs is being used?
   2. Determine if there are any physical changes present (e.g., needle track marks, swollen nasal mucous membranes, reddened conjunctivae).

B. ***Narcotic dependence.***

Example: *Opium, heroin, morphine, meperidine* ***(Demerol)****, codeine, fentanyl, methadone.*

   1. Street names: horse, junk, smack (heroin); black, poppy (opium); M (morphine); dollies (methadone); terp (terpin hydrate or cough syrup with codeine).
   2. Administration.
      a. Heroin: sniffed, smoked, injected IV (mainlining), injected SQ (skin popping).
      b. Other narcotics usually taken orally or injected.
   3. Symptoms of use.
      a. Drowsiness, decreased blood pressure, pulse and respiratory rate.
      b. Pinpoint pupils, needle tracks, scarring.
      c. Overdose effects: slow, shallow breathing, clammy skin, convulsions, coma, pulmonary edema, possible death.
   4. Withdrawal symptoms.
      a. Onset of symptoms approximately eight to twelve hours following the last dose.
      b. Lacrimation, sweating, sneezing, yawning.
      c. Gooseflesh (piloerection), tremor, irritability, anorexia.
      d. Dilated pupils, abdominal cramps, vomiting, involuntary muscle spasms.
      e. Symptoms generally subside within seven to ten days.

C. ***Sedative-hypnotic dependence.***

Example: *Barbiturates* ***(Nembutal, Seconal)*** *and the benzodiazepines* ***(Librium, Valium)****.*

   1. Street names: Peter (chloral hydrate); green and whites, roaches (**Librium**); red birds, red devils

(secobarbital); blue birds (**Amytal** capsules); yellow birds (**Nembutal**); downers, rainbow, 7145 (barbiturates; tranquilizer).

2. Administration: oral or injected.
3. Symptoms of use.
   a. Alterations of mood, thought, behavior.
   b. Impairment in coordination, judgment.
   c. Signs of intoxication: slurred speech, unsteady gait, decreased attention span or memory.
   d. Barbiturate use: often violent, disruptive, irresponsible behavior.
4. Withdrawal symptoms.
   a. Insomnia, anxiety, profuse sweating, weakness.
   b. Severe reactions of delirium, grand mal seizures, cardiovascular collapse.

D. ***Cocaine abuse.***

Example: *Cocaine.*

1. Street names: Cocaine, coke, toot, nose candy, snow, C, powder, lady.
2. Administration: intranasal ("snorting") or by IV or SQ injection, smoked in pipe (free-basing).
3. Symptoms of use.
   a. Euphoria and a sense of well-being.
   b. Amphetamine-stimulant-like effects such as increased blood pressure, racing of the heart, paranoia, anxiety.
   c. Taken regularly, may disrupt eating and sleeping habits, leading to irritability and decreased concentration.

NURSING PRIORITY: *Crack (rock) has been labeled the most addictive drug known to man. It is a potent form of cocaine hydrochloride mixed with baking soda and water, heated (cooked), allowed to harden, and then is broken or "cracked" into little pieces and smoked in cigarettes or glass water pipes. Cardiac dysrhythmias, respiratory paralysis, and seizures are some of the dangers associated with crack use.*

4. Withdrawal symptoms.
   a. Severe craving.
   b. Coming down from a "high" often leads to a severe "letdown," depressed feeling.
   c. Psychological dependence often leads to cocaine becoming a total obsession.

E. ***Amphetamine dependence.***

Example: *Amphetamine* ***(Benzedrine).***

1. Street names: crank, bennies, wake-ups, uppers, speed (amphetamines).
2. Administration: oral or injected.
3. Symptoms of use.
   a. Elation, agitation, hyperactivity, irritability.
   b. Increased pulse, respiration and blood pressure.
   c. Fine tremor, muscle twitching, and mydriasis (pupillary dilation).
   d. Large doses: convulsions, cardiovascular collapse, respiratory depression, coma, death.
4. Withdrawal symptoms.
   a. Appear within two to four days after the last dose.
   b. Depression, overwhelming fatigue, suicide attempts.

F. ***PCP-phencyclidine abuse.***

1. Street names: sernylan, hog, super pill, elephant tranquilizer, angel dust, rocket fuel, primo.
2. Administration: snorted, smoked, or orally ingested; usually smoked along with marijuana.
3. Symptoms of use.
   a. Euphoria, feeling of numbness, mood changes.
   b. Diaphoresis, eye movement changes (nystagmus), hypertension, catatonic-like stupor with eyes open.
   c. Seizures, shivering, decerebrate posturing, possible death.
   d. Synesthesia (seeing colors when a loud sound occurs).
4. Overdose symptoms ("bad trip"): psychosis, possible death.
   a. User may become violent, destructive, and confused.
   b. Users have been known to go berserk; may harm self and others.
   c. Intoxicating symptoms lighten and worsen over a period of forty-eight hours.

G. ***Hallucinogen abuse.***

Example: *LSD, psilocybin ("magic mushroom"), mescaline (peyote), DMT, MDA.*

1. Street name: acid.
2. Administration: usually oral, but LSD and mescaline can be injected.
3. Symptoms of use.
   a. Pupillary dilation, tachycardia, sweating.
   b. Visual hallucinations, depersonalization, impaired judgment and mood.
   c. "Flashbacks" and "bad trips".
   d. Usually no signs of withdrawal symptoms after discontinuing use.

H. ***Marijuana dependence.***

Example: *Marijuana, hashish, tetrahydrocannabinol (THC).*

1. Street names: joints, reefers, pot, grass, "shit", Mary Jane (marijuana); hash (hashish).
2. Administration: oral, sniffed, and smoked.
3. Symptoms of use.
   a. Euphoria, relaxation, tachycardia, and conjunctival congestion.
   b. Paranoid ideation; impaired judgment.
   c. Rarely, panic reactions and psychoses.
   d. Heavy use leads to apathy and general deterioration in all aspects of living.
   e. Overdose effects: flashbacks, bronchitis, personality changes.
4. Withdrawal symptoms.
   a. Anxiety, sleeplessness, sweating.
   b. Lack of appetite, nausea, general malaise.

I. ***Designer drugs.***

1. Street names: Ecstasy, (MDMA, Adam), MTPT (China White).
2. Called analog drugs because they retain the properties of controlled drugs (e.g., MTPT is an analog of **Demerol**).
3. Symptoms of use and side effects are similar to the controlled substance from which they are derived.

Nursing Intervention

✦ *Goal: to assess the drug use pattern.*

✦ *Goal: to assist in the medical treatment during detoxification or withdrawal.*

1. Narcotics.
   a. Narcotic antagonists, such as naloxone (**Narcan**), nalorphine (**Nalline**), or levallorphan (**lorfan**), are administered intravenously for narcotic overdose.
   b. Withdrawal is managed with rest and nutritional therapy.
   c. Substitution therapy may be instituted to decrease withdrawal symptoms using propoxyphene (**Darvon**) for longer effects.
2. Depressants.
   a. Substitution therapy may be instituted to decrease withdrawal symptoms using a long-acting barbiturate, such as phenobarbital (**Luminal**).
   b. Some physicians prescribe oxazepam (**Serax**) as needed for objective symptoms, gradually decreasing the dosage until the drug is discontinued.
3. Stimulants.
   a. Treatment of overdose is geared toward stabilization of vital signs.
   b. IV antihypertensives may be used, along with IV diazepam (**Valium**) to control seizures.
   c. Chlordiazepoxide (**Librium)** PO may be administered for the first few days while client is "crashing."
4. Hallucinogens and Cannabinols.
   a. Medications are normally not prescribed for withdrawal from the substances.
   b. In the event of overdose, diazepam (**Valium**) or chlordiazepoxide (**Librium**) may be given as needed to decrease agitation.
5. Awareness that gradual withdrawal, detoxification, or dechemicalization is necessary for clients addicted to barbiturates, narcotics, and tranquilizers.
6. Abrupt withdrawal, "cold turkey," is often dangerous and can prove fatal.
7. Maintain a patent airway-have oxygen available.
8. Provide a safe, quiet environment (i.e., remove harmful objects, use side rails).

✦ *Goal: to decrease problem behaviors of manipulation and "acting out."*

1. Set firm, consistent limits.
2. Confront client with manipulative behaviors.

✦ *Goal: to promote alternative coping methods.*

1. Encourage responsibility for own behavior.
2. Encourage the use of hobbies, exercise, or alternative therapies as a means to deal with frustration and anxiety.

✦ *Goal: to recognize complications of substance abuse.*

1. Obstetric implications.
   a. Narcotic addiction.
      (1) Increased risk of pregnancy-induced hypertension, malpresentation, and third trimester bleeding.
      (2) Maintain on methadone for the duration of the pregnancy, as withdrawal is not advisable due to risk to the fetus.
   b. Other use of drugs provides increased risk to mother and fetus.
2. Neonatal complications.
   a. Withdrawal symptoms depend on type of drug mother used.
   b. Restlessness, jitteriness, hyperactive reflexes, high-pitched shrill cry, feeds poorly.
   c. Maintain seizure precautions.

d. Administer phenobarbital or paregoric to treat withdrawal and prevent seizures.

e. Swaddle infant in snug-fitting blanket.

f. Increased risk for congenital malformations and prematurity.

3. Medical implications.

a. Increased risk of hepatitis, malnutrition, and infections in general.

✦ *Goal: to assist in the long-term process of client drug rehabilitation.*

1. Refer to drug rehabilitation programs.
2. Promote self-help residential programs which foster self-support systems and use ex-addicts as rehabilitation counselors.
3. Methadone maintenance programs.

a. Must be 18 years old and addicted for more than two years, with a history of detoxification treatments.

b. Methadone is a synthetic narcotic which appeases desire for opiates.

(1) Controlled substance given only under urinary surveillance.

(2) Administered PO; prevents opiate withdrawal symptoms.

4. 12-step self-help groups.

a. Narcotics Anonymous—support group for clients who are addicted to narcotics and other drugs.

b. Nar-Anon—support group for relatives and friends of narcotic addicts.

c. Families Anonymous.

AFFECTIVE DISORDERS

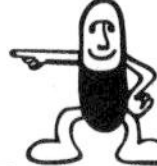

❑ **The major affective disorders are characterized by disturbances of mood.**

General Concepts

A. Incidence.

1. Approximately one percent of the adult population has had a bipolar disorder.
2. More prevalent among family members where there is a positive family history.
3. Major depression is more often seen in women.
4. More common in higher socioeconomic groups.

B. Causes.

1. Variety of theories which explain affective disorders.
2. Depressive: loss of significant others or objects; changes in levels of norepinephrine (decrease) and steroids (increase); loss of self-esteem leading to hopelessness, helplessness, and pessimism towards self and others.
3. Manic: unresolved diffuse anger and hostility; denial of depression; may develop from early childhood due to high parental expectations.

C. Personality characteristics associated with affective disorders.

1. Depressive: lacking in confidence, introverted, unassertive, dependent, pessimistic, feelings of inadequacy.
2. Manic: extroverted, confident, manipulative, obsessive.

Psychodynamics

A. *Manic.*

1. During infancy, needs and narcissistic goals are not met, which leads to impairment in the development of self-esteem.
2. Low self-esteem and helplessness lead to need for excessive attention, affection, warmth, and appreciation.
3. Usually a massive denial of depression.
4. The air of happiness and self-confidence are defenses against dependency feelings.

B. *Depressive..*

1. Loss, either real or perceived, of a loved person or object.
2. Turning aggressive feelings inward and displacing them onto the self; accompanied by feelings of guilt.
3. Ambivalent feelings toward the valued/lost object.
4. Repressive guilt, which leads to feelings of helplessness and hopelessness.

Assessment

A. *Bipolar disorder.*

1. Manic.

a. Onset before age thirty.

b. Mood: elevated, expansive, or irritable.

c. Speech: loud, rapid, difficult to interpret, punning, rhyming, clanging (using words that sound like the meaning rather than the actual word).

d. Cognitive skills: flight of ideas, grandiose delusions, easily distracted.

e. Psychomotor activity: hyperactive, decreased need for sleep, exhibitionistic, vulgar, profane, may make inappropriate sexual advances and be obscene.

f. Course of manic episode: begins suddenly, rapidly escalates over a few days, and ends more abruptly than major depressive episodes.

2. Depressive.
   a. Has had one or more manic episodes.
   b. Mood: dysphoric, depressive, despairing, loss of interest or pleasure in most usual activities.
   c. Cognitive process: negative view of self, world, and of the future; poverty of ideas; crying, and suicidal preoccupation.
   d. Psychomotor: may have either agitation or retardation in movements, feelings of fatigue, lack of appetite, constipation, sleeping disturbances (insomnia or early morning wakefulness), decrease in libido.
3. Mixed.
   a. Involves both manic and depressive episodes, either intermixed or alternating rapidly every few days.
   b. Depressive phase symptoms are prominent and last at least a full day.

B. *Major depression.*
1. May occur at any age.
2. Differentiated as either a single episode or a recurring type.
3. Symptoms the same as those listed under "Bipolar disorder-depressed".
4. Severity and type of depression vary with the ability to test reality.
   a. Psychotic: feels worse in the morning-better as the day goes on.
   b. Neurotic: wakes up feeling optimistic-mood worsens as the day passes.

C. Other disorders (not considered part of the major affective type classification).
1. Cyclothymic.
   a. Chronic mood disturbance of two-year duration.
   b. Numerous periods of mild depression and mania.
   c. Depressive mood periods: feelings of inadequacy, social withdrawal, sleeping too much, diminished work productivity.
   d. Hypomanic: inflated self-esteem, uninhibited people-seeking, decreased need for sleep, increased work productivity, and sharpened or unusually creative thinking.
2. Dysthymic disorder (depressive neurosis).
   a. Depressed mood with loss of interest in most usual daily activities.
   b. No delusions or hallucinations.
   c. Common disorder with an increased incidence in females; chronic course.

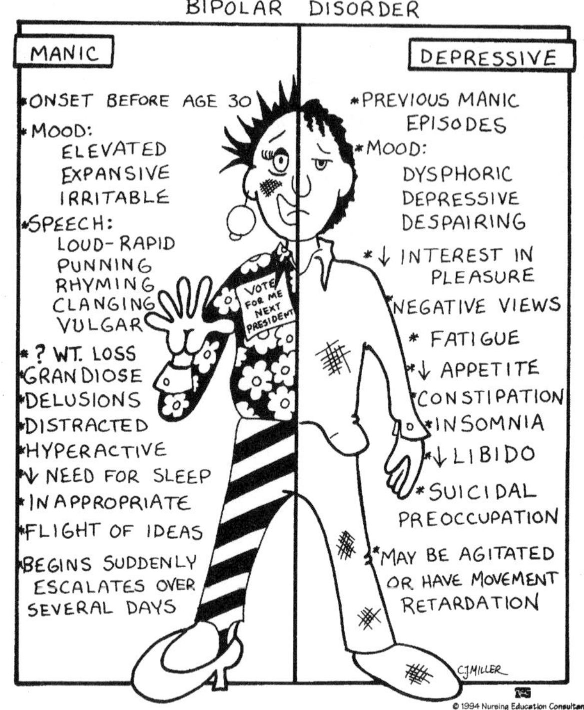

Figure 10-2: Bipolar Affective Disorder
Zerwekh, J. & Claborn, J. (2000). *Memory Notebook of Nursing*, Vol. 1, Dallas, TX: Nursing Education Consultants, Inc.

Nursing Intervention (manic episode)

✦ *Goal: to provide for basic human needs of safety and rest/activity.*
1. Reduce outside stimuli and provide a nonstimulating environment.
2. Monitor food intake—provide a high-calorie, high-vitamin diet with finger foods, to be eaten as the client moves about.

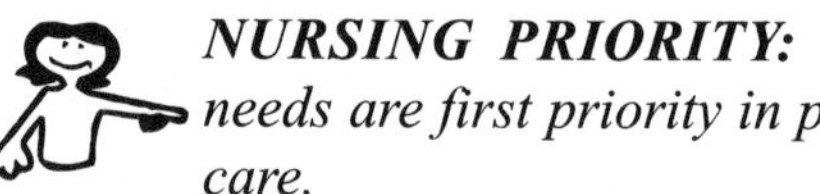
NURSING PRIORITY: *Physiological needs are first priority in providing client care.*

3. Encourage noncompetitive solitary activities—walking, swimming, and painting.
4. Assist with personal hygiene.

NURSING PRIORITY: *During the manic phase, the client's physical safety is at risk because the hyperactivity may lead to exhaustion and ultimately to cardiac failure.*

✦ *Goal: to establish a therapeutic nurse-client relationship.*
1. Use firm, consistent, honest approach.
2. Assess client's abilities and involve in his/her own care planning.

Table 10-6: SAD PERSONS SCALE

One of the most popular and easy-to-use tools available to help assess suicide risk. The more areas checked the higher the risk.

Sex (males are more likely to successfully commit suicide)
Age (younger than 19 or older than 45)
Depression

Previous suicide attempt
Ethanol (alcohol) abuse
Rational thinking (impaired)
Social support lacking (including recent loss of loved one)
Organized plan
No spouse
Sickness (especially chronic)

Total score ranges from O (lowest risk) to 10 (highest risk). This scale should be used as a guideline only; use your judgment and don't neglect unspecified factors.

3. Promote problem-solving abilities; recognize that false sense of independence is often demonstrated by loud, boisterous behavior.
4. Do not focus or discuss grandiose ideas.

✦ *Goal: to set limits on behavior.*

1. Instructions should be clear and concise.
2. Initiate regularly scheduled contacts to demonstrate acceptance.
3. Maintain some distance between self and client to allow freedom of movement and to prevent feelings of being overpowered.
4. Maintain neutrality and objectivity—realize that client can be easily provoked by harmless remarks, and may demonstrate a furious reaction but calm down very quickly.
5. Employ measures to prevent overt aggression (e.g., distraction, recognition of behaviors of increased excitement).

✦ *Goal: to promote adaptive coping with constructive use of energy.*

1. Do not hurry client, as this leads to anxiety and hostile behavior.

***NURSING PRIORITY:** In a hyperactive state, client is extremely distractible, and responses to even the slightest stimuli are exaggerated.*

2. Provide activities and constructive tasks that channel the agitated behavior (e.g., cleaning game room, going for a walk, gardening, playing catch).

✦ *Goal: to assist in the medical treatment.*

1. Administer lithium (**Lithane**).
2. Teach client about lithium medication instructions (Appendix 10-2).

Nursing Intervention (depressive episode)

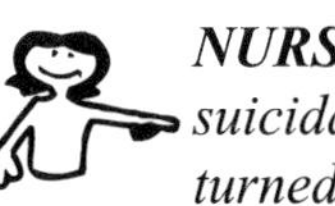

***NURSING PRIORITY:** Depression and suicidal behaviors may be viewed as anger turned inward on the self. If this anger can be verbalized in a non-threatening environment, the client may be able to resolve these feelings, regardless of the discomfort involved.*

✦ *Goal: to assess for suicide potential.*

1. Recognition of suicidal intent.
   a. Self-destructive behaviors are viewed as attempts to escape unbearable life situations.
   b. Anxiety and hostility are overwhelmingly present.
   c. There is the presence of ambivalence; living versus self-destructive impulses.
   d. Depression, low self-esteem, and a feeling of hopelessness are critical to evaluate, as suicide attempts are often made when the client feels like giving up.
   e. Assess for *indirect* self-destructive behavior—any activity that is detrimental to the physical well-being of the client where the potential outcome is death.
      (1) Eating disorders: anorexia nervosa, bulimia, obesity, and overeating.
      (2) Noncompliance with medical treatment (e.g., diabetic who does not take insulin).
      (3) Cigarette smoking, gambling, criminal, and socially deviant activities.
      (4) Alcohol and drug abuse.
      (5) Participation in high-risk sports (e.g., automobile racing and sky diving).
2. Suicide danger signs (Table 10-6: SAD Persons).
   a. The presence of a suicide plan: specifics relating to method, its lethality, and a likelihood for rescue.

Table 10-7: ADOLESCENT SUICIDE

Characteristics

History of suicide ideationPrevious suicide attemptChronic use of drugsActing-out behaviors—delinquency, stealing, vandalism, academic failure, promiscuity, loss of boyfriend/girlfriend

Family Characteristics

Unproductive, conflictual communication
Impaired problem-solving ability
Inconsistent positive reinforcements plus a greater number of negative reinforcements
Unstable home environment

b. Change in established patterns in routines (e.g., giving away of personal items, making a will, and saying good-bye).

c. Anticipation of failure: loss of a job, preoccupation with physical disease, actual or anticipated loss of a significant other.

d. Change in behavior, presence of panic, agitation, or calmness; usually, as depression lifts, client has enough energy to act on suicidal feelings.

e. Hopelessness: feelings of impending doom, futility, and entrapment.

f. Withdrawal and rejection of help.

3. Clients at risk (Table 10-7: Adolescent Suicide).

a. Adolescents and the elderly; males usually complete the suicide act.

b. Recent stress of a maturational or situational crisis.

c. Clients with chronic or painful illnesses.

d. Previous suicidal attempts or behavior.

e. Withdrawn, depressed, or hallucinating clients.

f. Clients with sexual identity conflicts and those who abuse alcohol and drugs.

✦ *Goal: to provide for basic human needs of safety and protection from self-destruction.*

1. Remove all potentially harmful objects (e.g., be[illegible] sharp objects, matches, lighters, strings, etc.).

2. Maintain a one-to-one relationship and close [illegible]servation.

NURSING PRIORITY: *Be aware of special times when client might be suicidal (e.g., when suddenly cheerful, when there is less staff available, upon arriving in the morning, or during a busy routine day).*

3. Have client make a written contract stating he will not harm himself, and provide an alternative plan of coping.

✦ *Goal: to provide for physical needs of nutrition and rest/activity.*

1. Assess for changes in weight (weight loss may indicate deepening depression).

2. Encourage increased bulk and roughage in diet along with sufficient fluids if constipated.

NURSING PRIORITY: *Depressed clients are particularly vulnerable to constipation, due to psychomotor retardation.*

3. Provide for adequate amount of exercise and rest; encourage client not to sleep during the day.

4. Assist with hygiene and personal appearance.

✦ *Goal: to promote expression of feelings.*

1. Encourage expression of angry, guilty, or depressed feelings.

2. Convey a kind, pleasant, interested approach to promote a sense of dignity and self-worth in the client.

3. Support the client in the expression of his/her feelings by allowing him/her to respond in his/her own time.

4. Seek out client; initiate frequent contacts.

5. Assist with decision-making when depression is severe.

✦ *Goal: to provide for meaningful socialization activities.*

NURSING PRIORITY: *The depressed client must have lots of structure in his or her life due to the impairment in decision-making/problem-solving ability. Devise a plan of therapeutic activities and provide client with a written time schedule.* ***Remember:*** *The client who is moderately depressed feels best early in the day, while later in the day is a better time for the severely depressed individual to participate in activities.*

1. Encourage participation in activities (e.g., plan a work assignment with client to do simple tasks: straightening game room, picking up magazines, etc.).

2. Assess hobbies, sports, or activities client enjoys, and encourage participation.

3. Encourage client to participate in small group conversation or activity; practice social skills through role playing and psychodrama.

4. Encourage activities that promote a sense of accomplishment and enhance self-esteem.

✦ *Goal: to assist in the medical treatment.*

1. Administer antidepressant medication (See Appendix 10-3).

2. Assist in electroconvulsive therapy (ECT) (See Table 10-8).

SCHIZOPHRENIC DISORDERS

NURSING PRIORITY: *The schizophrenic disorders constitute the largest group of psychotic disorders in society (approximately 1 percent of the U.S. population).*

Schizophrenia

❑ **Schizophrenia is a maladaptive disturbance characterized by a number of common behaviors involving disorders of thought content, mood, feeling, perception, communication, and interpersonal relationships. Onset of symptoms usually occurs before age 45, with a duration of symptoms for at least six months.**

General Concepts

A. Loss of ego boundaries.

B. May result from many possible factors:

1. Organic or physiologic-genetic, biochemical (overactivity of dopamine, an insufficiency of norepinephrine, or an imbalance of both; decreased MAO activity), immunological imbalance, or a structural deviation of brain tissue.
2. Psychosocial-individual adaptive patterns to stress, double-bind communication pattern, poor family relationships, past traumatic experiences, lack of ego strength, or a deficit in cognitive development due to perinatal, nutritional, and maturational factors.

C. Primary mental mechanisms are repression, regression, projection, and denial.

D. Failure or inability to trust self or others.

E. Security and identity are threatened, so client withdraws from reality.

Prepsychotic Personality Characteristics

A. Aloof, rejecting, and indifferent.

B. Social withdrawal, peculiar behavior.

C. Relatives and friends note a change in personality.

D. Unusual perceptual experiences, along with disturbed communication.

E. Lack of personal grooming.

Psychodynamics of Maladaptive Disturbances

A. Disturbance in thought processes.

1. Thoughts are confused, chaotic and disorganized.
2. Communication in symbolic language; all symbols have special meaning.
3. Feeling that thoughts or wishes can control other people (i.e., magical thinking).
4. Retreat to a fantasy world, rejecting the real world of painful experience while responding to reality in a bizarre or autistic manner.

B. Disturbance of affect.

1. Difficulty expressing emotions.
2. Affect is either absent, flat, blunted, or inappropriate.
3. Inappropriate affect makes it difficult to form close relationships.

C. Disturbance in psychomotor behavior.

1. Display of disorganized, purposeless activity.
2. Behavior may be uninhibited and bizarre; abnormal posturing (agitated or retardative catatonia), waxy flexibility.
3. Often appears aloof, disinterested, apathetic, and lacking motivation.

D. Disturbance in perception.

1. Hallucinations and delusions; auditory most common.
2. Abnormal bodily sensations and hypersensitivity to sound, sight, and smell.

E. Disturbance in interpersonal relationships.

Table 10-8: ELECTROCONVULSIVE THERAPY (ECT)

❑ **ECT is an electric shock delivered to the brain through electrodes that are applied to both temples. The shock artificially induces a grand mal seizure.**

Indications

1. Severly depressed clients who do not respond to medication.
2. High risk for suicide/starvation.
3. Overwehlming depression delusions or hallucinations.
4. Number of treatments: usually given in a series which varies according to the client's presenting problem and response to therapy; 2 - 3 treatments per week for a period of 2 -6 weeks.

Nursing Intervention

✦ *To prepare client for ECT.*

1. Assess client's record for routine preoperative type checklist for information.
2. NPO for 6 hours prior to treatment.
3. Remove dentures.
4. Administer preoperative medication.

✦ *To provide support and care immediately following treatment.*

1. Provide orientation to time.
2. Temporary memory loss is usually confusing; explain that this is a common occurrence.
3. Assess vital signs for 30 minutes to 1 hour after treatment.
4. De-emphasize preoccupation with ECT; promote involvement in regularly scheduled activities.

✦ *Long-term goal: To promote and develop a positive self-concept and realistic perception of self.*

1. Encourage problem-solving in social relationships; identify problem areas in relationships with others.
2. Acknowledge and encourage statements that reflect positive attributes and/or skills.
3. Reinforce new,, alternative coping methods,, especially if client uses a new method to handle sad situations and painful feelings.

1. Establishment of interpersonal relationships is difficult due to inability to communicate clearly and react appropriately.
2. Difficulty relating to others.
   a. Unable to form close relationships.
   b. Has difficulty trusting others and experiences ambivalence, fear, and dependency.
   c. "Need-fear dilemma"—withdraws to protect self from further hurt and consequently experiences lack of warmth, trust, and intimacy.
   d. "As if" phenomenon—feels rejected by others, which leads to increased isolation, perpetuating further feelings of rejection.

Types of Schizophrenia

A. Schizophrenia, disorganized (formerly called hebephrenic).
1. Inappropriate affect, giggling and silly laughter.
2. Regressive behavior.
3. Severe thought disturbance, incoherent speech, "word salad".
4. Withdrawn, fragmentary hallucinations and delusions.

B. Schizophrenia, catatonic.
1. Stupor and excitement phases of catatonic, bizarre posturing, waxy flexibility.
2. Negativism—rigidity and mutism.

C. Schizophrenia, paranoid.
1. Delusions of persecution and grandeur.
2. Extreme suspiciousness.
3. Anger, argumentativeness, and violence.
4. Doubts about gender identity.

D. Schizophrenia, undifferentiated.
1. Mixed psychotic symptoms.
2. Unclassifiable; either does not meet the criteria of one of the subtypes or meets the criteria of more than one.

E. Schizophrenia, residual.
1. History of exhibited psychotic symptoms of schizophrenia, but not psychotic at present.
2. Continued difficulty in thinking, mood, and perception.

Assessment

A. Four "A's"—Eugene Bleuler's classic symptoms.
1. Associative looseness—lack of logical thought progression resulting in disorganized and chaotic thinking.
2. Affect—emotion or feeling tone is one of indifference, flat, blunted, exaggerated, or socially inappropriate.
3. Ambivalence—conflicting, strong feelings (e.g., love and hate) that neutralize each other, leading to psychic immobilization and difficulty expressing other emotions.
4. Autism—extreme retreat from reality characterized by fantasies, preoccupation with daydreams, and psychotic thought processes of delusion and hallucination.
   a. Hallucinations—false sensory perception with no basis in reality; auditory, olfactory, tactile, visual, gustatory.
   b. Delusions—fixed, false beliefs, not corrected by logic; develop as a defense against intolerable feelings or ideas that cause anxiety.
      (1) Delusions of grandeur—related to feelings of power, fame, splendor, magnificence.
      (2) Delusions of persecution—people are out to harm, injure or destroy.
   c. Ideas of reference—actions and speech of others have reference to oneself; ideas symbolize feelings of guilt, insecurity, and alienation.
   d. Depersonalization—feeling alienated from oneself; difficulty distinguishing self from others; loss of boundaries between self and environment.

B. Additional characteristics.
1. Regression—extreme withdrawal and social isolation.
2. Negativism—doing the opposite of what is asked; typical behavior is to speak to no one and answer no one; used to cover feelings of unworthiness and inadequacy.
3. Religiosity—excessive religious preoccupation.
4. Lack of social awareness—crudeness and social insensitivity; neglectful of personal grooming and hygiene.

Nursing Intervention

✦ *Goal: to build trust.*

NCLEX ALERT: *Building trust is the primary goal for the schizophrenic client. Maintain a therapeutic milieu; stay with client to promote safety; reduce fear and assist client to communicate effectively are important nursing care measures.*

1. Encourage free expression of feelings (either negative or positive), without fear of rejection, ridicule, or retaliation.

2. Use nonverbal level of communication to demonstrate warmth, concern, and empathy, as client often distrusts words.
3. Consistency, reliability, acceptance, and persistence build trust.
4. Allow client to set pace; proceed slowly in planning social contacts.

✦ *Goal: to provide a safe and secure environment.*
1. Maintain familiar routines. Make sure persons who come in contact with the client are recognizable to the client.
2. Avoid stressful situations or increasing anxiety.

✦ *Goal: to clarify and reinforce reality.*
1. Involve client in reality-oriented activities.
2. Help client find satisfaction in the external environment and ways of relating to others.
3. Focus on clear communication and the immediate situation.

✦ *Goal: to promote and build self-esteem.*
1. Encourage simple activities with limited concentration and *no* competition.
2. Provide successful experiences with short-range goals realistic for client's levels of functioning.
3. Relieve client of decision-making until he/she is ready.
4. Avoid making demands.

✦ *Goal: to encourage independent behavior.*
1. Anticipate and accept negativism.
2. Avoid fostering dependency.
3. Encourage client to make his/her own decisions, using positive reinforcement.

✦ *Goal: to provide care to meet basic human needs.*
1. Determine client's ability to meet responsibilities of daily living.
2. Attend to nutrition, elimination, exercise, hygiene, and signs of physical illness.

✦ *Goal: to assist in the medical treatment.*
1. Administer antipsychotic medications (Appendix 10-4).
2. Assist with ECT; may be useful in some instances to modify behavior.

***NURSING PRIORITY:** As client's symptoms get under control, they often believe they can discontinue therapy and medication, which can lead to noncompliant behavior.*

✦ *Goal: to deal effectively with withdrawn behavior.*
1. Establish a therapeutic one-to-one relationship.
   a. Initiate interaction by seeking out client at every opportunity.
   b. Maintain a nonjudgmental, accepting manner in what is said and done.
   c. Attempt to draw client into a conversation without demanding a response.
2. Promote social skills by helping client feel more secure with other people.
   a. Accept one-sided conversations.
   b. Accept staff reaction toward client's negativism without remarks.
3. Attend to physical needs of client as necessary.
4. Have client focus on reality.
5. Protect and restrain client from potential destructiveness to self and others.

✦ *Goal: to deal effectively with hallucinations.*
1. Clarify and reinforce reality.
   a. Help client recognize hallucination as a manifestation of anxiety.
   b. Provide a safe, secure environment.
   c. Avoid denying or arguing with client when he/she is experiencing hallucinations.
   d. Acknowledge client's experience, but point out that *you* do not share the same experience.
   e. Do not give attention to content of hallucinations.
   f. Direct client's attention to real situations, such as singing along with music.
   g. Protect client from injury to self or others when prompted by "voices" or "visions."
2. Encourage social interaction to help client find satisfactory ways of relating with others.
   a. Increase interaction gradually.
   b. Respond verbally to anything real that client talks about.

Paranoid Disorder

❑ ***Paranoid disorders* are maladaptive disorders characterized by delusions, usually persecutory, and extreme suspiciousness.**

General Concepts

A. Primary mental mechanism is projection.

B. Onset of paranoid behavior may be precipitated by stressful events.
1. Loss of a real or imaginary love object.
2. Experience of failure leading to loss of self-esteem and feelings of inadequacy.

C. Delusional behavior.
1. An attempt to cope with stress and reality.
2. Associated with an extreme need to maintain self-esteem.

3. Delusions are a symbolic way to communicate with others.
4. Delusions are very real to client.
5. Delusional system usually entails denial of reality, followed by projection and rationalization.

Psychodynamics

A. Lack of security and trust is evident.
B. Inconsistency and failure to meet infant's basic needs lead to suspiciousness.
C. Conflicting messages and double-bind communication lead to low self-esteem.

Assessment

A. Extreme suspiciousness and withdrawal from emotional contact with others.
B. Aloof, distant, hypercritical of others.
C. Frequent complaining by letter-writing or instigating legal action.
D. Resentment, anger, possible violence.
E. Delusions of grandeur, persecution, and hypochondriases.
F. Misinterpretation or distortion of reality; may refuse food and medications; insists he are poisoned despite evidence or proof.

Nursing Intervention

✦ *Goal: to establish a trusting relationship.*

NCLEX ALERT: *Use therapeutic interventions to increase client understanding of behavior. This lack of trust in the paranoid client is often a focus of test questions surrounding the serving of meals or the administration of medications.*

---

1. Maintain calm, matter-of-fact attitude.
2. Keep promises made; be honest.
3. Avoid whispering or acting secretive.
4. Allow a choice of activities; involve in treatment plan.

✦ *Goal: to increase self-esteem by providing successful experiences.*

1. Allow client to set pace in closeness with others.
2. Avoid involvement in competitive, aggressive activities requiring physical contact (e.g., football, basketball).
3. Involve in solitary activities (e.g., drawing, photography, typing) and progress to intellectual activities with others using games (e.g., chess, bridge, word scrabble).
4. Reward completion of meaningful tasks.

✦ *Goal: to deal effectively with delusions.*

1. Clarify and focus on reality; use reality-testing.
2. Avoid confirming or approving false beliefs.
3. Point out that client's beliefs are not shared.
4. Divert attention from delusions to reality; focus on here and now.

Disorders of Impulse Control

❑ **With this group of disorders there is failure to resist an impulse, drive, or temptation to perform some act that may be harmful to others; usually preceded by an increasing amount of tension prior to committing the act, with an outcome of pleasure or gratification.**

Assessment

A. Pathologic gambling.
   1. Diagnostic criteria.
      a. A chronic and progressive failure to resist impulses to gamble.
      b. Disrupts, damages, or compromises family, personal, and vocational pursuits.
         (1) Evidence of forgery, fraud, embezzlement.
         (2) Unable to pay debts or other financial responsibilities.
         (3) Borrows money, either illegally or legally.
         (4) Frequent loss of work due to absenteeism.
   2. Additional characteristics.
      a. Overconfident, very energetic, "big spender."
      b. Often begins in adolescence.
B. Kleptomania.
   1. Recurrent impulse to steal objects.
   2. Characterized by increasing tension prior to stealing and a feeling of pressure or release after committing the act.
   3. Usually done without long-term planning.
C. Pyromania.
   1. Recurrent impulse to set fires.
   2. Usually, increased amount of tension prior to setting the fire, with subsequent release after committing the act.
D. Explosive disorder.
   1. A loss of control of aggressive impulses resulting in assault or destruction of property.
   2. Behavior is usually out of proportion to the precipitating stressor.
   3. Individual usually describes "spells" or "attacks;" usually regrets the display of aggression.

Nursing Intervention

✦ *Goal: to encourage client to develop alternative ways of dealing with stress.*

1. Refer client to self-help groups: Gamblers Anonymous (GAM-ANON).
2. Assist client in determining when anxiety and tension are increasing and provide a plan of action to prevent acts of stealing, setting fires, or destroying property.

Adjustment Disorders

Assessment

A. Can appear at any developmental stage and is related to the developmental task at hand.

B. Usually no underlying mental disorder or pathology.

C. Present behavior is usually disturbed and characterized by distortions in the situation and difficulty in decision making.

Nursing Intervention

✦ *Goal: to return client to homeostasis with the fullest possible functioning level.*

1. Provide empathetic understanding and support.
2. Encourage identification of specific problems and promote new problem-solving coping skills.
3. Enlist family and community support as necessary.⌘

Study Questions—Psychiatric Disorders

1. A client's depression has lifted and she says she feels much better. What is her suicide risk status?

① No longer a suicide risk.
② Less of a suicide risk than when she was deeply depressed.
③ More of a suicide risk than when she was deeply depressed.
④ A suicide risk only in the evening.

2. What is an important nursing intervention in caring for a client during a manic episode?

① Place the client in a quiet area, separate from others.
② Encourage the client to organize some physical activity.
③ Establish firm, set limits on behavior.
④ Include the client in the group's activities.

3. A client demonstrates inappropriate affect when she giggles while talking about her brain being destroyed. What purpose does this behavior serve?

① Convince the staff that her problem is physical and not psychological.
② Avoid the nurse's questions about the problems that resulted in her admission.
③ Deny that she is angry with her parents for bringing her to the hospital.
④ Protect herself against the painful emotional impact of what she fears is happening to her.

4. On admission, a depressed client states, "I feel like killing myself, but I wouldn't do that." After assessing the degree of the client's depression, what would be the initial focus of the nurse's intervention?:

① Exploring reasons why the client might want to take her life.
② Determining the severity of her suicidal risk.
③ Preventing the client from harming herself.
④ Guiding her to consider alternative ways of coping.

5. Which factor is most significant for the nurse working with the parents of an infant with Downs syndrome?

① Their response to the reactions of family and friends to their infant.
② Their ability to give physical care to their infant.
③ Their ability to talk about caring for their child and anticipated changes in their lifestyle.
④ Their understanding of the factors causing Down's syndrome.

6. A client with schizophrenia is incontinent and urinates on the floor? What is an appropriate nursing intervention?

① Ask her to clean up after herself.
② Tell her that ward privileges will be withheld if it happens again.
③ Ignore the client until her behavior improves.
④ Clean up the urine without communicating displeasure.

7. During the past month, a 55-year-old client has become increasingly agitated and hyperexcitable, with an increase in verbal and

physical activity. Considering all of these symptoms, which best describes the condition?

① Panic attacks.
② Paranoid behavior.
③ Free-floating anxiety.
④ Manic episode.

8. A client with a diagnosis of schizophrenia repeatedly states that flies are eating her brain and making her feel weird. What is the client experiencing?

① Ideas of reference.
② Grandiose delusion.
③ Somatic delusions.
④ Persecutory delusions.

9. What is the most common defect associated with Down syndrome?

① Deafness.
② Congenital heart disease.
③ Hydrocephaly.
④ Muscular hypertonicity.

10. What is a priority nursing task in establishing a relationship with a client with schizophrenia?

① Make emotional contact.
② Take a careful nursing history.
③ Increase voluntary motor activity.
④ Mutually agree to a contract.

11. Chlorpromazine (Thorazine) is ordered for a client. What should the nurse teach the client that may occur with this medication?

① Weight loss.
② Drowsiness.
③ Hypertension.
④ Insomnia.

12. What would be noted in an assessment on a client experiencing symptoms of lithium toxicity?

① Hypotension, bradycardia, polyuria.
② Tachycardia, hypertension, convulsions.
③ Diarrhea, ataxia, seizures, lethargy.
④ Urinary frequency, vomiting, fever.

13. A client who abuses cocaine is on a detoxification protocol. What is an important nursing measure?

① Increase fluid intake.
② Check vital signs.
③ Encourage a high sodium diet.
④ Check intake and output.

Answers and rationales to these questions are in the section at the end of the book entitled "Chapter Study Questions: Answers & Rationales.

Appendix 10-1:
ANTI-ANXIETY AGENTS

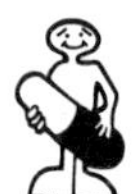

❖GENERAL NURSING IMPLICATIONS❖

—Withhold or omit one or more doses if excessive drowiness occurs.
—Assess for symptoms associated with a withdrawal syndrome in hospitalized clients—anxiety, insomnia, vomiting, tremors, palpitations, confusion, and hallucinations.
—When discontinuing, the drug dosage should be gradually decreased over a period of days depending upon the dose and length of time on the medication.
—Schedule IV drug requires documentation.
—Promote safety with the use of siderails and assisting with ambulation as necessary.
—Teach client and family not to drink alcohol while taking an antianxiety agent, and not to abruptly stop taking the medication.

MEDICATIONS	SIDE EFFECTS	NURSING IMPLICATIONS
BENZODIAZEPINES: Reduce anxiety by enhancing the action of the inhibitory neurotransmitter GABA on its receptor. Also promotes anticonvulsant activity and skeletal muscle relaxation.		
Chlordiazepoxide (**Librium**): PO, IM, IV Diazepam (**Valium**): PO, IM, IV Clonazepam (**Klonopin**):PO Chlorazepate dipotassium (**Tranzene**): PO Midazolam (**Versed**): IM, IV	Central nervous system depression, drowsiness (decreases with usage), ataxia, dizziness, headaches, dry mouth. ***Adverse effects:*** Leukopenia, tolerance commonly develops, physical dependency.	1. Alters liver function tests. 2. Assess for symptoms of leukopenia, such as sore throat, fever, and weakness. 3. Encourage client to rise slowly from a supine position and to dangle feet before standing. 4. **Librium**: Do not inject or add IV **Librium** to an existing IV infusion; inject directly into a large vein over a one-minute period. 5. Do not mix **Librium** or **Valium** with any other drug in a syringe or add to existing IV fluids. 6. **Versed** is commonly used for induction of anesthesia and sedation prior to diagnostic tests and endoscopic exams. 7. Flumazenil (**Rocmazicon**) is approved for the treatment of benzodiazepine overdose; has an adverse effect of precipitating convulsions, especially with clients who have a history of epilepsy. 8. ***Uses:*** anxiety and tension, muscle spasm, preoperative medication, acute alcohol withdrawal, and to induce sleep.
NONBENZODIAZEPINE AGENTS: Interact with serotonin and dopamine receptors in the brain to decrease anxiety. Lack muscle relaxant and anticonvulsant effects, doe not cause sedation or physical or psychological dependence, does not increase CNS depression of alcohol or other drugs.		
Buspirone (**Buspar**): PO	Dizziness, drowsiness, headache, nausea, fatigue, insomnia.	1. Not a controlled substance. 2. Some improvement can be noted in 7-10 days, however usually takes 3-4 weeks to achieve effectiveness. 3. ***Uses:*** short-term relief of anxiety and anxiety disorders.

Appendix 10-2: ANTIMANIC MEDICATIONS

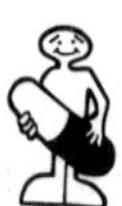

MEDICATION	SIDE EFFECTS	NURSING IMPLICATIONS
LITHIUM CARBONATE: Acts to lower concentrations of norepinephrine and serotonin by inhibiting their release; believed to alter sodium transport in both nerve and muscle cells. ***Uses:*** bipolar affective disorder—manic episode.		
(**Lithane, Lithobid**): PO	***High incidence:*** Increased thirst, increased urination (polyuria). ***Frequent:*** 1.5 mEq/L levels or less: Dry mouth, lethargy, fatigue, muscle weakness, headache, GI disturbances, fine hand tremors. ***Adverse effects:*** 1.5—2.0 mEq/L may produce vomiting, diarrhea, drowsiness, incoordination, coarse hand tremors, muscle twitching. 2.0—2.5 mEq/L may result in ataxia, slurred speech, confusion, clonic movements, high output of dilute urine, blurred vision, hypotension. ***Acute toxicity:*** Seizures, oliguria, coma, peripheral vascular collapse, death.	1. Monitor lithium blood levels: blood samples taken 12 hours after dosage. 2. Teach client the following: a. symptoms of lithium toxicity. b. the importance of frequent blood tests (every 2-3 days) to check lithium levels at the beginning of treatment (maintenance blood levels done every 1-3 months). c. the importance of dietary intake and taking dose at same time each day, preferably with meals or milk. 3. Encourage a diet containing normal amounts of salt and a fluid intake of 3 liters per day; avoid caffeine, due to its diuretic effect. 4. Report polyuria, prolonged vomiting, diarrhea,, or fever to physician (may need to temporarily reduce or discontinue dosage). 5. Do not crush, chew, or break the extended-release or film-coated tablets. 6. Assess clients at high risk of developing toxicity: postoperative, dehydrated, hyperthyroid, those with renal disease, or those clients on diuretics. 7. Blood levels: a. extremely narrow therapeutic range; 0.5—1.5 mEq/liter. b. toxic serum lithium level is greater than 2 mEq/liter. 8. Management of lithium toxicity: administration of osmotic diuretics(e.g., urea or mannitol); aminophylline and **Diamox**. 9. Long-term use may cause goiter; may be associated with hypothyroidism.
OTHER AGENTS: Both medications listed below were originally developed and used for seizure disorders. Both have mood-stabilizing abilities.		
Carbamazepine (**Tegretol**): PO	Drowiness, dizziness, visual problems (spots before eyes, difficulty focusing, blurred vision), dry mouth. ***Toxic reactions***: blood dyscrasias.	1. Used primarily for clients who have failed to respond to lithium or who cannot tolerate the side effects. 2. Avoid tasks that require alertness, motor skills until response to drug is established. 3. **Tegretol** — monitor CBC frequently during initiation of therapy and at monthly intervals thereafter. 4. **Depakene** — monitor liver function studies.
Valproic acid (**Depakene**): PO	Nausea, GI upsets, drowsiness, may cause hepatotoxicity.	

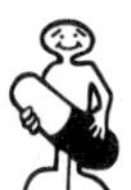

Appendix 10-3:
ANTIDEPRESSANT MEDICATIONS

MEDICATIONS	SIDE EFFECTS	NURSING IMPLICATIONS

❖GENERAL NURSING IMPLICATIONS❖

— SSRIs are overtaking TCAs as drug of choice for depression.
— MAOs are used as second-line drugs for the treatment of depression, due to their potential interactions with other drugs and certain foods.
— Therapeutic effect has a delayed onset of 7-21 days.
— Can potentially produce cardiotoxicity, sedation, seizures, and anticholingeric effects, as well as induce mania in bipolar clients (SSRIs less likely to cause these problems).
— Drugs are usually discontinued prior to surgery (10 days for MAOs; 2-3 days for TCAs) because of adverse interaction with anesthetic agents.

TRICYCLIC ANTIDEPRESSANTS (TCA): Prevent the reuptake of norepinephrine or serotonin, which results in increased concentrations of these neurotransmitters.

MEDICATIONS	SIDE EFFECTS	NURSING IMPLICATIONS
Imipramine hydrochloride (**Tofranil**): PO, IM Nortriptyline hydrochloride (**Aventyl**): PO Doxepin hydrochloride (**Sinequan**): PO Amitriptyline hydrochloride (**Elavil**): PO, IM	Drowsiness, dry mouth, blurred vision, constipation, and hypotension. ***Adverse reactions:*** Cardiac dysrhythmias, nystagmus, tremor, hypotension, restlessness.	1. Should not be given at the same time with an MAO inhibitor; a time lag of 14 days is necessary when changing from one drug group to the other. 2. Because of marked sedation, client should avoid activities requiring mental alertness (driving or operating machinery). 3. Instruct client to move gradually from lying to sitting and standing positions to prevent postural hypotension. 4. **Sinequan** is tolerated better by the elderly; has less effect on cardiac status; dilute the concentrate with orange juice. 5. Contraindicated in clients with epilepsy, glaucoma, and cardiovascular disease. 6. Usually given once daily at bedtime. ***Uses:*** depression; **Tofranil** also used to treat enuresis in children.

SELECTIVE SEROTONIN REUPTAKE INHIBITORS (SSRI): Causes selective inhibition of serotonin uptake and produces CNS excitation rather than sedation; has no effect on dopamine or norepinephrine.

MEDICATIONS	SIDE EFFECTS	NURSING IMPLICATIONS
Fluoxetine (**Prosac**): PO Sertraline (**Zoloft**): PO Paroxetine (**Paxil**): PO	Nausea, headache, anxiety, nervousness, insomnia, weight loss, skin rash.	1. Give medication in the morning. 2. ***Uses:*** depression, obsessive-compulsive disorder, bulimia, suppress appetite in obese clients.

MONOAMINE OXIDASE INHIBITORS (MAO): Inhibit the enzyme monoamine oxidase, which breaks down norepinephrine and serotinin, increasing the concentration of these neurotransmitters.

MEDICATIONS	SIDE EFFECTS	NURSING IMPLICATIONS
Isocarboxazid (**Marplan**): PO Phenelzine sulfate (**Nardil**): PO Tranylcypromine (**Parnate**): PO	Drowsiness, insomnia, dryness of mouth, urinary retention, hypotension. ***Adverse reactions:*** tachycardia, tachypnea, agitation, tremors, seizures, heart block, hypotension.	1. Potentiate many drug actions: narcotics, barbiturates, sedatives, and atropine-like medications. 2. Have a long duration of action; therefore, 2 - 3 weeks must go by before taking another drug while on an MAO inhibitor. 3. Interact with specific foods and drugs (ones containing tyramine or sympathomimetic drugs). May cause a severe hypertensive crisis characterized by marked elevation of blood pressure, increased temperature, tremors, and tachycardia. Foods to avoid: coffee, tea, cola beverages, aged cheeses, beer and wine, pickled foods, avocados, figs, and many over-the-counter cold preparations, hay fever medications, and nasal decongestants. 4. Monitor for bladder distention by checking urinary output. 5. **Parnate**: Most likely to cause hypertensive crisis and onset of action is more rapid. ***Uses:*** primarily psychotic depression and depressive episode of bipolar affective disorder.

MISCELLANEOUS ANTI-DEPRESSANTS

MEDICATIONS	SIDE EFFECTS	NURSING IMPLICATIONS
Trazodone (**Desyrel**): PO	Sedation, orthostatic hypotension, nausea, vomiting, can cause priapism (prolonged, painful erection of the penis).	1. See general nursing implications on previous page.
Bupropion (**Wellbutrin**): PO	Weight loss, dry mouth, dizziness.	

Appendix 10-4:
ANTIPSYCHOTIC (NEUROLEPTIC) MEDICATIONS

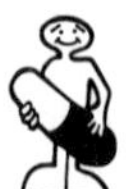

❖GENERAL NURSING IMPLICATIONS❖
— Use cautiously in elderly adults.
— Give daily dose 1-2 hours before betime.
— When mixing for parenteral use, do not mix with other drugs.
— Inject deep IM - client should stay in reclined position 30 - 60 minutes after dose.
— Caution against driving a car or operating machinery.

MEDICATIONS	SIDE EFFECTS	NURSING IMPLICATIONS
PHENOTHIAZINES: Block dopamine receptors and also thought to depress various portions of the reticular activating system; have peripherally exerting anticholinergic properties (atropine-like symptoms, dryness of mouth, stuffy nose, constipation, blurring of vision).		
Aliphatic types— Chloropromazine hydrochloride (**Thorazine**): PO, IM, IV, suppository Promazine hydrochloride (**Sparine**): PO, IM, IV *Piperazine types—* Prochlorperazine (**Compazine**): PO, IM, IV, suppository Fluphenazine hydrochloride (**Prolixin**): PO, IM Trifluoperazine (**Stelazine**): PO, IM *Piperidine types—* Thioridazine (**Mellaril**): PO Mesoridazine besylate (**Serentil**): PO, IM	***Extrapyramidal (movement disorder):*** occurs early in therapy and is usually managed with other drugs *acute dystonia* - spasm of muscles of the tongue, face, neck, or back, oculogyric crisis (upward deviation of the eyes), opisthotonus. *Parkinsonism* -muscle tremors, rigidity, spasms, shuffling gait, stooped posture, cogwheel rigidity. *akathisia* -motor restlessness, pacing. ***Tardive dyskinesia:*** (occurs late in therapy -symptoms are often irreversible) slow worm-like movements of the tongue is earliest symptom; later -fine twisting, writhing movements of the tongue and face, grimacing, lip-smacking, involuntary movements of the limbs, toes, fingers, and trunk. ***Neuroleptic malignant syndrome:*** rare problem, fever (> 41°C), "lead-pipe"muscle rigidity, agitation, confusion, delirium, respiratory and acute renal failure. **Endocrine:** amenorrhea, increased libido in women, decreased libido in men, delayed ejaculation, increased appetite, weight gain, hypoglycemia, and edema. ***Dermatologic:*** photosensitivity. ***Hypersensitivity reaction:*** jaundice, agranulocytosis.	1. Check blood pressure prior to administration; to avoid postural hypotension, encourage client to rise slowly from sitting or lying position. 2. Be aware of the antiemetic effect of the phenothiazines; may mask other pathology such as drug overdose, brain lesions, or intestinal obstruction. 3. Client teaching: protect skin from sunlight; wear long-sleeved shirts, hats, and sunscreen lotion when out in the sunlight. 4. Explain importance of reporting of sore throat, fever, or symptoms of infection. 5. Encourage periodic liver function studies to be done. 6. Teach that drug may turn urine pink or reddish brown. 7. Extrapyramidal symptoms treated with anticholinergics, (i.e., **Cogentin**). 8. ***Uses:*** severe psychoses; schizophrenia, manic phase of bipolar affective disorder, personality disorders, and severe agitation and anxiety; also an adjunct to preoperative anesthesia (e.g., **Compazine, Phenergan**).
BUTYROPHENONES: Same as for phenothiazine.		
Haloperidol (**Haldol**): PO, IM	Significant extrapyramidal effects; low incidence of sedation, orthostatic hypotension; does not elicit photosensitivity reaction.	1. May reduce prothrombin time. 2. Often used as the initial drug for treatment of psychotic disorders. ***Uses:*** tics, vocal disturbances, and psychotic schizophrenia.
THIOXANTHENES: Similar to phenothiazine.		
Thiothixene (**Navane**): PO, IM	Frequent Parkinson-like symptoms; dystonia, atropine-like effects.	1. Same as for phenothiazine. ***Uses:*** same as for phenothiazine.

INTEGUMENTARY SYSTEM 11

PHYSIOLOGY OF THE SKIN

A. Glands on the skin.
  1. Sebaceous glands—secrete sebum, which is an oily secretion that is emptied into the hair shaft.
  2. Apocrine glands—secrete an odorless fluid from the hair shaft which produces a distinctive body odor.
    a. Located in the axillary, anal region, scrotum, and labia majora.
    b. Become more active at the time of puberty.
    c. Eccrine glands—sweat glands that are stimulated by elevated temperature and emotional stress.
      (1) Located all over the body especially the forehead, palms of the hands, and soles of the feet.
      (2) Under control of the sympathetic nervous system.

B. Functions of the skin.
  1. Protection—primary function.
  2. Sensory—major receptor for general sensation.
  3. Water balance.
    a. 500 to 900 ml of water is lost daily through insensible perspiration.
    b. Forms a barrier that prevents loss of water and electrolytes from the internal environment.
  4. Temperature regulation.
  5. Involved in the activation of vitamin D.

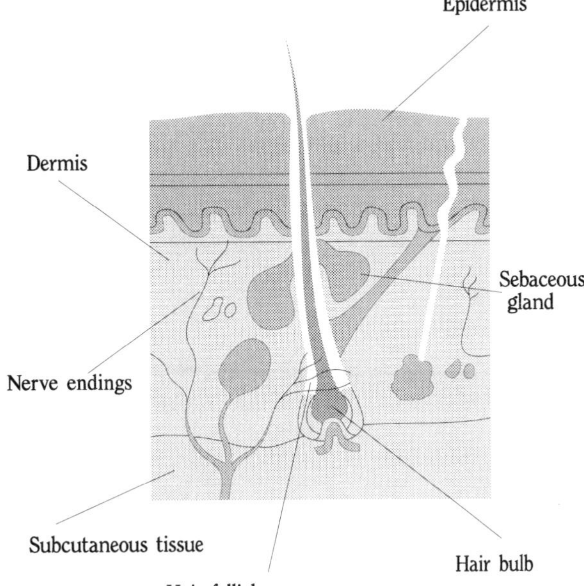

Figure 11-1: Skin Anatomy

  6. Involved in wheal and flare reaction.
    a. Wheal—swelling.
    b. Flare—diffused redness.
    c. These responses are due to local edema secondary to increased capillary permeability and dilatation of the surrounding arterioles.
    d. Reaction is initiated by the release of histamine and the kinins.

System Assessment

A. Health history.
  1. How long has the particular rash, lesion, been present?
  2. Is there any itching, burning, or discomfort associated with the problem?
  3. Has the client been in contact with any irritants, sun, unusual cold, or unhygienic conditions?
  4. Has anyone in the family ever had this same type of problem with their skin?
  5. Is the client taking any medications?
  6. What is the diet history? Does the client have any food allergies?

B. Physical assessment.
  1. Inspection.
    a. Assess the skin for color.
      (1) Jaundice.
      (2) Vitiligo—loss of melanin, resulting in white, depigmented area.
      (3) Areas to assess include the sclera, conjunctiva, nail beds, lips, and buccal mucosa.
    b. Assess for vascularity.
      (1) Determine if there are areas of bruising, purpura, or petechiae.
      (2) Determine if skin blanches on direct pressure.
    c. Assess lesions for type, color, size, distribution and grouping; location and consistency.
      (1) Use metric rulers to measure the size of the lesion.
      (2) Use appropriate specific terminology to describe and report type of lesion.
    d. Common dermatological lesions.
      (1) Macule—flat, circumscribed area of color change in the skin without surface elevation.

(2) Papule—circumscribed, solid, and elevated lesion.

(3) Nodule—raised, solid lesion that is larger and deeper than a papule.

(4) Vesicle—small elevation in skin, usually filled with serous fluid or blood; bulla—larger than a vesicle; pustule—vesicle or bulla filled with pus.

(5) Wheal—elevation of the skin caused by edema of the dermis.

(6) Cyst—mass of fluid-filled tissue that extends to the subcutaneous tissue or dermis.

2. Palpation.
   a. Determine temperature, tissue turgor, and mobility.
   b. Evaluate moisture and texture.

C. Diagnostic skin testing.

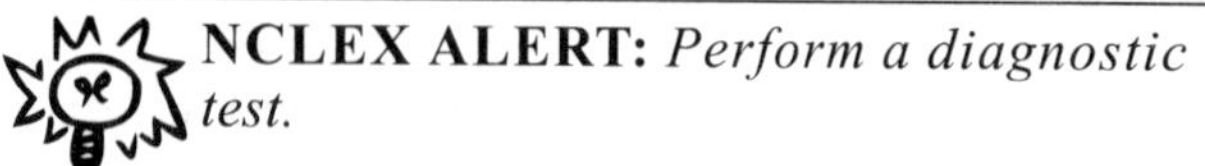

NCLEX ALERT: *Perform a diagnostic test.*

1. Purpose—confirm sensitivity to a specific allergen by placing antigen on or directly below skin (intradermal) to check for presence of antibodies.
   a. Three methods.
      (1) Scratch test (also known as a tine or prick test)—allergen applied to a superficial scratch on skin.
      (2) Patch test—antigen applied to skin and covered with a gauze.
      (3) Intradermal test—injecting a small amount of the antigen in the intradermal layer of the skin; most accurate; high risk of severe allergic reaction.
   b. Interpreting results.
      (1) Immediate reaction—appears within 15-20 minutes after the injection; marked by erythema and a wheal; denotes a positive reaction.
      (2) Positive reaction—indicate an antibody response to previous exposure.
      (3) Negative reaction—is inconclusive; may indicate antibodies have not formed, yet; or antigen was deposited to deep in skin (not an intradermal injection); or immunosuppression.
2. Complications—minor itching to anaphylaxis (see Chapter 7).

DISORDERS OF THE SKIN

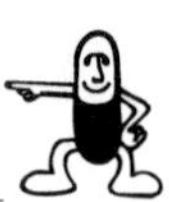

Acne Vulgaris

❑ ***Acne*** **is an inflammatory disorder of the sebaceous glands and their hair follicles.**

Data Collection

1. More common in teenagers; may persist into adulthood.
2. Under hormonal influence during puberty; affected by presence of androgen; which stimulates the sebaceous glands to secrete sebum.
3. Inflammatory lesions or pustules.
4. Cysts, deep nodules that may produce scarring.

Treatment

1. Medical - Topical therapy.

✦ *Goal: to promote psychological adjustment related to body image and appearance.*

1. Counsel and assure that problem is not related to uncleanliness, dietary intake, masturbation, or sexual activity.
2. Encourage verbalization with someone client can talk to about problem.
3. Make sure client recognizes that picking and squeezing lesions will worsen condition.

Self-Care

1. Instruct to cleanse face twice daily - avoid over-cleansing.
2. May use a polyester sponge pad to cleanse, as it provides a mechanical removal of the epidermal layer.
3. Instruct to keep hands away from face and to avoid any friction or trauma to the area; avoid propping hands against face, rubbing face, etc.
4. Emphasize the importance of a nutritious diet - encourage adequate food intake and vitamin A.
5. Avoid the use of cosmetics, shaving creams, and lotion, as they may aggravate acne; if cosmetics are to be used, a water-base make-up is preferable.
6. Instruct the client to administer medication - topical application, avoidance of sunlight while on medications, etc.

Psoriasis

❑ ***Psoriasis*** **is a chronic inflammatory disorder of the skin.**

Data Collection

1. Scaling, plaques on the elbow, scalp and knees.
2. If scales are scraped away, a dark red base of the lesion is seen, which will produce multiple bleeding points.

3. May improve, but often reoccurs throughout life.
4. Bilateral symmetry of symptoms is common.

Treatment

1. Medical.
   a. Topical therapy.
      (1) Coal tar preparation (Anthralin).
      (2) Corticosteroids.
   b. Photo chemotherapy (PUVA therapy) - psoralen, ultraviolet A therapy.
   c. Occlusive dressing - medication applied to the skin, followed by wrapping of the affected area, then covering with a plastic bag.

Home/Self Care

1. Encourage verbalization of anxiety regarding appearance.
2. Instruct client to use a soft brush to remove scales while bathing.
3. Assess client to determine factors that may trigger skin condition (i.e., emotional stress, trauma, seasonal changes).
4. Make sure client understands treatment and implications of care related to occlusive dressings, PUVA therapy, and other treatments.

Pressure Ulcer

❑ **A *pressure ulcer* (decubitus ulcer, bedsore) is a localized area of infarcted tissue characterized by erythematous area that does not blanche, is warm to the touch, and finally, leads to a break in the skin.**

NCLEX ALERT: *Identify potential for skin breakdown - the ulcer can be and should be prevented. Identify those clients at increased risk for ulcer development and begin preventative care as soon as possible. Do not wait for the reddened area to occur before preventative measures are initiated.*

Data Collection

1. Risk factors/etiology.
   a. Prolonged pressure due to immobility.
   b. Malnutrition, hypoproteinemia, vitamin deficiency.
   c. Infection.
   d. Skin dryness, maceration, excessive skin moisture.
   e. Advancing age.
   f. Equipment such as casts, restraints, tractions, etc.
2. Clinical manifestations.
   a. First indication usually erythema, which will not blanche on pressure.
   b. Four stages of ulcer formation (Table 11-1).

Treatment

1. Medical & Surgical.
   a. Debridement (initial care is to remove moist, devitalized tissue).
      (1) Sharp debridement—use of a scalpel or other instrument; used primarily, especially with cellulitis or sepsis.
      (2) Mechanical debridement—wet-to-dry dressings, hydrotherapy, wound irrigation, and dextranomers (small beads poured over secreting wounds to absorb exudate).
      (3) Enzymatic and autolytic debridement—use of enzymes or synthetic dressings that cover wound and self-digest devitalized tissue.
   b. Wound cleansing (use normal saline for most cases).
      (1) Use minimal mechanical force when cleansing to avoid trauma to the wound bed.
      (2) Avoid the use of antiseptics (i.e., Dakin's solution, iodine, hydrogen peroxide).
   c. Dressings (should protect wound, be biocompatible, and hydrate).
      (1) Moistened gauze.
      (2) Film (transparent).
      (3) Hydrocolloid (moisture and oxygen retaining).

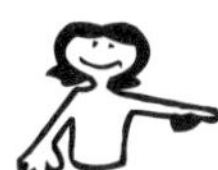

***NURSING PRIORITY:** Keep the ulcer tissue moist and the surrounding intact skin dry.*

2. Dietary.
   a. Increased carbohydrates and protein.
   b. Increased vitamin C and zinc.

Nursing Intervention

✦ *Goal: to prevent or relieve pressure and stimulate circulation.*

1. Frequent change of position - turn client every 1 to 2 hours.
2. Special beds with mattresses that provide for a continuous change in pressure across the mattress.
3. Silicone gel pads placed under the buttocks of wheelchair clients.
4. Sheepskin pads to provide a soft surface to protect the skin from abrasion.

5. Eggcrate mattress to allow circulation under the body and keep the area dry.
6. Active and passive exercises to promote circulation.
7. Gentle skin massage with lotion.

✦ *Goal: to keep skin clean and healthy and prevent the occurrence of a pressure sore.*

1. Wash skin with mild soap and blot completely dry with soft towel.
2. Inspect skin frequently, especially over bony prominences.

NURSING PRIORITY: *Avoid massage over bony prominences. When the side-lying position is used in bed, avoid positioning directly on the trochanter. Do not use donut-type devices. Limit the time the head of the bed is elevated. Avoid uninterrupted sitting in any chair or wheelchair.*

3. Remove any foreign material from the bed, as it may serve as a source of irritation; keep sheets tightly stretched on bed to prevent wrinkles.

✦ *Goal: to promote healing of decubitus ulcer.*

1. Utilize methods discussed to decrease the pressure on the area of the decubitus ulcer.
2. Keep the ulcer area dry.
   a. Minimize skin exposure to moisture due to incontinence, perspiration, or wound drainage.
   b. Use only underpads or briefs that are made of materials that absorb moisture and provide a quick-drying surface to the skin.
   c. Position the client with the ulcer exposed to air; may use light to increase the drying and promote healing.
3. Utilize skin barriers to decrease contamination and increase healing in a non-infected ulcer.
4. Observe the ulcer for signs of infection. Infected ulcers will have to be debrided, if healing is to occur.

Table 11-1: STAGES OF PRESSURE ULCERS

Stage 1
- Skin is intact.
- Area is red and *does not blanche* with external pressure.

Stage 2
- Skin is not intact.
- There is partial thickness skin loss of the epidermis or dermis.
- The ulcer is superficial and presents as an abrasion, blister, or shallow crater.

Stage 3
- Full thickness skin loss occurs.
- Damage or necrosis of subcutaneous tissue extends down to, but not through, fascia.
- Ulcer presents as a deep crater with or without undermining of adjacent tissue.

Stage 4
- Full thickness skin loss with extensive tissue destruction,, tissue necrosis or damage to muscle,, bone,, or supporting structures (e.g., tendon or joint capsule).
- Undermining and sinus tracts may develop.

Source: U.S. Department of Health and Human Services (1992): Pressure ulcers in adults: Prediction and prevention. *Clinical Practice Guidelines,* No.3. Rockville, MD: Health Care Policy and Research.

Atopic Dermatitis

❑ ***Atopic dermatitis (also called eczema)*** **is a superficial, inflammatory disorder of genetically hypersensitive skin—condition occurs primarily during infancy, usually between 2 and 6 months of age; usually spontaneous and permanent remissions by 3 years of age.**

Data Collection

1. Reddened lesions.
2. Discomfort from itching (worse at night).
3. Lesions tend to occur on the cheeks, arms, and legs.
4. As the child gets older, the lesions tend to be dry with a thickening of the skin.
5. Infants with eczema are more likely to have allergies as children and adults.

Treatment

1. Food allergies are not associated with adult atopic dermatitis; milk, eggs, wheat, and peanuts are the most common suspicious foods in children.
2. Pruritus is treated with Benadryl and topical steroids.
3. Systemic steroids, if condition is severe.

Home/Self-Care

1. Teach parents about dietary restrictions; provide them with written guidelines.
2. Keep fingernails and toenails cut short.
3. Feed the child when he is well-rested and is not itching.
4. Assist parents to identify foods that contain eggs and other "hidden" allergic foods.
5. Avoid overheating, decrease perspiration (no nylon clothing).
6. Child should avoid contact with the chicken pox virus and herpes simplex.
7. Avoid immunizations with live vaccines due to the possibility of severe reactions.
8. Non-irritating clothing; avoid wool or abrasive fabrics.

Contact Dermatitis

❑ ***Contact dermatitis* is an inflammatory skin reaction which results because the skin has come in contact with a specific irritant (irritant contact dermatitis that occurs immediately after injury to skin) or allergen (allergic contact dermatitis, which is usually a symptom of delayed hypersensitivity).**

Data Collection

1. Causes.
   a. Poison ivy and poison oak.
   b. Fabric—wool, polyester.
   c. Cosmetics.
   d. Household products such as detergents, soap, hair dye.
   e. Industrial substances—paints, dyes, insecticides, rubber compounds, etc.
2. Clinical manifestations.
   a. Pruritus and discomfort.
   b. Hive-like papules, vesicles, and plaques (more chronic).
   c. Edema.
   d. Sharply circumscribed areas (with occasional vesicle formation) that crust and ooze.

Treatment

1. Medical.
   a. Topical steroids, oral steroids for severe cases.
   b. Antihistamines and antipruritic agents.
   c. **Aveeno** (oatmeal) baths and topical soaks.
2. Skin testing to determine allergen; skin lesions usually appear within 12 to 48 hours after contact with allergen.

Home/Self Care

1. Teach importance of washing exposed skin with cool water and soap as soon as possible after exposure (within 15 minutes is best).
2. Provide cool, tepid bath; trim fingernails, and utilize measures to control itching.
3. Teach about fallacy of blister fluid spreading the disease.

Impetigo

❑ ***Impetigo* is a bacterial skin infection caused by invasion of the epidermis by pathogenic *Staphylococcus aureus* and/or group A beta-hemolytic *streptococcus.***

Data Collection

1. Pustule-like lesions with moist honey-colored crusts surrounded by redness.
2. Pruritus.
3. Appears more commonly on the face, especially around the mouth.
4. Spreads to surrounding areas.

Treatment

1. Medical.
   a. Local—topical treatment.
      (1) Gentle washing 2-3 times a day to remove crust.
      (2) Topical mupirocin (**Bactroban**) antibiotic cream, if only a couple of lesions found.
   b. Systemic antibiotic therapy is the treatment of choice with extensive lesions.

Home/Self Care

1. Teach the client and family the importance of good hand washing.
2. Encourage adherence to therapeutic regime, especially taking the full course of antibiotics.
3. Untreated impetigo may result in glomerulonephritis.

Fungal (Dermatophyte) Infections

Data Collection

1. Types.
   a. Tinea corporis (ringworm)—temporary hair loss, if scalp is affected.
   b. Tinea cruris ("jock itch")—small, red, scaly patches in the groin area.
   c. Tinea pedis (athlete's foot)—scaling, maceration, erythema, blistering, and pruritus; usually found between the toes.

Treatment

1. Topical antifungal creme (Appendix 11-1).
2. Systemic therapy —Griseofulvin - used primarily for extensive cases.

Home/Self Care

1. To prevent athlete's foot, client should be instructed to keep feet as dry as possible and use socks of absorbent cotton.
   a. Talcum powder or antifungal powder; **Tinactin** may be applied twice daily.
   b. Encourage aeration of shoes, to allow them to completely dry out.
2. Client should maintain hygienic measures to prevent the spread of fungal diseases, specifically ringworm of the scalp.
   a. Family members should avoid using the same comb.

b. Scarves and hats should be washed thoroughly.

c. Examine family and household pets frequently for symptoms of the disease.

3. Client should avoid infection.

a. Any activity that allows heat, friction, and maceration to occur may lead to skin breakdown and infection.

b. Loose-fitting clothing and cotton underwear are to be encouraged.

Parasitic Infestations

A. **Pediculosis.**

1. Types.

a. *Pediculus humanus capitis*—head lice.

b. *Pediculus humanus corporis*—body lice.

c. *Phthirus pubis*—pubic lice or crabs.

2. Clinical manifestations.

a. Intense pruritus which may lead to secondary excoriation and infection.

b. Tiny, red, noninflammatory lesions.

c. Eggs (nits) are often attached to the hair shaft in both head and body lice.

d. Pubic lice are often spread by sexual contact.

B. **Scabies** (mites)—an infestation of the skin by itch mites.

1. Intense itching, especially at night.

2. Burrows are seen, especially between fingers, on the surface of wrists, and in axillary folds.

3. Redness, swelling, and vesicular formation may be noted.

Treatment

1. Pediculosis

a. Permethrin 1% (**NIX**) - effective against nits and lice with just one application.

b. Pyrethrin compounds (**RID**).

2. Scabies - Permethrin 5% cream (**Elimite**) Cream applied to the skin from head to soles of feet and left on for 8-14 hours, then washed off. Second application in 48 hours is recommended.

Home/Self Care.

1. All family members and close contacts need to be treated for parasitic disorders; nits can survive up to 3 weeks when removed from host.

2. Bedding and clothing that may have lice or nits should be washed or dry cleaned; furniture and rugs should be vacuumed or treated.

3. When shampooing hair, use a fine-tooth comb to remove remaining nits.

Viral Infections

1. **Herpes simplex virus** (fever blister, cold sore) - herpes virus Type I (HSV-1).

a. Painful, local reaction of vesicles with an erythematous base; most often occur around the mouth.

b. Contagious by direct contact, is recurrent; there is no immunity.

c. Chronic disorder which may be exacerbated by stress, trauma, menses, sunlight, fatigue, or systemic infection.

d. Recurrent episodes are characterized by appearance of lesions in the same place.

e. Not to be confused with Type II herpes virus (HSV-2) that primarily occurs below the waist (genital herpes).

f. It is possible for the Type I herpes to cause genital lesions, and for the Type II to cause oral lesions (See Sexually Transmitted Diseases in Chapter 17).

2. **Herpes zoster** (shingles).

a. Related to the chicken pox virus - varicella.

b. Contagious to anyone who has not had chicken pox or who may be immunosuppressed.

c. Linear patches of vesicles with an erythematous base are located along spinal and cranial nerve tracts.

d. Often unilateral and appears on the trunk; however, may appear on the face.

e. Pain, burning, and neuralgia occur at the site prior to outbreak of vesicles.

f. Often precipitated by the same factors as *herpes simplex* infection.

3. **Herpetic whitlow**—occurs on fingertips and around nail cuticle; often seen in medical personnel.

Treatment

1. Usually symptomatic - soothing moist compresses.

2. Analgesics.

3. Antiviral agents (Appendix 11-1).

Home/Self Care

1. Alleviate pain by administering analgesics.

Melanomas tend to have

A Asymmetry
B Border irregularity
C Color variegation
D Diameter greater than 6mm.

2. Antihistamines may be administered to control the itching.
3. Usually lesions heal without complications; *herpes simplex* usually heals without a scar, whereas *herpes zoster* may scar.
4. If hospitalized, contact precautions with *herpes zoster.*

Cancer of the Skin

Data Collection

1. Risk factors.
   a. Overexposure to sunlight.
   b. Exposure to chemicals.
   c. Clients who have scars due to severe burns.
2. Types.
   a. **Actinic keratosis** - premalignant type.
      (a) Small macules or papules with a dry, rough, adherent yellow or brown scale.
      (b) Appears on face, neck, back of hand, and forearm.
      (c) May slowly progress to squamous cell carcinoma.
   b. **Basal cell carcinoma** - most common type of skin cancer.
      (1) Appears as a small, waxy nodule with a translucent pearly border.
      (2) Appears more frequently on the face, usually between the hairline and upper lip.
   c. **Squamous cell carcinoma** - malignant proliferation arising from the epidermis; usually on sun-damaged skin or skin that has been irradiated or excessively scarred.
      (1) May metastasize.
      (2) Appears as a firm nodule with an indistinct border; may be opaque.
   d. **Malignant melanoma** - has the highest mortality rate of any form of skin cancer.
      (1) Often appears in pre-existing moles in the skin.
      (2) Common sites include back and legs.

Treatment

1. Surgical.
   a. Excisional surgery.
   b. Cryosurgery.
   c. Electrodesiccation and curettage.
2. Medical.
   a. X-ray therapy.
   b. Topical chemotherapy - fluorouracil (**5-FU**).

Nursing Intervention

✦ *Goal: to assist client to understand disease process, importance of follow-up treatment, and measures to maintain health.*

1. Teach the importance of avoiding unnecessary exposure to sunlight.
2. Apply protective sun screen when outside.
3. Teach the warning signals of cancer.
4. Have moles treated that are in areas where there is friction or repeated irritation.

✦ *Goal: to support the client and promote psychological homeostasis.*

1. Allow for verbalization of fear and anxiety.
2. Encourage verbalization relating to altered body image when large, wide, full-thickness excisions must be made to treat malignant melanoma.
3. Point out client's resources and support effective coping mechanisms.
4. Teach the importance of examining and checking moles and any new lesions.

BURNS

A. Types of burns.
   1. ***Chemical injury***—results from contact with a corrosive substance.
   2. ***Electrical injury***—intense heat is generated from electrical current and causes coagulation necrosis as it flows through the body.
   3. ***Thermal injury***—most common type of burn injury results from flames, flash (explosion), scald, or direct contact.

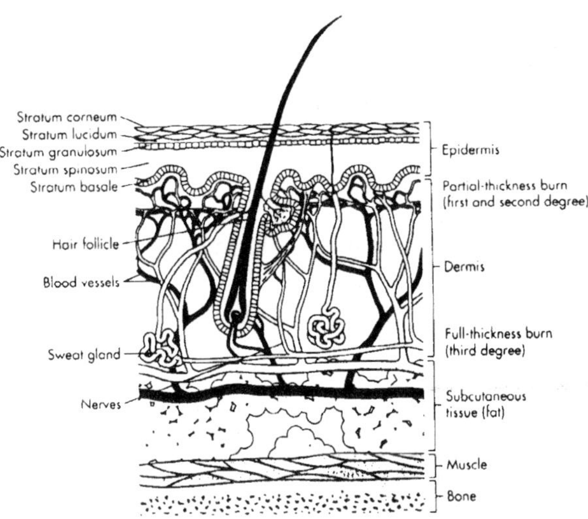

Figure 11-2: Levels of human skin involved in burns.
Reprinted with permission: Phipps, WJ, Sands, JK, & Marek, JF (1999). *Medical Surgical Nursing: Concepts & Clinical Practice,* 6th ed. Philadelphia: Mosby, p. 2110

4. ***Inhalation injury***—results from inhalation of smoke and asphyxiates. The respiratory system frequently sustains two types of burn injuries:
   a. Smoke inhalation and upper airway burns may precipitate airway edema and obstruction within 24 to 48 hours post-burn.
5. Inhalation of carbon monoxide combines with hemoglobin, thereby decreasing oxygen availability to cells.

B. Fluid considerations.
   1. Fluid shift and edema formation occurs within 24 to 48 hours post-burn. Fluid mobilization occurs within approximately 18-36 hours post burn.
   2. Serum potassium levels increase, and hematocrit levels increase due to hemoconcentration.
   3. The increased capillary permeability and histamine released from the injured cells precipitate a decrease in fluid volume.

Assessment

A. Pulmonary function assessment.
   1. Findings.
      a. Patent airway.
      b. Presence of adequate breath sounds.
      c. Symptoms of hypoxia.
      d. Criteria suggesting pulmonary damage.
         (1) History of burn occurring within a confined area.
         (2) Burns around the face, neck, mouth, or in the oral mucosa.
      e. Circulatory status.
         (1) Tachycardia, hypotension may occur early.
         (2) Evaluate urine output.
      f. Identify when client ate last; check GI function.
      g. Evaluate response to fluid therapy; observe for:
         (1) Presence of hematuria.
         (2) Urine output should be at least 30 cc per hour.
         (3) Hypotension (below 90/60).
         (4) Confusion, disorientation.
      h. Evaluate circulatory status of the extremities.

NURSING PRIORITY: *The burned client is often awake, mentally alert and cooperative at first. The level of consciousness may change as respiratory status changes or the fluid shift occurs, precipitating hypovolemia. If the client is unconscious or confused, assess him for possibility of a head injury.*

Table 11-2: DEPTH OF BURN

✦ ***Superficial or first degree burn*** - area reddened and blanches with pressure; no edema present; area is generally painful to touch.

✦ ***Partial thickness or second degree*** - Dermis and epidermis affected; formation of large, thick-walled blisters; underlying skin is erythematous.

✦ ***Full thickness or third degree*** - All of the skin is destroyed; may have damage to the subcutaneous tissue and muscle; usually has a dry appearance, may be white or charred; will require skin grafting to cover area.

✦ ***Fourth degree burn*** - Full thickness burn in which underlying structures (fascia, tendons, and bones) are severely damaged, usually blackened.

   2. Determine the severity of the burn injury (Table 11-2 and Figure 11-2).
      a. Extent of burn surface (burn surface area—BSA).
         (1) Rule of nines—generally used for adults (Figure 11-3).
         (2) Pediatric burns are calculated taking into the client's age in relation to proportion of body parts.
      b. Area of burn.
         (1) Burns around the neck and face may cause enough edema formation to precipitate mechanical occlusion of the airway.
         (2) Circumferential burns (burns surrounding an entire extremity) may cause severe reduction of circulation to an extremity, due to edema formation and lack of elasticity of the eschar.
      c. Age.
         (1) Infants have an immature immune system and poor body defense.
         (2) Elderly clients heal more slowly and are more likely to have wound infection problems and pulmonary complications.
      d. Presence of other health problems - diabetes and peripheral vascular disease delay wound healing.

Treatment

1. Respiratory status takes priority over the treatment of the burn surface area.
2. If the burned area is small, apply cold compresses or immerse injured area in cool water to decrease heat; ice should not be directly applied to the burn area.
3. Administer tetanus injection.
4. Do not put any ointment or salves on the burn area.
5. If the cause of the burn is chemical, thoroughly rinse the area with large amounts of cool water.

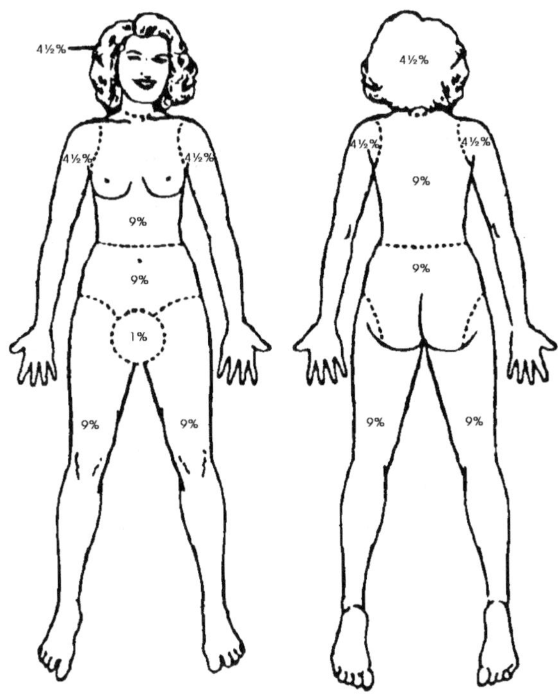

Figure 11-3: Rule Of Nines

6. Fluid resuscitation.
   a. Utilized in clients with 20 percent or greater burn surface area.
   b. Fluid replacement is determined by:
      (1) Size and depth of burn.
      (2) Age.
      (3) Pre-existing burn conditions (dehydration, CHF, etc.).
7. Maintain NPO, assess need for nasogastric tube.
8. Analgesics are give IV; IM, sub-q; PO medications may not absorbed effectively.
9. Methods of wound care (area is cleaned and debrided of necrotic burned tissue).
   a. Open method (exposure)—burn is covered with a topical antibiotic cream and no dressing is applied.
   b. Closed method of dressing—fine mesh is used to cover the burned surface; may be impregnated with antibiotic ointment or ointment may be applied prior to dressing.
   c. Escharotomy—procedure involves excision through the eschar to increase circulation to an extremity with circumferential burns.
   d. Wound grafting—as eschar is debrided and granulation tissue begins to form, grafts are utilized to protect the wound and to promote healing.
10. Nutritional support.
    a. Diet is high in calories and protein.
    b. In clients who sustain large burned areas, supplemental gastric tube feedings or hyperalimentation may be utilized.

Nursing Intervention

✦ *Goal: to maintain patent airway and prevent hypoxia.*

1. Assess circumstances surrounding the burn.
2. As edema phase begins, evaluate respiratory status.
3. ET intubation or tracheotomy may be necessary.
4. Assess for ongoing respiratory complications.
5. Anticipate transfer to burn unit if greater than 20% BSA.

✦ *Goal: to evaluate fluid status and determine circulatory status and adequacy of fluid replacement.*

1. Obtain client's weight on admission.
2. Assess status and time frame of fluid resuscitation.
3. Evaluate renal status and urine output.

✦ *Goal: to prevent or decrease infection.*

1. Implement infection control procedures to protect the client.
2. After eschar sloughs or is removed, assess wound for infection. Infection is difficult to identify prior to the eschar sloughing.

✦ *Goal: to maintain nutrition and promote positive nitrogen balance for healing.*

1. Work with dietitian to maintain nutritional intake.
2. Tube feedings as indicated.
3. Care of hyperalimentation as indicated. (Appendix 18-7)
4. Daily weight.

✦ *Goal: to prevent contractures and scarring.*

1. Assist client to attempt mobilization and ambulation as soon as possible.
2. Passive and active range of motion should be initiated from the beginning of burn therapy and throughout therapy.
3. Position client to prevent flexion contractures; position of comfort for the client may increase contracture formation.
4. Utilize splints and exercises to prevent flexion contractures.

✦ *Goal: to promote acceptance and adaptation to alterations of body image*

1. Utilize counselors and resource team members.
2. Maintain open communication and encourage expression of feelings.

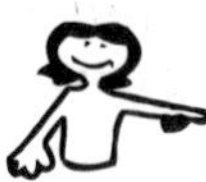

NURSING PRIORITY: It is important to recognize that the client's anger is not a direct attack on the care provider; it is an expression of grief and sorrow.

3. Anticipate depression as a normal consequence of burn trauma; it should decrease as condition improves.

Self-Care

1. Physical therapy.
2. Continue high calorie, high protein diet.
3. Wound care management.
4. Avoid direct sunlight to burn area.⌘

Questions—Integumentary System

1. A client has extensive burns on the anterior trunk with eschar. What is the nurses primary concern regarding the eschar formation?

① It prevents fluid remobilization in the first 48 hours post burn trauma.
② Infection is difficult to assess prior to the eschar sloughing.
③ It restricts the ability of the client to move about.
④ Circulation to the extremities is diminished due to edema formation.

2. A client comes to the outpatient clinic with impetigo on his left arm. What information would the nurse give this client?

① Apply antibiotic ointment to the dried lesion.
② Wash the lesions with soap and water then apply a steroid ointment.
③ Soak the scabs off the lesion and apply an antibiotic ointment.
④ Wash the lesions with hydrogen peroxide and apply an antifungal creme.

3. A teacher notifies the school nurse that many of the students in her third grade class have been scratching their heads and complaining of intense itching of the scalp. The nurse notices tiny white material at the base of the hair shaft. What condition does this assessment reflect?

① Tinea capitis.
② Pediculosis capitis.
③ Dandruff.
④ Scabies.

4. In which situation would it be appropriate for the nurse to administer a skin test?

① A toddler with a possible diagnosis of cystic fibrosis.
② A client who has a transdermal patch ordered.
③ A client scheduled for a electromyography.
④ A child who is to receive ampicillin for the first time.

5. What is the type of skin cancer that is most difficult to treat?

① Oat cell.
② Malignant melanoma.
③ Basal cell epithelioma.
④ Squamous cell epithelioma.

6. A client has a pressure ulcer which appears infected and the subcutaneous tissue is necrotic. The ulcer also has foul-smelling, purulent drainage present. What is the classification of this ulcer?

① Stage 1.
② Stage 2.
③ Stage 3.
④ Stage 4.

7. The nurse understands that scaling around the toes, blistering, and pruritus is characteristic of what condition?

① Eczema.
② Psoriasis.
③ Tinea pedis.
④ Pediculosis corporis.

8. What are the physical characteristics of a client who is most susceptible to develop malignant melanoma?

① Light to pale skin, blond hair, blue eyes.
② Olive complexion, oily skin, dark eyes.
③ Dark skin with freckles, dry flaky skin, hazel eyes.
④ Coarse skin, ruddy complexion, brown eyes.

9. Herpes zoster has been diagnosed in an elderly client. What will the nursing management include?

① Apply antifungal creme to the areas daily.
② Place client on contact precautions.
③ Administer a herpes zoster immunization.
④ Expect to find lesions in the perineal area.

10. What is considered a priority in a teaching plan for a client with pruritus?

① Use of medications to decrease level of anxiety.
② Measures to keep the client from scratching.
③ Teaching warning signs and symptoms of infection.
④ Obtaining daily skin assessments.

11. The nurse is teaching self-care to an elderly client. What would the nurse encourage the client do for his dry, itchy skin?

① Apply a moisturizer on all dry areas daily.
② Shower twice a day with a mild soap.
③ Use a pumice and exfoliating sponge on areas to remove dry scaly patches.
④ Wear protective pads on areas which show the most dryness.

12. What is the priority assessment finding for client who has sustained burns on the face and neck?

① Spreading, large, clear vesicles.
② Increased respirations.
③ Difficulty with vision.
④ Increased thirst.

13. A client has suffered a third degree burn. What would the nursing assessment findings indicate?

① Area reddened, blanches with pressure, no edema.
② Blackened skin and underlying structures.
③ Thick, clear blisters, underlying skin edematous and erythematous.
④ Dry white, charred appearance, damage to subcutaneous tissues.

Answers and rationales to these questions are in the section at the end of the book entitled "Chapter Study Questions: Answers & Rationales."

Appendix 11-1: MEDICATIONS USED IN SKIN DISORDERS

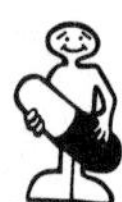

MEDICATIONS	SIDE EFFECTS	NURSING IMPLICATIONS

❖ GENERAL NURSING IMPLICATIONS ❖

— Topical medications are used primarily for local effects when systemic absorption is undesirable.
— For topical application:
Apply after shower or bath for best absorption, as skin is hydrated.
Apply small amount of medication and rub in well.

ANTI-FUNGAL: Inhibits or damages fungal cell membrane, either altering permeability or disrupting cell mitosis.

MEDICATIONS	SIDE EFFECTS	NURSING IMPLICATIONS
Clotrimazole (**Lotrimin**): topical Nystatin (**Mycolog**): topical Ketoconazole (**Nizoral**): PO, topical Griseofulvin (**Fulvicin**): PO	Nausea, vomiting, abdominal pain. Hypersensitivity reaction— rash, urticaria, pruritus. Hepatotoxicity. Gynecomastia (ketoconozole).	1. Monitor hepatic function (when on oral medication). 2. Avoid alcohol due to potential liver problems. 3. Check for local burning, irritation, or itching with topical application. 4. Prolonged therapy (weeks or months) is usually necessary, especially with griseofulvin (Fulvicin). 5. Take griseofulvin (Fulvicin) with foods high in fat, (e.g., milk, ice cream) to decrease GI upset and assist in absorption. 6. Uses: Tinea infections, fungal infections, candidiasis diaper dermatitis.

ANTI-VIRAL: Reduces viral shedding, pain, and time to heal.

MEDICATIONS	SIDE EFFECTS	NURSING IMPLICATIONS
Acyclovir (**Zovirax**): topical, PO, IV. Vidarabine (**Ara-A, Vir-A**): IV, ophthalmic	IV: phlebitis, rash, hives PO: nausea, vomiting Topical: burning, stinging, pruritus. Anorexia, nausea, vomiting. Ophthalmic: burning, itching.	1. Apply topically to affected area six times per day. 2. Avoid auto-inoculation; wash hands frequently; apply with gloved hand. 3. Avoid sexual intercourse during duration of genital lesions. 4. Drink adequate fluids. 5. Infuse IV preparations over 1 hour; use an infusion pump for accurate delivery. 6. ***Uses:*** herpes infections.

ANTI-INFLAMMATORY: Decreases the inflammatory response.

MEDICATIONS	SIDE EFFECTS	NURSING IMPLICATIONS
Triamcinolone adetonide (**Aristocort**): topical	Skin thinning, superficial dilated blood vessels (teleangiectasis), acne-like eruptions, adrenal suppression.	1. Triamcinolone and hydrocortisone cremes come in various strengths and potency. Watch the percent strength. 2. Applied 2-3 times a day. 3. Use an occlusive dressing only if ordered. 4. Encourage client to use the least amount possible and for the shortest period of time.

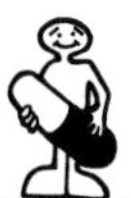

Appendix 11-2: TOPICAL ANTIBIOTICS FOR BURN TREATMENT

MEDICATIONS	SIDE EFFECTS	NURSING IMPLICATIONS
TOPICAL ANTIBIOTICS: Prevent and treat infection at the burn site.		
Silver sulfadiazine **(Silvadene)**	Pain, burning on application. Hypersensitivity: rash, itching, or burning sensation in unburned skin.	1. Liberal amounts are spread topically with a sterile, gloved hand or on impregnated gauze rolls over the burned surface. 2. If discoloration occurs in the **Silvadene** cream, do not use. 3. A thin layer of cream is spread evenly over the entire burn surface area, reapplication every 12 hours. 4. Client should be bathed or tubbed daily to aid in debridement. 5. Medication does not penetrate eschar. 6. On extensive burns, monitor urine output and renal function; a significant amount of sulfa may be absorbed.
Mafenide acetate **(Sulfamylon 10%)**	Pain, burning or stinging at application sites; excessive loss of body water; excoriation of new tissue; may be systemically absorbed and cause metabolic acidosis.	1. Bacteriostatic medication diffuses rapidly through burned skin and eschar and is effective against bacteria under the eschar. 2. Dressings are not required, but are frequently utilized. A thin layer of cream is spread evenly over the entire burn surface. 3. Monitor renal function, as medication is rapidly absorbed from the burn surface and eliminated via the kidney. 4. Pain occurs on application.

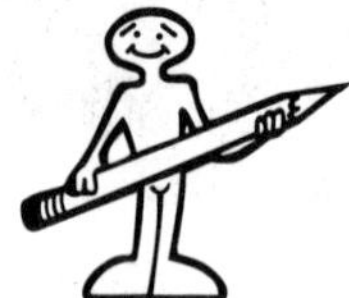

Notes

12 SENSORY SYSTEM

PHYSIOLOGY OF THE EYE

A. Eyeballs.
  1. External layer.
    a. Sclera—tough, protective covering of the outside of the eye.
    b. Cornea—transparent tissue over the pupil.
  2. Middle layer.
    a. Choroid—pigmented layer; contains large amount of blood vessels.
    b. Ciliary muscle—muscular body that allows the eye to focus through contraction and relaxation.
    c. Iris—controls the amount of light; gives the eye the characteristic color.
  3. Inner layer.
    a. Retina—contains millions of nerve cells to coordinate and transmit signals via the optic nerve to the brain.
    b. Aqueous humor—fluid that fills anterior and posterior chambers; circulates through the pupil and empties into canal of Schlemm.
    c. Vitreous humor—fluid that fills the cavity posterior to the lens.
    d. Crystalline lens—provides for the convergence and refraction of light rays and images onto the retina; enables vision to be focused.
    e. Optic nerve—leaves the eyeball through the retina at the location of the optic disc.

B. Eyelids — protective coverings of the eye.
  1. Conjunctiva—inner lining of the eyelid.
  2. Lacrimal gland—excretes lacrimal fluid (tears) to lubricate, clean, and protect the outer surface of the eye.

System Assessment

A. External assessment.
  1. Assess position and alignment of the eyes—both eyes should fixate on one visual field simultaneously.
  2. Evaluate for presence of ptosis.
  3. Inspect lids and conjunctiva for discharge or inflammation.
  4. Assess color of sclera—normally thin coating, may have a yellowish color with aging.
  5. Evaluate size and equality of pupils—should be equal in size and shape.
  6. Evaluate pupillary reaction to light.
    a. Direct light reflex—constriction of pupil when stimulated with light.
    b. Consensual reflex—constriction of opposite pupil when stimulated with light.

B. Evaluate visual acuity and for refractory errors. (Appendix 12-1)
  1. Myopia—(nearsightedness) vision for near objects is better than far.
  2. Hyperopia—(farsightedness) vision for distant objects is better than near.
  3. Determine any problems with double vision.

C. Assess for presence of pain, and any recent change in vision.

NCLEX ALERT: *Assist clients to cope with sensory impairment (e.g., hearing, sight, etc.).*

DISORDERS OF THE EYE

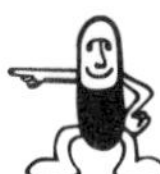

Glaucoma

❑ ***Glaucoma* is a condition characterized by an increase in intraocular pressure and progressive loss of vision. It is a chronic disease and a leading cause of blindness.**

Types

1. Primary open-angle glaucoma— most common form. Flow of aqueous humor is slowed or stopped by obstruction, thus increasing intraocular pressure. Characterized by a slow onset.
2. Primary angle-closure glaucoma (acute glaucoma)—caused by a blockage in the flow of aqueous humor, thus increasing pressure; characterized by rapid onset.

Assessment

1. Risk factors.
  a. Familial tendency.
  b. Over 40 years of age.
  c. Diabetic.
  d. History of injury or eye surgery.
  e. Severe nearsightedness.
  f. Damage to vision is permanent.
2. Diagnostics— pressure is above 22 mm Hg. (Appendix 12-1)

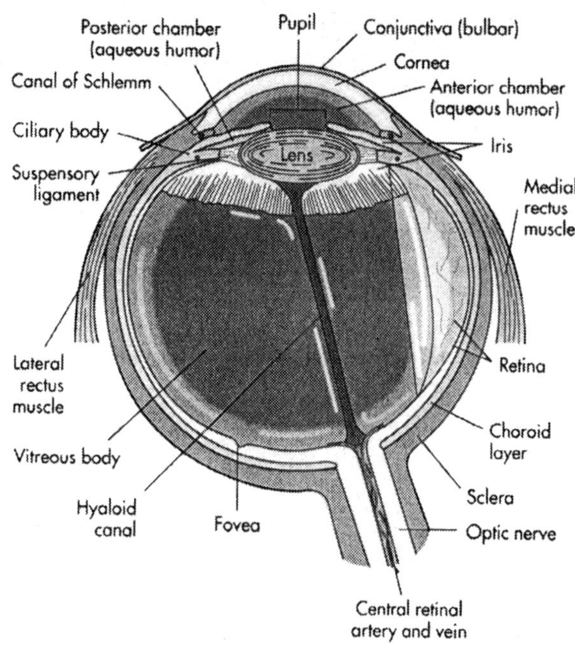

Figure 12-1: Horizontal Section of the Eye
Reprinted with permission: Phipps, WJ, Sands, JK, & Marek, JF (1999). *Medical Surgical Nursing: Concepts & Clinical Practice,* 6th ed. Philadelphia: Mosby, p. 1812

3. Clinical manifestations of primary open-angle glaucoma.
   a. Gradual loss of peripheral vision (i.e., tunnel vision).
   b. Vague headache.
   c. Halos around lights.
   d. Transient blurred vision.
   e. Blindness will eventually occur if untreated.
   f. Generally painless, symptoms occur late.

Treatment

1. Medications (Appendix 12-2).
   a. Topical miotics.
   b. Topical beta-blockers (ophthalmic).
   c. Oral glycerin preparations to promote diuresis and lower intraocular pressure.
2. Surgical intervention.
   a. Laser trabeculoplasty—usually done outpatient with a topical anesthetic.
   b. Filtering procedures—trabeculectomy.

Nursing Intervention

✦ *Goal: to teach client and significant others about the problems of increased pressure, treatment to control problem, and consequences of failure to follow prescribed regimen.*

1. Teaching plan.
   a. Explanation of the problem of increased intraocular pressure.
   b. Visual damage cannot be corrected, but further damage can be prevented.
   c. Correct utilization of prescribed medications; client must remain on medication in order to control disease.
   d. Importance of continued follow-up medical care.
   e. Importance of wearing medical alert identification.

✦ *Goal: to decrease intraocular pressure.*

1. Client should avoid straining at stool, lifting, stooping.
2. Administer medications to decrease intraocular pressure.

✦ *Goal: to provide appropriate preoperative nursing measures if surgery is indicated.*

1. If surgery is required, it is frequently done on an outpatient basis and with a local anesthetic. Orient the client to the surroundings and sounds that will occur during the procedure.
2. For outpatient surgery, client should wear comfortable clothes and arrange for someone to provide transportation home.

✦ *Goal: to prevent client from experiencing postoperative complications (surgery frequently done under local anesthesia).*

1. Tell client to avoid activities that increase intraocular pressure.
2. Administer medications—miotic, antibiotics, and steroids.
3. Be sure medication is administered in the eye it is ordered for, as the unaffected eye may be treated with a different medication.
4. Client may eat and ambulate as desired after the initial sedative effect is gone.

Self-Care

1. The eye should remain patched with a plastic or metal shield until the client returns to the physician for a follow-up visit, usually within two days postoperative.
2. Teach the client not to rub his eyes, because it could damage the healing tissue.
3. Demonstrate client correct administration of eye medication and have client return demonstrate.

Cataract

❑ **A complete or partial opacity of the lens is known as a *cataract*. It may occur at birth (congeni-**

tal cataract); however, it occurs most commonly in adults past middle-age (senile cataracts).

Assessment

1. Clinical manifestations.
   a. Painless.
   b. Gradual decrease in visual acuity.
   c. Pupil appears gray to milky white.
   d. Red light reflex is distorted on direct opthalmoscope examination.
2. Diagnostics (Appendix 12-1).
   a. Decrease in visual acuity.
   b. Ophthalmoscopic exam.
   c. Slit lamp examination.

Treatment

Surgical treatment is only method of correcting problem; surgery is usually performed when client begins to experience problems in activities of daily living.

1. Intracapsular extraction—the lens is removed intact in the lens capsule.
2. Extracapsular extraction—the lens material is removed without removing the posterior lens capsule.
3. Since surgery removes the lens, the client will require some type of lens correction. Surgery is most often an out-patient procedure and is done under conscious sedation.
   a. Intraocular lens implant is frequently placed during the original surgical procedure.
   b. Contact lens also achieves the visual correction but is frequently difficult for the elderly client to clean and handle.
   c. Eyeglasses are usually very thick and do not provide as high a quality of vision correction as the intraocular lens implant (see Box 12-1).

Nursing Intervention

✦ *Goal: to provide appropriate teaching and nursing care.*

1. Orient the client to the surroundings and sounds that will occur during the procedure.
2. For outpatient surgery, client should wear comfortable clothes and arrange for someone to provide transportation home.
3. Prior to surgery, the nurse will instill mydriatic eye drops and frequently, cycloplegic drops as well.
4. Determine if client has any questions regarding replacement lens.

Box 12-1: Elderly Care Focus
Promoting Independent Activities of Daily Living for the Client with Diminished Vision

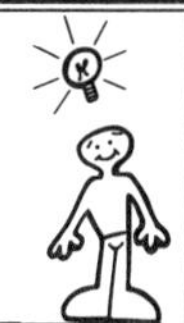

➻ *MEDICATIONS*

- Use different shapes of containers with lids (square, round, triangular) when client has to take medications more than once a day.
- Obtain medication boxes with raised letters or numbers on them for the days of the week.
- Obtain a "talking clock" which states the time.

➻ *SAFETY*

- Remove throw rugs.
- Use non-breakable dishes, cups, and glasses.
- Keep appliance cords short and out of walkways.
- Avoid footstools in favor of recliner with a built-in foot-rest.
- Cleansers, cleaning fluids, and caustic chemicals should be labeled with large, raised lettering.
- Have hand grips installed in bathrooms.
- Put nonskid stripping on tub floor surface.
- Encourage use of an electric razor.

➻ *COMMUNICATION*

- Use telephones that have programmed, automatic dialing features. Be sure to include emergency phone numbers, such as fire department, police, relatives, friends, and 911 (or whatever emergency number is available).

➻ *DAILY LIVING CONSIDERATIONS*

- Provide information on "Meals on Wheels" for assistance in having cooked, ready-to-eat meals delivered.
- Find out which local grocery stores provide a "shop by phone" or delivery service.
- Encourage use of a microwave for cooking, as it is safer than using a standard stove.
- Encourage the use of large-print books, newspapers, and magazines for reading. Also, many of these are available on audio tape at local libraries and vision aid services.

5. General preoperative teaching regarding anticipated activities and care.

Self- Care

1. Maintain client's orientation to surroundings.
2. Eye patch is is used for about 24 hours, or until the client returns to the physician for a follow-up visit.
3. Client should avoid stooping, lifting, or straining in the early postoperative period.
4. Teach the client to avoid sleeping on the affected side.
5. Teach the client to avoid rubbing the eye; there should be minimal discomfort, and this is generally relieved by acetaminophen.

6. Client should report any pain that is not easily relieved.
7. Teach client how to administer eye drops (antibiotic and steroid eye drops); have client demonstrate procedure.
8. Provide the client with written instructions; make sure the type is large enough for him to read.

Retinal Detachment

❑ **A separation of the two layers of the retina is called *retinal detachment.* When separation occurs, vitreous humor seeps between the layers and detachment of the retina from the choroid occurs.**

Assessment

1. Risk factors.
   a. Severe myopia.
   b. Diabetic retinopathy.
   c. Trauma.
   d. Degenerative changes in the retina.
   e. Previous cataract surgery.
2. Diagnostics.
   a. Ophthalmoscopic examination.
   b. Evaluation of visual acuity.
3. Clinical manifestations.
   a. Sudden onset.
   b. Flashes of light in visual field.
   c. Sensation of a veil over the eye.
   d. Floating spots.
   e. May experience area of blank vision.
   f. Area of lost vision correlates with location of retinal detachment.
   g. Eventually results in greater loss of vision.

Treatment

There is no medical treatment. The surgical repair may be done on an outpatient basis or may require hospitalization.

1. or laser photocoagulation—used to seal the area if complete detachment has not occurred.
2. Scleral buckling—the sclera is depressed from the outside to place the retina in contact with the choroid.

Nursing Intervention

✦ *Goal: to enable client and significant others to discuss problem associated with detachment of the retina, the rationale for surgery, and anticipated preoperative and postoperative activities.*

1. Discourage client from jerky head movements, stooping or straining; may be placed on activity restrictions, depending on degree of detachment.
2. If scleral buckling procedure is performed, client is usually placed under general anesthesia.
3. The client should not expect immediate return of vision after surgery; inflammation and eye drops will interfere with vision.

✦ *Goal: to prevent postoperative complications.*

1. Prevent nausea and vomiting.
2. Cover affected eye, or both eyes may remain covered postoperatively.
3. Orient client to surroundings.
4. Postoperative pain may require narcotic analgesic.
5. Client may experience redness and swelling of the lids; of the lids may also occur.
6. Warm or cool compresses may be used to promote comfort.
7. If an air bubble was injected during surgery, there will be specific postoperative positioning so the bubble will enhance pressure on the affected area.
8. Postoperative medications usually include antibiotic eye drops, ophthalmic steroid drops, and agents.

✦ *Goal: to help client understand and perform own eye care.*

1. Activities requiring visual acuity may be restricted for several weeks (reading, driving, etc.).
2. Discourage any straining, lifting or stooping in the postoperative period.
3. If an air bubble was injected to facilitate pressure on the retina, client should avoid air travel until advised by physician.
4. Make sure client understands symptoms of detachment and importance of seeking immediate attention if it occurs again (increased risk of it occurring again).

Visual Impairment in Children

A. Refractory problems—same as an adult (Appendix 12-1).

B. Amblyopia—"lazy eye," reduced vision in one eye. Preventable if primary problem is corrected prior to 6 years old.

C. of eyes. May result in amblyopia if not corrected.
   1. Corneal light reflex—when light is shone directly into both eyes, the light reflex should be symmetrical; if light falls off-center, then eyes are .
   2. Cover —uncover test is screening test for problem.
   3. Treatment may involve patching the unaffected eye to increase muscle strength of the affected eye.

4. Surgical correction can be done if due to muscle imbalance.

D. Conjunctivitis—an inflammation of the conjunctiva.

1. Characterized by redness, tearing and exudate.
2. Treatment with antibiotic eye drops.
3. Contagious, encourage good hand washing.

Nursing Intervention.

1. Assess child's development level.
2. Encourage early testing of vision in the community.
3. Parent education regarding importance of therapy and continued medical follow-up.
4. Assess client's home environment to determine if further referral is necessary.
5. Assist parents to encourage independence appropriate for age.
6. Postoperative care is similar to that of the adult.

EYE TRAUMA

❑ **May include surface, imbedded or impaled objects. History is usually compatible with eye injury.**

A. Treatment and assessments are often carried out at the same time.

B. As soon as the eye injury is determined, the client should be seen by a physician (ophthalmologist).

Assessment.

1. Determine in which trauma occurred.
2. Determine if client has a contact lens in the affected eye.
3. Pain, inability to open the eye.
4. Decreased visual acuity — may be unable to determine light and images.
5. If there is visible trauma, gently apply dressing soaked with normal saline to prevent drying during transport.

Treatment

1. Any suspected or known corneal abrasion should be examined with fluorescein, followed by ocular irrigation with normal saline (Appendix 12-2).
2. Nonpenetrating foreign objects may be removed by normal saline irrigation.
3. Penetrating foreign bodies must be removed by a physician (ophthalmologist) as soon as possible.
4. Do not attempt to stop bleeding from the eye or the eye lid with direct pressure.
5. For chemical eye burns, immediately irrigate the eye with copious amounts of normal saline. May require short acting opthalmic anesthetic drops.
6. Severe trauma may require an (surgical removal of the entire eyeball).

Nursing Intervention

✦ *Goal: to prevent further eye damage.*

1. Do not put any pressure on the outside of the eyelid.
2. Do not attempt to remove a penetrating foreign object in the eye.
3. Irrigate eyes with normal saline from inner canthus to outer canthus so solution does not flow into unaffected eye.
4. Eye may remain irritated after foreign body is removed. Physician will frequently order an eye patch.
5. If penetrating eye injury is present, decrease activities that cause increased pressure.
6. Immobilize the client, keep them until they can be evaluated by an ophthalmologist.

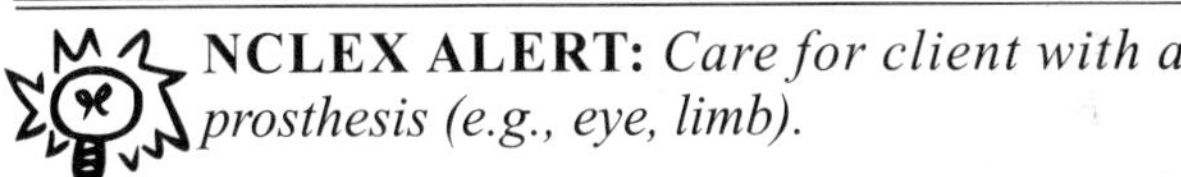

NCLEX ALERT: *Care for client with a prosthesis (e.g., eye, limb).*

✦ *Goal: to care for a client with an enucleation.*

1. Immediate — VS, monitor for bleeding.
2. Apply antibiotic—steroid ophthalmic eye ointment until prosthesis is fitted.
3. Prosthesis usually fitted one month postop to allow time for the ball implant area to heal to provide a firm base or the socket prosthesis.
4. Insertion and removal of prosthesis.
   a. Insertion—notched end of prosthesis should be closet to the client's nose; lift upper eyelid (using nondominant hand) and insert saline-rinsed prosthesis into socket area with top edge slipping under upper lid, gently retract lower lid until bottom edge of prosthesis slips behind it.
   b. Removal—client in sitting position with head slightly downward; pull lower lid down and laterally; prosthesis should slide into hand; store in container filled with saline.

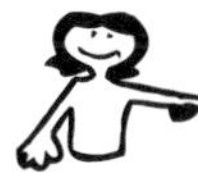

NURSING PRIORITY: *Important to teach client to report any of the following symptoms: progressive dimming of vision, "floaters" or specks, partial/complete loss of vision.*

PHYSIOLOGY OF THE EAR

A. External ear.

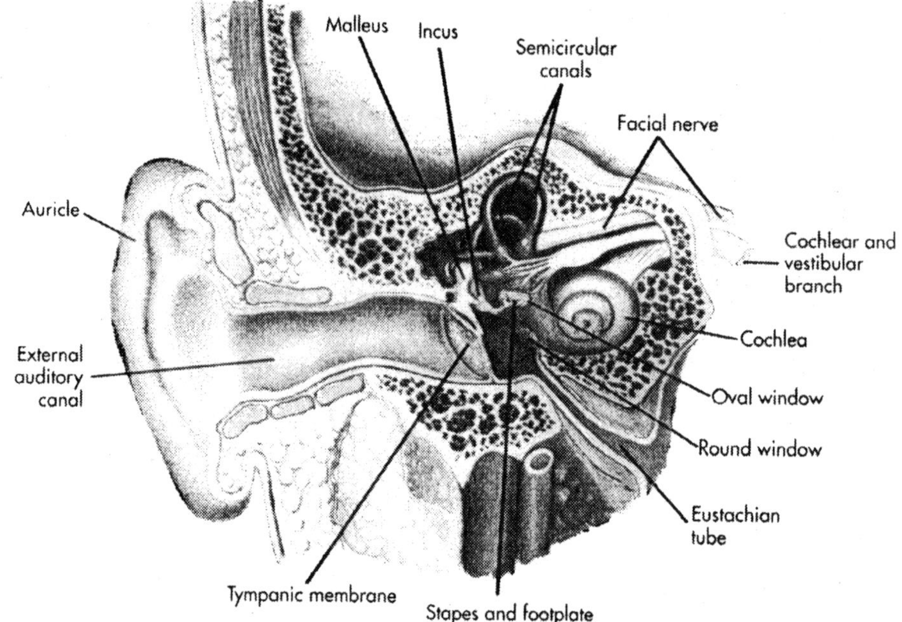

Figure 12-2: Structures of the Ear
Reprinted with permission: Phipps, WJ, Sands, JK, & Marek, JF (1999). *Medical Surgical Nursing: Concepts & Clinical Practice,* 6th ed. Philadelphia: Mosby, p.1852.

1. External auditory canal—function is to transmit the collected sound waves to the tympanic membrane; outer half of canal secretes cerumen, or wax, which provides a protective function.
2. Tympanic membrane—a tough membrane separating the external and middle ear; transmits vibrations from external ear to the malleus of the middle ear; normally a pearly gray color.

B. Middle ear.
   1. Middle ear is filled with air at atmospheric pressure by means of the eustachian tubes; the eustachian tube in infants and young children is shorter and wider than in adults.
   2. The external and middle ear functions to conduct and magnify sound waves by air conduction.
   3. Problems in the external and middle ear cause conductive hearing loss.

C. Inner ear.
   1. Bony labyrinth.
      a. Vestibule—central area contains oval window and is bathed in fluid.
      b. Semicircular canals—open into the vestibule and are concerned with maintaining equilibrium.
      c. Cochlea—contains organ of Corti, which is the receptive end organ for hearing.
   2. Pathology of the inner ear or nerve pathway can result in sensorineural hearing loss.

System Assessment

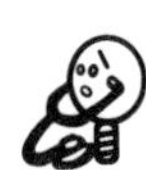

A. External assessment of the ear.
   1. Assess placement of the ears—low-set ears may be indicative of overlooked congenital anomalies.
   2. Movement of the auricle should not elicit pain.
   3. Note presence of any discharge in the external canal.
   4. With an otoscope examine tympanic membrane for landmarks, color, and intactness.

B. Middle ear and inner ear cannot be examined directly.

C. Assessment of bone and air conduction (Appendix 12-1).

D. Assess for vertigo—ask client to close eyes and stand on one foot; have client walk with eyes closed; client may fall to one side or complain of the room spinning.

DISORDERS OF THE EAR

Acute Otitis Media

❑ **This is an acute infection of the middle ear. Infants and young children are predisposed to the development of otitis media because of the physiological characteristics of the ear: the eustachian tube is shorter, wider, and straighter than in the adult ear. Common organisms are: H.influenza, Streptococcus, and Staphylococcus.**

Assessment

A. Acute media (purulent, suppurative) is characterized by a rapid and short onset of symptoms.

B. Chronic media is characterized by repeated infections and rupture of tympanic membrane.

C. Otitis media with effusion is characterized by a collection of fluid in the middle ear that may persist for weeks to months.

1. Risk factors.
   a. Age.
   b. History of upper respiratory infection.
   c. Less common in breast fed infants.
   d. Increase incidence in infants who are fed in the supine position.
   e. Increased incidence in infants who are exposed to passive smoke.
2. Reveals tympanic membrane bright red and bulging, with no light reflex.
3. Clinical manifestations.
   a. Pain from pressure in the middle ear.
      (1) Infants—irritable, pull at their ears, sucking aggravates pain.
      (2) Young children verbally complain of severe ear pain.
   b. Fever as high as 104° F. is not uncommon.
   c. Postauricular and cervical lymph node enlargement.
   d. If tympanic membrane ruptures, purulent drainage may be present in the outer ear; pain will decrease temporarily.
   e. Conductive hearing loss mar occur with recurrent rupture.
   f. Otitis with effusion is frequently asymptomatic.
   g. Mastoiditis or infection in the mastoid cavity is very rare if the infection is adequately treated.

Treatment

1. Medications.
   a. Antibiotics.

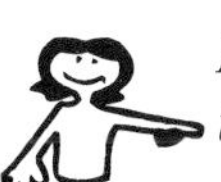

NURSING PRIORITY: It is important to teach the parents to administer the full course of the antibiotic.

   b. Analgesics.
   c. Antipyretic.
   d. Ear drops (antibiotic and steroid combination).
   e. Decongestants and antihistamines.
2. Surgical—myringotomy; drainage of the middle ear with insertion of myringotomy tube, for recurrent cases which do not respond to medication.

Nursing Intervention

✦ *Goal: to enable parents of clients to describe problem, handle medication schedule, and cope with home care.*

1. Recurrent infections cause an increased risk of permanent hearing loss.
2. Antibiotics should be continued until all prescribed medication is taken, even after all symptoms are relieved.
3. Administer acetaminophen or ibuprofen for pain and fever. There should be relief of symptoms within 24 to 72 hours; if not, the physician should be contacted.
4. Control of allergies and upper respiratory congestion.
5. The child should be discouraged from blowing his nose, or holding his nose closed when sneezing.
6. Decrease risk of recurrence by preventing fluids from pooling around eustachian tube.
   a. Hold or elevate infant's head while feeding.
   b. Do not prop bottle and allow infant to fall asleep with a bottle.
   c. Encourage water prior to sleeping.
7. Child should not go swimming or get water in the ears.
8. Increased risk of hearing loss with repeated, and untreated infections.

Hearing Loss

❑ **Hearing loss results from an impairment of the transmission of sound waves.**

1. Conductive — results from an impairment in transmission of sound from the outer or middle ear or both. Client will be able to benefit from a hearing aid.
2. Sensorineural (perceptive) — results from a problem in the inner ear or nerve pathway. Incoming sound cannot be analyzed correctly. Client will not benefit from a hearing aid.
3. is a gradual sensorineural hearing loss that occurs with aging.
4. Impacted cerumen can lead to conductive hearing loss; occurs often in the elderly.
5. Otosclerosis is an immobilization of the small bones in the inner ear; it occurs most often in women and has an autosomal dominant trait; is usually bilateral.

Box 12-2: Elder Care Focus
Improving Communication with Hearing Impaired Clients

- Standing in front of client at eye level to speak with light on your face helps with speech reading, (i.e., reading lips).
- Get client's attention by raising your hand or arm.
- Do not walk back and forth in front of client while speaking.
- Speak clearly and in an even tone; do not shout.
- Do not chew gum, cover mouth, or smile excessively while talking.
- Because clients rely on visual cues, watch your facial expressions.
- Encourage professional counseling in speech and sign language.
- Assist client in obtaining hearing aid, if appropriate promote social interaction appropriate for elderly adult.
- Do not avoid conversation with the client, do not depend on family to interpret information.

Assessment

1. Risk factors.
   a. Prolonged exposure to high intensity sound waves.

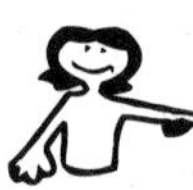

***NURSING PRIORITY:** Earplugs should be worn when the potential for loud noise exists.*

   b. Repeated, chronic ear infections.
   c. Prenatal problems of rubella and eclampsia.
   d. Premature birth.
   e. Ototoxic medications.
   f. Female with family history of otosclerosis.
2. Diagnostics (Appendix 12-1).
   a. Audiometric tests to determine hearing and comprehension.
   b. Weber and tests to differentiate between conductive and sensorineural loss.
3. Clinical manifestations.
   a. Speech problems—deterioration of present speech, or delayed speech development.
   b. Fails to respond to oral communication, or responds inappropriately.
   c. Excessively loud speech.
   d. General indifference to sound.
   e. Tinnitus.
   f. Responds more to facial expressions than to verbal ones.
   g. Inappropriate emotional response.

Treatment

1. Hearing aid, most effective with conductive loss.
2. Speech therapy.
3. Sign language.
4. Stapedectomy for otosclerotic lesions.

Nursing Intervention

✦ *Goal: to promote communication and socialization of the hearing-impaired client (see Box 12-2).*

1. Provide information concerning a TDD (telephone device for the deaf), which transmits typed words over the phone line.
2. Suggest light-activated devices rather than sound-activated devices—connecting doorbell, smoke, and security alarms to an electrical device which causes lights to flicker on and off.
3. Avoid crowded, noisy environments (such as restaurants) especially if a hearing aid is used, since it amplifies the background sound.
4. Teach how to care for hearing aid (Box 12-3).
5. Teach client how to remove ear wax, if impacted cerumen is a problem; may need an ear irrigation (Appendix 12-3).

✦ *Goal: to ensure that client who undergoes will not experience complications postoperatively.*

1. Appropriate preoperative teaching regarding postoperative activities.
2. Outer dressing may be reinforced or changed; do not disturb the inner ear dressing.
3. Assess for dizziness, maintain safety measures.
4. Position client on the side with head of bed slightly elevated.
5. Instruct client not to blow nose.
6. Administer medications.
   a. Analgesics.
   b. Antibiotics.
7. Instruct client that hearing may not improve for several weeks because of edema in the operative area.

Self-Care

1. Do not shampoo for about a week, keep the ear dry for 4-6 weeks after surgery.
2. Avoid flying for at least a month after surgery.
3. Report unusual sensations or feelings in the ear, or any ear drainage.
4. Avoid contact with people with upper respiratory infections.

NCLEX ALERT: *Hearing loss is very common in geriatric clients. Watch for questions about hearing loss to be incorporated into test situations pertaining to other chronic health care problems.*

Ménière's Disease

❑ **Ménière's Disease is caused by excess endolymph in the vestibular and semicircular canals. The etiology is thought to be involved with the over production or under absorption of endolymph fluid. Usually only one ear is involved.**

Assessment

1. Diagnostics (Appendix 12-1).
   a. Weber test and auditory testing indicate hearing loss.
   b. Vestibular test (caloric) indicates decreased function; may precipitate an acute attack.
2. Clinical manifestations.
   a. Vestibular vertigo — sense of environment spinning.
   b. Tinnitus may mask the progressive hearing loss.
   c. Fluctuating hearing loss.
   d. Violent paroxysmal attacks may occur.
      (1) Severe nausea, vomiting.
      (2) Nystagmus.
      (3) Loss of balance.
      (4) No pain or loss of consciousness.
   e. Client may proceed normally between attacks.
   f. Manifestations become less severe with time.

Treatment

1. Medications.
   a. Tranquilizers (to control vertigo) diazapam (**Valium**).
   b. Antihistamines.
   c. Diuretics (to decrease endolymph fluid).
   d. (Antivert)
2. Diet—low-sodium or low-salt.

Box 12-3: Elderly Care Focus

Hearing Aid Care

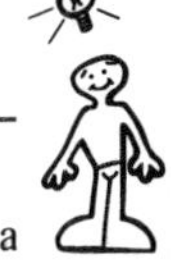

- Keep the hearing aid dry; do not wear it while bathing, swimming, or allow it to get wet during a rain shower.
- Avoid using hair spray, cosmetics, or oils around the ear.
- Always keep extra batteries on hand.
- When not using hearing aid, turn it off and remove the battery to store it.
- Avoid dropping the hearing aid (has delicate electronics) or exposing it to extremes in temperatures (i.e., leaving it on a window ledge in the sunlight).
- Clean ear mold part with a mild soap and water; do not get it excessively wet.
- Clean any debris or, cerumen from the hole in the middle part that goes in the ear by using a toothpick or pipe cleaner.
- If the hearing aid does not work, change the battery or check the on-off switch, check the connection between the ear mold and receiver, clean it using the steps described above, or take it in to an authorized hearing aid service center.

Nursing Intervention

✦ *Goal: to provide emotional and physical support during an acute attack.*

1. Maintain bedrest in a quiet, dimly lit room.
2. Client may assume a position of comfort.
3. Disturb or move the client only when necessary. Avoid unnecessary nursing procedures.
4. Administer medications parenterally, due to severe nausea.
5. Keep side rails up to protect client from falling.

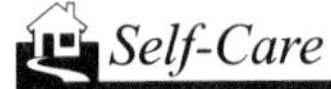

Self-Care

1. Identify activities that precipitate an attack.

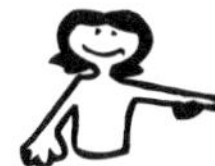

NURSING PRIORITY: *As a safety precaution, be sure to instruct the client to lie down immediately if an attack feels imminent.*

2. Stop smoking.
3. Avoid alcohol.
4. Maintain a low-sodium diet.
5. Cope appropriately with hearing loss.

Study Questions—Sensory System

1. The nurse would discuss which medication with the physician before administering to a client with open-angle glaucoma?

① Atropine (**Atropisol**) eye gtts.
② Hydrochlorothiazide (**Diruril**).
③ Propranolol (**Inderal**).
④ Carbamyl choline (**Isoptocarbachol**) eye gtts.

2. A client tells you she has heard that glaucoma may be a hereditary problem and she is concerned about her children. What is the best response?

① "There is no need for concern; glaucoma is not a hereditary disorder."
② "Screening for glaucoma should be included in an annual eye exam for everyone over 50."
③ "There may be a genetic factor with glaucoma and your children should be screened yearly."
④ "Are your grandchildren complaining of any eye problems? Glaucoma generally skips a generation."

3. What is included in the nursing care for the client with angle-closure glaucoma?

① Evaluation of medications to determine if any of them cause an increase in pressure as a side effect.
② Observation for an increase in loss of vision; it can be reversed if promptly identified.
③ Control blood pressure to decrease the client's potential loss of peripheral vision.
④ Evaluation of discomfort, since the client will experience considerable pain until the optic nerve atrophies.

4. A 2-year-old is scheduled for a myringotomy. What is the goal of this procedure that the nurse will discuss with the parents?

① Promote drainage from the ear.
② Irrigate the eustachian tube.
③ Correct a malformation in the inner ear.
④ Equalize pressure on the tympanic membrane.

5. A client comes to the clinic with decreased hearing. Examination of the ear canal reveals a large amount of ear wax. What is the best manner in which to remove the wax?

① Forceps.
② Normal saline irrigation.
③ D/5/W irrigation.
④ Cotton swab applicator.

6. Which is *not* considered a risk factor for hearing loss?

① Prenatal problem of rubella.
② Repeated, chronic ear infections.
③ Taking penicillin and cephalosporin medication.
④ Exposure to high-intensity sound waves.

7. After a client's eye has been anesthetized, what instructions will the nurse provide to the client?

① Not to watch television for at least one day.
② Not to rub the eye for 15 to 20 minutes.
③ To irrigate the eye every hour till sensation is felt.
④ To wear an eye patch for two days.

8. A child is diagnosed with conjunctivitis. Which statement reflects that the child understood the nurse's teaching?

① "It's okay for me to let my friends use my sunglasses while we are playing together."
② "It's okay for me to softly rub my eye, as long as I use the back of my hand."
③ "I can pick the crusty stuff out of my eyelashes with my fingers when I wake up in the morning."
④ "I will use my own washrag and towel while my eyes are sick."

9. What drug would the nurse expect to give to a client with Ménière's Disease?

① Antihypertensive.
② Antibiotic.
③ Vasoconstrictor.
④ Diuretic.

10. When teaching a family and a client about the use of a hearing aid, the nurse will base the teaching on what information regarding the hearing aid?

① Provides mechanical transmission for the damaged part of the ear.
② Stimulates the neural network of the inner ear to amplify sound.
③ Amplifies sound but does not improve the ability to hear.
④ Tunes out extraneous noise in the lower frequency sound spectrum.

Answers and rationales to these questions are in the section at the end of the book entitled "Chapter Study Questions: Answers & Rationales."

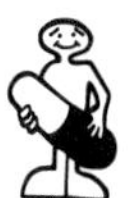

Appendix 12-1: OPHTHALMIC AND HEARING DIAGNOSTICS

OPHTHALMIC DIAGNOSTICS

SNELLEN CHART is used in screening for visual acuity problems. Client is placed 20 feet from the chart and visual acuity is expressed in a ratio of what he/she should see at 20 feet to what he/she can see at 20 feet. A ratio of 20/50 means that the client can see at 20 feet what he/she should see at 50 feet.

GLAUCOMA TESTS
Non-contact tonometer—a nonivasive method to measure intraocular pressure. Normal pressure is 12-22 mm Hg. pressure. A puff of air is directed toward the cornea, which causes indentation and allows measurement of intraocular pressure.

DIRECT OPHTHALMOSCOPY examination of the fundus or backportion of the interior of the eyeball with a hand held ophthalmoscope.

BIOMICROSCOPY (Slit-lamp exam) is used for assessment of the anterior eye for problems of the cornea, iris, lens, and to evaluate the depth of the anterior chamber.

REFRACTIVE ERROR EVALUATION determines what refractive errors have occurred because light is not correctly focused on the retina. Conditions that occur in refractive errors are:

(a) **myopia** (nearsightedness)—when the light ray is focused in front of the retina;
(b) **hyperopia** (farsightedness)— when the light ray is focused behind the retina;
(c) **presbyopia**—when there is a decrease in the elasticity of the lens which causes poor accommodation for near vision (common in older adults);
(d) **astigmatism**—when there is an uneven curvature of the cornea and light rays do not focus on the retina at the same time.

HEARING DIAGNOSTICS

AUDIOGRAM is a graphic outline of an individual's hearing as measured by various tones. Tones introduced into the external auditory opening will measure air conduction. Tones introduced over the mastoid bone will measure appropriate nerve conduction.

RINNE TEST is conducted by holding a vibrating tuning fork about two inches from the external ear. When the client can no longer hear the sound, the tuning fork is placed on the mastoid bone. When the tone is louder through air than through bone, the test is positive and indicates normal hearing, or a sensorineural hearing loss. A negative test, or when bone conduction is louder than air conduction, is indicative of a conductive loss. In the client who hears normally, it will demonstrate that air conduction will last longer than bone conduction.

WEBER TEST is conducted by placing a vibrating tuning fork on top of the client's head or in the middle of the forehead; the sound should be heard equally well in each ear. The tone is louder in an ear with unilateral conductive loss, and quieter in sensorineural loss.

OTOSCOPY is the examination of the external ear and the tympanic membrane utilizing an otoscope.

Appendix 12-2: OPHTHALMIC MEDICATIONS

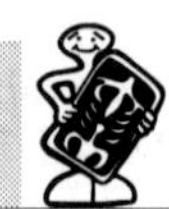

MEDICATIONS	SIDE EFFECTS	NURSING IMPLICATIONS

❖ GENERAL NURSING IMPLICATIONS ❖

— To decrease systemic absorption, teach client to apply gentle pressure (punctal occlusion) to the lacrimal duct (tear duct) during and immediately following instillation of drops.

— Instruct client or family in proper administration of eye drops or ointment, (i.e., maintain sterile technique and prevent dropper contamination, and store away from heat).

— Expect some blurriness from ointments and apply at bedtime, if possible, to avoid safety problems from diminished vision.

— Instruct client to report changes in vision, blurring, difficulty breathing, or flushing.

MEDICATIONS	SIDE EFFECTS	NURSING IMPLICATIONS
CARBONIC ANHYDRASE INHIBITORS: Restricts actions on enzyme necessary for production of aqueous humor.		
Acetazolamide (**Diamox**): PO, IV Dichlorphenamide (**Daranide**): PO	Metabolic acidosis. GI disturbances. CNS disturbances. GI Distress. Acidosis. Tingling of extremities.	1. Use with caution in clients with acidosis, diabetes. 2. Assess for hypokalemia. 3. Administer drug in AM because of diuretic effect. 4. Monitor I and O.
Methazolamide (**Neptazanel**)	Drowsiness. Fatigue. Malaise.	
MIOTICS: Contraction of ciliary muscle (pupillary constriction), thus increasing flow of aqueous humor.		
Pilocarpine hydrochloride (**Isopto carpine, Pilocar**): 1 percent to 6 percent solutions, topical Carbamylcholine (**Ccarbecel, Miostat, Isopto carbachol**): 1.5 percent to 3 percent solutions, topical	Conjunctive irritation. Provocation of asthma. Headache. Ciliary spasm. Inflammation of conjunctiva. Nausea/vomiting.	1. Contraindicated in inflammatory eye conditions.
BETA-BLOCKERS: Reduce intraocular pressure by decreasing formation of aqueous humor.		
Timolol maleate (**Timoptic**) Betazolol HCl (**Betoptic**)	Eye irritation. Insomnia Bradycardia	1. Same as with miotics. 2. A decrease in the resting heart rate may occur if there is systemic absorption.
MYDRIATICS: Block response of sphincter muscle of iris, produces dilation of pupil; may cause paralysis of accommodation.		
Epinephrine HCl (**Epitrate**): 0.1 percent solution, topical Atropine sulfate (**Atropisol**): 0.25 percent to 2 percent solution, topical Cyclopentolate HCl (**Cyclogyl**): 0.5 percent to 1 percent topical Tropicamide (**Mydriacyl**)	Headache. Hyperemia. Stinging. Flushing, sweating, dry mouth, dizziness.	1. Contraindicated in glaucoma client. 2. Dark glasses may be worn to decrease discomfort from photophobia. 3. Use only ophthalmic preparations.
DIAGNOSTICS: Surface of eye absorbs dye, thus demonstrating corneal abrasions.		
Fluorescein sodium (**Fluoresite, Fluor-L-Strip**)	Stinging, burning sensation.	1. Avoid touching eye with tip of dropper. 2. Used to diagnose corneal lacerations in clients with eye trauma. 3. Aqueous humor will stain green, indicating a leak from the anterior chamber.

Appendix 12-2: OPHTHALMIC MEDICATIONS

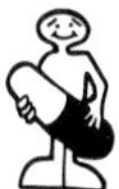

MEDICATIONS	SIDE EFFECTS	NURSING IMPLICATIONS
ADRENERGICS (Sympathomimetics): Decrease production of aqueous humor and enhance outflow.		
Dipivefrin HCl (**Propine**)	Transient burning and stinging.	1. May increase heart rate. 2. Instruct client to perform punctal occlusion to prevent systemic absorption.

Appendix 12-3: NURSING PROCEDURE ■ EAR AND EYE IRRIGATION ■

EAR IRRIGATIONS

COMMON SOLUTIONS

Warm tap water or normal saline
2-4% boric acid
0.8% bicarbonate of soda
Glycerin and water.

✓ Key Points: Irrigation

- Temperature of irrigating solution should be near body temperature (37(C, approximately 98(F). If too cold or hot, can cause dizziness and nausea.
- To soften cerumen, add a few drops of warm mineral oil or hydrogen peroxide to the ear.
- A rubber bulb syringe or a water pressure device may be used.
  Straighten the ear cannal by either pulling the outer ear up for adults or down for children under 3.
- Direct water flow toward the top of the ear cannal to create a circular motion.
- Teach the client how to irrigate his own ears.
- Do not forcefully push fluid into the ear canal, as this may rupture the eardrum. If nausea, vomiting, or dizziness develop, stop the irrigation immediately.

EYE IRRIGATIONS

COMMON SOLUTIONS

Normal Saline
Ringers Lactate

✓ Key Points: eye irrigation

- Place client in position where solution does not run into unaffected eye.
- Small amount of fluid - use a cotton ball moistened in solution.
- Moderate amount of fluid - a plastic squeeze bottle to direct fluid along conjunctiva and over the eyeball from inner to outer canthus.
- Large amount of fluid - bags of IV solutions may be used to provide constant stream and flushing of chemical from the eye.
- Do not allow tip of irrigating equipment to touch the eye.

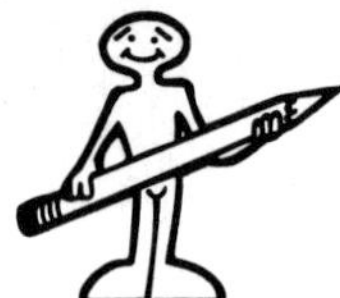

Notes

PHYSIOLOGY OF THE PITUITARY GLAND

A. Often referred to as the "master gland," as it secretes hormones which in turn control the level of hormone secretion of other endocrine glands (Figure 13-1).

B. Located within the skull; connected to the hypothalamus.

C. Lobes.
   1. Anterior pituitary—secretes hormones affecting other glands (Table 13-1).
   2. Posterior pituitary—hormones are produced in the hypothalamus and subsequently secreted by the posterior pituitary.

System Assessment

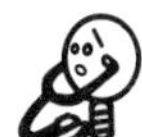

A. Assess for growth imbalance.
   1. Evaluate overall growth pattern of child.
   2. Assess for excessive or retarded growth.
      a. In adults, assess for excessive growth of small bones and soft tissue.
      b. In children, assess for excessive or retarded growth in height.
   3. Evaluate excessive weight gain or loss.

B. Evaluate familial tendencies.
   1. Parents who displayed slower growth patterns.
   2. Compare rate of growth of siblings at comparable age of clients.
   3. Assess for specific characteristics and/or genetic traits in the adults of the immediate family.

C. Assess for secondary sexual characteristics appropriate to age.

D. Assess intellectual development and mental changes appropriate to physical development and age.
   1. Intelligence.
   2. Increased excitability.
   3. Mental confusion, apathy.

DISORDERS OF THE PITUITARY GLAND

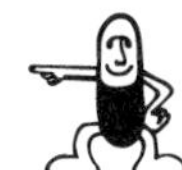

Hyperpituitary - Acromegaly

❑ **Acromegaly is most often the result of a benign pituitary tumor that secretes growth hormones. Occurs after the closure of epiphysis of the long bones.**

Assessment

1. Clinical manifestation:
   a. Enlargement the hands and feet.
   b. Changes in facial features—protruding jaw, slanting forehead, and an increase in the size of the nose.
   c. Severe enlargement of the pituitary gland may cause pressure on the optic nerve, resulting in changes in vision and headache.
2. Diagnostics.
   a. Increased serum growth hormone.
   b. X-rays, CAT scan, MRI.
   c. Physical examination.
3. Complications.
   a. Increased intracranial pressure.
   b. Diabetes insipidus.
   c. Meningitis.

Treatment

Surgical intervention is primary method of correcting problem; hypophysectomy may be accomplished by the transsphenoidal approach.

Nursing Intervention

✦ *Goal: to provide supportive preoperative care (Chapter 3).*

✦ *Goal: to ensure that client will not experience complications following hypophysectomy.*
   1. Elevate the head 30 degrees.
   2. Discourage coughing, sneezing, or straining at stool, to prevent cerebrospinal fluid leak.
   3. Assess for symptoms of increasing intracranial pressure (Chapter 20).
   4. Evaluate urine for excessive increase, above 200 cc/hr. or specific gravity <1.005. (i.e., development of diabetes insipidus).
   5. Frequent oral hygiene with non irritating solutions.

✦ *Goal: to assist client to reestablish hormone balance following hypophysectomy. (adrenal insufficiency and hypothyroid are most common complications).*
   1. Administer corticosteroids.
   2. If output becomes excessive (due to decrease in ADH), anticipate administration of ADH-regulating medications (Appendix 13-2).
   3. Evaluate serum glucose levels for significant changes.

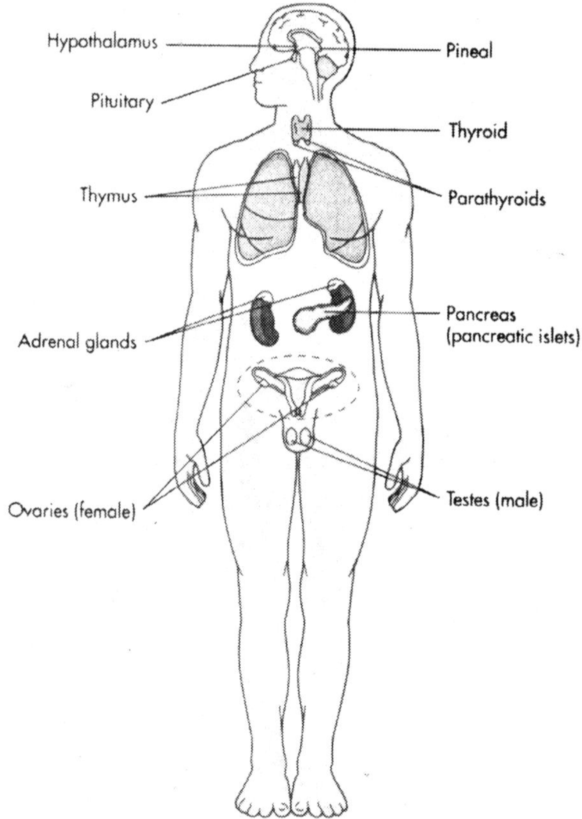

Figure 13-1: Selected Glands and Conditions of the Endocrine System

4. Monitor for problems related to hypothyroid.

✦ *Goal: to cope with changed body image.*

1. Frequently will experience infertility due to hormone changes.
2. Skeletal changes prior to surgery are not reversible.
3. Medication
   a. Cortisone replacement throughout lifetime.
   b. ADH regulating medications
   c. Medication to support target organs involved (pancreas, thyroid, gonads).

Disorders of the Posterior Pituitary

❑ **Diabetes insipidus (DI) is characterized by a deficiency of the antidiuretic hormone (ADH). When it occurs, it is most often secondary to neurological conditions - surgery, tumors, head injury, or inflammatory problems.**

❑ **The syndrome of inappropriate antidiuretic hormone (SIADH) is a condition in which there is continued release of ADH, regardless of the level of plasma osmolarity.**

A. When there is a decrease in the serum osmolarity, the normal body response is to decrease the secretion of ADH.

B. When the normal feedback mechanism for ADH fails and the level of ADH is sustained, there is excessive water retention in the body.

C. When there is a decreased or inadequate amount of ADH, the body is unable to concentrate urine, there is excessive water loss from the body.

Assessment

1. Risk factors/etiology—Both conditions frequently have predisposing pathology.
2. Clinical manifestations- DI
   a. Excretion of excessive amounts urine (>200cc hour).
   b. Polydipsia.
   c. Low urine specific gravity (1.001 to 1.005).
   d. Severe dehydration.
   e. Increase in serum sodium.
3. Clinical manifestations - SIADH

Table 13-1: SUMMARY OF PITUITARY GLAND HORMONE PRODUCTION

HORMONE PRODUCED	SITE OF ACTION	FUNCTION
ANTERIOR LOBE		
Adrenocorticotropic hormone (ACTH)	Adrenal cortex	Growth and secretion activity of adrenal cortex.
Thyroid-stimulating hormone (TSH)	Thyroid gland	Controls secretion of thyroid gland.
Follicle-stimulating hormone (FSH)	Testes Ovaries	Male - stimulates development of seminiferous tubules. Female - stimulates development of follicles and secretion of estrogen.
Luteinizing hormone (LH)	Testes Ovaries	Ovulation, development of corpus luteum, secretion of progesterone, secretion of testosterone.
Luteotropic hormone (LTH, prolactin)	Mammary glands	Secretion of milk, maintenance of corpus luteum.
Growth hormone (GH, somatotropin)	General	Growth and maturation of bones, muscles, and other organs.
POSTERIOR LOBE		
Antidiuretic hormone (ADH)	Renal tubules	Increases reabsorption of water, thereby decreasing urinary output.
Oxytocin	Smooth muscle (particularly wall of uterus)	Contraction of uterus at end of gestation. Initiates let-down response of milk during lactation.

NOTE: Pituitary gland secretions are controlled primarily by the hypothalamus.

a. Low urinary output with weight gain and no obvious edema.
b. Decreased (dilutional) serum sodium and potassium.
c. GI disturbances,
d. Cerebral edema—altered mental status, headaches, seizures.
e. High specific gravity (above 1.030).

4. Diagnosis based on the characteristic clinical manifestations.

Treatment

1. Diabetes insipidus - administration of ADH regulating medications (Appendix 13-2).
2. SIADH
   a. IV of normal saline.
   b. Fluid restriction.
   c. Limit fluid intake.

Nursing Intervention

✦ *Goal: to maintain fluid and electrolyte balance (Chapter 6).*

1. Encourage intake of fluids containing electrolytes in DI, restrict fluids in SIADH.
2. Monitor intake and output carefully.
3. Evaluate urine specific gravity for changes.
4. Assess hydration status.
5. Correlate hydration status with weight gain or loss.
6. Closely monitor sodium and potassium levels with fluid shifts.(Low sodium in SIADH, and increased sodium in DI).

✦ *Goal: to understand implications of the condition.*

1. Diabetes insipidus secondary to other problems is usually self-limiting.
2. Correction of SIADH is based on identification and correction of the predisposing condition

PHYSIOLOGY OF THE THYROID GLAND

A. Location in the anterior portion of the neck.
B. Anterior pituitary gland controls secretions of the thyroid-stimulating hormone (TSH).
C. Release of TSH is controlled by the level of the thyroid hormone in the blood.
D. Primary function of the thyroid hormone is to control the level of the cellular metabolism by secreting thyroxin (T_4), and triiodothyronine (T_3) (Table 13-2).
E. An inadequate secretion of hormone during fetal life and neonatal development will depress meta-

Table 13-2: SUMMARY OF THYROID GLAND HORMONE PRODUCTION

HORMONE PRODUCED	SITE OF ACTION	FUNCTION
Thyroxine (T_4)	General	Controls metabolic rate, growth and development
Triiodothyronine (T_3) Thyrocalcitonin	Bone	Inhibits bone resorption, lowers serum calcium levels

NOTE: Thyroid gland hormone secretion is controlled by the TSH secretion of the pituitary gland.

bolic activity and result in stunted physical and mental growth.

F. Disorders of the thyroid gland result in hyperfunction and hypofunction or simple enlargement of the gland.

System Assessment

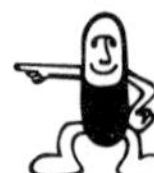

A. Assess for changes in metabolism.
   1. Significant increase weight or decrease in weight.
   2. Diarrhea or constipation
   3. Increase or decrease in appetite.
   4. Changes in vital signs.
   5. Changes in texture and appearance of skin.

B. Assess for intellectual development and mental changes.
   1. Intellectual level appropriate for age.
   2. Increased irritability, excitability, nervousness.
   3. Mental confusion, lethargy.

DISORDERS OF THE THYROID GLAND

Hyperthyroidism

❑ **This condition results in Graves' disease or thyrotoxicosis. It is characterized by excessive output of thyroid hormones.**

Assessment

1. Risk factors.
   a. More prevalent in women.
   b. Peak incidence in third or fourth decade of life.
   c. Probably autoimmune.
2. Clinical manifestations.
   a. Increased rate of body metabolism.
      (1) Intolerance to heat.
      (2) Significant weight loss, despite increased appetite and food intake.
      (3) Tachycardia.
      (4) Increase in systolic blood pressure.
      (5) Increased peristalsis leading to diarrhea.
      (6) Hand tremors at rest.
   b. Visual problems.
      (1) Exophthalmos (bulging eyeballs).
      (2) Changes in vision.
      (3) Eyelid retraction (lid lag).
   c. Changes in menstrual cycle.
   d. Enlarged, palpable thyroid glands.
   e. Labile emotional state.
3. Diagnostics (Appendix 13-1).
   a. Increase in T_3, T_4.
   b. Thyroid stimulating hormone (TSH).
   c. Increase in uptake of I^{131}.
   d. Client's physical appearance and symptoms.

Complications.

1. Thyroid storm or crisis—may occur after surgery or treatment with radioactive iodine.
   a. Systolic hypertension.
   b. Tachycardia.
   c. Increased temperature.
   d. Increased agitation and anxiety.
2. Calcium deficit may occur due to trauma to
3. the parathyroid. (See Hypoparathyroid)

Treatment

1. Surgical—thyroidectomy.
2. Medical.
   a. Reduce thyroid tissue—irradiation of thyroid gland with radioactive iodine (I^{131}), eventually resulting in hypothyroid state.
   b. Decrease thyroid synthesis and release (Appendix 13-2).

Nursing Intervention

✦ *Goal: to decrease effects of excess thyroid.*
1. Decrease environmental stress (lights, visitors, noise etc).
2. Cool environment.
3. Sedatives if appropriate.
4. Well-balanced meals (high in calories and high in vitamins); small meals served four to six times per day.

✦ *Goal: to protect eyes of client experiencing complication due to eye changes.*
1. Eye drops or ointment.
2. Assess for excess tearing, a sign of dry cornea.

3. Eye patches or mask may be necessary at night.

✦ *Goal: to prevent complications of thyroid storm (or crisis).*

1. Identify risk factors precipitating thyroid crisis.
   a. Inadequate preoperative preparation.
   b. Infection.
   c. Increased emotional lability.
   d. Surgical removal of thyroid gland.
2. Assess for increase in hyperthyroid state.
   a. Increase in temperature.
   b. Dehydration.
   c. Tachycardia (above 130).
   d. Pulmonary edema.
   e. Nausea, vomiting, diarrhea.
   f. Increase in agitation.

✦ *Goal: to maintain homeostasis in client experiencing thyroid storm (or crisis).*

1. Decrease body temperature and heart rate.
   a. Hypothermia blanket.
   b. Acetaminophen to decrease fever.
   c. Propranolol (**Inderal**) to reduce cardiac rate.
2. Oxygen to meet increased metabolic demands.
3. IV fluids.
4. Hydrocortisone for shock and adrenal insufficiency.
5. Iodine preparations to decrease thyroxin output.
6. Assess for cardiac tachy-dysrhythmias.

✦ *Goal: to provide preoperative nursing measures if surgery is indicated.*

1. Demonstrate to client how to provide neck support postoperatively.
2. Iodine preparations to decrease vascularity of the thyroid gland.
3. Establish baseline data for postoperative comparison.

✦ *Goal: to maintain homeostasis postoperative thyroidectomy.*

1. Maintain semi-Fowler's position to avoid tension on the suture line.
2. Analgesics for pain.
3. IV fluids until nausea and swallowing difficulty subside.
4. Check dressings on the side and back of the neck for bleeding.
5. Assess for hematoma around the wound.
6. Ice collar to decrease edema.
7. Evaluate calcium levels; parathyroid may have been damaged or accidentally removed.
8. Evaluate temperature elevations; temperature increase may be early indication of thyroid storm.

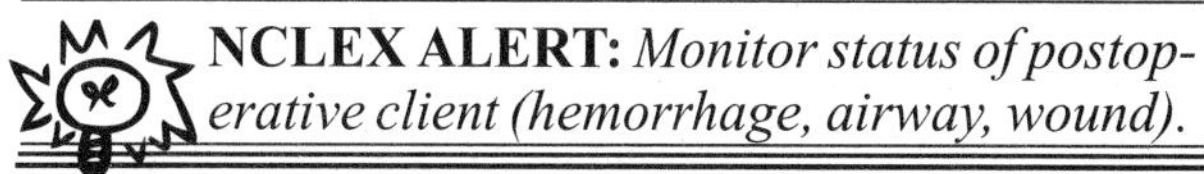
NCLEX ALERT: *Monitor status of postoperative client (hemorrhage, airway, wound).*

✦ *Goal: to prevent complication of respiratory distress following thyroidectomy.*

1. Assess client frequently for noisy breathing and increased restlessness.
2. Evaluate voice changes; increasing hoarseness may be indicative of laryngeal edema.
3. Keep tracheotomy set easily available.

✦ *Goal: decrease radiation exposure in client being treated with radioactive iodine (I^{131}).*

1. All body secretions are contaminated because this is a systemic type of radiation.
2. Urine is highly contaminated. Flush commode 2-3 times, or store urine in containers in room until radioactivity decreases.
3. Advise family members to avoid oral contact because saliva is contaminated.
4. For any body fluid spills (urine, vomitus, etc.) contact the Radiation Safety Officer for the facility. Do not clean up the spill.
5. General guideline is to maintain 1 meter (a little over 3 feet) distance from the client unless direct contact is necessary.
6. Infants and pregnant women should avoid contact with client for approximately 2 days.
7. All health care personnel providing direct care to client should wear a radiation badge.

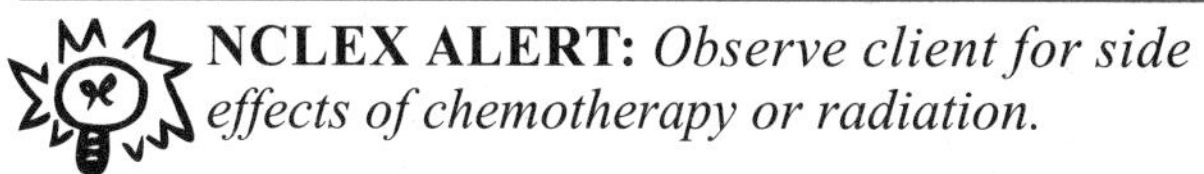
NCLEX ALERT: *Observe client for side effects of chemotherapy or radiation.*

Self-Care

1. Thyroid levels checked annually.
2. Lifelong thyroid replacement.
3. If excessive fatigue or tachycardia and tremors become a consistent problem, notify health care provider.

Hypothyroidism (Myxedema)

❑ **This condition is characterized by a slow deterioration of the thyroid function. It occurs primarily in older adults and five times more frequently in women than in men.**

Assessment

1. Early clinical manifestations.
   a. Extreme fatigue.
   b. Menstrual disturbances.
   c. Hair loss, brittle nails, and dry skin.
   d. Intolerance to cold.
   e. Anorexia.
   f. Constipation.
   g. Apathy.
2. Late clinical manifestations.
   a. Subnormal temperature.
   b. Bradycardia.
   c. Weight gain and edema.
   d. Change or decrease in level of consciousness.
   e. Thickened skin.
   f. Cardiac complications (bradycardia).
3. Diagnostics.
   a. Decrease in serum T_3, T_4.
   b. Increase in TSH.

Treatment

1. Medical management.
   a. Replacement of thyroid hormone.
   b. Low-calorie diet to promote weight loss.
   c. Decrease in cholesterol intake.

Complications

1. Replacement thyroid will increase the workload of the heart and increase myocardial oxygen requirements.
2. Observe client for development of cardiac failure.

Nursing Intervention

✦ *Goal: to assist the client to return to hormone balance.*

1. Begin thyroid replacements and evaluate client response; advise client it will be about 7 days before he/she begin to feel better.
2. Provide a warm environment.

NURSING PRIORITY: *Administer sedatives and hypnotics with caution, due to increased susceptibility. These medications tend to precipitate respiratory depression in the hypothyroid client.*

---

3. Prevent and/or treat constipation.
4. Assess progress.
   a. Decrease in body weight.
   b. Intake and output balance.
   c. Decrease in visible edema.
   d. Energy level and mental alertness should increase in seven to fourteen days and continue to rise until normal.
5. Evaluate cardiovascular response to medication.

✦ *Goal: to assist client to understand implications of disease and requirements for health maintenance.*

1. Need for lifelong drug therapy.
2. Diabetic client needs to evaluate blood sugar more frequently, thyroid preparations may alter hypoglycemics.
3. Continue to reinforce teaching information as client begins to progress; early in the disease the client may not comprehend importance of information.

Congenital Hypothyroidism (Cretinism)

❑ **A deficiency of thyroid hormones present at birth. Symptoms depend on the amount of thyroid present at birth.**

Assessment

1. Condition is not generally evident in the newborn, due to thyroid received through the maternal circulation; may become evident at three to six months of age.
2. Early clinical manifestations.
   a. Thick, dry, mottled skin.
   b. Bradycardia.
   c. Hypotonia, hyporeflexia.
   d. Poor feeding.
   e. Hypotonic abdominal musculature.
      (1) Constipation.
      (2) Protruding abdomen (umbilical hernia).
3. Diagnostics.
   a. Filter-paper, blood-spot thyroxin (T_4), if result is low, then a TSH is done.
   b. Mandatory test in all states, should be done within 24 to 48 hours after birth.

Treatment

Medical management includes replacement of thyroid hormones. (If replacement is accomplished shortly after birth, it is possible that the child will have normal physical growth and intellectual development.)

Nursing Intervention

✦ *Goal: to identify neonates experiencing the problem.*

✦ *Goal: to assist parents to understand the implications of the disease and requirements for continued health maintenance.*

1. Child will require lifelong medication.
2. Continue medical care to evaluate changes in thyroid replacement as the child grows.

PHYSIOLOGY OF THE PARATHYROID

Four small parathyroid glands are located near or embedded in the thyroid gland. The hormone secreted is parathyroid hormone (PTH), which is primarily involved in the control of serum calcium levels.

A. Function of PTH.
 1. Facilitates the mobilization of calcium and phosphorous from the bone.
 2. Promotes the resorption of calcium from the bone to maintain normal serum calcium levels.
 3. Promotes absorption of calcium in the GI tract.

B. Function of calcium.
 1. Maintains normal muscle and neuromuscular response.
 2. Necessary component of blood coagulation mechanisms.

C. Control of the parathyroid hormone is by way of the negative feedback system involving the level of serum calcium. When serum calcium levels are low, there is an increase mobilization of calcium from the bone resulting in an increase in serum calcium levels.

System Assessment

A. History of problems of calcium metabolism and or thyroid surgery.

B. Assess for changes in mental or emotional status.

C. Evaluate reflexes and neuromuscular response to stimuli.

D. Evaluate serum and urine calcium levels.

DISORDERS OF THE PARATHYROID

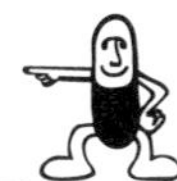

Hyperparathyroidism

❑ **This condition is characterized by an excessive secretion of PTH resulting in hypercalcemia.**

A. Normal function of PTH is to maintain serum calcium and phosphate levels.

B. Excessive PTH leads to bone damage, hypercalcemia and kidney damage.

Assessment

1. Risk factors—more common in women after menopause.
2. Clinical manifestations.
 a. Bone cysts and pathologic fractures due to lack of resorption of calcium in the bone. Calcium is released into the blood causing hypercalcemia.
 b. Secondary hyperparathyroidism is frequently due to chronic renal failure.
  (1) Renal calculi.
  (2) Azotemia.
  (3) Hypertension secondary to renal failure.
  (4) Repeated urinary tract and renal infections.
 c. CNS problems of lethargy, stupor, psychosis.
 d. GI problems.
  (1) Anorexia.
  (2) Nausea and vomiting.
  (3) Constipation.
  (4) Development of peptic ulcer.
3. Diagnostics.
 a. Increased level of serum calcium, decreased level of serum phosphorous.
 b. X-ray shows demineralized cystic areas in the bone.
 c. Increased urine calcium and phosphorous.

Treatment

1. Decrease level of circulating calcium.
2. Parathyroidectomy.

Nursing Intervention

✦ *Goal: to decrease level of serum calcium.*

1. High fluid intake to dilute serum calcium and urine calcium levels.
2. If IV is necessary, generally administer normal saline.
3. Furosemide (**Lasix**) a loop diuretic may be used to increase excretion of calcium.
4. Encourage mobility, as immobility increases demineralization of bones.
5. Limit foods high in calcium.

✦ *Goal: to assess client's tolerance of and response to increased PTH.*

1. Assess for skeletal involvement.
2. Assess for renal involvement.
 a. Strain urine for stones.
 b. Evaluate for low back pain (renal).
 c. Check for hematuria.

d. Assess intake and output carefully.
3. Assess for presence of bone pain.
4. Assess cardiac response to increased level of calcium.

✦ *Goal: to provide appropriate preoperative measures if surgery is indicated (Chapter 3).*

✦ *Goal: to prevent postoperative complications of parathyroidectomy.*

1. Care of parathyroidectomy client is same as for a thyroidectomy client.
2. Bone pain is relieved shortly after surgery; bone lesions frequently heal; serious renal disease may not be reversible.

Hypoparathyroidism

❑ **This condition is characterized by a decrease in PTH, resulting in hypocalcemia. Severe hypocalcemia results in tetany.**

Assessment

1. Risk factors or precipitating causes.
   a. Adults—inadvertent removal of parathyroid gland during thyroidectomy or radical neck dissection.
   b. Children primary cause is idiopathic or unknown.
2. Clinical manifestations.
   a. Chronic onset.
      (1) Muscle weakness.
      (2) Loss of hair; dry skin.
   b. Overt/acute tetany (potentially fatal).
      (1) Bronchospasm, laryngospasm.
      (2) Seizures.
      (3) Cardiac dysrhythmias.
      (4) Circumoral paresthesia.
      (5) Positive Chvostek's sign (sign is positive when sharp tapping over the facial nerve elicits mouth, nose, and eye twitching).
      (6) Positive Trousseau's sign (sign is positive when carpopedal spasm is precipitated by occluding blood flow of the upper portion of the upper extremity).
   c. Pediatrics
      (1) Carpopedal spasms.
      (2) Muscle cramps, twitching.
      (3) Seizures - generalized or absence.
      (4) Brittle hair, thin nails.
3. Diagnostics.
   a. Decreased serum calcium.
   b. Increased serum phosphate.
   c. Low PTH levels.

Treatment

1. Vitamin D to enhance calcium absorption.
2. Increased calcium in the diet.

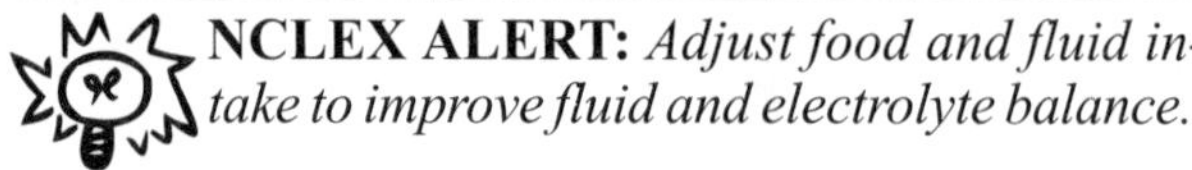

NCLEX ALERT: *Adjust food and fluid intake to improve fluid and electrolyte balance.*

3. Acute.
   a. Replace calcium through slow IV drip (calcium gluconate, calcium chloride).
   b. Sedatives, anticonvulsants.

Nursing Intervention

✦ *Goal: to assist client to increase serum calcium levels.*

1. Administer calcium preparations.
2. Evaluate increases in serum calcium and decreases in serum phosphate.
3. Client will require lifelong medical care to maintain homeostasis.

✦ *Goal: to prevent complications of neuromuscular irritability.*

1. Quiet environment.
2. Low lights.
3. Seizure precautions.

✦ *Goal: to help client avoid complications of respiratory distress.*

1. Bronchodilators.
2. Tracheotomy set easily available.
3. Frequent assessment of respiratory status.

✦ *Goal: to prevent complications of cardiac problems.*

1. Assess client for history of cardiac problems.
2. Assess frequently for dysrhythmias.
3. Calcium will potentiate digitalis; use cautiously together.

PHYSIOLOGY OF THE PANCREAS

❑ **The pancreas is located in the upper left aspect of the abdominal cavity. The pancreas produces the enzymes trypsin, amylase, and lipase, which are secreted into the duodenum and are necessary for the digestion and absorption of nutrients. Located within the pancreas are the islets of Langerhans, which contain beta cells; these cells are responsible for the production of insulin. Insulin is necessary in**

Table 13-3: PROFILE OF INSULINS

TYPE	ONSET OF ACTION	PEAK ACTION	DURATION OF ACTION	NURSING IMPLICATIONS
RAPID ACTING				
Insulin lispro (**Humalog**): SQ	< 15 min	1 hr	3-5-4.5 hr	***NURSING PRIORITY:*** *Because of quick onset of action, client must eat immediately.*
Regular insulin[R] (**Humulin R, Novolin R**) SQ, IV	1/2 to 1 hr	2 to 4 hrs	6 to 8 hrs	***NURSING PRIORITY:*** *Administer injections - 1. May mix regular insulin with other insulins. 2. Only regular insulin may be given IV.*
INTERMEDIATE ACTING				
Isophane insulin suspension [NPH] (NPH, Lente, Novolin N): SQ	1 to 2 hr	6 to 12 hrs	18 to 24 hrs	1. Hypoglycemia tends to occur in mid-to late-afternoon. 2. Never give IV. 3. May be mixed with regular insulin.
LONG ACTING				
Insulin zinc suspension [L] (Ultralente): SQ	1 to 3 hrs	6 to 12 hrs	18 to 24 hrs	1. Slow onset may require readjustment of carbohydrate intake. 2. Prolonged action may require more between-meal and bedtime snacks. 3. May be mixed with regular insulin.
MIXTURE				
NPH 70u and regular insulin 30 u (**Humulin 70/30, Novolin 70/30**):SQ	1/2 hr	2 to 12 hrs	24 hrs	1. Eliminates problem of mixing different types. 2. Do not give IV. 3. NPH 70/30 - regular insulin will peak in 2-4 hours, NPH in 6-12 hours, the overlap of the two types is 4-6 hours after administration.
NPH 50u and regular insulin 50u (**Humulin 50/50**):SQ	1/2 hr	3-5 hrs	24 hrs	4. Response to insulin mixtures vary with individuals.

NCLEX ALERT: *Intervene to control hypo/hyperglycemia. Know various insulins and nursing implications. Specifically, know when to anticipate reaction and what to teach the client about his insulin.*

maintaining normal carbohydrate metabolism and glucose utilization.

System Assessment

A. Evaluate changes in weight, particularly increase in weight in the adult and decrease in weight in a child.

B. Evaluate alterations in fluid balance.

C. Evaluate changes in mental status.

D. Evaluate serum glucose levels.

E. Evaluate pancreatic enzyme studies.

F. Evaluate the abdomen for epigastric pain and abdominal discomfort.

DISORDERS OF THE PANCREAS

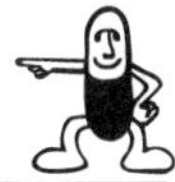

Diabetes Mellitus

❑ **A complex, multi-system disease characterized by the absence of or a severe decrease in the secretion or utilization of insulin.**

A. Pathophysiology.

1. The primary function of insulin is to decrease the blood glucose level.
   a. Necessary for transport of glucose into the muscle.
   b. Regulates the rate of carbohydrate metabolism and conversion to glucose.

2. Insulin is secreted by the beta cells in the islets of Langerhans in the pancreas.
3. The body uses carbohydrates more effectively for conversion of glucose for energy.
   a. Adequate intake of carbohydrate.
   b. Available insulin to facilitate the movement of the glucose into the cell.
   c. Adequate reserves of glucagon.
4. If carbohydrates are not available to be utilized for energy, the cell will begin to oxidize the fats and protein stores.
   a. Breakdown of the fat results in the production of ketone bodies.
   b. Protein is wasted during insulin deficiency. Protein is broken down and converted to glucose by the liver, thus contributing to the increase in circulating glucose.
   c. When fats are used for the primary energy source, the serum lipid level rises and contributes to the accelerated development of atherosclerosis.
5. When the circulating glucose cannot be utilized for energy, the level of the serum glucose will increase (hyperglycemia).
   a. Hyperglycemia will cause an increase in the osmotic gradient; water moves out of the cell into the circulating volume to decrease the osmolarity. This results in an increase in urinary output.
   b. The increase in the circulating glucose exceeds the renal threshold and glucose spills into the urine.
6. Pathophysiologic bases for symptoms.
   a. Polyuria—due to the increased serum osmolarity there is more circulating volume; water is not reabsorbed from the renal tubules and there is a significant increase in urine output.
   b. Polydipsia—increased loss of fluids precipitates dehydration, causing thirst.
   c. Polyphagia—tissue breakdown and wasting cause hunger.
   d. Weight loss (Type 1)—glucose is not available to the cells; body begins to break down fat and protein stores for energy.

B. Classification.

1. Type 1—insulin-dependent diabetes mellitus.
   a. Absence of insulin production; client is dependent on insulin to prevent ketoacidosis and maintain life.
   b. Onset frequently in childhood, most often diagnosed prior to age 18. Most common age range is 10-15 years old.
   c. Previously called juvenile diabetes, or insulin dependent diabetes mellitus (IDDM).
   d. Familial tendencies in transmission.
   e. Client will remain Type 1 diabetic for rest of his life.
2. Type 2 —Non-insulin dependent diabetes mellitus.
   a. Insulin deficiency caused by defects in insulin production, or by excessive demands for insulin; client is not dependent on insulin.
   b. Ketoacidosis generally not a problem due to limited amounts of insulin production.
   c. Onset predominately in adults, generally over age 40, but may occur at any age.
   d. Previously called adult onset diabetes (AODM), or non-insulin dependent diabetes mellitus (NIDDM).
   e. Associated with obesity; overweight people require more insulin.
   f. If not associated with obesity, there is usually a strong family history.
   g. May require insulin for control.
3. Gestational Diabetes.
   a. Develops during pregnancy; onset may be in second trimester.
   b. Glucose tolerance usually returns to normal soon after delivery.
   c. May not occur again; client should be evaluated for development of Type 2 diabetes.
   d. Infant may be large for gestational age and may experience hypoglycemia shortly after birth.

Assessment

1. Clinical manifestations.
   a. Types 1 and 2.
      (1) Three Ps—polyphagia, polydipsia, polyuria.
      (2) Fatigue.
      (3) Increased frequency of infections.
   b. Type 1.
      (1) Weight loss.
      (2) Excessive thirst.
      (3) Bed-wetting.
      (4) Onset is rapid, generally over days to weeks.
      (5) Complaints of abdominal pain
   c. Type 2.
      (1) Weight gain (obese).
      (2) Visual disturbances.
      (3) Onset is slow; may occur over months.
      (4) Onset usually after age 40, peaks around 45-50 years.
      (5) Fatigue and malaise.

2. Diagnostics (the criterion for diagnosis is two or more abnormal tests with two or more values outside the normal range) (See Appendix 13-1).
   a. Fasting blood glucose is above 125 mg/dl on two or three consecutive tests.
   b. Glucose tolerance test—2 hour glucose values are greater than 200mg/dL.
   c. Impaired glucose tolerance — two hours post-prandial plasma glucose is > 140mg/dl, and less than or equal to 200mg.dl during an oral glucose tolerance test.
   d. Glycosylated hemoglobin (HbA_{1c}) is increased. (less than 7% is considered good control for diabetic).

NURSING PRIORITY: *The glycosylated hemoglobin will indicate the overall glucose control for approximately the past 120 days. This allows evaluation of control of the blood sugar regardless of increases or decreases in blood sugar immediately prior to drawing the sample.*

Treatment

1. Factors in diabetes management:
   a. Regular physical activity.
   b. Diet.
   c. Pharmacological intervention.
2. Hypoglycemia agents.
   a. Insulin—may be used in both types of diabetes. Primary function of insulin is to transport glucose into the muscle and fat cells (Table 13-3).
   b. Oral hypoglycemics for non-insulin-dependent clients.
3. Insulin requirement increases when:
   a. Client is seriously ill.
   b. An infection develops.
   c. Surgery is performed.
   d. Client suffers trauma.
   e. During adolescence and puberty.
4. Diabetic diet (See Chapter 3).
   a. Decrease calories for weight loss.
   b. Diet to meet nutritional needs and maintain optimum glucose level. Avoid simple sugars.
   c. Decrease in cholesterol.
5. Exercise.
   a. Planned exercise; sporadic exercise is discouraged.
   b. Glucose for exercising muscles comes from the liver.
   c. The counter-regulatory hormones increase the delivery of glucose to the muscles.

NCLEX ALERT: *Intervene to control symptoms of hypoglycemia or hyperglycemia.*

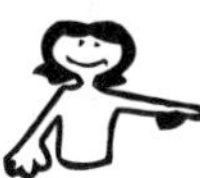

NURSING PRIORITY: *Metabolic effects of exercise: ◆ Reduces insulin needs by reducing the blood glucose. ◆ Contributes to weight loss or maintenance of normal weight. ◆ Assists the body to metabolize cholesterol more efficiently. ◆ Promotes less extreme fluctuations in blood glucose. ◆ Decreases blood pressure.*

Complications—Insulin Therapy

1. Hypoglycemia (Table 13-4).
2. Lipodystrophy (tissue atrophy and hypertrophy).
   a. Associated with administration of cold insulin.
   b. May result from poor rotation of injection sites.
3. Somogyi effect.
   a. Physiologic reflex: A rebound hyperglycemia from an unrecognized hypoglycemic state.
   b. Most often occurs at night.
   c. May be treated by decreasing the evening insulin or by increasing the bedtime snack.
4. Hormones that counteract insulin.
   a. Glucagon.
   b. Epinephrine.
   c. Cortisol.
   d. Growth hormone.

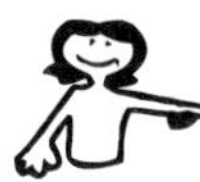

NURSING PRIORITY: *Intensive control of blood glucose in Type 1 diabetics can prevent or ameliorate the complications.*

Complications Associated with Poorly Controlled Diabetes

1. Diabetic ketoacidosis (DKA).
   a. A severe increase in the hyperglycemia state.
   b. An increase in the mobilization of fat and protein for an energy source.
   c. Metabolism of fat results in the production of fatty acids, which are converted to ketone bodies.
   d. An increase in circulating ketone bodies precipitates the state of acidosis.
   e. Occurs predominately in Type 1.
2. Clinical manifestations of diabetic ketoacidosis (Table 13-4).

Table 13-4: COMPARISON OF DKA, HHNC, HYPOGLYCEMIA

	DKA	HHNC	HYPOGLYCEMIA
Age	All ages, increased incidence in children.	Adult	All ages
GI	Anorexia, nausea, vomiting, diarrhea	Normal	Normal—may be hungry.
Mental state	Dull, confusion increasing to coma	Dull, confusion increasing to coma	Difficulty in concentrating, coordinating; eventually coma
Skin temperature	Warm, dry, flushed	Warm, dry, flushed	Normal
Pulse	Tachycardia	Tachycardia	Tachycardia
Respirations	Initially deep and rapid; leads to Kussmaul	Normal	Shallow
Breath odor	Fruity, acetone	Normal	Normal
Urine output	Increased	Increased	Normal
Lab Values - Serum			
Glucose ⇒	High, 300 to 1,500 mg/dl	Very high, up to 3,000 mg/dl	Below 60 mg/100 cc
Ketones ⇒	High/large	Normal	Normal
pH ⇒	Acidotic (below 7.25)	Normal	Normal
Hematocrit ⇒	High due to dehydration	High due to dehydration	Normal
Lab Values - Urine			
Sugar	High	High	Negative
Ketones	High	Negative	Negative
Onset	Slow	Slow	Rapid
Classification of diabetes	Primarily Type 1; Type 2 in severe distress	Type 2	Type 1 and Type 2.

a. Onset.

(1) May be acute or occur over several days.

(2) May result from stress, infection, surgery, or lack of effective insulin control.

(3) Results from poorly controlled diabetes.

b. Severe hyperglycemia (300 mg.% or higher).

c. Presence of metabolic acidosis.

d. Hyperkalemia.

e. Urine ketones and sugar are increased.

f. Excessive weakness, increased thirst.

g. Nausea, vomiting.

h. Fruity (acetone) breath.

i. Kussmaul respirations.

j. Decreased level of consciousness.

k. Dehydration.

l. Increased temperature due to dehydration.

3. Hyperosmolar hyperglycemia nonketotic coma (HHNC).

a. Occurs in the adult with Type 2.

b. Condition is characterized by enough insulin production to prevent the breakdown of fat for cellular function, but severe hyperglycemia exists.

c. Severe electrolyte imbalance and dehydration exist in the absence of the acidotic state.

d. Characterized by extreme hyperglycemia (700-2000 mg/100dL).

e. Occurs primarily in Type 2 geriatric clients.

f. Due to the ability of the body to maintain a low level of insulin production, the breakdown of fat and the production of ketone bodies does not occur. This prevents the client from developing acidosis.

g. Osmotic diuresis occurs due to the hyperglycemia; the client becomes dehydrated very rapidly.

4. Clinical manifestations of HHNC (See Table 13-4).

a. Warm, flushed skin.

b. Lethargic.

c. Decreased level of consciousness.

d. Weak, thirsty.

e. Increased temperature from dehydration.

f. Tachycardia.

g. Generally does not experience GI problems.

h. Decrease in blood pressure.

i. No acetone odor to breath.

j. Severe hyperglycemia (700mg %).

k. Serum pH is normal.

l. Urine output is increased.

m. Glycosuria.

5. Electrolyte imbalance.

a. As acidosis develops, the potassium ion moves out of the cell; this leaves the cell potassium depleted, but the serum potassium is normal due to excessive excretion.

b. As osmotic diuresis occurs from the hyperglycemia/hyperosmolar state, serum potassium is excreted.

c. As the client becomes more dehydrated, the serum potassium becomes concentrated and does not reflect the potassium loss.

d. As the osmolarity and acidosis are corrected, along with the administration of insulin, the potassium will move back into the cell and result in severe hypokalemia.

Box 13-1: Elderly Care Focus

Diabetic Care

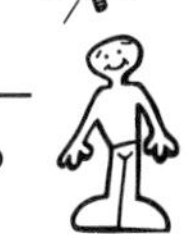

- Determine mental status and manual dexterity to handle injections.
- Determine if client can access the injection sites.
- Is client alert and mentally capable of making judgments on medications?
- Determine if the client can pay for supplies.
- What is the client's attitude about needles and injections?
- Assess how many other medications is the client taking; problems with "polypharmacy" (too many medications).
- Determine family's or client's ability to accurately perform serum glucose testing.
- What is the client's support system?

Complications—Long-term diabetes

1. Angiopathy—premature degenerative changes in the vascular system.

a. May affect the large vessels (macroangiopathy, early onset of atherosclerosis, and arteriosclerotic vascular problems).

b. May affect the small vessels (microangiopathy); problems are specific to diabetes.

2. Peripheral vascular disease—combination of both types of angiopathy.

3. Hypertension.

4. Diabetic gastroparesis - delayed gastric emptying.

5. Cerebrovascular disease.

6. Coronary artery disease.

7. Ocular complications.

a. Cataracts.

b. Retinopathy.

c. Glaucoma.

8. Nephropathy.

a. Microangiopathy primarily affects the glomerular capillaries, resulting in thickening and increased permeability of the glomerular basement membrane, will progress to end-stage renal disease.

b. Recurrent pyelonephritis, particularly in females.

c. Diabetic effects on the kidney are the single most common cause of end stage renal failure.

9. Neuropathy—inadequate blood supply to the nerve tissue and high blood sugar levels cause metabolic changes within the neuron.

a. Peripheral neuropathy—may be general pain and tingling, may progress to painless neuropathy.

NURSING PRIORITY: *Painless peripheral neuropathy is a very dangerous situation for the diabetic. Severe injury may occur to the lower extremities and the client will not be aware of it. Clients should be taught to visually inspect their feet and legs.*

b. Autonomic nerve damage—diarrhea or constipation, urinary incontinence or retention, decreased sweating, orthostatic hypotension, and impotence in the male. Interferes with the client's ability to recognize hypoglycemia episode.

c. Approximately 60% of diabetics experience neuropathy, it is the most common chronic complication.

10. Infections—an alteration in immune system response results in impairment of white cells for phagocytosis. Persistent glycosuria potentiates urinary tract infections.

Clinical Implications of Diabetes in Pregnancy

1. Effects of pregnancy on diabetes (Table 13-5).

a. During the first trimester of the pregnancy, there is an increase in fetal need for glucose and amino

Table 13-5: MODIFIED WHITE'S CLASSIFICATION OF DIABETES MELLITUS FOR PREGNANCY

CLASS	DESCRIPTION
A	Chemical diabetes diagnosed *before* pregnancy; managed by diet *alone*; any age of onset of duration.
B	Insulin treatment necessary *before* pregnancy; onset after age 20; duration of less than 1to 10 years.
C	Onset at age 10-19; or duration of 10-19 years.
D	Diabetic of long duration, over 20 years; onset before age 10; evidence of vascular disease. Complications - intrauterine fetal death, neonatal death.
F	Renal disease.
H	Coronary artery disease.
R	Proliferative retinopathy
T	Renal transplant.

acids; this lowers the maternal blood glucose and decreases her need for additional insulin.

b. During the second and third trimester, the need for insulin will increase, due to insulin antagonism by placental hormones.

c. Oral hypoglycemics will not be used to control pregnant client.

2. Effects of diabetes on pregnancy.

a. Increase in size and number of islets of Langerhans in the Type 2 client.

b. Increased tendency toward the development of metabolic acidosis, due to an increase in metabolic rate.

c. Placental antagonist to insulin will decrease the effectiveness of the insulin.

d. Fetal antagonists to insulin decrease the utilization of glucose.

3. Influence of pregnancy on diabetic control.

a. Decrease in insulin requirements during the first trimester of pregnancy.

b. Increase in insulin requirements during the second and third trimester of pregnancy to as much as 70% to 100% over pre-pregnancy amounts.

c. Tendency to intensify the existing complications of diabetes.

4. Monitoring fetal and maternal well-being during pregnancy, labor, and delivery.

a. Antepartum.

(1) Assess stability of mother's blood sugar control.

Table 13-6: IMPLICATIONS IN THE ADMINISTRATION OF INSULIN

1. Do not administer cold insulin; it increases lipodystrophy and pain at site.
2. A 10 ml vial of unrefrigerated insulin should be discarded after 30 days, regardless of how much was used.
3. Regular, NPH, and lente insulin does not need refrigeration if kept away from heat and sunlight.
4. Insulin pens (NPH and 70/30) should be discarded after one week of storage at room temperature. Regular cartridges, which don't contain preservatives, may be left unrefrigerated for up to one month.
5. Extreme temperatures (less than 36°F or greater than 86°F) should be avoided.
6. Shaking the vial (especially NPH and lente) decreases the risk of an inconsistent concentration of insulin, because rolling the vial does not adequately mix the suspension .
7. The abdomen is the primary site for subcutaneous injections of insulin. Rotate injection sites; injection sites should be one inch apart.
8. Abdomen area provides most rapid insulin absorption.
9. Use only insulin syringes to administer insulin.
10. Check expiration date on insulin bottle.
11. When drawing up regular insulin with a long acting insulin, draw up the regular (clear) before the longer acting (cloudy) insulin.
12. Regular insulin is used for administration by sliding scale and periods when blood sugar is unstable and difficult to control.
13. Insulin may be injected through lightweight clothing.

(2) Weekly or biweekly blood glucose levels, to maintain optimum level of control.

(3) Third trimester evaluation of fetal/placental function by determining twenty-four-hour urinary estriol levels.

(4) 36 to 38 weeks' gestation non-stress or oxytocin challenge tests (stress test), to determine ability of fetus to withstand stress.

(5) Amniocentesis to obtain fluid samples to determine L/S ratio (lecithin/sphingomyelin).

b. Intrapartum.

(1) As long as there is evidence of adequate placental function, and the infant's response to stress is appropriate, the pregnancy is allowed to progress to term, with an anticipated vaginal delivery.

(2) During labor, blood glucose levels are maintained with IV glucose and regular insulin.

(3) Fetal monitoring during labor.

c. Postpartum.

(1) Endocrine and metabolic changes will occur rapidly after delivery.

(2) Insulin requirements for mother will be markedly decreased and will fluctuate over next few weeks.

(3) Mother must go through a period of diabetic re-regulation.

5. Presence of diabetes predisposes the client to an increased incidence of:
   a. Pregnancy induced hypertension (PIH).
   b. Hemorrhage.
   c. Polyhydramnios.
   d. Vaginal and urinary tract infections.
   e. Premature delivery.
   f. Intrauterine death in third trimester.
   g. Compromised newborn.
      (1) Respiratory distress syndrome.
      (2) Hypoglycemia.
      (3) Hyperbilirubinemia.
      (4) Congenital anomalies—are directly associated with the degree of maternal hyperglycemia in the first trimester.

Nursing Intervention (All types)

NURSING PRIORITY: *Evaluating Client's Control of Diabetes.* ***1.*** *Normal fasting blood sugar 110-115 mg/dL.* ***2.*** *2 hours after meals or after glucose load, blood sugar is no higher than 140 mg/dL.* ***3.*** *Client is in good general health and is of normal weight.* ***4.*** *Glycoslyated hemoglobin is less then 7%.*

✦ *Goal: to return serum glucose to normal level.*

1. Initially administer regular insulin on a proportional basis according to need (Table 13-6).
2. Administer insulin 30 minutes prior to eating.
3. Maintain adequate fluid intake.
4. Evaluate serum electrolytes.
   a. Do not administer potassium unless client is voiding or if urine output begins to drop.
   b. Generally begin potassium replacement within 1-2 hours after starting insulin therapy.
   c. Serum potassium levels will be misleading if the client is dehydrated or in ketoacidosis.
5. Evaluate hydration status.
6. Evaluate for clinical manifestations of hypoglycemia and hyperglycemia.

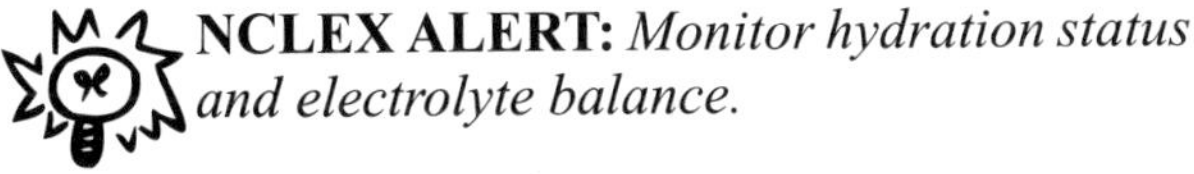
NCLEX ALERT: *Monitor hydration status and electrolyte balance.*

✦ *Goal: plan and implement a teaching regimen.*

Table 13-7: DIABETIC "SICK DAY" GUIDELINES

1. If you do not feel well (not eating regularly, fever, lethargy, nausea and vomiting, etc.) call your health care provider.
2. Check your blood glucose every 2 hours and urine ketones when voiding.
3. Increase your intake of fluids that are high carbohydrate; every hour drink fluids that replace electrolytes - fruit drinks, sports drinks, regular soft drinks (not diet beverages).
4. If you cannot eat and you have replaced 4 to 5 meals with liquids, notify your health care provider.
5. Get plenty of rest; if possible, have someone stay with you.
6. Do not omit or skip your insulin injections or oral medications unless specifically directed to do so by your health care provider.
7. Follow your health care provider's instructions regarding blood glucose levels and insulin or oral hypoglycemics.
8. Stay warm, stay in bed and do not overexert yourself.

1. Assess current level of knowledge regarding diabetes (See Box 13-1).
2. Evaluate cultural and socioeconomic parameters.
3. Evaluate client's support system (family, significant others).

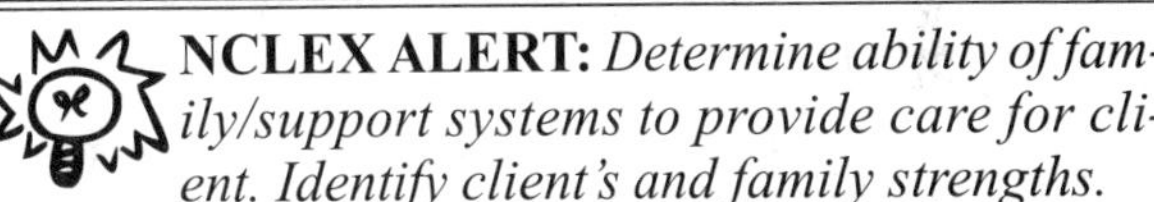
NCLEX ALERT: *Determine ability of family/support systems to provide care for client. Identify client's and family strengths.*

4. Administration of insulin. (Table 13-6).
   a. Correct injection techniques.
   b. Rotate injection site.
   c. Insulin may be injected through light clothing.
   d. Check expiration date on the insulin.
   e. Duration and peak action of prescribed insulin.
   f. Allow for ample practice time.
   g. Administer at the same time each day.
   h. Clients following an intensive diabetes therapy program may choose to use an insulin pump or to monitor blood glucose levels 4-6 times a day and take injections at those times.
   i. Disposable needles and syringes may be used for up to 3 days. Good hand washing is critical, needle should be recapped and stored in refrigerator to decrease bacterial growth.
5. Oral hypoglycemic agents.
   a. Take medication as scheduled; do not skip or add dose.
   b. Signs and symptoms of hypoglycemia.
   c. Anticipate change in medication with pregnancy.
6. Exercise.
   a. Establish an exercise program.
   b. Avoid sporadic exercise.

c. Review instructions regarding adjustment of insulin and food intake, to meet increased activity.

d. Extremities involved in activity should not be used for insulin injection (i.e., arms when playing tennis).

7. Diet (See Box 13-2).

a. Regularly scheduled mealtimes.

b. Understanding of food groups and balanced nutrition.

c. Incorporate family tendencies and cultural patterns into prescribed dietary regimen.

d. Provide client and family with written instructions regarding dietary needs.

8. Infection control.

a. Report infections promptly.

b. Insulin requirements may increase with severe infections.

c. Increased problems with vaginitis, UTI, and skin irritation.

9. Avoid injury.

a. Decreased healing capabilities especially in lower extremities.

b. Maintain adequate blood supply to extremities; avoid tight-fitting clothing around the legs.

c. Proper foot care (Chapter 16).

✦ *Goal: to prepare the diabetic client for surgery.*

1. Obtain base serum laboratory values for comparison postoperatively.
2. Surgery should be scheduled in early AM to decrease problems with diet and insulin replacement.
3. Oral hypoglycemics should not be given the morning of surgery.
4. For clients that are NPO requiring insulin, an IV of D_5W is frequently started.
5. Obtain a blood glucose reading about an hour prior to sending the client to surgery to make sure he is not developing hypoglycemia.

✦ *Goal: to maintain control of diabetic condition in the postoperative surgical client.*

1. IV fluids and regular insulin until client is able to take PO fluids.
2. Obtain blood sugar level 4 to 6 times a day to determine fluctuations.
3. After glucose levels stabilize, the client can usually resume his preoperative diabetic medication.
4. Observe for hypoglycemia immediately postoperatively.
5. Avoid urinary bladder catheterization.
6. Evaluate peripheral circulation and prevent skin breakdown.

Box 13-2: Elderly Care Focus

Guidelines for Food Selection

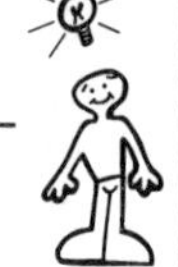

- Avoid canned fruits that are in heavy syrup, select ones packed in water.
- Include fresh fruits and vegetables, whole grain cereals and breads to provide adequate dietary fiber to prevent constipation.
- Avoid casseroles, fried foods, sauces and gravies, and sweets.
- Fats (oils, margarines) that are liquid at room temperature are better than those that are solid.
- Read food labels - the highest content ingredient is listed first.
- Select foods where the majority of calories do not come from a fat source.

7. Assess for development of postoperative infections.

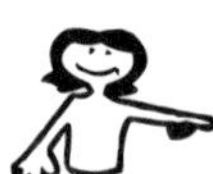

NURSING PRIORITY: *Evaluate intake, do not give NPO client insulin unless IV is in place.*

✦ *Goal: to identify DKA and assist client to return to homeostasis.*

1. Establish an IV access.
2. Anticipate rapid infusion of normal saline or plasma expanders initially, then maintenance rate. Administer with caution in clients with cardiac condition.
3. Administer insulin—IV during the acute phase, then subcutaneous as blood glucose begins to decrease.
4. Frequent monitoring of vital signs.
5. Frequent serum glucose checks.
6. Hourly urine measurements—do not administer potassium if urine output is low or dropping.
7. Monitor blood glucose levels frequently.
8. May utilize cardiac monitor.
9. Monitor serum electrolytes, particularly potassium levels.
   a. Hyperkalemia may occur initially in response to the acidosis.
   b. Hypokalemia occurs about 4 to 6 hours after treatment, as the acidosis is resolving.
10. Evaluate acid-base status.

✦ *Goal: to identify HHNC; to assist client to return to homeostasis.*

1. Establish an IV access.
2. IV infusion to rehydrate client; normal saline is frequently used.
3. Low-dose insulin IV initially to decrease blood glucose slowly.

4. Evaluate urine output.
5. Monitor serum glucose level.
6. Evaluate acid-base status.
7. Assess client for presence of other chronic health problems.

Self-Care

1. Maintain optimum weight.
2. Remain on long-term medical care.
3. Notify all health care providers of diagnosis of diabetes; wear a medical alert identification.
4. Recognize problems of the cardiovascular system.
   a. Peripheral vascular disease.
   b. Decreased healing.
   c. Increased risk of stroke.
   d. Increased risk of MI.
   e. Presence of retinopathy.
   f. Increased risk of renal disease.
5. Recognize problems of peripheral neuropathy.
6. Assist client to understand problems diabetes imposes on pregnancy and the subsequent development of a high-risk pregnancy.
7. Assist client to understand the problem of increased susceptibility to infections.

✦ *Goal: (pregnancy) to assist the client to maintain homeostasis throughout pregnancy.*

1. Prevent infection.
2. Frequent evaluation of glucose levels.
3. Physicians will change client from oral hypoglycemic agents to regular insulin.
4. Maintain optimum level of weight gain; may be induced for labor or have cesarean section if complications are evident.

✦ *Goal: (pregnancy) to assist the client to maintain homeostasis throughout labor and delivery.*

1. IV D_5W and insulin or Ringer's lactate to maintain homeostasis during labor.
2. Fetal monitoring to identify early stages of fetal distress.
3. X-ray pelvimetry to identify cephalopelvic disproportion (CPD).
4. Increased incidence of dystocia due to large infants.
5. Frequent evaluation of serum glucose levels (every 2 to 3 hours).

✦ *Goal: (pregnancy) to assist the client to return to homeostasis during the postpartal period.*

1. Anticipate fluctuation in insulin requirements due to:
   a. Loss of fetal insulin.
   b. Removal of placental influence on insulin.
   c. Changes in metabolic activity.
2. Monitor for fluctuations in serum glucose levels.
3. Prevent postpartal infection.

Hypoglycemia (Insulin Reaction)

❑ **Hypoglycemia is a condition characterized by decreased serum glucose level, which results in decreased cerebral function.**

Assessment

1. Risk factors.
   a. Poorly controlled diabetic.
      (1) Too little food.
      (2) Increase in exercise without adequate food.
      (3) Increase in insulin intake.
   b. Excessive alcohol intake with poor nutrition.
   c. Gastroenteritis, or gastroparesis which may impede absorption of food.
   d. Reflex action of insulin due to increased carbohydrate intake (Somogyi effect).
2. Clinical manifestations.
   a. Lability of mood.
   b. Emotional changes, confusion.
   c. Headache.
   d. Impaired vision.
   e. Tachycardia.
   f. Nervousness, tremors.
   g. Diaphoresis.
3. Diagnostics.
   a. Serum glucose below 50 mg per 100 dL.
   b. Negative urine acetone.
   c. Normal pH.

Treatment

1. Carbohydrates by mouth if client is alert and can swallow.
   a. Milk preferred in children with a mild reaction; it provides immediate lactose as well as protein and fat for prolonged action.
   b. Simple sugars for immediate response—orange juice, honey, candy, glucose tablets.
2. Glucagon IV if client is unconscious.

Nursing Intervention

✦ *Goal: to increase serum glucose level.*

1. Glucose/carbohydrate preparations as indicated.

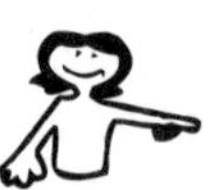

***NURSING PRIORITY:** When in doubt of diagnosis of hypoglycemia versus hyperglycemia, administer carbohydrates; severe hypoglycemia can rapidly result in permanent brain damage.*

2. Thorough assessment of the diabetic client for the development of hypoglycemia.

✦ *Goal: to assist client to identify precipitating causes and activities to prevent the development of hypoglycemia.*

1. Instruct the diabetic client to carry simple carbohydrates.
2. Administer between-meal snacks at the peak action of the insulin.
3. Between-meal snacks should limit simple carbohydrates and increase complex carbohydrates and protein.
4. Evaluate client's understanding of insulin and diabetic control; reteach as appropriate.

Pancreatitis

❑ **Pancreatitis is an inflammatory condition of the pancreas.**

A. Acute—characterized by an acute inflammatory process; problems range from mild edema to severe hypotension and severe hemorrhagic necrosis.

B. Chronic—characterized by progressive destruction and fibrosis of the pancreas; condition may follow acute pancreatitis, but also may occur alone.

Assessment

1. Risk factors/etiology.
   a. Biliary tract obstructive disease, causing reflux of bile secretions.
   b. Alcohol intake precipitating an increase in the secretion of pancreatic juices.
2. Clinical manifestations.
   a. Severe epigastric pain.
      (1) Radiates to the back or the flank area.
      (2) Aggravated by eating.
   b. Acute.
      (1) Persistent vomiting.
      (2) Low-grade fever.
      (3) Hypotension.
      (4) Jaundice if common bile duct is obstructed.
      (5) Abdominal distention.
   c. Chronic.
      (1) Decrease in weight.
      (2) Mild jaundice.
      (3) Steatorrhea.
      (4) Abdominal distention and tenderness.
      (5) Hyperglycemia.
3. Diagnostics.
   a. Increase in serum amylase, lipase.
   b. Increase in urine amylase.
   c. Hyperglycemia.
   d. Ultrasound.

Treatment

1. Medications.
   a. Analgesics (**Demerol**).
   b. Antibiotics.
2. Decrease pancreatic stimulus.
   a. NPO, IV fluids.
   b. Nasogastric suction
   c. Bed rest.
      (1) Diet - low fat, high carbohydrate.
3. Surgical intervention to eliminate precipitating cause (biliary tract obstruction).

Nursing Intervention

(Nursing intervention is the same for acute pancreatitis and for the client with chronic pancreatitis experiencing an acute episode).

✦ *Goal: to relieve pain.*

1. Administer analgesics, do not give Morphine.
2. Position on side in knee chest or in semi-Fowler's.
3. Evaluate precipitating cause.

✦ *Goal: to decrease pancreatic stimulus.*

1. Bed rest.
2. Maintain NPO initially.
3. Maintain nasogastric suctioning.
4. Small frequent feedings when food is allowed.

✦ *Goal: to prevent complications.*

1. Identify electrolyte imbalances, especially hypocalcemia.
2. Maintain adequate hydration.
3. Maintain respiratory status—problems occur due to pain and ascites.
4. Assess for hypoglycemia and development of diabetes.

Self-Care

1. Avoid all alcohol intake.
2. Signs of development of diabetes and return checkup for evaluation of blood sugar.
3. Low fat diet, high protein, moderate carbohydrates.
4. Replacement pancreatic enzymes.

Table 13-8: SUMMARY OF ADRENAL HORMONES

HORMONE	SITE OF ACTION	FUNCTION
Mineralcorticoids* (Aldosterone)	Renal tubule	1. Reabsorption of water, Na, Cl. 2. Decrease reabsorption of K. 3. Conditions which cause increase in aldosterone secretion: a. Decrease in serum Na. b. Shock.
Glucocorticoids† (Cortisol, hydrocortisone)	Metabolism of all food; enable individual to withstand stress	1. Increased rate of gluconeogenesis. 2. Catabolic effect on protein metabolism. 3. Antiinflammatory effect. 4. Increased secretion during times of increased body stress.
Androgens—sex hormones‡ Females—estrogen and progesterone (ovaries)	Stimulate reproduction organs to secrete gonadal hormones.	1. Responsible for secondary sexual characteristics. 2. Phases of menstrual cycle. 3. Uterine changes in pregnancy.
Males—testosterone (testes)		1. Development and maintenance of secondary sex characteristics. 2. Spermatogenesis.
Adrenal medulla§ Epinephrine	Smooth muscle Cardiac muscle	1. Stimulation of sympathetic nervous system. 2. Produces increase in systolic blood pressure.
Norepinephrine	Organs innervated by sympathetic nervous system	1. Increase peripheral resistance (i.e., increase in blood pressure).

*Mineralcorticoids are primarily controlled by the renin-angiotensin system.
†Glucocorticoids are primarily controlled by secretion of ACTH from the anterior pituitary.
‡Androgens are primarily controlled by secretions from the pituitary gland.
§Adrenal medulla hormones are primarily controlled by the sympathetic division of the autonomic nervous system.

Cancer of the Pancreas

❑ **The majority of tumors occur in the head of the pancreas. As the tumor grows, the bile ducts are obstructed, thereby causing jaundice. Tumors in the body of the pancreas frequently do not cause symptoms until growth is advanced. Cancer of the pancreas has a poor prognosis, 90% die within the first year after diagnosis.**

Assessment

1. Risk factors/etiology.
   a. Higher in males 45 to 65 years old.
   b. History of chronic pancreatitis is common.
2. Clinical manifestations.
   a. Dull, aching abdominal pain.
   b. Ascites
   c. Nausea, vomiting.
   d. Anorexia and progressive weight loss.
   e. Jaundice.
   f. Clay colored stools.
   g. Dark frothy urine.
3. Diagnostics.
   a. Increased carcinoembryonic antigen (CEA).
   b. Ultrasonography.

Treatment

1. Surgery—Whipple's procedure (radical pancreaticduodenectomy).
2. Radiation therapy.
3. Chemotherapy.

Nursing Intervention

✦ *Goal: to maintain homeostasis (see nursing intervention for pancreatitis).*

✦ *Goal: to provide preoperative nursing measures if surgery is indicated.*

1. Maintain nasogastric suctioning, assess for adequate hydration.
2. Control hyperglycemia.
3. Assess status of cardiac respiratory stability.
4. Assess for development of thrombophlebitis.

✦ *Goal: to promote comfort, prevent complications, and maintain homeostasis postoperative Whipple's.*

1. General postoperative care (Chapter 3).
2. Evaluate for bleeding tendencies caused by decreased prothrombin activity.
3. Monitor for fluctuation in serum glucose levels.
4. Maintain NPO and nasogastric suction until peristalsis returns.
5. Encourage adequate nutrition when appropriate.
   a. Decrease fats, increase carbohydrates.
   b. Small, frequent feedings.

Self-Care

1. Evaluate for bouts of anxiety and depression due to severity of illness and prognosis. (See Chapter 8)
2. Assist client in setting realistic goals.
3. Encourage ventilation of feelings.
4. Discuss methods for pain control.

PHYSIOLOGY OF THE ADRENALS

The adrenal glands are located at the apex of each kidney.

A. Adrenal medulla—secretes catecholamines, epinephrine and norepinephrine; under the influence of the sympathetic nervous system.

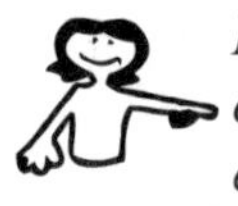

NURSING PRIORITY: *Clients experiencing problems of the adrenal medulla experience severe fluctuations in blood pressure related to the levels of catecholamines.*

B. Adrenal cortex—main body of the adrenal gland; responsible for the secretion of glucocorticoids, mineralocorticoids, and adrenal sex hormones; adrenal cortical function is essential for life (Table 13-8).

C. Function of the adrenal cortex is controlled by the negative feedback mechanisms regulating hormone release; pituitary gland secretes ACTH, which in turn regulates hormone release of the adrenal cortex.

System Assessment

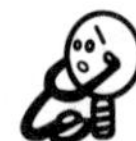

A. Adrenal medulla.
   1. Evaluate changes in blood pressure.
   2. Assess for changes in metabolic rate.

B. Adrenal cortex.
   1. Evaluate changes in weight.
   2. Evaluate changes in the skin color and texture, as well as the in presence and distribution of body hair.
   3. Assess cardiovascular system for instability, as evidenced by a labile blood pressure and cardiac output.
   4. Evaluate GI discomfort.
   5. Assess fluid and electrolyte changes due to effect on mineralcorticoids and glucocorticoids.
   6. Assess for changes in glucose metabolism.
   7. Assess for changes in reproductive system and in sexual activity.
   8. Evaluate changes in muscle mass.

DISORDERS OF THE ADRENALS

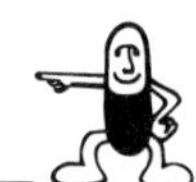

Pheochromocytoma

❑ **This tumor of the adrenal medulla secretes an excess of epinephrine and norepinephrine.**

A. An increase in these catecholamines produces vasoconstriction, with a precipitant increase in blood pressure, glycogenolysis, and cardiac workload.

B. Condition may become evident during pregnancy, as increasing uterine pressure precipitates problems.

Assessment

1. Clinical manifestations.
   a. Persistent or paroxysmal hypertension.
   b. Palpitations, tachycardia.
   c. Hyperglycemia
   d. Diaphoresis
   e. Nervousness, apprehension.
   f. Headache.
2. Diagnostics (See Appendix 13-1).
   a. Increase in urinary excretion of catecholamine.
   b. Increase in urinary excretion of vanilly lmandelic acid (VMA).
   c. Serum assay of catecholamine.
   d. MRI, CAT scan.
3. Treatment
   a. Medications.
      (1) Antihypertensive medications.
      (2) Antidysrhythmic medications.
   b. Surgery—removal of the tumor is the treatment of choice.

Nursing Intervention

✦ *Goal: to decrease client's hypertension and provide preoperative nursing measures as appropriate. (See Chapter 3).*

1. Decrease intake of stimulants.
2. Sedate as indicated.
3. Maintain calm, quiet environment.
4. Assess vital signs frequently.

✦ *Goal: to assist client to return to homeostasis postoperative adrenalectomy.*

1. Maintain normal blood pressure the first 24 to 48 hours postoperatively; client is at increased risk of developing hemorrhage or severe hypotensive episode.
   a. Assess for blood pressure changes due to catecholamine balance (both hypertension and hypotension).
   b. Administer analgesics judiciously.
   c. Administer corticosteroids as indicated.
   d. Maintain quiet, cool environment.
   e. Maintain IV fluid intake.
2. Assess for hypoglycemia.
3. Tendency toward hemorrhagic problems.
4. Monitor renal perfusion and urinary output.
5. Assess for problems of adrenal insufficiency.

✦ *Goal: to maintain health postoperative adrenalectomy.*

1. Continued medical follow-up care.
2. If both adrenals are removed, client will remain on corticosteriods.

Addison's Disease

❑ **This disorder is caused by a decrease in secretion of the adrenal cortex hormones.**

A. Decreased physiologic response to stress, vascular insufficiency, and hypoglycemia.

B. Decrease in aldosterone secretions (mineralcorticoids), which normally promote concentration of sodium and water and excretion of potassium.

C. May cause an alteration in adrenal androgen secretion necessary for secondary sex characteristics.

Assessment

1. Risk factors/etiology.
   a. An autoimmune induced problem.
   b. Occurs after bilateral adrenalectomy.
   c. Abrupt withdrawal from long-term corticosteroid therapy.
   d. Adrenal crisis may be precipitated by failure of the client to take medications.
   e. AIDS is increasingly being identified as a cause of adrenal insufficiency.
   f. Increased emotional stress without appropriate hormone replacement.
2. Clinical manifestations (development of symptoms requires loss of 90% of both adrenal cortices).
   a. Onset is insidious, client may go for weeks to months before diagnosis.
   b. Fatigue, weakness.
   c. Weight loss.
   d. Gastrointestinal disturbances.
   e. Bronze pigmentation of the skin.
   f. Postural hypotension.
   g. Hyponatremia, hyperkalemia.
   h. Hypoglycemia.
   i. Adrenal crisis.
      (1) Profound fatigue.
      (2) Dehydration.
      (3) Vascular collapse.

NCLEX ALERT: *Determine if vital signs are abnormal (e.g. hypotension, hypertension), notify others for change in client's condition.*

3. Diagnostics (Appendix 13-1).
   a. ACTH stimulation test.
   b. Decreased serum sodium and increased serum potassium.
   c. Plasma ACTH.

Treatment

Replace corticosteroids.

Nursing Intervention

✦ *Goal: to return to homeostasis.*

1. Initiate and maintain IV infusion of normal saline.
2. Administer large doses of corticosteroids through IV bolus initially, then titrate in a diluted solution.
3. Frequent evaluation of vital signs.
4. Assess sodium and water retention.
5. Evaluate serum potassium levels.
6. Keep client immobilized and quiet.

***NURSING PRIORITY:** If any client is experiencing difficulty with maintaining adequate blood pressure, do not move him unless absolutely necessary. Avoid all unnecessary nursing procedures until the client is stabilized.*

✦ *Goal: to safely take steroid replacements. (See Appendix 6-8).*

1. Administer steroid preparations with food or an antacid.
2. Evaluate for edema and fluid retention.
3. Assess serum sodium and potassium levels.
4. Check daily weight.
5. Increase protein and carbohydrates.
6. Evaluate for hypoglycemia.
7. Observe for Cushingoid symptoms.

Self Care

1. Lifelong steroid therapy is necessary.
2. Dosage of steroids may need to be increased in times of additional stress.
3. Infection, diaphoresis, and injury will necessitate an increase in the need for steroids and may precipitate a crisis state.
4. Report gastric distress as it may be due to steroids.
5. Carry a medical identification card.

Cushing's Syndrome

❑ **This disorder occurs as a result of excess levels of adrenal cortex hormones (primarily glucocorticoids) and, to a lesser extent, androgen and aldosterone (See Table 13-8).**

NCLEX ALERT: *Evaluate client's use of medications. Implement procedures to counteract adverse effects of medication. The most common cause of Cushing's syndrome is the long-term use of steroid therapy in treatment of chronic conditions. There are many chronic conditions that necessitate the use of long-term steroid therapy.*

Assessment

1. Risk factors/etiology.
   a. More common in women.
   b. Pituitary hypersecretion.
   c. A benign pituitary tumor.
   d. Iatrogenic- most often a result of long-term steroid therapy.
2. Clinical manifestations.
   a. Marked change in personality.
   b. Changes in appearance.
      (1) Moon face.
      (2) Deposit of fat on the back.
      (3) Thin skin, purple striae.
      (4) Thin extremities.
      (5) Bruises and petechiae.
   c. Persistent hyperglycemia.
   d. GI distress from increased acid production.
   e. Osteoporosis.
   f. Increased susceptibility to infection.
   g. Sodium and fluid retention, potassium depletion.
   h. Hypertension.
   i. Changes in secondary sexual characteristics.
      (1) Amenorrhea (females).
      (2) Hirsutism (females).
      (3) Gynecomastia (males).
3. Diagnostics (See Appendix 13-1).
   a. Increased serum sodium and decreased serum potassium levels.
   b. Hyperglycemia.
   c. Increased plasma cortisol levels.
   d. Loss of diurnal variation of cortisone levels.
   e. Dexamethasone suppression test.
4. Complications.
   a. Congestive heart failure.
   b. Hypertension.
   c. Pathologic fractures.
   d. Psychosis.

Treatment

Depends of the etiology of the problem.

Nursing Intervention

✦ *To assist return to hormone balance.*

1. Restrict sodium and water intake.
2. Monitor fluid and electrolyte levels.
3. Evaluate for hyperglycemia.
4. Assess for GI disturbances.
5. Prevent infection.

✦ *Goal: to prevent complications.*

1. Excessive sodium and water retention— monitor for edema, hypertension, CHF.
2. Potassium depletion— monitor for cardiac arrhythmias.
3. Evaluate client's ability to cope with change in body image.
4. Evaluate for thromboembolic problems.
5. Predisposed to fracture; promote weight bearing; monitor for joint and bone pain, promote home safety.

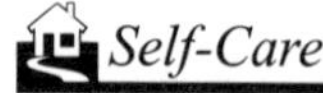
Self-Care

1. Stress the need for continuous health care.
2. Encourage continuation of activities.

3. Have client demonstrate an understanding of the medication regimen.
4. Assist client to identify methods of coping with problems of therapy.
5. Have client demonstrate an understanding of specific problems for which he/she needs to notify the physician.⌘

Study Questions—Endocrine

1. A client is receiving NPH insulin 20 units subq at 7 a.m. daily. At 3 p.m. the nurse finds the client apparently asleep. How would the nurse know if the client were having a hypoglycemic reaction?

① Feel the client and bed for dampness.
② Observe client for Kussmaul respirations.
③ Smell client's breath for acetone odor.
④ Check client's pupils for dilatation.

2. Postoperative thyroidectomy nursing care includes which measures?

① Have the client speak every 5 to 10 minutes if hoarseness is present.
② Provide a low-calcium diet to prevent hypercalcemia.
③ Check the dressing at the back of the neck for bleeding.
④ Apply a soft cervical collar to restrict neck movement.

3. What would the nurse note as typical findings on the assessment of a client with acute pancreatitis?

① Steatorrhea, abdominal pain, fever.
② Fever, hypoglycemia, dehydration.
③ Melena, persistent vomiting, hyperactive bowel sounds.
④ Hypoactive bowel sounds, decreased amylase and lipase.

4. A client is found to be comatose and hypoglycemic with a blood sugar of 50 mg. What nursing action is implemented first?

① Infuse 1,000 cc D_5W over a 12-hour period.
② Administer 50 percent glucose intravenously.
③ Check the client's urine for the presence of sugar and acetone.
④ Encourage the client to drink orange juice with added sugar.

5. Which medication will the nurse have available for emergency treatment of tetany in the client who is postoperative thyroidectomy?

① Calcium chloride.
② Potassium chloride.
③ Magnesium sulfate.
④ Sodium bicarbonate.

6. What is the primary action of insulin in the body?

① Enhance the transport of glucose across the cell wall.
② Aid in the process of gluconeogenesis.
③ Stimulate the pancreatic beta cells.
④ Decrease the intestinal absorption of glucose.

7. What will the nurse teach the diabetic client regarding exercise in his treatment program?

① During exercise the body will use carbohydrates for energy production, which in turn will decrease the need for insulin.
② With an increase in activity, the body will utilize more carbohydrates, therefore more insulin will be required.
③ The increase in activity results in an increase in the utilization of insulin, therefore the client should decrease his carbohydrate intake.
④ Exercise will improve pancreatic circulation and stimulate the islets of Langerhans to increase the production of intrinsic insulin.

8. The nurse is caring for a client who has exophthalmos secondary to her thyroid disease. What is the cause of exophthalmos?

① Fluid and edema in the retro-orbital tissues, which forces the eyes to protrude.
② Impaired vision, which causes the patient to squint in order to see.
③ Increased eye lubrication, which makes the patient blink less.
④ Decrease in extraocular eye movements, which results in the "thyroid stare."

9. What is a characteristic symptom of hypoglycemia that should alert the nurse to an early insulin reaction?

① Diaphoresis.
② Drowsiness.
③ Severe thirst.
④ Coma.

10. A client is scheduled for a routine glycosylated hemoglobin test (HbA_{1c}). What is important for the nurse to tell the client prior to this test?

① Drink only water after midnight and come to the clinic early in the morning.
② Eat a normal breakfast and be at the clinic two hours later.
③ Expect to be at the clinic for several hours due to the multiple blood draws.
④ Come to the clinic at the earliest convenience to have blood drawn.

11. A client has been on inhalation *Vasopressin* therapy. What will the nurse evaluate to determine the therapeutic response of this medication?

① Urine specific gravity.
② Blood glucose.
③ Vital signs.
④ Oxygen saturation levels.

Answers and rationales to these questions are in the section at the end of the book entitled "Chapter Study Questions: Answers & Rationales."

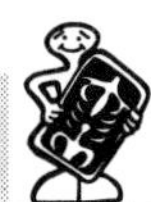

Appendix 13-1: ENDOCRINE DIAGNOSTICS

DIAGNOSTIC TEST	NORMAL	CLINICAL/NURSING IMPLICATIONS
THYROID		
Thyroxine (T_4)	5 - 12 mg/dl	
Triiodothyronine (T_3 uptake)	70-220ng.dL	1. Stimulation of the thyroid gland by TSH will initiate the release of stored thyroid hormone. 2. When T_3 & T_4 are low, TSH secretion increases. 3. T_3 &T_4 are used to confirm abnormal TSH.
Thyroid-stimulating hormone (TSH)	Increased in hypothyroidism. Decreased in primary hyperthyroidism.	
Neonatal thyroxine (T_4)	Normal levels vary with age from 1 day to 120 days	1. Positive test is associated with hypothyroidism. 2. Procedure is done by means of a heel puncture on infant. 3. Levels of neonatal thyroxine are not interpreted in same terms as serum T_4 values; this is a completely different test.
PANCREAS		
Serum glucose	115 mg/100 cc	1. Test is timed to rule out diabetes by determining rate of glucose absorption from serum. 2. In normal person, insulin response to large dose of glucose is immediate. 3. Insulin and oral hypoglycemics should not be administered before test.
Oral glucose tolerance test	1 hr - <150 mg/dl 2 hr - <120 mg/dl	
Glucose fasting blood sugar (FBS)	<115mg/dl	1. Utilized as a screening test for problems of metabolism. 2. Maintain client in fasting state 12 hours until blood drawn. 3. If client is a known diabetic and experiences dizziness, weakness, fainting, draw blood sugar.
Glycosolated hemoglobin (HbA_{1c})	Nondiabetic usually is 5-8%. 2-6% considered good diabetic control. >8% is considered poor diabetic control.	1. More accurate test of diabetic control, because it measures glucose attached to hemoglobin (indicates overall control for past 90- 120 days which is the lifespan of the RBC).

NCLEX ALERT: *Frequently the level of the FBS is given in a question and it is necessary to evaluate the level and determine appropriate nursing intervention.*

DIAGNOSTIC TEST	NORMAL	CLINICAL/NURSING IMPLICATIONS
Postprandial blood sugar	Less than 120 mg/dl	1. Involves measuring the serum glucose two hours after a meal, results are significantly increased in diabetic.
Serum amylase	60 to 200 Somogyi units/100 ml	1. Used to evaluate pancreatic cell damage. 2. Other intestinal conditions and inflammatory conditions cause increase.
Serum lipase	Normal values vary with method; elevated is abnormal	1. Appears in serum following damage to pancreas.
Urine sugar (Clinistix, Clinitest, Labstix)	Negative for glucose	1. Use fresh double-voided specimen. 2. A rough indicator of serum glucose levels. 3. Results may be altered by various medications.
Ketone bodies (Acetone)	Negative	1. Ketone bodies occur in the urine before there is significant increase in serum ketones. 2. Use freshly voided urine.
Urinary amylase	5-50 U/hr	1. In pancreatic injury more amylase enters blood and is excreted in urine. 2. May be done on a 2 hour or a 24-hr urine specimen.

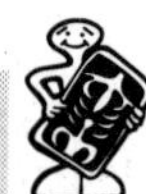

Appendix 13-1: ENDOCRINE DIAGNOSTICS

DIAGNOSTIC TEST	NORMAL	CLINICAL/NURSING IMPLICATIONS
PITUITARY		
Growth Hormone (GH)	Below 10 mg/ml	1. NPO midnight. 2. Maintain bed rest until serum sample is drawn.
Osmolarity urine Osmolarity serum	300 to 800 mOsm/kg 285 to 295 mOsm/kg	1. Used in evaluating ADH. 2. Do serum and urine tests at same time and compare results. 3. Normally, urine osmolarity should be higher than serum.
ADRENAL MEDULLA		
Urinary vanillylmandelic acid (VMA)	Increased with pheochromocytoma.	1. Nursing implications: depending on how test is measured, there may be dietary and medication restrictions. 2. 24-hr urine collection.
Urine catecholamines: Epinephrine, norepinephrine Metanephrine Normetanephrine	Increased in conditions that precipitate increase in catacholamine secretion	(Same as for VMA).
ADRENAL CORTEX		
ACTH stimulation test	Increase in plasma cortisol levels	1. ACTH is infused over a period of hours to evaluate ability of adrenal glands to secrete steroids.
Dexamethasone suppression test	Normal suppression 50% decrease in cortisone production	1. An overnight test - a small amount of dexamethasone is administered in the evening, and serum and urine are evaluated in the AM, or extensive test may cover 6 days. 2. Cushing's is ruled out if suppression is normal.
Plasma cortisol levels for diurnal variations	Secretion high in early morning, decreased in evening. 8 AM - 10 to 25 ug/dl 8 PM - <10 ug/dl	1. Elevation in plasma cortisol levels occurs in the morning and significant decrease in evening and night - a diurnal variation.
24-hr urine for hydroxycorticosteroids and ketosteroids	Normal values vary with method and age of client	1. Increase in urine levels indicates hyperadrenal function.

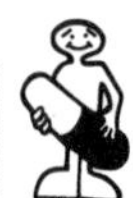

Appendix 13-2:
MEDICATIONS USED IN ENDOCRINE DISORDERS

MEDICATIONS	SIDE EFFECTS	NURSING IMPLICATIONS
ADH REPLACEMENT		
Desmopressin **(DDAVP)**: nasal spray, PO, IV, SQ Vasopressin (**Pitressin**): IM, SC Lypressin (**Diapid**): nasal spray	Excessive water retention, headache, nausea, flushing.	1. Monitor daily weight, correlate with intake and output. 2. Vasopressin more likely to cause adverse cardiovascular and thromboembolic problems.
ANTITHYROID: Inhibits production of thyroid hormone; does not inactivate thyroid in circulating blood. Medications are not reliable for long term inhibition of thyroid production.		
Propylthiouracil (**PTU**):PO Methimazole (**Tapazole**): PO	Agranulocytosis; abdominal discomfort; nausea, vomiting, diarrhea, crosses placenta (Same; crosses placenta more rapidly)	1. May increase anticoagulation effect of heparin and oral anticoagulants. 2. May be combined with iodine preparations. 3. Monitor CBC. 4. Store **Tapazole** in light-sensitive container. 5. May be used prior to surgery or treatment with radioactive iodine.
Lugol's solution: PO Saturated solution of potassium iodide **(SSKI)**	Inhibits synthesis and release of thyroid hormone	1. Administer in fluid to decrease unpleasant taste. 2. May be used to decrease vascularity of thyroid gland prior to surgery.
RADIOACTIVE IODINE: Accumulates in the thyroid gland; causes partial or total destruction of thyroid gland through radiation.		
Iodide, (**I^{131}**): PO	Discomfort in thyroid area; bone marrow depression; permanent hypothyroidism.	1. Check that antithyroid drugs are discontinued 2 to 4 days prior to administering I^{131}. 2. Radiation precautions on body secretions—3 days. 3. Client should avoid contact with women who are pregnant and small children. 4. Increase fluids immediately after treatment, as radioactive isotope is excreted in the urine. (See Chapter 8 for radiation safety).
THYROID REPLACEMENTS: Replacement of thyroid hormone.		
Levothyroxine sodium **(Levothyroid, Levoxyl, Synthroid)**: PO, IM, IV Liothyronine **(Cytomel)**	Overdose may result in symptoms of hyperthyroidism: tachycardia, heat intolerance, nervousness	1. Be careful in reading exact name on label of medications; micrograms and milligrams are used as units of measure. 2. Generally taken once a day before breakfast. 3. Within 3-4 days begin to see improvement, maximum effect in 4-6 weeks.
PANCREATIC ENZYMES: Replacement enzyme to aid in digestion of starch, protein and fat.		
Pancreatin: PO Pancrelipase **(Pancrease. Cotazym, Vioplase)**: PO	GI upset and irritation of the mucous membranes.	1. Client is usually on a high-protein, high-carbohydrate, low-fat diet. 2. Enteric-coated tablets should not be crushed or chewed. 3. Pancreatin may be given before, during, or within one hour after meals. 4. Pancrelipase is given just before or with each meal or snack.
ANTIHYPOGLYCEMIC: Increases plasma glucose levels and relaxes smooth muscles.		
Glucagon: IM, IV, SQ	None significant.	1. Watch for symptoms of hypoglycemia and treat with food first, if conscious. 2. Client usually awakens in 5-20 min. after receiving glucagon. 3. If client does not respond, anticipate IV glucose to be given.

Appendix 13-2:
MEDICATIONS USED IN ENDOCRINE DISORDERS

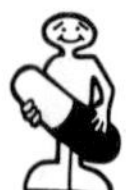

MEDICATIONS	SIDE EFFECTS	NURSING IMPLICATIONS
ORAL HYPOGLYCEMIA AGENTS: Stimulate beta cells to secrete more insulin; biguanides enhance body utilization of insulin. (See Table13-1 for Insulin)		
❖ **GENERAL NURSING IMPLICATIONS** ❖ — Dose should be decreased for elderly. — Use with caution in clients with renal and hepatic impairment. — All oral hypoglycemics are contraindicated in pregnant clients. — All clients should be carefully observed for symptoms of hypo-and hyperglycemia. — Medications should be taken in the morning. — Long-term therapy may result in decreased effectiveness.		
SULFONYLUREAS: stimulate the pancreas to make more insulin.		
Glipizide (**Glucotrol**): PO Glyburide (**Micronase, Diabeta**): PO Glimepiride (**Amaryl**): PO Tolbutamide (**Orinase**): PO Tolazamide (**Tolinase**): PO	Hypoglycemia, jaundice, GI disturbance, skin reactions	1. Tolbutamide has shortest duration of action, requires multiple daily doses. 2. Glyburide has a long duration of action. 3. Interact with: calcium channel blockers oral contraceptives glucocorticoids phenothiazines thiazide diuretics
BIGUANIDES: decrease sugar production in the liver and help the muscles use insulin to breakdown sugar.		
Metformin (**Glucophage**): PO	Dizziness, nausea, back pain, possible metallic taste	1. Metformin is administered with meals. 2. Metformin has a beneficial effect on lowering lipids. 3. Weight gain may occur.
ALPHA GLUCOSIDASE INHIBITOR: slows down how the body absorbs sugar after eating.		
Acarbose (**Precose**): PO Miglitol (**Glyset**): PO	Diarrhea, flatulence, abdominal pain	1. Take at beginning of meals; not effective on an empty stomach. 2. Acarbose is contraindicated in clients with inflammatory bowel disease. 3. Frequently given with sulfonylureas to increase effectiveness of both medications.

PHYSIOLOGY OF THE BLOOD

A. Components.
1. Plasma—90 percent water; accounts for about half of the total blood volume.
2. Formed elements (cells)—account for about half of the volume.
a. Erythrocytes (red cells).
b. Leukocytes (white cells).
c. Thrombocytes (platelets).

B. Characteristics of plasma (See Table 14-1).
1. Plasma is clear, straw colored, and does not contain cellular elements.
2. Liquid portion of the circulating volume; consists of 91 percent to 92 percent water.
3. Protein—6 percent to 8 percent of the plasma.
a. Albumin—most abundant protein, maintains normal colloid osmotic pressure of the plasma.
b. Globulins.

Table 14-1: CHARACTERISTICS OF NORMAL BLOOD

PLASMA	
Albumin	3.5 to 5.5 gm/dL
Glucose	70 to 110 mg/dL
NITROGENOUS WASTE	
BUN	5 to 20 mg/dL
Creatinine	0.7 to 1.5 mg/dL
Bilirubin	Total 0.3 to 1.3 mg/dL Direct unconjugated - 0.1 to 0.4 mg/100 dL Newborn - 1 to 12 mg/dL
LIPIDS	
Cholesterol	below 200 mg/dL
LDL	60-180 mg/dL
HDL	30-80 mg/dL
Triglycerides	40 to 150 mg/dL
CELLULAR CONCENTRATION	
Hemoglobin	Female 12 to 16 gm/dL Male 14 to 18 gm/dL Newborn 14 to 20 gm/dL
Hematocrit	Female 37% to 47% Male 40% to 50% Newborn 50% to 62%
Platelets	150,000 to 400,000 cu mm
Leukocytes	5,000 to 10,000 cu mm
Erythrocytes	4.5 to 5.5 mill/cu mm

(1) Gammaglobulins (immunoglobulins) consist primarily of antibodies produced by the plasma cells.
(2) Alpha and beta globulins are essential factors in the clotting mechanism.

c. Fibrinogen—necessary element in normal clot formation; produced in the liver.
d. Prothrombin— necessary element for normal coagulation.
(1) Produced in the liver.
(2) Normal production is dependent on availability of adequate vitamin K.
e. Normal body nutrients are carried by way of the plasma.
(1) Carbohydrates in the form of glucose.
(2) Proteins in the form of amino acids.
(3) Fat in the form of lipids.
f. Metabolic waste products are carried to organs of excretion by way of the plasma.
(1) Urea.
(2) Uric acid.
(3) Lactic acid.
(4) Creatinine.

C. Characteristics of erythrocytes (red blood cells).
1. Formed in the red bone marrow (reticuloendothelial system); erythropoiesis is production of red blood cells.
2. In early childhood, all bones contain red marrow; as child grows older, red marrow is replaced with fatty yellow marrow.
3. In the adult, only specific bones contain red marrow (humerus, proximal end of the femur, iliac crest).
4. In situations causing low oxygen tension, the kidney initiates the formation of erythropoietin, which in turn stimulates erythrocyte production.
5. Vitamin B_{12} and folic acid are necessary for the production of normal erythrocytes.
6. Functions of erythrocytes—primary function is transportation of oxygen and carbon dioxide.
a. Hemoglobin is the primary component of the red cell.
(1) Serves as a buffer in the acid-base balance.
(2) Hemoglobin combines easily with oxygen to form oxyhemoglobin.

(3) Iron is a major component of hemoglobin and is necessary for normal oxygen transport.

(4) Reduced hemoglobin has given up its oxygen component.

b. Hematocrit is fraction of the blood occupied by the erythrocytes. As a "rule of thumb," the hematocrit is usually 3 times the hemoglobin value.

7. When red cells are exposed to hypotonic solutions, water enters the cells, thus precipitating cellular wall rupture and destruction or hemolysis of the red cell.

8. Hemolysis also occurs when cellular membrane is damaged, as in trauma.

9. The life span of an erythrocyte is approximately 120 days or four months.

10. Old erythrocytes are removed from circulation by the liver, spleen, and bone marrow; iron is salvaged and returned to the bone marrow; the remainder of the cell is converted to bile pigments, which are excreted by the liver.

D. Characteristics of the leukocytes (white blood cells).

1. Primary work of the leukocytes is accomplished when the cells leave the circulating volume and enter the body tissue.

2. Types of cells.

a. Granulocytes (polymorphonuclear leukocyte—PMNs) originate in the bone marrow.

(1) Consist of neutrophils, eosinophils, and basophils.

(2) Primary function is to destroy bacteria (phagocytosis).

b. Agranular leukocytes (mononuclear) originate primarily in the lymphatic tissue.

(1) Consist of lymphocytes and monocytes.

(2) Assist in the removal of broken down tissue cells.

(3) Release substances which enhance the activity of the granulocytes.

3. Life span of the leukocyte is variable.

4. Leukocytosis refers to an overall increase in the leukocytes: leukopenia refers to an overall decrease in the leukocytes.

E. Characteristics of thrombocytes (platelets).

1. Smallest of the formed cells in the circulating volume.

2. Function—primarily involved with hemostasis; when vessel wall is damaged, platelets adhere to the area and eventually form a platelet plug to decrease bleeding.

3. Thrombocytosis refers to a marked abnormal increase in thrombocytes; thrombocytopenia refers to a marked abnormal decrease in thrombocytes.

F. Hemostasis.

1. Extrinsic mechanisms—clotting process is initiated by tissue damage and blood loss.

2. Intrinsic mechanism—clotting mechanism within the vessel where blood loss and tissue trauma are not present.

3. Both mechanisms produce the same result— clot formation.

4. Three phases of hemostasis (coagulation).

a. First phase—tissue injury precipitates release of platelet factor; in presence of calcium and accessory factors, thromboplastin is formed.

b. Second phase—conversion of prothrombin to thrombin; thromboplastin in Phase 1 initiates the conversion of prothrombin.

c. Third phase—action of thrombin in conversion of soluble fibrinogen to insoluble fibrin (fibrin is an insoluble protein which appears like a fine network of thread or like a web).

5. Erythrocytes are not part of the actual coagulation process; red cells are essentially trapped in the fibrin mesh and give the clot its characteristic color.

6. Fibrinolysis—process by which clots, formed in tissue and small vessels, are dissolved by fibrinolysin.

G. Blood classification.

1. Major blood groups—A, B, AB, and O.

a. Blood compatibility and systems of classification are based on the presence or absence of specific antigens present on red cells, as well as specific antibodies in the plasma.

b. There are two antigens or agglutinable substances present on red cells: A and B.

(1) Neither antigen is present in O.

(2) A is present in A.

(3) B is present in B.

(4) A and B are present in AB.

c. There are two antibodies present in the plasma: anti-A and anti-B.

(1) Both antibodies are present in O.

(2) Anti-B is present in A.

(3) Anti-A is present in B.

(4) Neither is present in AB.

d. If the antigen A on the red cells of the donors comes in contact with the antibody A of the recipi-

Box 14-1: Elderly Care Focus
Age Related Assessment Findings For The Hematologic System

Assessment Area	Hematologic System Findings	Elderly Changes & Significance
• Nail beds (check for capillary refill)	Pallor, cyanosis, and decreased capillary refill is often noted in hematologic disorders.	Nails are typically thickened and discolored. Need to use another body area, such as the lips to assess capillary refill.
• Hair distribution	Thin or absent hair on trunk and extremities may indicate poor oxygenation and blood supply to area.	Older adults are losing body hair, but often in an even pattern distribution that has occurred slowly over time. Lack of hair on lower legs and toes may indicate poor circulation.
• Skin moisture and color	Skin dryness, pallor, and jaundice may occur with anemia, leukemia, etc.	Dry skin is a normal aspect of aging and thus becomes a unreliable indicator of skin moisture. Pigment loss and skin changes along with some yellowing occurs with aging. Pallor may be noted in older adults that is not associated with anemia, as they tend not to go outdoors as often as younger adults and get exposed to sunlight.

ent and vice versa, agglutination and clumping will occur. (Example: type A blood transfused into type B recipient).

e. O negative is called the universal donor because there are no antigens on the red blood cells and the Rh factor is not present.

f. AB positive is called the universal recipient because there are no antibodies in the serum, and the Rh factor is present.

g. In agglutination and clumping of red cells, hemolysis occurs; hemolysis releases hemoglobin into the plasma.

h. Therefore, the problem that occurs is the destruction of the donor's red cells by the plasma of the recipient's cells.

2. Rh factor.

a. Rh factor is present on the red cell.

b. Rh is positive, or factor is present, in 85 percent to 95 percent of the population.

c. Rh is negative, or factor is absent, in 5 percent to 15 percent of the population.

d. Normal plasma does not contain Rh antibodies. Antibodies are formed in Rh negative blood if transfused with Rh positive blood; thus, the recipient is sensitized to the Rh factor and subsequent Rh positive blood might result in severe transfusion reaction.

e. Problems of sensitization occur in the newborn when the mother is Rh negative and the infant is Rh positive (Chapter 26).

System Assessment

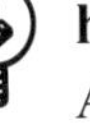

A. Evaluate history.

1. History of disease of bone marrow or bone producing organs.
2. History of treatment which depressed bone marrow activity (especially chemotherapy or radiation therapy).
3. Family history of problems (inheritance pattern).
4. History of blood transfusion.

B. Bleeding problems occurring during pregnancy, labor and delivery, or immediately after birth in both mother and infant.

C. Presence of disorders or disease processes other than the hematologic disorders; effect of aging (Box 14-1).

D. Evaluate effect hematologic disorder has on client's life style and daily living (ADL).

1. How long has client experienced symptoms?
2. What are current activities and metabolic requirements of the client?
3. Presence or absence of bleeding episodes.
4. Ability to control pain.
5. Presence of appropriate coping/defense mechanisms.

E. Assess client's current nutritional status.

F. Evaluate current blood values.

G. Evaluate status of respiratory and cardiovascular systems in maintaining homeostasis.

Anemias

❑ **Anemia is characterized by a low red cell count and a decrease to below normal of hemoglobin and hematocrit.**

A. Origin.

1. Defect in bone marrow production of red cells.

2. Loss of red cells.
   a. Hemorrhage.
   b. Chronic bleeding.
   c. Hemolytic processes.
3. Hereditary disorders of the red cells.
4. Inadequate nutritional intake of iron, folic acid.

B. The more rapidly an anemia occurs, the more severe the symptoms.

C. Normal term infants have adequate iron storage for the first 5-6 months, premature infants may need iron supplement at 2-3 months.

D. Common goal in treatment of all anemias is to identify the origin and correct the problem.
1. Assessment.
   a. Pale skin, delayed wound healing, sore mouth and tongue.
   b. Shortness of breath, dyspnea on exertion.
   c. Tachycardia, palpitations- cardiac complications can progress to cardiac decompensation.
   d. Chronic fatigue and weakness.
   e. Anorexia, nausea, weight loss, constipation and diarrhea.
   f. Beefy red tongue, hematemesis.
   g. Headache, dizziness, tingling in extremities.
   h. Chronic fatigue malaise.
   i. Chronic anemia may result in growth retardation in infants and children.

E. Iron Deficiency Anemia—characterized by inadequate intake of dietary iron or excessive loss of iron.
1. Risk factors/etiology.
   a. Common in adolescents.
   b. Common in infants whose primary diet is milk.
   c. May occur in pregnancy.
   d. Heavy flow during menses.
2. Elderly are more prone to anemia due to poor dietary intake and decreased absorption in the small intestine.
3. Diagnostics—decreased hemoglobin and hematocrit.
4. Clinical manifestations.
   a. May be asymptomatic.
   b. General symptoms of anemia.
5. Treatment - supplemental iron intake is necessary for 6 months to replenish body storage.
   a. Supplemental iron (Appendix 14-2).
   b. Increased dietary iron intake (Chapter 3).
   c. Supplemental folic acid.

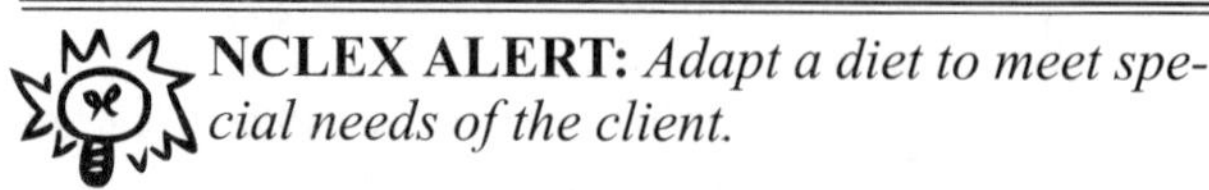
NCLEX ALERT: *Adapt a diet to meet special needs of the client.*

F. Pernicious anemia—condition characterized inability to absorb vitamin B_{12} (cyanocobalamin). It may be associated with loss of intrinsic factor (gastric resection), or it may be an autoimmune problem.
1. Risk factors/etiology.
   a. Generally not associated with inadequate dietary intake.
   b. More common in elderly.
   c. Familial tendency.
   d. May be precipitated by gastric resection.
2. Diagnostics.
   a. Schilling test for B_{12} absorption.
   b. Reduced and abnormal red blood cells.
   c. Gastric analysis for free hydrochloric acid.
3. Clinical manifestations.
   a. General symptoms of anemia.
   b. Confusion.
   c. Paresthesia in the extremities.
   d. Loss of sense of balance.
4. Treatment
   a. Injections of vitamin B_{12} may be required indefinitely.
   b. Supplemental iron and folic acid to prevent iron deficiency problems.

G. Aplastic anemia—characterized by depression of the bone marrow in production of red cells.
1. Risk factors/etiology.
   a. Examples of medications precipitating aplastic anemia.
      (1) Chemotherapeutic agents.
      (2) Benzene.
      (3) Chloramphenicol.
      (4) Anticonvulsant medications (Dilantin)
   b. Radioactive therapy.
   c. May be of idiopathic origin.
2. Diagnostics—bone marrow biopsy reveals severe decrease in all marrow elements (pancytopenia—Appendix 14-1).
3. Clinical manifestations.
   a. General symptoms of anemia.
   b. Fever.
   c. Infections.

d. Bleeding problems secondary to thrombocytopenia.

4. Treatment.

a. Bone marrow transplants (Appendix 14-4).

b. Androgenic hormone therapy.

c. Corticosteroids.

H. Folic acid deficiency anemia—very common anemia associated with decreased dietary intake of folic acid.

1. Risk factors/etiology. (origin very similar to B12 deficiency)

a. Diet lacking in folic acid.

b. Malabsorption syndromes.

c. Deficiency may occur with increased demands for folic acid—infancy, adolescence, and pregnancy.

2. Clinical manifestations.

a. Slow, insidious onset

b. Weight loss, emaciated.

c. May appear ill with malnourishment.

3. Diagnostics.

a. Differentiate between folic acid deficiency and vitamin B_{12} deficiency.

b. Serum folate levels <4ng/ml.

4. Treatment—Folic acid injections may be necessary initially, then oral replacement.

Nursing Intervention

For clients with anemia.

✦ *Goal: to assist in establishing a diagnosis.*

1. Complete nutritional evaluation.
2. History of possible causes.

✦ *Goal: to decrease body oxygen needs.*

1. Assess client's tolerance to activity.
2. Provide diversional activities, but provide for adequate rest.
3. May need supplemental oxygen.

✦ *Goal: to prevent infections.*

1. Decrease exposure.
2. Frequent evaluation of temperature elevations.
3. Observe for leukocytosis.
4. Maintain adequate hydration.

✦ *Goal: to assess for complications of chronic anemic state.*

1. Evaluate ability of cardiovascular system to maintain adequate cardiac output.
2. Evaluate for symptoms of hypoxia (Chapter 15).

✦ *Goal: to assist client to understand implications of disease and measures to maintain health.*

1. Medical regimen.
2. Importance of continuing medical follow-up.
3. Side effects of medications.
4. Identify foods high in iron and folic acid (Chapter 2).

Sickle Cell Anemia

❑ **Sickle Cell Anemia is a problem which is characterized by the sickling effect of the erythrocytes.**

A. Basic defect of the erythrocyte is in the globulin portion of the hemoglobin.

B. Sickling problem is not apparent until around six months of age; the increased levels of fetal hemoglobin up to that age prevent serious sickling problems.

C. Predominantly a problem of children. The child may be asymptomatic between crises.

D. Pathologic changes of sickle cell disease result from:

1. Increased blood viscosity.
2. Increased red cell destruction.
3. Increased viscosity eventually precipitates ischemia and tissue necrosis due to capillary stasis and thrombosis.
4. Cycle of occlusion, ischemia, and infarction to vascular organs.

E. Conditions precipitating sickling effect.

1. Hypoxia
2. Acidosis.
3. Dehydration.
4. Temperature elevation.

F. Pathologic effects of sickle cell disease on pregnancy.

1. Mother.

a. Increased anemia problems.

b. Increase in thromboembolic problems.

c. Increased risk of preeclampsia.

2. Infant.

a. SGA.

b. Spontaneous abortion.

c. Fetal distress due to hypoxia.

G. Multiple body systems are involved.

Assessment

1. Risk factors/etiology.

a. Autosomal recessive disorder (See Chapter 24).

(1) Presence of HgbS indicates active sickle cell disease.

(2) Presence of HgbAS indicates sickle cell trait.

b. Predominantly in the black population.

c. People with sickle cell trait have the same basic defect, but only 35-45% of total hemoglobin is HgbS.

2. Clinical manifestations—primarily the result of obstruction cause by the sickled RBC's and by the increased RBC destruction.
   a. Splenomegaly—caused by congestion and engorgement with sickled cells, decreases immune response.
   b. Liver failure, hepatomegaly, and necrosis from severe impairment of hepatic blood flow.
   c. Kidney damage caused by the congestion of glomerular capillaries and tubular arterioles.
   d. Skeletal changes caused by hyperplasia and congestion of bone marrow.
3. Crisis—often precipitated by an infection, or can occur spontaneously.
   a. Vaso-occlusive crisis—severe bone pain, acute abdominal pain, priapism, and arthralgia.
      (1) Hand-foot syndrome—occlusions in the small distal bones of the hands and the feet, characterized by pain and swelling.
      (2) Liver infarctions will affect metabolism; client may be jaundiced.
      (3) CNS occlusions that alter sensorium and coordination; may produce paralysis if occlusion is large enough.
   b. Splenic sequestration crisis.
      (1) Pooling of large amounts of blood in the spleen and liver.
      (2) May develop circulatory shock.

NCLEX ALERT: *Recognize occurrence of a hemorrhage - bleeding in this client would present different symptoms than bleeding in a surgical client.*

   c. Aplastic crisis—a severe anemia develops because of the decreased production of RBC's.
   d. Chest syndrome—very similar to pneumonia.
   e. Stroke—may occur suddenly with no warning, results in cerebral infarction.
4. Diagnostics (See Appendix 14-1)—early diagnoses, prior to 3 months assists to minimize complications.
   a. Hemoglobin electrophoresis indicates the presence and percentage of Hemoglobin S.
   b. Sickle-turbidity tests (Sickledex).

Treatment

1. Prevention of the sickling problem.
   a. Adequate hydration.
   b. Prevent infections, especially respiratory.
   c. No specific medication; clients generally do not require iron, due to increased resorption.
   d. Daily folic acid supplement when red blood cells are low.
2. Treatment of crisis.
   a. Bed rest.
   b. Hydration.
   c. Analgesic for pain.
   d. Antibiotics.
   e. Promote adequate oxygenation.
   f. Blood transfusions (Appendix 14-3).
3. Surgery - splenectomy for severe splenic sequestration.

Nursing Intervention

✦ *Goal: to prevent sickle cell disease.*
1. Participate in community screening programs and education.
2. Refer persons who are trait carriers to genetic counseling (autosomal recessive) (Figure 24-1).

✦ *Goal: to prevent sickling crisis.*
1. Maintain adequate hydration, IV fluids may be necessary.
2. Promote tissue oxygenation.
3. Prevent infection.

✦ *Goal: to control pain.*
1. Assessment of involved area.
2. Appropriate analgesics—meperidine (**Demerol**) is not recommended, morphine, hydromorphone, methadone may be used, PCA's are frequently used to control pain.
3. Position for comfort.
4. Maintain bed rest.

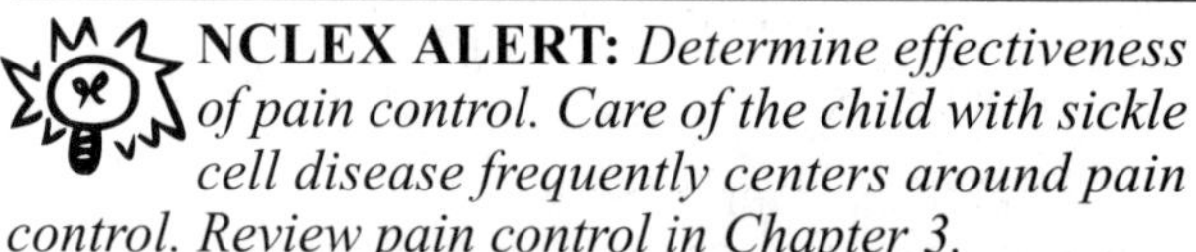

NCLEX ALERT: *Determine effectiveness of pain control. Care of the child with sickle cell disease frequently centers around pain control. Review pain control in Chapter 3.*

✦ *Goal: to maintain adequate hydration and oxygenation.*
1. Evaluate adequacy of hydration.
2. Low specific gravity may not be indicative of fluid balance if there is renal involvement.
3. Monitor IV fluid carefully, accurate I&O.
4. Evaluate electrolyte balance.
5. Administer O_2 as indicated.
6. Good pulmonary hygiene.

7. Assess for acidosis.

✦ *Goal: to identify complication of affected organs - systematic evaluation of client to identify problems discussed in clinical manifestations.*

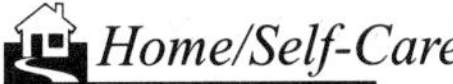

Home/Self-Care

1. Increase fluids with physical activity.
2. Report temperature elevations, vomiting, diarrhea, pain.
3. Encourage normal growth and developmental activities as tolerated by the child.
4. Client with sickle cell disease should avoid situations which may precipitate hypoxia.
   a. Traveling to high-altitude areas.
   b. Flying in an unpressurized aircraft.
   c. Participating in strenuous exercise.
5. Inform all significant health personnel, child should wear medical identification.

NCLEX ALERT: *Compare physical development of client to normal. Chronically ill children frequently are slower in growth and development, care is provided for the developmental level not the chronological age.*

Polycythemia Vera (Primary)

❑ **This blood disorder is characterized by a proliferation of all red marrow cells.**

Assessment

1. Risk factors—usually develops in middle ages.
2. Diagnostics.
   a. Increased erythrocytes.
   b. Increased leukocytes in the bone marrow.
   c. Excessive production of platelets.
3. Clinical manifestations.
   a. Ruddy complexion.
   b. Headaches.
   c. Hepatosplenomegaly.
   d. Problems of decreased blood flow.
      (1) Angina.
      (2) Claudication (pain in muscles during activity).
      (3) Thrombophlebitis.

Treatment

1. Phlebotomy.
2. Decreased iron intake.

Table 14-2: BLEEDING PRECAUTIONS

Clients diagnosed with leukemia, hemophilia, or any condition that causes bleeding, clients who are receiving anticoagulants or thrombolytic medications.

Limit number of venipunctures and IM injections.Guaiac stools as necessary.

✦ Oral hygiene -
  —discourage flossing
  —soft toothbrush or no toothbrush, may need to use Q-tips while gums are friable.
  —avoid harsh mouthwashes.
  —frequent mouth rinse with mild mouthwash.

✦ Electric razor for shaving.

✦ Assess perianal area for fissures and bleeding.

✦ Discourage client from blowing his nose.

✦ Avoid aspirin products, evaluate NSAIDs for bleeding properties.

✦ Avoid catheters when possible - urinary and suctioning.

✦ Avoid overinflation of blood pressure cuff or leaving cuff inflated for prolonged period of time.

✦ Provide safe environment and prevent injury according to age (pad siderails, soft toys, house shoes, etc).

✦ Monitor for bleeding episode - nosebleed, hematuria, increased bruising.

Nursing Intervention

✦ *Goal: to assist client in understanding dietary implications.*

✦ *Goal: to help client understand implications of the disease in long-term health care.*

Leukemia

❑ **Leukemia is an uncontrolled proliferation of abnormal white cells; eventual cellular destruction occurs, due to the infiltration of the leukemic cells into the body tissue.**

A. High vascular organs of the reticuloendothelial system (RES) are primarily affected; spleen, liver, and lymph show marked infiltration, enlargement, and eventually fibrosis.

B. Invasion of the bone marrow by the leukemic cells precipitates pathologic fractures.

C. Three primary consequences of leukemia.
   1. Anemia from red cell destruction and bleeding.
   2. Infection secondary to neutropenia.
   3. Bleeding tendencies, due to decreased platelets.

D. Types of leukemia.
   1. Acute lymphocytic leukemia (ALL, blast or stem cell).
      a. Peak occurrences around four years of age, then again around 65 years.
      b. Favorable prognosis with chemotherapy.
      c. Leukemic cells will infiltrate the meninges, precipitating increased intracranial pressure.

d. Onset may be acute to insidious.

2. Chronic myelogenous leukemia (CML).
   a. Uncommon before age 20.
   b. Onset is generally slow.
   c. Symptoms are less severe than acute stages of disease.
3. Acute non-lymphocytic leukemia (ANLL) (previously known as acute myelogenous leukemia AML) and chronic lymphocytic leukemia (CLL) are less common.

Assessment

1. Clinical manifestations.
   a. Anemia, infection and bleeding tendencies occurring together.
   b. Anorexia, weight loss.
   c. Fatigue, lethargy.
   d. Headache, confusion.
   e. Petechiae, bruises easily.
   f. Complaints of bone and joint pain.
   g. Hepatomegaly and splenomegaly.
2. Diagnostics (See Appendix 14-1).
   a. Complete blood count.
      (1) Anemia.
      (2) Thrombocytopenia.
      (3) Increased numbers of immature white cells.
   b. Bone marrow aspiration—increased numbers of blast (immature) cells.
   c. Lumbar puncture to identify presence of leukemic cells in spinal fluid.
   d. Studies to evaluate liver and renal function; most chemotherapy agents are detoxified in the liver and excreted by way of the renal system; these systems need to be evaluated prior to beginning chemotherapy.

Treatment

1. Medications.
   a. Corticosteroids.
   b. Antineoplastic agents (See Appendix 8-1).
   c. Xanthine-oxidase inhibitor — allopurinol (**Zyloprim**) decreases uric acid levels in clients on chemotherapy.
   d. Chemotherapy usually involves an induction phase, consolidation phase, and a maintenance phase.
   e. A combination of chemotherapy agents are used initially to promote a remission.
   f. Majority of children will go into remission during the induction phase.
2. Bone marrow transplant (Appendix 14-4).
3. Radiation therapy.
4. A remission is characterized by absence of leukemia cells and disorders, and disappearance of all disease symptoms.

Nursing Intervention (see Chapter 8)

✦ *Goal: to prevent infection.*

1. Systematically assess for evidence of infection—fever, inflammation, pain.
2. Monitor temperature elevation closely—notify doctor for increase over 100.5° F (38°C).
3. Meticulous skin care, especially oral hygiene and around perianal area.
4. Protect client from exposure to infection; degree of restriction depends on immunosuppression.
5. Isolate child from communicable childhood diseases, especially chicken pox.
6. Polio, varicella, and MMR are not given to children during immunosuppression.
7. Avoid urinary catheterization if possible.
8. Encourage adequate protein and calorie intake, low bacteria diet.
9. Maintain adequate hydration.

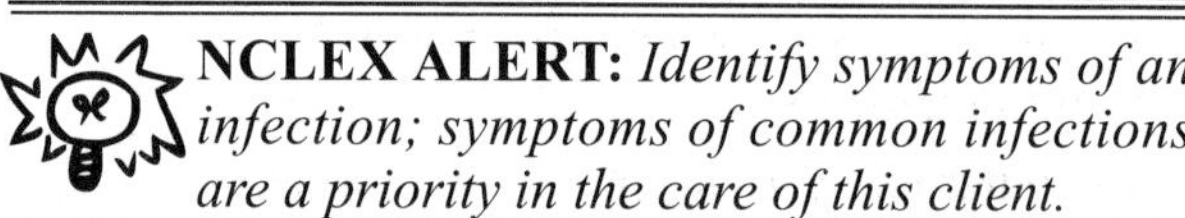

NCLEX ALERT: *Identify symptoms of an infection; symptoms of common infections are a priority in the care of this client.*

✦ *Goal: to prevent or limit bleeding episodes.(Table 14-2).*

1. Use local measures to control bleeding.
2. Restrict strenuous activity.
3. Involve client in evaluating level of activity; decrease activity when platelet counts are low.
4. Avoid IM injections.
5. Soft toothbrush or toothettes for oral hygiene.
6. Evaluate for hematuria.
7. No aspirin compounds.

✦ *Goal: to prevent renal complications secondary to chemotherapy.*

1. Maintain adequate hydration to flush the chemicals from the kidney.
2. Monitor levels of uricemia.
3. Monitor renal function before and during treatment.

✦ *Goal: to provide pain relief.*

1. Use acetaminophen rather than aspirin.
2. Maintain environment conducive to rest.
3. Position carefully; may coordinate with analgesics.

4. Evaluate effectiveness of pain relief; administer analgesic prior to pain becoming severe.

✦ *Goal: to decrease effects of chemotherapy and radiation therapy (Chapter 8).*

✦ *Goal: to prevent complications of transfusions (Appendix 14-3).*

✦ *Goal: to demonstrate an understanding of the disease, and its prognosis, and display an ability to cope with the diagnosis.*

1. Assist client and family to maintain realistic expectations.
2. Be honest in discussion of the outcome of possible side effects of anticipated therapy.
3. Provide emotional support and encourage ventilation of feelings.

NCLEX ALERT: *Care of client receiving chemotherapy, blood transfusions, client and family teaching, and pain relief are all components of the exam.*

Self/Home Care

1. No aspirin compound.
2. Monitor weight gain or loss.
3. Counseling to determine effect of child's illness on family members.
4. Encourage family involvement in client's care.
5. Discourage pets, such as fish, birds and cats, due to bacteria and virus transmission.
6. Teach family methods to stop bleeding.
7. Assist parents to prepare for child's return to school.
8. Teach the importance of good hand washing.
9. Teach family members early signs of infection and importance of reporting them as soon as observed.

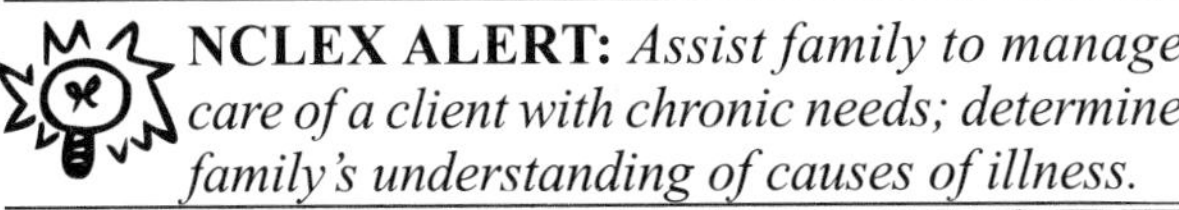
NCLEX ALERT: *Assist family to manage care of a client with chronic needs; determine family's understanding of causes of illness.*

Hodgkin's Disease

❑ **Characterized by painless enlargement of lymph nodes with progression to involve the liver and spleen.**

A. Common metastatic sites are the spleen, liver, bone marrow, and lungs.

B. Staging of Hodgkin's disease

1. Stage I: Lesions limited to one lymph node or to one extralymphatic site.
2. Stage II: Involves two or more nodes on same side of the diaphragm; may involve one extralymphatic site on the same side.
3. Stage III: Lymph nodes on both sides of the diaphragm are involved; may have spleen involvement and another extralymphatic site.
4. Stage IV: Diffuse involvement of extralymphatic organs.

Assessment

1. Risk factors/etiology.
   a. Unknown etiology.
   b. Increased incidence in young adults.
   c. History of immunosuppression.
2. Clinical manifestations.
   a. Initially, painless enlargement of the lymph node on one side of the neck.
   b. Mediastinal lymph node enlargement causing pressure on.
      (1) Trachea—dyspnea.
      (2) Esophagus—dysphagia.
      (3) Veins—edema of upper extremities.
      (4) Nerves—laryngeal edema.
   c. Obstruction of bile ducts.
   d. Hepatomegaly, splenomegaly.
   e. Low-grade fever, night sweats.
   f. Weight loss.
   g. Renal failure secondary to urethral obstruction.
   h. Severe pruritus.
3. Diagnostics.
   a. Lymph node biopsy—presence of Reed-Sternberg cells.
   b. Exploratory laparotomy for staging purposes.

Treatment

1. Radiation and supplemental chemotherapy.
2. Chemotherapy.
   a. Induction - achieves initial remission.
   b. Intensification or consolidation therapy - further decreases the malignancy.
   c. Central nervous system prophylactic therapy - prevents leukemic cells from invading the CNS.
   d. Maintenance - maintains the remission phase.

Nursing Intervention

✦ *Goal: to maintain physiological equilibrium.*

1. Maintain hydration and nutrition.
2. Maintain good pulmonary hygiene.

3. Evaluate for shortness of breath, maintain in semi-Fowler's position.
4. Decrease body needs for oxygen.
5. Assess ability of cardiovascular system to maintain cardiac output.

✦ *Goal: to prevent infection (See Goal to prevent infection, Leukemia).*

✦ *Goal: to decrease side effects of chemotherapy and radiation therapy (See Chapter 8).*

✦ *Goal: to assist client to understand implications of the disease, its prognosis, and display ability to cope with diagnosis (See Goal to help client and parents demonstrate an understanding of the disease, Leukemia).*

Multiple Myeloma

❑ **This disorder is a malignancy of plasma cells, with infiltration into bones and soft tissues. The client may be totally incapacitated, due to severe pain.**

Assessment

1. Clinical manifestations.
   a. Back pain, bone pain.
   b. Pathologic fractures.
   c. Hypercalcemia
2. Diagnostics.
   a. Bone marrow biopsy (See Appendix 14-1).
   b. X-ray showing typical punched-out appearance of the bones from demineralization.

Treatment

1. Chemotherapy and palliative radiation therapy.
2. Glucocorticoids, calcitonin to decrease hypercalcemia and reduce bone destruction.

Nursing Intervention

✦ *Goal: to maintain physical equilibrium.*

1. Careful ambulation to decrease hypercalcemia and improve pulmonary status.
2. Adequate hydration to prevent calcium from precipitating in the kidneys, carefully monitor hydration status.
3. Comfort measures and analgesics for pain.
4. Safety measures to prevent pathologic fractures.

✦ *Goal: to assist client to understand implications of the disease and measures to maintain health (See related Goal, Leukemia).*

DISORDERS OF COAGULATION

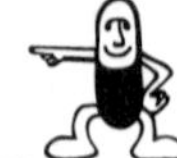

Hemophilia

❑ **Hemophilia is a defect in the clotting mechanism. Classically, there are two types, distinguishable only by lab tests. Clinically, the two types are the same, but both may occur in varying degrees of severity. The disease is generally recognized during the toddler stage.**

A. Hemophilia A—Factor VIII deficiency (factor VIII concentrate).

B. Hemophilia B—Factor IX deficiency (Christmas factor).

Assessment

1. Risk factors/etiology—both are sex-linked traits.
   a. Primarily affects males.
   b. Females are carriers.
2. Clinical manifestations.
   a. Excessive bleeding from an injury—bleeding may not be obvious initially.
   b. Spontaneous bleeding into joints.
   c. Hematuria.
   d. Recurring joint bleeding leads to severe restriction of joint mobility.
   e. Intracranial hemorrhage may be fatal.
   f. Hemorrhage into the gastrointestinal tract.
   g. Petechiae are uncommon, since platelet count is normal.
3. Diagnostics.
   a. History of bleeding episodes.
   b. Family inheritance pattern.
   c. Identification of deficient factor.

Treatment

1. Fresh frozen plasma.
2. IV administration of deficient factor.
   a. Factor VIII concentrate—must be reconstituted with sterile water immediately prior to administration.
   b. DDAVP - synthetic vasopressin used to treat mild cases.
3. Treatment may be carried out at home.

Nursing Intervention

✦ *Goal: to prevent spontaneous bleeding episodes.*

1. Decrease risk of injury.
   a. Make environment as safe as possible without hampering motor development.
   b. Avoid contact sports.

c. Regular exercise and physical therapy to promote muscle strength around joints and decrease bleeding episodes.
2. Good dental care, especially when deciduous teeth become loose.
3. Maintain normal weight; increased weight causes increased strain on the joints.
4. Avoid any aspirin compounds.
5. Administer clotting factors prior to invasive medical procedures.

✦ *Goal: to recognize and treat bleeding episodes.*
1. Apply pressure to the area.
2. Immobilize and elevate the joints involved.
3. Apply cold pack to promote vasoconstriction.
4. Observe for internal bleeding—tarry stools, slurred speech, headache.

✦ *Goal: to prepare client and family to administer clotting factors IV at home.*
1. Correct technique for venipuncture.
2. Indications for utilization.
3. Encourage child to learn self-administration, generally around age 9 to 12.

✦ *Goal: to prevent permanent joint degeneration.*
1. Elevate joint and immobilize during acute bleeding.
2. Initiate passive range of motion after acute phase.
3. Physical therapy after the acute phase.
4. Maintain pain relief during physical therapy.

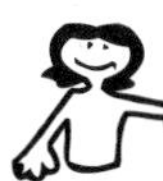
***NURSING PRIORITY:** RICE the affected joints—rest, ice, compression, elevation.*

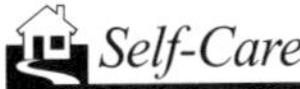
Self-Care
1. Have client and family demonstrate ability to perform IV puncture.
2. Have client and family discuss situations for utilization of IV infusion of deficient factor - endoscopy, dental work , etc.
3. Have family member demonstrate the ability to carry out range of motion on affected joints.
4. Discuss with family importance of routine prophylactic dental checkups.
5. Encourage ventilation of feelings regarding diagnosis of the disease.
6. Encourage counseling for parents regarding concern and guilt over hereditary disorder.

NCLEX ALERT: *Determine family's understanding of the causes/consequences of client's illness.*

Disseminated Intravascular Coagulation (DIC)

❑ **This is a secondary coagulation disorder involving widespread clotting in the small vessels, leading to consumption of clotting factors, thereby precipitating a bleeding disorder.**

Assessment
1. Risk factors/etiology
   a. Increase in release of coagulation factors into circulation - hemolytic processes, extensive tissue damage.
   b. Damage to the vascular endothelium.
   c. Stagnant blood flow - shock.
   d. Infection - sepsis.
   e. Obstetrical complications. - hemorrhage.
2. Clinical manifestations.
   a. Petechiae, ecchymoses on skin and mucous membrane.
   b. Prolonged bleeding from multiple body areas.
   c. Hypotension.
   d. Dysfunction of organs due to infarction.
3. Diagnostics (See Appendix 14-1).
   a. Low fibrin levels.
   b. Prolonged prothrombin time.
   c. Severe thrombocytopenia.
   d. Ineffective clotting of the blood.

Treatment
1. Correction of the underlying problem.
2. Platelets, fresh frozen plasma transfusions.
3. Heparin.
4. Treatment of shock if indicated.

Nursing Intervention
✦ *Goal: to identify the problem early and to decrease potential effects.*
1. Thorough assessment of bleeding problems in clients severely compromised by other problems.
2. Nursing measures to prevent bleeding episodes.
3. Assess and support all vital systems.

✦ *Goal: to assist client's family to understand implications of the disease and demonstrate appropriate coping behaviors.*
1. Provide emotional support and encourage visiting as intensive care policies and patient condition allow.
2. Encourage ventilation of feelings regarding critical illness of family member.
3. Be available to family members during visiting time.⌘

Study Questions—Hematological System

1. A client and her husband are positive for the positive sickle cell trait. The client asks the nurse about the chances of her children having the sickle cell disease. The nurse understands this genetic problem will reflect what pattern in the client's children?

① One of her children will have sickle cell disease.
② Only the male children will be affected.
③ Each pregnancy carriers a 25% chance of the child being affected.
④ If she had four children, one of them will have the disease.

2. The nurse is performing a well baby checkup on a 12 month old infant. What finding would be of most concern?

① He cannot walk yet.
② Takes a longer afternoon nap.
③ Has increased bruising.
④ Doesn't eat as much as he used to.

3. A client is experiencing a sickle cell crisis during labor and delivery, what is the best nursing action?

① Maintain IV fluid infusion and assess adequacy of hydration.
② Administer high concentration of oxygen.
③ Insert a Foley catheter and monitor hourly urine output.
④ Provide continuous sedation for pain relief.

4. The nurse identifies which problem as most likely to lead to a sickle cell crisis?

① Slight weight loss.
② Fatigue after mild exercise.
③ Perspiring in a warm room.
④ Recurrence of respiratory infection.

5. What does the pathophysiology of sickle cell crisis involve?

① Altered metabolism and dehydration.
② Tissue hypoxia and vascular occlusion.
③ Increased bilirubin levels and hypertension.
④ Decreased clotting factors and white cells increase.

6. A 25 year old female comes to the clinic complaining of dizziness, weakness, and palpitations. What will be important for the nurse to initially evaluate when obtaining the health history?

① Activity and exercise patterns.
② Nutritional patterns.
③ Family health status.
④ Coping and stress tolerance.

7. An child with leukemia is being discharged after beginning chemotherapy. What instructions will the nurse provide the parents of this child?

① Provide a diet low in protein and high in carbohydrates.
② Avoid fresh vegetables that are not cooked or peeled.
③ Notify the doctor if the child's temperature exceeds 101° F (39°C).
④ Increase the use of humidifiers throughout the house.

8. Which client is most likely to develop iron deficiency anemia?

① A cancer client on radiation therapy twice a week.
② A toddler whose primary nutritional intake is milk.
③ A peptic ulcer client who is 6 weeks postoperative.
④ A 15-year-old client in sickle crisis.

9. A hemophiliac client comes to the ER after bumping his knee, the knee is rapidly swelling. What is the first nursing action?

① Administer cryoprecipitate.
② Type and cross match for transfusion.
③ Have hemoglobin and hematocrit drawn for comparison.
④ Apply ice pack and compression dressings to the knee.

10. A client has an order for one unit of whole blood. What is a correct nursing action?

① Initiate the IV with D5W to maintain a patent access.

② Initiate the transfusion within 30 minutes of receiving the blood.

③ Monitor the client's vital signs for the first five minutes.

④ Monitor vital signs every 2 hours during the transfusion.

11. The nurse is caring for a client who is receiving a blood transfusion. The transfusion was started 30 minutes ago at 100cc per hour. The client begins to complain of low back pain, headache, and is increasingly restless. What is the first nursing action?

① Slow the infusion and evaluate the vital signs and client's history of transfusion reactions.

② Stop the transfusion, disconnect the blood tubing and begin a primary infusion of normal saline.

③ Stop the infusion of blood, begin the normal saline infusion from the Y connector.

④ Recheck the unit of blood for correct identification numbers and cross match information.

Answers and rationales to these questions are in the section at the end of the book entitled "Chapter Study Questions: Answers & Rationales."

Appendix 14-1: HEMATOLOGIC DIAGNOSTICS

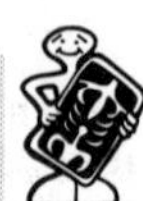

TEST	NORMAL	CLINICAL AND NURSING IMPLICATIONS
Bone Marrow Aspiration or Biopsy	All formed cell elements within normal range (erythrocytes, leukocytes, and platelets).	1. Evaluates presence, absence, or ratio of cells characteristic of a suspected disease. 2. Preferable site is posterior iliac crest. 3. Client preparation: a. local anesthetic used as well as analgesics. b. feeling of pressure when bone marrow is entered; pain occurs as marrow is being withdrawn. 4. Post test: a. observe for bleeding at site. b. apply pressure to site. c. bed rest for approximately 30 minutes afterward. d. analgesics as indicated.
Sickle Cell Test (Sickledex)	No hemoglobin S present.	1. Routine screening test for sickle cell trait or disorder; does not distinguish between them. 2. False negative in infants under 3 months. 3. False positive can occur for up to four months after a transfusion of red cells that are positive for the trait.
Hemoglobin Electrophoresis	Separates various hemoglobins and allows for identification of specific problem.	1. Differentiates between trait or disorder in sickle cell anemia. 2. Diagnosis of thalassemia and hemolytic anemia.
Activated Partial Thromboplastin Time (aPTT)	Normal 30-45 seconds.	1. Sensitive in monitoring heparin; draw 1 hour prior to next heparin dose. 2. May be used to detect circulating anticoagulants.
Prothrombin Time (PT)	10 to 13 seconds or 100 % (each client will have a control value).	1. Production of prothrombin depends on adequate intake and utilization of vitamin K. 2. Used in management of **Coumadin** therapy.
Fibrin Split Products	Increased destruction in DIC	1. Fibrinolysis occurs in intravascular coagulation. 2. Abnormally high levels in DIC.
Schilling Test	Normal excretion is 10-40% of oral dose of the radioactive B_{12}.	1. Stage 1 is a 24-hour urine test after a dose of radio labeled B_{12}. 2. Stage 2 is a second 24-hour urine to determine response to intrinsic factor; distinguishes between pernicious anemia and malabsorption.

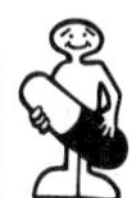

Appendix 14-2: HEMATOLOGIC MEDICATIONS

MEDICATIONS	SIDE EFFECTS	NURSING IMPLICATIONS
IRON PREPARATIONS: Replacement		
Ferrous fumarate **(Feostat, Span 77, Femiron)**: IM, PO Ferrous gluconate **(Fergon, Ferralet)** PO Ferrous sulfate **(Feosol, Fer-In-Sol)** PO **Iron dextran injection (Imferon)**: IV, IM	GI irritation Nausea Constipation Toxic reactions: Fever Urticaria	1. Absorbed better on empty stomach; however, may give with meals if GI upset occurs. 2. Liquid preparations should be diluted and given through a straw to prevent staining of the teeth. 3. Tell client stool may be black. 4. If given IM, use Z- track method to prevent tissue staining and trauma. 5. Eggs, milk, cheese and antacids inhibit oral iron absorption. 6. IM iron preparations are not recommended. 7. Inhibit tetracycline absorption.
VITAMIN K: Necessary for normal prothrombin activity		
Vitamin K (**Aquamephyton**): PO, SQ, IM, IV	GI upset, rash Hypersensitivity reaction if given IV: rash, urticaria	1. Pain, hematoma formation at injection site. 2. Antidote for **Coumadin**. 3. Observe bleeding precautions.

Appendix 14-3: BLOOD TRANSFUSIONS

BLOOD COMPONENTS FOR TRANSFUSIONS

Component	Purpose Of Administration	Charting
PACKED RED CELLS	Increases oxygen carrying capacity. Decreases risk of incompatible antibodies from the plasma.	1. Type and amount of blood product infused. 2. Vital signs immediately prior to infusion, at 5 minutes and 15 minutes into transfusion, every hour during transfusion, and at completion of transfusion. 3. Time started and time completed. 4. Rate of infusion. 5. Blood unit identification number. 6. Client observations during the transfusion.
PLATELETS	Given to clients with thrombocytopenia.	
FRESH FROZEN PLASMA	Administered for clotting factors, proteins, fluid volume.	

NCLEX ALERT: *Administer blood or blood products.*

NURSING GUIDELINES FOR BLOOD TRANSFUSIONS

1. Informed consent and alternatives should be explained to the client. Autologous, (using client's own blood), and designated donors are options. If client is unable to give consent, then consent should be obtained from family.

2. Obtain the type and crossmatch records and the unit of blood to administer. Check:
   a. The ABO group on the unit against the crossmatch records.
   b. The Rh type of the blood against the crossmatch record.
   c. Have two RNs independently or one RN and a physician check the records, and sign that they have checked.
   d. Check the client's name and hospital number on the unit of blood and on the crossmatch records.
   e. If any of the above do not match - DO NOT GIVE THE BLOOD.
   f. Check the expiration date on the unit of blood.

3. Administer the blood immediately after receiving it from the blood bank; blood should NEVER be stored in a unit refrigerator or allowed to sit out at room temperature. The maximum amount of time out of monitored storage is 30 minutes.

4. Do not add any medications to blood products.

5. Do not warm blood prior to transfusion, unless there are several units to be infused rapidly and client is in danger of developing a hypothermic response. If blood must be warmed, equipment specifically designed for the procedure must be used.

6. Inspect the blood bag for leaks, abnormal color, excessive air or bubbles.

7. DO NOT use a microwave to warm the blood.

Box 14-2: Elderly Care Focus:
Blood Transfusion

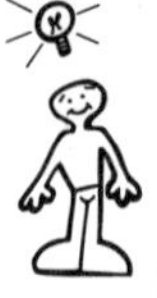

- Obtain baseline renal, hydration and circulatory status prior to initiating the transfusion.
- Monitor vital signs more frequently during administration phase.
- Try to use a 19 gauge needle.
- Administer blood over ordered time, closely monitor client at increased risk for volume overload.
- Symptoms of overload: rapid, bounding pulse; increased blood pressure; distended peripheral veins; dyspnea; moist crackles in the lungs.

Appendix 14-3:
BLOOD TRANSFUSIONS

8. The usual rate of transfusion in an adult is 1 unit of blood over about 3 to 4 hours, depending on the condition of the client.

9. The blood administration set should be changed every 4-6 hours to reduce the risk of septicemia.

10. It is not recommended to use an infusion pump to administer red blood cells. The pump causes red cell hemolysis.

***NURSING PRIORITY**: The majority of major adverse transfusion reactions are due to improper identification of the blood product and the recipient.*

Key Points: Guidelines For Performance Phase Of Transfusion

- Check the doctor's order, check the labels on the blood bag with the client identification at the bedside.
- Baseline vital signs must be obtained prior to hanging the blood; if the client has a temperature above 101°, advise the physician prior to starting the transfusion.
- Initiate the infusion with an #18 or #20 gauge needle and begin infusing normal saline.
- Do NOT use D_5W to initiate the transfusion; it causes the blood to hemolyze and precipitate.
- Always use a standard blood administration set with a filter; DO NOT use straight IV tubing.
- Initiate infusion (rate of approximately 100 cc per hour) and remain with the client, the first 10-15 minutes is the most critical time; the majority of transfusion reactions occur with in the first 50cc.
- During the transfusion, continue to monitor for circulatory overload or transfusion reaction.
- Blood deteriorates rapidly after about two hours or exposure to room temperature; a unit of blood should not hang longer than 4 hours.
- Components that contain few red cells may be administered rapidly.

TRANSFUSION REACTIONS	NURSING MANAGEMENT
Hemolytic Transfusion Reaction: 1. Low back pain, kidney region. 2. Hypotension, tachycardia. 3. Apprehension, sense of impending doom 4. Fever, chills, flushing. 5. Chest pain. 6. Headache. 7. Immediate onset. 8. Dyspnea.	1. Stop transfusion immediately and notify physician. 2. Change the IV tubing; do not allow blood in the tubing to infuse into the client, maintain IV access. 3. Obtain first voided urine specimen to test for blood in the urine. 4. Anticipate blood samples to be drawn by the lab. 5. With suspected renal involvement, treatment with diuretics is initiated to promote diuresis.
Allergic Reaction: 1. Urticaria (hives). 2. Pruritus. 3. Facial flushing. 4. Severe-shortness of breath, bronchospasm.	1. If client has a history of allergic reactions, **Benadryl** (PO or IM) may be given prior to starting the infusion. 2. Stop transfusion until status of reaction may be determined, if symptoms are mild and transient, the transfusion may be resumed.
Febrile Reaction: 1. Chills and fever. 2. Headache, flushing. 3. Nausea and vomiting. 4. Increased anxiety.	1. Keep client covered and warm during transfusion. 2. Administer antipyretic medication to persons known to have this reaction. 3. Transfusion with leukocyte-poor red blood cells or frozen washed packed cells may prevent this reaction in persons susceptible to fever.

Appendix 14-4: BONE MARROW TRANSPLANT

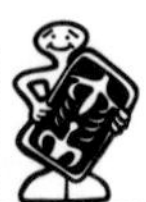

✦ *GOAL: To restore hematological and immunological function in clients with immunological deficiencies, leukemia, congenital or acquired anemias.*

PROCEDURE: In the adult client, approximately 400-800 cc of bone marrow may be aspirated from the donor's iliac crest; marrow is then processed and transfused into the recipient.

INDICATIONS:

1. Leukemia clients who have experienced relapse after aggressive chemotherapy.
2. Aplastic anemia clients, especially those who have not been sensitized by previous blood transfusions.
3. Thalassemia, especially beta thalassemia, when client does not respond to conventional therapy.
4. In infants with severe combined immunodeficiency.

COMPLICATIONS:

1. Infection from immunosuppressed state.
2. Severe thrombocytopenia resulting in bleeding problems.
3. Graft-versus-host disease (GVHD, rejection).
   a. Acute rejection generally occurs in 7-30 days post-transplant, chronic in 100 days.
   b. Maculopapular rash on the palms and feet, spreading to rest of body, may be an early symptom.
   c. Altered liver enzyme profiles with liver tenderness and jaundice.
   d. GI disturbances -nausea, vomiting, diarrhea.

STAGES:

1. Typing:
   a. Allogenic - matching of a histocompatible donor, preferably a relative.
   b. Autologous - utilizes client's own bone marrow collected from disease-free tissue and frozen.
   c. Syngeneic -donors are identical twins with perfect tissue match.
2. Immunoablative preparation - chemotherapy and radiation to produce immunologically suppressed state prior to marrow transfusion.
3. Complications posttransplant -graft versus host disease (GVHD).
   a. Most often occurs within 7-30 days.
   b. Stage I occurs in majority of allogenic transplants: intestine-mild gastrointestinal upset; skin-maculopapular rash over less than 25% of the body; mild to moderate liver dysfunction.
   c. Stage II and III are characterized by increasing problems of skin, intestine and liver.

NURSING IMPLICATIONS:

1. Preparation of the client for immunosupression with chemo-and radiation therapy.
2. Confirmation of rejection is by skin or oral mucosal biopsy.
3. Successful engraftment is indicated by formation of erythrocytes, leukocytes, and platelets, usually 2 to 5 weeks post-transplant.
4. Care of the immunosuppressed client (Chapter 7).

❑ The respiratory unit focuses on pathophysiologic conditions which interfere with gas exchange. When problems of gas exchange occur, regardless of the precipitating cause, a hypoxic state is frequently the result. A thorough understanding of hypoxia and appropriate nursing interventions for the hypoxic client are necessary for an understanding of the disease processes and ensuing nursing interventions.

PHYSIOLOGY OF THE RESPIRATORY SYSTEM

Organs of the Respiratory System

A. Bronchial tree.
   1. Trachea divides into the right and left main stem bronchi which extend into the lung.
   2. The right main stem bronchus is shorter and wider than the left; therefore, foreign objects are more likely to enter the right side.
   3. Secondary bronchi—branches from the primary bronchi.
   4. Terminal bronchioles—branches from the secondary bronchi.

B. Lungs (organs of respiration).
   1. Lungs are located within the thoracic cavity (Figure 15-1).
   2. Pleura—the transparent serous membrane around the lungs.
      a. Each lung is sealed within its own compartment by the pleura.
      b. Visceral pleura—adheres to the surface of the lung.
      c. Parietal pleura—covers the inner wall of the chest.
      d. Pleural cavity—potential space between the pleura membrane; normally pleural layers are in close contact.
   3. Lungs.
      a. Divided into lobes.
         (1) Right lung—three lobes.
         (2) Left lung—two lobes.
      b. Each terminal bronchus branches into respiratory bronchioles.
      c. The alveolar ducts are located at the end of the terminal respiratory bronchioles.
      d. Alveoli—area of gas exchange; diffusion of O_2 and CO_2 between the blood and the lungs occurs across the alveolar membrane.
      e. Surfactant is produced in the alveoli; primary function is to reduce surface tension, which facilitates alveolar expansion, and to prevent collapse.
   4. Premature infants frequently have inadequate production of surfactant.
   5. Blood supply to the lungs.
      a. Pulmonary arteries to pulmonary capillaries to alveoli, where exchange of gas occurs.
      b. Bronchial arteries supply the nutrients to the lung tissue and do not participate in gas exchange.

Physiology of Respiration

External respiration is a process by which gas is exchanged between the circulating blood and the inhaled air.

A. Atmospheric pressure—that pressure exerted on all body parts by surrounding air.

B. Intrapulmonic pressure—the pressure within the bronchial tree and alveoli.

C. Gases flow from an area of high pressure to an area of low pressure; pressure below atmospheric pressure is designated as negative pressure.

D. Inspiration.
   1. Stimulus to the diaphragm and the intercostal muscles by way of the CNS.
   2. Diaphragm moves down, intercostal muscles move outward, thereby increasing the capacity of the thoracic cavity and decreasing intrapulmonary pressure to below atmospheric pressure.
   3. Through the airways, the lungs are open to atmospheric pressure; air will flow into the lungs to equalize that of atmospheric pressure.

E. Expiration.
   1. Diaphragm and intercostal muscles relax and return to a resting position, therefore lungs recoil and capacity is decreased.
   2. Air will flow out until intrapulmonic pressure is again equal to atmospheric pressure.

F. Negative pressure is greater during inspiration, therefore air flows easily into the lungs.

G. Compliance describes how elastic or how easily the lungs can be inflated; when compliance is decreased, the lungs are more difficult to inflate.

H. Respiratory volumes.
   1. Tidal volume—amount of air moving in and out of the lungs in one normal breath.

Figure 15-1: Respiratory System
Reprinted with permission: Phipps, WJ, Sands, JK, & Marek, JF (1999). *Medical Surgical Nursing: Concepts & Clinical Practice*, 6th ed. Philadelphia: Mosby, p. 838

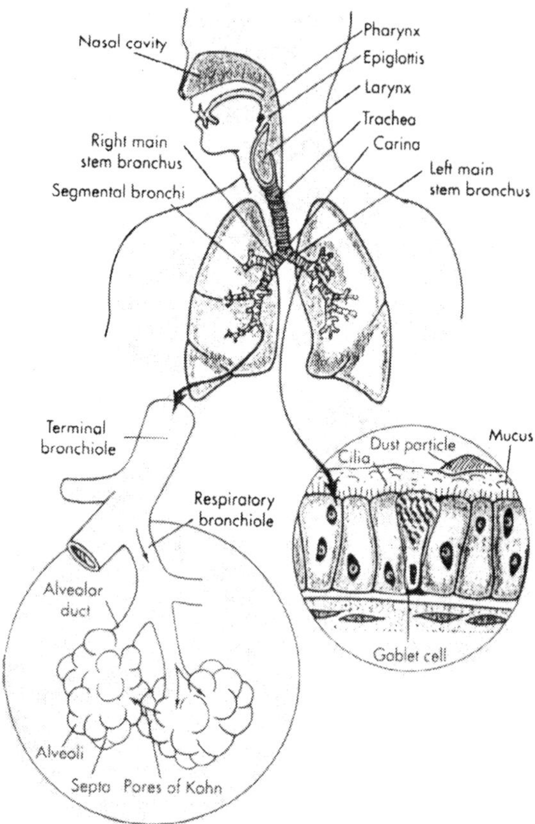

2. Vital capacity—amount of air inhaled and forcibly exhaled in one breath.
3. Residual volume—air remaining in the lungs at the end of a forced expiration.

I. Control of respiration.
   1. Movement of the diaphragm and accessory muscles of respiration is controlled by the respiratory center located in the brain stem (medulla and pons). The respiratory center will control respirations by way of the spinal cord. The diaphragm is innervated by the phrenic nerve, which comes from the spinal cord between C-3 and C-5; the intercostal muscles are innervated by nerves from the spinal cord between T-2 and T-11. Activity of the respiratory center is regulated by chemoreceptors. These receptors respond to a change in the chemical composition of the blood, especially blood gases and blood pH.
   2. The medulla contains chemoreceptors responsive to changes in CO_2 blood levels.
      a. CO_2 diffuses into cerebral spinal fluid (CSF), thus increasing hydrogen ion concentration of CSF, which has a direct stimulative effect on the chemoreceptors in the medulla.
      b. CO_2 saturation of the blood regulates ventilation through its effect on the pH of the CSF, and the effects of the CSF on the respiratory center in the medulla.

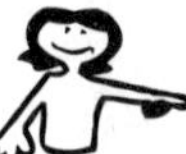

***NURSING PRIORITY:** The primary respiratory stimulus is CO_2; when the $PaCO_2$ is increased, ventilation is initiated.*

   3. Carotid and aortic bodies contain chemoreceptors for arterial O_2 levels.
      a. Primary function is to monitor arterial O_2 levels; maintain little control over normal ventilation.
      b. When arterial O_2 decreases to below 60 mm mercury pressure, stimulation to breathe is initiated by the chemoreceptors.
      c. In a person whose primary stimulus to breathe is hypoxia, this becomes the mechanism of ventilatory control.

J. The process of gas exchange.
   1. Ventilation - the process of moving air between the atmosphere and alveoli.
   2. Diffusion.
      a. The process of moving oxygen and carbon dioxide across the alveolar capillary membrane.
      b. Links the processes of ventilation and perfusion.
      c. Gas diffuses across the alveolar capillary membrane from an area of high concentration to an area of low concentration.
      d. Factors affecting diffusion: surface area of the lung, thickness of the alveolar capillary membrane, characteristics of the gases.

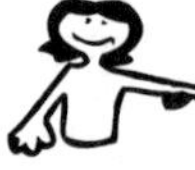

***NURSING PRIORITY:** When mucus is retained and pools in the lungs gas diffusion is affected.*

   3. Perfusion.
      a. The process of linking the blood system to the alveoli.
      b. Dependent on the volume of blood flowing through the pulmonary circulation.
   4. Transport.
      a. The process by which oxygen is delivered to the tissue by the circulatory system.
      b. Dependent upon the cardiac output.
      c. Oxygen is carried either chemically (bound to the hemoglobin) or physically (dissolved in plasma).

Oxygen and Carbon Dioxide Transport

Internal respiration is the exchange of gases between the blood and interstitial fluid. The gases are measured by an analysis of arterial blood (Table 15-1).

A. Oxygen.

1. Transported as a dissolved gas, PaO_2 refers to the partial pressure of the O_2 in arterial blood.
2. O_2 is primarily transported through the hemoglobin; when hemoglobin leaves the pulmonary capillary bed, it is usually 95 percent to 100 percent saturated with O_2. It may be referred to as the SaO_2
3. Oxygenated hemoglobin moves through the arterial system into the cellular capillary bed, where O_2 is released from the hemoglobin and made available for cellular metabolism.
4. Venous blood contains about 75 percent O_2 as it returns to the right heart.

B. Oxygen—hemoglobin dissociation.

1. Oxygen that remains bound to hemoglobin does not contribute to cellular metabolism.
2. Affinity of hemoglobin refers to the capacity of hemoglobin to bind to O_2.
3. The affinity of hemoglobin for O_2 is influenced by the pH.
   a. Hemoglobin binds tightly together with O_2 in an alkaline condition.
   b. Hemoglobin releases O_2 in an acid condition.
   c. As CO_2 moves into the serum at the capillary bed, it decreases the pH (acidotic), thereby enhancing O_2 release.
   d. As CO_2 moves out of the venous system into the lungs, the pH (alkalotic) is increased in the blood, thereby enhancing hemoglobin affinity for O_2.
4. If both the SaO_2 and the PaO_2 are decreased, the client in a state of hypoxemia.

C. Effects of altitude on oxygen transport.

1. At high levels (above 10,000 feet), there is reduced oxygen in the atmosphere.
2. Body compensatory mechanisms.
   a. Increase in the number of red cells or hematocrit from body storage areas, thereby increasing the total amount of hemoglobin- and oxygen-carrying capacity of the blood.
   b. Hyperventilation.
   c. Renal erythropoietic factor is released, thereby enhancing the production of red cells (secondary polycythemia). It takes approximately 4 to 5 days to actually increase red cell production.
3. Extended exposure to high altitudes will result in an increased vascularization of the lungs, thus increasing the capacity of the blood to carry oxygen.
4. Problem with oxygenation at high altitudes.

Table 15-1: NORMAL ARTERIAL BLOOD GAS VALUES

Acidity index	pH	7.35 - 7.45
Partial pressure of dissolved 0_2	PaO_2	80 to 100 mm Hg
Percentage of Hgb saturated with O_2	SaO_2	95 percent or above
Partial pressure of dissolved CO_2	$PaCO_2$	35 to 45 mm Hg
Bicarbonate	HCO_3	22 to 28 mEq/L

   a. Decrease in oxygen supply (loss of cardiac output or inadequate hemoglobin).
   b. Increase in body's demand.

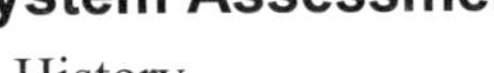

System Assessment

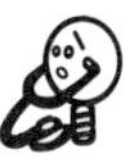

A. History.

1. History of childhood and adult illnesses.
2. Family history.
3. Status of immunizations.
   a. Tuberculin skin test.
   b. Pertussis.
   c. Polio.
4. Medication.
5. Occupational environment.
6. Habits.
   a. Smoking.
   b. Alcohol intake.

B. Physical Assessment.

NCLEX ALERT: *Determine changes in the client's respiratory status. The primary indicators of respiratory disorders are sputum production, cough, dyspnea, hemoptysis, chest pain and wheezing.*

1. Initially observe client's resting position.
   a. Appearance - comfortable or distressed?
   b. Assess client in the sitting position if possible.
   c. Any dyspnea or respiratory discomfort?
2. Evaluate vital signs (Table 15-2).
   a. Appropriate for age level?
   b. Establish data base and compare with previous data.
   c. Assess client's overall response.

(1) Normal vital signs vary greatly from one individual to another.

(2) A blood pressure of 90/60 may be normal for one person, but may be hypotensive for another person.

3. Assess upper airway passages and patency of the airway.
4. Inspect the neck for symmetry; check to see if the trachea is in midline and observe for jugular vein distention.
5. Assess the lungs.

a. Visually evaluate the thoracic cavity.

(1) Do both sides move equally?

(2) Observe characteristics of respirations and presence of retractions.

(3) Note chest wall configuration. (barrel chest, kyphoscoliosis, etc.).

b. Palpate chest for tenderness, masses, and symmetry of motion.

c. Auscultate breath sounds; begin at posterior base and compare each area side to side. Breath sounds should be present and equal bilaterally.

d. Determine presence of tactile fremitus - when client says "ninety-nine" there should be equal vibrations palpated bilaterally. Over areas of consolidation, there will be an increase in the vibrations.

e. Determine presence of adventitious breath sounds.

(1) Crackles - usually heard during inspiration and do not clear with cough, occurs when airway contain fluid (previously also known as "rales").

(2) Rhonchi - usually heard on expiration and may clear with cough, occurs as air moves through fluid filled passages.

(3) Wheezes - may be heard during inspiration and/or expiration, is caused by air moving through narrowed passages.

(4) Pleural friction rub - heard primarily on inspiration over an area of pleural inflammation, may be described as a grating sound.

NCLEX ALERT: *Identify changes in respiratory status - (Cheyne Stokes respirations, postoperative respiratory complications, abnormal lung sounds, etc)*

6. Assess cough reflex and sputum production.

a. Is cough associated with pain?

Table 15-2: NORMAL VITAL SIGNS

Neonate:	
Respiration	30 to 60
Pulse	110 to 160
Child 2 to 4 years:	
Respiration	24 to 32
Pulse	90 to 130
Child 6 to 10 years:	
Respiration	20 to 26
Pulse	100
Blood Pressure	80/40 to 110/80
Adult:	
Respiration	12 to 18
Pulse	60 to 100
Blood Pressure	90/60 to 140/90

NCLEX ALERT: *Know the range of normal for vital signs at different age levels. This is critical in identifying abnormals as well as being specific criteria for medication administration.*

b. What precipitates coughing episodes?

c. Is cough productive or nonproductive?

d. Characteristics of sputum.

(1) Consistency.

(2) Amount.

(3) Color (should be clear or white).

e. Presence of hemoptysis.

(1) Duration.

(2) Amount.

7. Assess for and evaluate dyspnea.

a. Onset of dyspnea.

b. Orthopnea.

c. Adventitious breath sounds.

d. Noisy expiration.

e. Level of tolerance of activity.

f. Correlate vital signs with dyspnea.

g. Cyanosis.

(1) Darkly pigmented clients, assess the areas that are less pigmented (oral cavity, nailbeds, lips, palms).

(2) Darkly pigmented clients may exhibit cyanosis as a gray hue to skin color rather than blue.

(3) Capillary refill time should be less than 3 seconds.

8. Assess for and evaluate chest pain.
   a. Location of pain.
   b. Character of pain.
   c. Pain associated with cough.
   d. Pain either increased or decreased with breathing.
9. Evaluate extremities for clubbing (characteristic in clients with chronic respiratory disorders).
10. Evaluate lab data. (See Appendix 15-1.)
   a. Hemoglobin and hematocrit (presence of polycythemia or anemia).
   b. Electrolyte imbalances.
   c. Arterial blood gases.

ACUTE RESPIRATORY DISORDERS

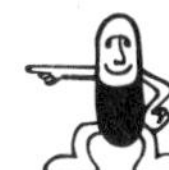

Hypoxia

❑ **Hypoxia is a condition characterized by an inadequate amount of oxygen available for cellular metabolism.**

NCLEX ALERT: *It is essential to know how to care for the client in respiratory distress. Problems with respiratory status occur in all nursing disciplines. There will be questions regarding nursing priority of airway and nursing interventions in the client with respiratory difficulty. The questions may arise from any client situation—obstetrics, newborn, surgical, etc.*

A. Hypoxia—decreased oxygen saturation of the blood; mild is PaO_2 is below 80 mm Hg, severe is PaO_2 below 50mm Hg.
   1. Decreased oxygen in inspired air.
   2. Disorders causing respiratory obstruction and alveolar hypoventilation.

B. Hypoxia may be caused by inadequate circulation.
   1. Shock.
   2. Cardiac failure.

C. Anemia precipitates hypoxia due to decrease in oxygen-carrying capacity of the blood.
   1. Inadequate red cell production.
   2. Deficient or abnormal hemoglobin.

Assessment

1. Risk factors/etiology.
   a. Chronic hypoxia.
      (1) COPD.
      (2) Cystic fibrosis.
      (3) Cancer of the respiratory tract.
      (4) CHF.
      (5) Chronic anemia.
   b. Inflammatory problems affecting alveolar surface area, and membrane integrity (i.e., pneumonia, bronchitis).
   c. Acute hypoxia.
      (1) Acute respiratory failure.
      (2) Sudden airway obstruction.
      (3) Conditions affecting pulmonary expansion (i.e., respiratory paralysis).
      (4) CHF.
      (5) Hypoventilation (sedation, anesthesia, etc.).
2. Clinical manifestations—underlying respiratory problem either chronic or acute (Table 15-3).
3. Diagnostics.
   a. ABGs.
   b. Pulmonary function tests.
   c. Hemoglobin and hematocrit levels.
   d. Clinical manifestations.
   e. History of underlying problems.
4. Compensatory mechanisms.
   a. Increase cardiac output (tachycardia).
   b. Increase extraction of oxygen from capillary blood.
   c. Increase in amount of hemoglobin.
5. Complications.
   a. Acute.

Table 15-3: SYMPTOMS OF RESPIRATORY DISTRESS AND HYPOXIA

Early Symptoms	Late Symptoms
Restlessness	Extreme restlessness to stupor
Tachycardia	Dyspnea
Tachypnea, exertional dyspnea	Depressed respiration
Anxiety	Bradycardia
Diaphoresis	Cyanosis (peripheral or central)
Poor judgment	
Disorientation	
Confusion	
Headache	
Specific to pediatric:	
Flaring nares	
Sternal retractions	
Expiratory grunt	
Inspiratory stridor	
Feeding difficulty	

Table 15-4: EFFECTIVE COUGHING

- Increase activity prior to coughing - walking, or turning from side to side.
- Place client in sitting position, preferably with feet on the floor.
- Client should turn his shoulders inward and bend his head slightly forward.
- Take a gentle breath in through the nose and breathe completely.
- Take two deep breaths through the nose and mouth and hold for five seconds.
- On the third deep breath, cough to clear secretions.
- Sips of warm liquids (coffee, tea, or water) may stimulate coughing.
- Demonstrate to client how to splint chest or incision during cough to decrease pain.

(1) Cardiac decompensation.

(2) Progression to chronic hypoxia.

b. Chronic.

(1) CO_2 narcosis.

(2) Cor pulmonale.

(3) Cardiac failure.

c. Treatment—Depends on underlying problem.

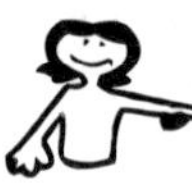

NURSING PRIORITY: *Oxygen should never be withheld from a severely hypoxic client for fear of increasing the* PaO_2 *levels.*

Nursing Intervention

✦ *Goal: to maintain good pulmonary hygiene and prevent hypoxic episode.*

1. Position client to maintain patent airway.
   a. Unconscious client—position on side with the chin extended.
   b. Conscious client—elevate the head of the bed and may position on side as well.
2. Encourage coughing and deep breathing (Table 15-4).
3. Suction client as indicated by amount of sputum and ability to cough.
4. Maintain adequate fluid intake to keep secretions liquefied.
5. Encourage exercises and ambulation as indicated by condition.
6. Administer expectorants.
7. Administer O_2 if dyspnea is present.

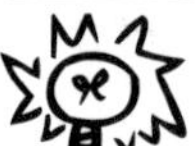

NCLEX ALERT: *Administer fluids very cautiously to a client who is having difficulty breathing. Begin with small sips of water to determine if he can swallow effectively. Do not begin with fluids that contain any fat (milk) or caloric value, due to the increased risk of the client aspirating.*

✦ *Goal: implement nursing measures to decrease hypoxia.*

1. Assess patency of airway (first priority).
   a. Can client speak? If not, initiate emergency procedures. (Appendix 15-3).
   b. If speaking is difficult because of level of hypoxia, notify physician and remain with client.
   c. If client is able to speak in sentences and is coherent, continue with assessment of the problem.
   d. Evaluate amount of secretions and ability to cough. Suction and administer O_2 as indicated.
2. Assess use of accessory muscles.
3. Maintain calm approach, as increasing anxiety will potentiate hypoxia.

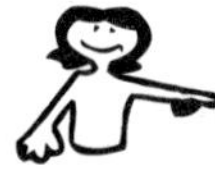

NURSING PRIORITY: *Increasing anxiety will accelerate the dyspnea in a client who is experiencing severe difficulty breathing.*

4. Position adult and older children in semi-Fowler's if not contraindicated.
5. Place infant in an infant seat, or elevate the mattress.

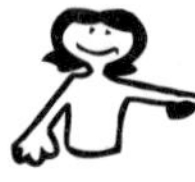

NURSING PRIORITY: *Position a dyspneic client with a pillow lengthwise behind his back and head. Do not flex his head forward or backward.*

6. Assess color, presence of retractions, and diaphoresis.
7. Evaluate vital signs: are there significant changes from previous readings?
8. Evaluate for dysrhythmias.
   a. If on a monitor, check for presence of premature ventricular contractions (PVCs).
   b. Evaluate level of tachycardia.
9. Evaluate chest movements: are they symmetrical?
10. Evaluate anterior and posterior breath sounds.
11. Assess client for chest pain with dyspnea.
12. Notify physician of significant changes in respiratory function.

13. Remain with client experiencing acute dyspnea or hypoxic episodes.
14. Assess response to oxygen therapy, report PaO_2 levels above 100mm Hg.
15. Evaluate diagnostic information.
   a. ABG.
   b. Chest X-ray.
   c. EKG.
   d. Pulse oximetry.

Pneumothorax

❑ **Air in the pleural cavity results in the collapse or atelectasis of that portion of the lung. This condition is known as *pneumothorax*.**

A. Tension pneumothorax—the development of a pneumothorax that allows excessive buildup of pressure in the pleural space, causing a shift in the mediastinum toward the unaffected side.

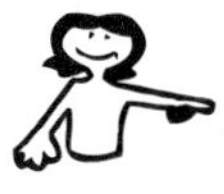

***NURSING PRIORITY:** A tension pneumothorax can very rapidly become an emergency situation. It is much easier to treat the client if the pneumothorax is identified before it begins to exert tension on the mediastinal area.*

Assessment

1. Risk factors/etiology.
   a. Ruptured bleb (spontaneous).
   b. Thoracentesis.
   c. Secondary to infection.
   d. Trauma.
2. Clinical manifestations.
   a. Diminished or absent breath sounds on the affected side.
   b. Dyspnea, hypoxia.
   c. Tachycardia, tachypnea.
   d. Sudden onset of persistent chest pain.
   e. Anxiety.
   f. Asymmetrical chest wall expansion.
   g. Hyperresonance on percussion of affected side.
   h. Possible development of a tension pneumothorax.
      (1) Decreased cardiac filling—leading to decreased cardiac output.
      (2) Tracheal shift from midline toward unaffected side.
      (3) Increasing problems of hypoxia.
3. Diagnostics.
   a. Chest X-ray.
   b. ABGs (PaO_2, $PaCO_2$).

Box 15-1: Elderly Care Focus

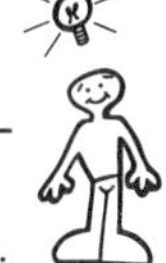

Respiratory Care Priorities

- Elderly client may not present with respiratory symptoms, but with confusion and disorientation.
- Provide adequate rest periods between activities, such as bathing, going for treatments, eating, etc.
- Increase compliance with medications by scheduling medications with routine activities.
- Encourage annual flu shot for individuals over age 65 and determine if older adult has received pneumococcal vaccination.
- Frequent evaluation of client's response to changes in activity and therapy.
- Administer oxygen with caution; evaluate response to increased levels of O_2 saturation.

NCLEX ALERT: *When atmospheric pressure is allowed to disrupt the negative pressure in the pleural space, it will cause the lung to collapse. This requires chest tube placement in order to reestablish negative pressure and reinflate the lung.*

Treatment

Placement of chest tubes connected to water-sealed drainage (Appendix 15-4).

Nursing Intervention

✦ *Goal: to recognize problem and prevent severe hypoxic episode (see Nursing Intervention, Hypoxia).*
1. Notify physician.
2. Begin oxygen therapy.
3. Prepare client for insertion of chest tubes.

✦ *Goal: to reinflate lung without complications.*
1. Have client cough and deep breathe every two hours.
2. Encourage exercise and ambulation.
3. Establish and maintain water-seal chest drainage (Appendix 15-4).

Pleural Effusion

❑ **A collection of fluid in the pleural space causes pleural effusion. It is generally secondary to other disease processes.**

Assessment

1. Etiology.
   a. Increased capillary oncotic pressure (liver or renal failure).
   b. Increased pulmonary capillary pressure (left-sided heart failure).

c. Decreased capillary oncotic pressure from the loss of circulating protein (renal or hepatic failure).

d. Obstruction in the lymphatic system (tumor).

e. If the pleural fluid becomes purulent, the condition is referred to as empyema.

2. Clinical manifestations.

a. Symptoms of an underlying problem.

b. Large quantities of fluid will cause shortness of breath and dyspnea.

c. Decreased breath sounds.

d. Pleuritic pain on inspiration.

e. Asymmetrical chest expansion.

3. Diagnostics.

a. Chest X-ray.

b. Clinical manifestations.

c. Malignancy may be determined by a cytology study of the aspirated fluid.

d. Culture and sensitivity on aspirated fluid.

Treatment

1. Thoracentesis (Appendix 15-1).
2. If empyema develops, area may have to be opened and allowed to drain.
3. Chest tube if there is rapid fluid buildup requiring removal to facilitate respirations.

Nursing Intervention

✦ *Goal: to recognize problem and prevent acute episode of hypoxia (see Nursing intervention, hypoxia).*

Self-Care

1. Demonstrate to client and family the prescribed method of managing wound care.
2. Client is at increased risk for respiratory infections.
3. The purulent fluid is localized and will not be hazardous to other family members if the basic concepts of hand washing and good technique for dressing change are utilized.

Open Chest Wound

❑ **An open or sucking chest wound is frequently caused by a penetrating injury of the chest, as in a gunshot or knife wound. If a chest tube is inadvertently pulled out of the chest, a sucking chest wound may be created.**

Assessment

1. Clinical manifestations.

a. Increase in dyspnea

b. A chest wound with evidence of air moving in and out via the wound.

Treatment

1. Have the client take a deep breath, hold it and bear down against a closed glottis. Apply a light occlusive dressing over the wound.

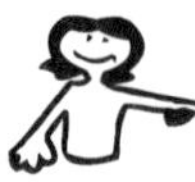

***NURSING PRIORITY:** Immediately occlude the chest wound; do not leave the client to go find a dressing. If necessary, place a towel, or whatever is at hand over the wound to stop the flow of air.*

2. Prepare for insertion of chest tubes and water-sealed drainage.
3. After covering the wound with an occlusive dressing, carefully evaluate the client for development of a tension pneumothorax. If respiratory distress increases, remove the occlusive dressing and allow the air to escape.

Nursing Intervention

✦ *Goal: to prevent problems of hypoxia.*

✦ *Goal: to assess for development of tension pneumothorax.*

Flail Chest

❑ **The loss of stability of the chest wall with respiratory impairment due to multiple rib fractures.**

Assessment

1. Clinical manifestations.

a. Paradoxical respirations—the movement of the fractured area (flailed segment) inward during inspiration and outward during expiration, or opposite to the other areas of the chest wall.

b. Symptoms of hypoxia.

2. Diagnostics.

a. X-ray of the chest wall.

b. Arterial blood gases.

Treatment

1. Maintain patent airway.
2. Adequate pain medication to enable client to breath deeply.
3. Oxygen.
4. Endotracheal intubation with mechanical ventilation for severe respiratory distress (Appendix 15-5 and 15-8).
5. Chest tubes if pneumothorax occurs due to puncture of the lung by the fractured rib.

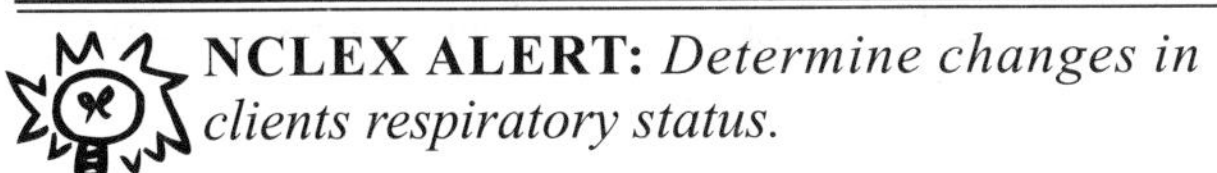

NCLEX ALERT: *Determine changes in clients respiratory status.*

Nursing Intervention

✦ *Goal: to stabilize the chest wall and prevent complications.*

1. Prepare client for endotracheal intubation and mechanical ventilation (Appendix 15-5 and 15-8).
2. Assess for symptoms of hypoxia.
3. Assess for symptoms of pneumothorax.

Pulmonary Embolus

❑ **This is an obstruction of a pulmonary artery, most often due to an embolism caused by air, fat, amniotic fluid, or emboli. The severity of the problem depends on the size of the embolus.**

A. The right lobe is most frequently involved; of the clients who die, three-fourths die within two hours.

B. The majority of emboli arise from thrombi in the deep veins of the thigh or pelvic cavity.

C. A pulmonary embolus must originate from the venous circulation, or the right side of the heart.

Assessment

1. Risk factors/etiology.
   a. Conditions predisposing to venous stasis: surgery, immobility, pregnancy, obesity, etc.
   b. Hypercoagulation - dehydration, malignancy, pregnancy or normal birth, oral contraceptives.
   c. Vascular injury - intravenous catheters, thrombophlebitis, varicose veins, leg fractures.
2. Clinical manifestations.
   a. Dyspnea.
   b. Sudden, unexplained, pleuritic chest pain.
   c. Tachypnea.
   d. Tachycardia.
   e. Hemoptysis.
   f. Apprehension.
   g. Hypotension and syncope.
   h. May result in sudden death if pulmonary embolus is large.
3. Diagnostics.
   a. Pulmonary angiogram (definitive study).
   b. Ventilation/perfusion radioisotope lung scan (best non invasive test).
   c. EKG (nonspecific).
   d. Chest X-ray (nonspecific).
   e. Arterial blood gases (decreased PaO_2, normal or low $PaCO_2$).

Treatment

1. Bed rest.
2. Respiratory support - oxygen, ventilator, etc.
3. Anticoagulants (Heparin) to prevent further thrombi formation.
4. IV access for fluids and medications to maintain blood pressure.
5. Small doses of morphine sulfate to decrease anxiety, alleviate chest pain, or to improve tolerance to endotracheal tube.

NCLEX ALERT: *Assess clients for complications due to immobility. Immobilized clients are at an increased risk for development of a pulmonary embolus. Questions require an understanding of principles for prevention of thrombophlebitis and subsequent embolus formation. It is far easier to prevent the problem than it is to treat the pulmonary embolus.*

Nursing Intervention

✦ *Goal: to identify problem and implement nursing measures to alleviate hypoxia (see Nursing intervention, hypoxia).*

✦ *Goal: monitor client's respiratory function and response to treatment.*

Croup

❑ **The term *croup* describes a group of conditions characterized by edema and inflammation of the respiratory tract.**

A. Acute epiglottitis—a severe infection of the epiglottis, characterized by rapid inflammation and edema of the area; generally occurs in children 2 to 4 years old; may rapidly cause airway obstruction.

1. Etiology—*H. Influenza.*
2. Clinical manifestations - hypoxia (Table 15-3).
   a. Rapid, abrupt onset.
   b. Sore throat, swallowing difficulty.
   c. Inflamed epiglottis.
   d. Symptoms of increasing respiratory obstruction.
      (1) Characteristic position—sitting with the neck hyperextended and mouth open, drooling.
      (2) Inspiratory stridor (crowing).
      (3) Retraction.
      (4) Increased restlessness.
   e. High fever (above 102°).

NURSING PRIORITY: *The absence of spontaneous cough, presence of drooling and agitation are cardinal signs distinctive to epiglottis.*

3. Treatment
   a. Endotracheal intubation for obstruction (Appendix 15-5).
   b. Humidification.
   c. Antibiotics.

B. Acute laryngotracheobronchitis (LTB)—inflammation of the vocal cords, subglottic tissues, trachea; occurs in children 3 months to 3 years of age.
1. Etiology—viral agents (parainfluenza, respiratory syncytial virus.)
2. Clinical manifestations (Table 15-3).
   a. Slow onset.
   b. Frequently preceded by upper respiratory infection (URI).
   c. Respiratory distress.
      (1) Inspiratory stridor.
      (2) Flaring of nares
      (3) Retractions - substernal, intercostal, suprasternal with activity.
   d. Slight temperature elevation (usually below 102°).
   e. Signs of increasing respiratory distress (hypoxia).
      (1) Retractions at rest.
      (2) Increasing inspiratory stridor.
      (3) Respiratory rate above 60.
      (4) Restlessness and tachycardia.
3. Treatment
   a. Maintain patent airway.
   b. Bronchodilators, racemic epinephrine by inhalation.
   c. Cool mist humidification.
   d. No sedatives.
   e. Oxygen.

C. Acute spasmodic laryngitis—mildest form of croup; generally occurs in small children 1 to 4 years old.
1. Etiology—unknown.
2. Clinical manifestations.
   a. Characterized by paroxysmal attacks.
   b. Occurs at night.
   c. Mild respiratory distress.
      (1) Noisy inspiration.
      (2) Utilizes accessory muscles of respiration.
      (3) Anxious.
   d. No fever.
   e. After the attack, the child appears well.
3. Treatment - the child is generally cared for at home.

Nursing Intervention

✦ *Goal: to maintain patent airway in hospitalized child.*

1. Tracheotomy set readily available.

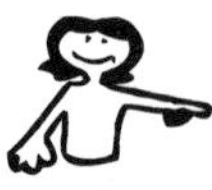

NURSING PRIORITY: *Epiglottitis - do not examine child's throat, as it may precipitate airway spasm.*

2. Suction airway as indicated with endotracheal tube.
3. Position of comfort, do not force child to lay down.
4. If child is intubated, do not leave unattended.
5. If obstruction is impending, maintain ventilation by mechanical ventilation (ambu bag) until child can be intubated.

✦ *Goal: to evaluate and maintain adequate ventilation.*

1. Assess for increasing hypoxia.
2. Humidified oxygen, closely evaluate because cyanosis may be masked.
3. Conserve energy.
4. Assess pulse oximetry for adequate oxygenation.

✦ *Goal: to maintain hydration and nutrition*

1. Do not give po fluid until danger of aspiration is past.
2. IV fluids during acute episodes.
3. High caloric liquids when danger of aspiration is over.
4. Suction nares of infant prior to feeding.
5. Assess for adequate hydration.

Home Care.

1. Teach parents to recognize symptoms of increasing respiratory problems and when to notify physician.
2. Child should sleep in a warm or cool humidity until cough subsides.
3. Maintain adequate fluid intake.
4. Immunization of *H. Influenza* type B (HIB).

NCLEX ALERT: *Evaluate client/family's use of home remedies and over the counter drugs.*

Bronchiolitis Respiratory Syncytial Virus (RSV)

❑ **Inflammation of the bronchioles, alveoli are usually normal.**

A. Most common in winter and spring in children under 2 years old.

B. Transmitted by direct contact with respiratory secretions.

C. Considered the single most important respiratory pathogen of infancy and early childhood.

Assessment

1. Etiology—Respiratory syncytial virus (RSV), usually begins with an URI
2. Peak time is in the winter and spring.
3. Clinical manifestations.
   a. Initial—copious nasal drainage, decreased appetite, coughing and low grade fever.
   b. Acute phase
      (1) Rhinorrhea.
      (2) Chest retractions.
      (3) Tachypnea, air hunger
      (4) Paroxysmal wheezy cough.
      (5) Low grade fever
4. Diagnostics- RSV nasal prep for antigens.

Treatment

1. Rest, fluids, and high humidity.
2. Oxygen.
3. Ribavirin (antiviral agent) for hospitalized infants.
4. RSV immune globulin (RSV-IGIV, RespiGam) may be given to high risk infants and toddlers.

Nursing Intervention

✦ *Goal: to promote effective breathing patterns.*

1. Frequent assessment for development of hypoxia (Table 15-3). Close monitoring of O2 saturation (oximetry)
2. Increase in respiratory rate and audible crackles in the lungs are indications of cardiac failure and should be reported immediately.
3. Monitor response to humidified oxygen (pulse oximetry, ABG's).
4. Maintain adequate hydration to facilitate removal of respiratory secretions.
5. Conserve energy, avoid unnecessary procedures but encourage parents to console and cuddle infant.

✦ *Goal: to prevent transmission of organism.*

1. If hospitalized, the child should be placed in a private room, with contact isolation.
2. Nasal mucosa and conjunctive harbor the organisms.
3. Nurses assigned to care for these children should not be assigned the care of other children that are at a high risk for respiratory infections.
4. Consistent hand washing.

Home Care.

1. Decrease energy level, will tire easily.
2. Small frequent feedings.
3. Teach parents how to assess for respiratory difficulty.
4. Consult physician before obtaining live virus vaccines for about 9 months after receiving RespiGam.

Tonsillitis

❑ **Tonsillitis is an inflammation and infection of the palatine tonsils.**

Assessment

1. Clinical manifestations.
   a. Edematous, enlarged tonsils, exudate on tonsils.
   b. Difficulty swallowing and breathing.
   c. Petechiae on soft palate.
   d. Frequently precipitates *otitis media.*
   e. Fever.
2. Diagnostics.
   a. Confirm by visualization of the oropharynx.
   b. Throat culture for group A beta hemolytic streptococcus.

Treatment

1. Appropriate antibiotic for identified organism.
2. Surgery—tonsillectomy for severe repeated episodes of tonsillitis resulting in difficulty breathing and eating..

Nursing Intervention

✦ *Goal: to promote comfort and healing in home environment.*

1. Soft or liquid diet.
2. Cool mist vaporizer to maintain moisture to mucous membranes.
3. Throat lozenges, warm gargles to soothe the throat.
4. Antibiotics—important to give child all of the medication prescribed in order to prevent reoccurrence.
5. Analgesics, antipyretic (acetaminophen).

✦ *Goal: to provide preoperative nursing measures if surgery is indicated (Chapter 3).*

✦ *Goal: to maintain patent airway and evaluate for bleeding postoperative tonsillectomy.*

1. Restrict fluids until child is fully awake; administer cool, clear liquids initially.
2. Evaluate for frequent or continuous swallowing due to bleeding.
3. Suction equipment available.
4. Evaluate for tachycardia.
5. Ice collar to decrease edema.
6. Evaluate voice for increasing hoarseness.
7. Check throat with flashlight for bleeding.
8. Oral codeine or acetaminophen for pain, aspirin is contraindicated.
9. Avoid coughing.

NURSING PRIORITY: *Before the child is fully awake, they should be positioned on the side or on the abdomen, to prevent aspiration from bloody drainage or vomitus. Always consider the tonsillectomy client to be nauseated due to swallowing of blood.*

Home/Self-Care

1. Child will have sore throat for several days.
2. Symptoms of bleeding, especially significant on the fifth to tenth postoperative days when tissue sloughing may occur due to infection.
3. Maintain adequate hydration; encourage bland juices and fluids.
4. A gray membrane on the sides of the throat is normal, should disappear in 1-2 weeks.

Pneumonia

❑ **Pneumonia is an acute inflammatory process involving the lung parenchyma. This includes the small airways and alveoli.**

Assessment

1. Predisposing conditions.
   a. Chronic upper respiratory infection.
   b. Postoperative.
   c. Immobility.
   d. Smoking.
   e. Decreased immune state.
   f. Aspiration of foreign material or gastric contents.
   g. Most frequent cause of death by infection in clients over 65 years old..
2. Etiology.
   a. Viral - parainfluenza, respiratory syncytial virus (primarily infants and young children).
   b. Bacterial - *Streptococcus pneumoniae* and *Mycoplasma pneumoniae.*
   c. Fungal (increase in immunosuppressed clients).
3. Clinical manifestations.
   a. Fever, chills.
   b. Tachycardia.
   c. Tachypnea, dyspnea.
   d. Productive cough—thick, blood streaked, yellow, purulent sputum.
   e. Pleuritic chest pain.
   f. Malaise.
   g. Respiratory distress (hypoxia) (Table 15-3).
   h. Diminished breath sounds, wheezing, crackles, tactile fremitus.
   i. Feeding difficulty in infants.
4. Diagnostics.
   a. Culture of organism from sputum.
   b. Chest X-ray.
   c. CBC for increased leukocytes.
   d. Arterial blood gases, pulse oximetry

GERIATRIC PRIORITY: *An elderly client may initially present with mental confusion and volume depletion rather then respiratory symptoms and fever.*

Treatment

1. Antibiotic according to organism identified (Appendix 6-10).

NCLEX ALERT: *Administration of medications. Do not start antibiotics until a good sputum specimen has been collected. An accurate culture and sensitivity cannot be done if client has already been started on antibiotics.*

2. Respiratory precautions - transmitted via air borne droplets.
3. Inhalation therapy.
   a. Cool oxygen mist.
   b. Postural drainage.
   c. Bronchodilators.

Nursing Intervention

✦ *Goal: to teach client and family how to provide home care when appropriate.*

1. Antibiotics as directed.
2. Cool mist humidification.
3. Maintain high PO fluid intake.
4. Antipyretic - acetaminophen.

5. Frequent change of position.
6. Understand symptoms of increasing respiratory problems and when to notify physician.

✦ *Goal: to decrease infection and remove secretions to facilitate oxygen and carbon dioxide exchange.*

1. Antibiotics.
2. Have client turn, cough, and deep breathe.
3. Liquefy secretions.
   a. Adequate hydration.
   b. Cool mist inhalation.
4. Evaluate changes in sputum.
5. Position of comfort or semi-Fowler's.
6. Nursing measures to prevent and evaluate levels of hypoxia (see Nursing interventions, hypoxia).

Tuberculosis (TB)

❑ **Tuberculosis is a reportable communicable disease that is characterized by pulmonary pathology.**

A. Characteristics.

1. Organism is primarily transmitted through respiratory droplets; it is inhaled and implants on alveolar surface.
2. A client in good health is frequently able to resist the primary infection and does not develop an active disease, these clients will continue to harbor the bacilli.
3. The primary site or tubercle may undergo a process of degeneration or caseation, this area can erode into the bronchial tree and be coughed up in the sputum.
4. The area may never erode but calcify and remain dormant after the primary infection. However, the tubercle may contain living bacilli that can reactivate several years later.
5. The majority of people with a primary infection will harbor the TB bacilli in a tubercle in the lungs and will not exhibit any symptoms of an active infection.
6. An opportunistic infection in clients who are HIV positive.

Assessment

1. Predisposing conditions.
   a. Frequent close contact with infected individual.
   b. Debilitating conditions and diseases.
   c. Poor nutrition and crowded living conditions.
   d. Increasing age
2. Etiology—Mycobacterium tuberculosis, a gram-positive, acid-fast bacillus.
   a. Primary infection—the first time the client is infected, primary sites may remain latent for years.
   b. Secondary infection—reinfection that leads to an active form of TB.
3. Clinical manifestations (client may be asymptomatic).
   a. Fatigue, malaise.
   b. Anorexia, weight loss.
   c. May have a chronic cough progressing to more frequent and productive cough.
   d. Long term, low-grade fever.
   e. Night sweats.
   f. Hemoptysis is associated only with advanced condition.
   g. Pleuritic chest pain.
4. Diagnostics (Appendix 15-1).
   a. Tuberculin skin testing. (Mantoux, purified protein derivative -PPD)
      (1) Positive reaction means the individual has been infected, does not differentiate between primary, active or dormant infection.
      (2) Generally is 2-6 weeks after exposure to develop sensitivity and positive skin test.

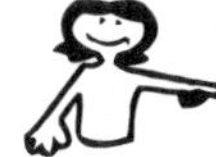

NURSING PRIORITY: *A positive reaction to a TB skin test means that the person has at some time been infected with the TB bacillus, developed a primary infection and has developed antibodies. It does not mean that the person has an active TB infection.*

   b. Chest X-ray—may demonstrate presence of calcified lesions or tubercle.
   c. Bacteriologic studies to identify acid-fast bacilli in the sputum (Appendix 15-1).
5. Complications.
   a. Pleural effusion.
   b. Pneumonia.
   c. Other organ involvement.

Treatment

1. Chemotherapy (Appendix 15-2).
   a. Medical regimen involves simultaneous administration of three or more medications; this increases the therapeutic effect of medication and decreases development of resistant bacteria.
   b. Course of treatment averages 6-12 months, is considered to be non-infectious after 2-3 weeks of continuous therapy.
   c. Preventive chemotherapy is utilized for:
      (1) Close contact with a newly diagnosed client.
      (2) Newly infected with positive skin test.

(3) Positive skin test with conditions that decrease immune response (HIV, steroid therapy, diabetes).

(4) Isoniazid is used for prophylaxis.

2. Most often treated on an outpatient basis.

Nursing Intervention

✦ *Goal: to understand implications of the disease, measures to protect others and maintain own health.*

1. Evaluate client's lifestyle and identify needs regarding compliance with treatment and long-term therapy.
2. Identify community resources available for client.

NCLEX ALERT: *Identify community/home services which would facilitate a client's independent living.*

3. Understand medication schedule.
   a. To prevent the development of a resistant bacteria, the client must take his medication in correct amounts and on schedule.
   b. Medications may be administered on directly observed therapy (DOT) to guarantee compliance.
   c. Medications may be taken at bedtime to decrease side effects.

NCLEX ALERT: *Evaluate client's compliance with prescribed therapy.*

4. Return for sputum checks every 2-4 weeks during therapy.
5. Balanced diet and good nutritional status.
6. Avoid excessive fatigue, endurance will increase with treatment.
7. Identify family and close contacts who need to report to the Public Health Department for TB screening.
8. Offer client HIV testing.

✦ *Goal: to prevent transmission of the disease.*

1. When sputum is positive for the organism, maintain respiratory isolation, use HEPA respirator mask for all people in close contact with client. (Appendix 6-10).
2. Cover mouth and nose when sneezing or coughing.
3. Careful hand washing routine.
4. Wear a mask when in contact with other people.
5. Discard all secretions (nose and mouth) in plastic bags.
6. Periodic reevaluation for active disease or secondary infection.

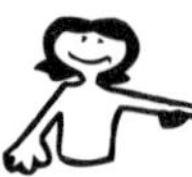

NURSING PRIORITY: *TB is most likely to be spread by clients who have active undiagnosed TB.*

Chronic Obstructive Pulmonary Disease

❑ **Chronic airflow limitation or chronic obstructive pulmonary disease (COPD) is a group of chronic respiratory diseases characterized by obstruction of air flow.**

A. Although each of the disorders may occur individually, it is more common for two or more problems to coexist and the symptoms to overlap.

B. Clinical manifestations common to chronic airflow limitation.
   1. Distended neck veins.
   2. Orthopnea
   3. Barrel chest
   4. Prolonged expiratory time
   5. Diminished breath sounds.
   6. Thorax is hyperresonant to percussion.
   7. Exertional dyspnea progressing to dyspnea at rest.
   8. Increased respiratory rate.

C. Due to a chronic increase in $PaCO_2$ levels, normal respiratory center in the medulla may be altered; if this occurs, hypoxia will become the primary respiratory stimulus.

D. Emphysema—primarily a problem with the alveoli that is characterized by a loss of alveolar elasticity, over distention and destruction, with severe impairment of gas exchange across alveolar membrane.
   1. Clinical manifestations.
      a. Cough is not common.
      b. Sensation of air hunger.
      c. Use of accessory muscles of respiration.
      d. Thin in appearance.
      e. Generally do not have any cardiac enlargement; cor pulmonale is late in disease.
      f. ABG's are often normal until late in disease.
      g. Characteristic position is leaning forward with arms braced on knees.

E. Chronic bronchitis—primarily a problem of the airway that is characterized by excessive mucus production, impaired ciliary function which decreases mucus clearance. Client may develop polycythemia secondary to the low PaO_2.
   1. Clinical manifestations.

a. Excessive, chronic sputum production (generally not discolored unless infection is present).

b. Impaired ventilation resulting in decreased PaO_2 and cyanosis.

c. Respiratory symptoms: productive cough, exercise intolerance, wheezing and shortness of breath.

d. Dependent edema.

e. Generally normal or over weight.

f. Cardiac enlargement with cor pulmonale.

Assessment

1. Risk factors/etiology.
   a. Cigarette smoking.
   b. Chronic infections.
   c. Inhaled irritants.
2. Diagnostics.
   a. Pulmonary function studies (See Appendix 15-1).
      (1) Normal to increased total lung capacity.
      (2) Increased residual volume (air trapping).
   b. Decreased vital capacity.
   c. ABGs - (See Table 15-1).
      (1) Changes in $PaCO_2$ - most often increased.
      (2) Low PaO2 more prominent in bronchitis clients.
      (3) Decompensated condition—decreased PaO_2, increased $PaCO_2$, decreased pH.

Treatment

1. Prevention or treatment of respiratory infections.
2. Bronchodilators (See Appendix 15-2).
3. Mucolytics and expectorants (See Appendix 15-2).
4. Chest physiotherapy (postural drainage, nebulized bronchodilators).
5. Breathing exercises.
6. Exercise to maintain cardiovascular fitness, most common is walking.
7. Low flow humidified oxygen.
8. Corticosteriods (See Appendix 6-8).

NCLEX ALERT: *Administer oxygen - low flow oxygen administration for patients with emphysema. High concentrations of oxygen would eliminate the patient's hypoxic drive and cause respiratory distress*

Nursing Intervention

✦ *Goal: to improve ventilation.*

1. Teach pursed-lip breathing - inhale through the nose and exhale against "pursed" lips.
2. Avoid activities that increase dyspnea.
3. Humidified oxygen, low flow via nasal cannula at 1 to 3 liters per minute—utilized when clients are experiencing exertional or resting hypoxemia.
   a. Monitor for hypercapnia and hypoxia.
   b. A significant increase in PO_2 may decrease respiratory drive.
   c. Administer oxygen via nasal prongs or Venturi mask.

NCLEX ALERT: *Administer oxygen - the risk of inducing hypoventilation should not prevent the administration of oxygen in low levels to the COPD client experiencing respiratory distress.*

4. Assess breath sounds before and after coughing.
5. Avoid cough suppressants.
6. High-Fowler's or sitting position.
7. Maintain adequate hydration to facilitate removal of secretions.

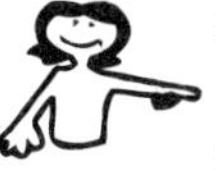

NURSING PRIORITY: *The optimum amount of oxygen is the concentration that reverses the hypoxemia without causing adverse side effects.*

✦ *Goal: Improve activity tolerance.*

1. Balance activities and dyspnea.- gradually increase activities, wear O_2 when walking, avoid respiratory irritants.
2. Pursed lip and diaphragmatic breathing during exercise.
3. Schedule activities after respiratory therapy.
4. Assess for negative responses to activity.

✦ *Goal: to maintain adequate nutrition.*

1. Soft, high-protein, high calorie diet, decreased carbohydrates (by product of carbohydrate metabolism is CO_2).
2. Postural drainage at least 45 minutes prior to meals.
3. Good oral hygiene after postural drainage.
4. Small frequent meals.

Self-Care

1. Encourage client and family to verbalize feelings about condition and lifelong restriction of activities.

2. Include client in active planning for home care.
3. Instruct client regarding community resources.
4. Instruct client regarding medication schedule and side effects of prescribed medications.
5. Recognize signs and symptoms of upper respiratory infection and when to call physician.

NCLEX ALERT: *Administer medications: administer narcotics, tranquilizers, and sedatives with caution; instruct client about self-administration of prescribed medications.*

Asthma

❑ **Asthma is an intermittent, reversible, obstructive airway problem. It is characterized by exacerbations and remissions. Between attacks the client is generally asymptomatic. It is a common disorder of childhood that may continue to cause problems throughout adult life.**

A. A chronic inflammatory process that produces mucosal edema, mucus secretion, and airway inflammation.

B. Intermittent narrowing of the airway is caused by:
   1. Constriction of the smooth muscles of the bronchi and the bronchiole.
   2. Excessive mucus production.
   3. Mucosal edema of the respiratory tract.

C. Constriction of the smooth muscle causes significant increase in airway resistance, thereby trapping air in the lung.

D. Emotional factors are known to play an important role in precipitating childhood asthma attacks.

E. Exercise induced asthma - initially after exercise there is an improvement in the respiratory status, followed by a significant decline; occurs in the majority of clients.

Assessment

1. Risk factors/etiology.
   a. Familial tendencies.
   b. Hypersensitivity.
   c. Pediatric implications.
      (1) Reactive airway disease is the term used to describe asthma in children.
      (2) General onset before age 3 years.
      (3) Children are more likely to have airway obstruction.
2. Diagnostics.
   a. Family history.
   b. History of hypersensitivity reactions (history of eczema in children).
   c. Increased eosinophil count in the sputum and in the serum.
   d. Clinical manifestations.
   e. ABGs.
   f. Pulmonary function tests.
3. Clinical manifestations—*early phase reactions* occur immediately and last about an hour, *late phase reactions* do not begin until 4-8 hours after exposure and may last for hours or days.
   a. Episodic wheezing, chest tightness, shortness of breath, cough.
   b. Use of accessory muscles in breathing.
   c. Symptoms of hypoxia, cyanosis occurs late.
   d. Increased anxiety, restlessness.
   e. Exercise intolerance.
   f. Excessive sputum production.
4. Complications—Status asthmaticus: severe asthma, unresponsive to initial treatment.

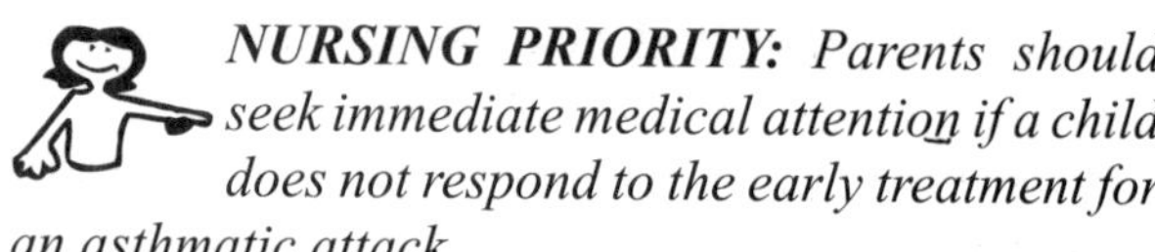

***NURSING PRIORITY:** Parents should seek immediate medical attention if a child does not respond to the early treatment for an asthmatic attack.*

Treatment

1. Medications (see Appendix 15-2).
   a. Beta adrenergic medications by nebulizer or metered dose inhalers.
   b. Epinephrine.
   c. Antibiotics, if infection is present.
   d. Bronchodilator.
   e. Expectorants.
   f. Inhalation steroids to prevent edema.
   g. Supplemental oxygen for hypoxemia.
2. Status asthmaticus.
   a. NPO.
   b. IV fluids for hydration.
   c. May require intubation and mechanical ventilation.
   d. IV bronchodilators and steroids.
3. Medications to avoid in the asthmatic client.
   a. Beta adrenergic blockers.
   b. Cough suppressants.

Nursing Intervention

(See Nursing Intervention, Hypoxia)

✦ *Goal: to relieve asthmatic attacks.*

1. Position of comfort - usually high-Fowler's or sitting with chest forward.
2. Assess response to supplemental oxygen.
3. Assess response to bronchodilators and aerosol therapy.
4. Maintain adequate fluid intake to liquefy secretions.

NCLEX ALERT: *Determine changes in a client's respiratory status: the inability to hear wheezing breath sounds in the asthmatic client with acute respiratory distress may be an indication of impending respiratory obstruction.*

Self Care

1. Assess emotional factors precipitating asthmatic attack.
2. Educate regarding identifying and avoiding allergens.
3. Implement therapeutic measures before attack becomes severe.
4. Purpose of prescribed medications and how to use them correctly (See Appendix 15-2).
5. Administer bronchodilators prior to postural drainage.
6. Bronchodilators and good warm up exercises prior to exercise to prevent exercise induced asthma.
7. Encourage participation in activities according to developmental level.

Cystic Fibrosis

❑ **This disorder is a generalized dysfunction precipitated by an obstruction of the exocrine gland ducts. The disease primarily affects the pulmonary and gastrointestinal systems.**

A. The factor responsible for the multiple clinical manifestations of the disease process is the mechanical obstruction caused by thick mucous secretions.

B. Effects of disease process.
   1. Pulmonary system—bronchial and bronchiolar obstruction by thick mucus, causing atelectasis and reduced area for gas exchange; the thick mucus provides excellent medium for bacterial growth and secondary respiratory infections.
   2. GI tract—decreased absorption of nutrients due to the obstruction of pancreatic ducts and lack of adequate enzymes for digestion.

Assessment

1. Risk factors/etiology.
   a. Inherited as an autosomal recessive trait.
   b. Present in all races and socioeconomic groups; however, is less prevalent in blacks.
2. Clinical manifestations.
   a. Wide variation in severity and extent of manifestations as well as period of onset.
   b. GI tract.
      (1) May present with meconium ileus in the newborn.
      (2) Increased bulk in feces from undigested foods.
      (3) Increased fat in stools (steatorrhea); foul smelling.
      (4) Decreased absorption of nutrients—weight loss or failure to thrive.
      (5) Increased appetite due to decreased absorption of nutrients.
      (6) Abdominal distention.
      (7) Rectal prolapse related to the large bulky stools and loss of supportive tissue around rectum.
   c. Genital tract.
      (1) Increased viscosity of cervical mucus in females may lead to decreased fertility due to blockage of sperm.
      (2) Males are generally sterile due to the blockage or obstruction of the vas deferens.
   d. Respiratory tract.
      (1) Evidence of respiratory involvement generally occurs in early childhood.
      (2) Increasing dyspnea, tachypnea.
      (3) Paroxysmal, chronic cough.
      (4) Repeated URIs.
      (5) Symptoms of chronic hypoxia: clubbing, barrel chest.
      (6) Sputum production generally occurs after treatment and mucus is expectorated.
   e. Excessive salt on the skin: "salty taste when kissed."
3. Diagnostics.
   a. Family history.
   b. Sweat chloride test—chloride concentration above 60 mEq/L is diagnostic; chloride concentration 40 to 60 mEq/L is suspicious.
   c. Pancreatic enzymes—decrease or absence of trypsin and chymotrypsin.
   d. Fat absorption in intestines is impaired.
   e. Pulmonary function test show decreased vital capacity and tidal volume.

4. Complications.
   a. Cor pulmonale.
   b. Frequent pulmonary infections.

Treatment

(Child generally cared for at home unless complications are present).

1. Diet—high calorie, high protein, fats as tolerated or decrease in fats, increased salt intake.
2. Fat soluble vitamins A,D,E, and K in a water soluble preparation.
3. Pancreatic enzyme replacement - (Appendix 13-2).
4. Pulmonary therapy.
   a. Physical therapy: postural drainage, breathing exercises.
   b. Aerosol therapy: nebulization in conjunction with postural drainage.
   c. Percussion and vibration.
   d. Expectorants (Appendix 15-2).
5. Antibiotics prophylactically and when there is evidence of infection.

Nursing Intervention

✦ *Goal: to promote optimum home care for child. (See Chapter 3 for care of chronically ill child).*

1. Identify community resources for family.
2. Assist family to identify problems and solutions congruent with their lifestyle.
3. Encourage verbalization regarding impact of child's problem on the family, their ability to cope with the child at home, and the possibility of the child's death.

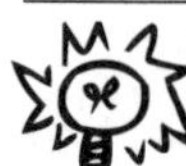

NCLEX ALERT: *Determine needs of family, evaluate family's emotional response and adaptation.*

4. When appropriate, teach child about disease and treatment and encourage active participation in planning of care.
5. Assist parents to identify activities to promote normal growth and development.

✦ *Goal: to maintain nutrition.*

1. Minimum restriction of fats, need to increase intake of pancreatic enzyme with increased fat.
2. Pancreatic enzymes with meals and snacks.
3. Vitamins A, D, E, and K in about twice the normal dosage due to poor absorption.
4. Good oral hygiene after postural drainage.
5. Postural drainage one to two hours prior to meals.

✦ *Goal: to prevent or minimize pulmonary complications.*

1. Assist child to mobilize secretions.
   a. Postural drainage, breathing exercises, nebulization treatments.
   b. Encourage active exercises appropriate to child's capacity and developmental level.
2. Prevent respiratory infections.
3. Maintain adequate PO fluid intake.

Adult Respiratory Distress Syndrome

❑ **ARDS, also referred to as "shock lung" and "white lung," or non-cardiogenic pulmonary edema is a condition characterized by increased capillary permeability in the alveolar capillary membrane, resulting in fluid leaking into the interstitial spaces and into the alveoli.**

Assessment

1. Risk factors/etiology -damage or trauma to the lung tissue, indirectly damage occurring in other parts of the body.
   (1) Aspiration of gastric contents.
   a. Fluid overload.
   b. Smoke inhalation.
   c. Hypoalbuminemia (nephrotic syndrome, liver disease).
2. Clinical manifestations.
   a. Tachypnea and dyspnea.
   b. Increasing hypoxia that does not respond to increased levels of FIO_2.
   c. Hypoxia, cerebral hypoxia.
   d. Tachycardia.
   e. Crackles.
3. Diagnostics.
   a. Preexisting compromised state.
   b. X-ray—diffuse alveolar infiltration bilaterally.
   c. ABGs—decrease in PaO_2 with increased levels of FIO_2

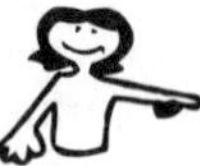

NURSING PRIORITY: *It is essential to closely monitor the ABGs in a client with ARDS. A decreasing PaO_2 and increasing difficulty breathing are indications that the client's condition is deteriorating.*

   d. Ventilation perfusion imbalance indicating a shunt.

Treatment

(Generally cared for in an intensive care setting).

1. Maintain oxygenation.

a. Endotracheal (ET) intubation.
b. Mechanical ventilation.
2. Positive end expiratory pressure (PEEP)—used to decrease the effects of shunting and to improve pulmonary compliance.
3. Hemodynamic monitoring.
4. Treatment of underlying condition.
5. Supportive medications.
a. Prophylactic antibiotics.
b. Diuretics.
c. Sedatives.
d. Bronchodilator.
e. Neuromuscular blocking agents.
6. Nutritional support.

NCLEX ALERT: *Monitor client's gas exchange, increasing levels of CO_2 are generally not a problem with the ARDS client; the problem exists with the diffusion of oxygen and the availability of the oxygen to the circulating hemoglobin.*

Nursing Intervention

✦ *Goal: to maintain airway patency and improve ventilation.*
1. Frequent assessment for increasing respiratory difficulty; anticipate intubation or tracheotomy (See Appendix 15-5).
2. ET or tracheotomy suctioning.
3. Evaluate ABG reports.
4. Sedate as necessary for client to tolerate the ventilator (Appendix 15-8).
5. Maintain hemoglobin levels and PaO_2 saturation levels.

✦ *Goal: to maintain fluid balance.*
1. Fluid balance is maintained with IV hydration.
2. Evaluate serum electrolytes.
3. Strict intake and output.

✦ *Goal: to assess and maintain cardiac output.*
1. Assess for dysrhythmias.
2. Correlate vital signs with other changes.
3. Evaluate cardiac output in relation to fluid intake.
4. Evaluate cardiac output when PEEP is initiated, because it will decrease venous return.

✦ *Goal: to provide emotional support to client and family.*
1. Careful repeated explanation of procedures to client.
2. Calm, gentle approach to decrease anxiety.
3. Be available to family at visiting times to explain procedures and equipment.
4. If endotracheal tube or tracheotomy is in place, explain to family and client that speech is only temporarily interrupted.
5. Assist client to maintain communication.

Pulmonary Edema

❑ **This condition is caused by an abnormal accumulation of fluid in the lung, both in the interstitial and in the alveolar spaces.**

A. Origin is cardiac - pulmonary congestion occurs when the pulmonary vascular bed receives more blood from the right heart than the left heart can accommodate.
B. Pulmonary edema results from severe impairment of the left heart function, thereby precipitating engorgement of the pulmonary vascular bed.

Assessment

1. Risk factors/etiology.
a. Hypertension.
b. Aortic valve problems.
c. Cardiac myopathy.
2. Clinical manifestations (Table 15-3).
a. Problem may occur at night or in clients on bed rest. The supine position increases venous return and promotes reabsorption of edema from the legs, thus precipitating an increase in cardiac work load and an increase in circulating volume.
b. Sudden onset of dyspnea.
c. Severe anxiety, restlessness, irritability.
d. Cool, moist skin.
e. Tachycardia.
f. Jugular vein distention (JVD).
g. Severe coughing.
h. Noisy, wet respirations that do not clear with coughing.
i. Frothy, blood-tinged sputum.

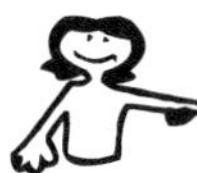

GERIATRIC PRIORITY: *Pulmonary edema can occur very rapidly become a medical emergency.*

3. Diagnostics.
a. Clinical manifestations.
b. Predisposing condition.

Treatment

(Condition demands immediate attention, medications are administered IV).
1. O_2 in high concentration.

2. Sedation (morphine) to allow controlled ventilation.
3. Diuretics to reduce the myocardial workload.
4. Dopamine to facilitate myocardial contractility.
5. Cardiac glycoside (**Digitalis**) to increase cardiac output.
6. Vasodilators to decrease afterload.

Nursing Intervention

✦ *Goal: to assess and decrease hypoxia (see Nursing Intervention, Hypoxia).*

✦ *Goal: to improve ventilation.*

1. Position in high-Fowler's with legs dependent.
2. Administer high levels of O_2.
3. Evaluate level of hypoxia and dyspnea; may need ET intubation and mechanical ventilation.
4. IV sedatives/narcotics.
   a. To decrease anxiety and dyspnea, and to decrease pressure in pulmonary capillary bed.
   b. Closely observe for respiratory depression.

NCLEX ALERT: *One of the few circumstances in which a client with respiratory distress will be given a narcotic. The fear of not being able to breathe is so strong that the client cannot cooperate. When a sedative/narcotic is administered, the nurse must be ready to support ventilation if respirations become severely depressed.*

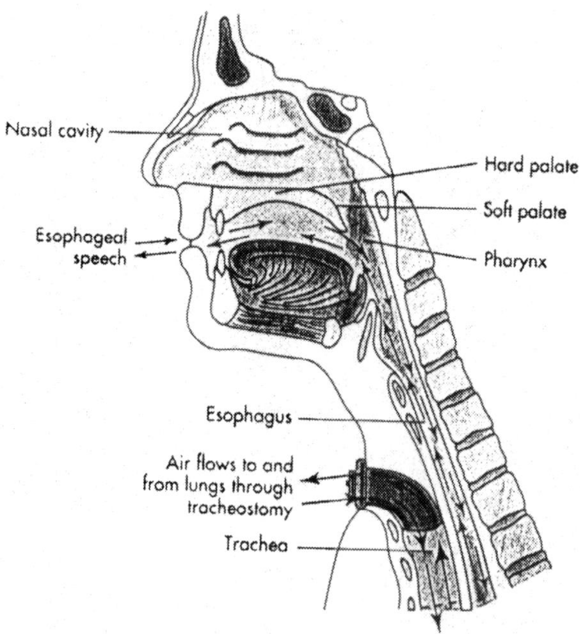

Figure 15-2: Permanent Tracheostomy.
Reprinted with permission: Phipps, WJ, Sands, JK, & Marek, JF (1999). *Medical Surgical Nursing: Concepts & Clinical Practice*, 6th ed. Philadelphia: Mosby, p. 892

5. Administer bronchodilators and evaluate client response as well as common side effects.

✦ *Goal: to reduce circulating volume and cardiac work load.*

1. Diuretics (Appendix 16-5).
2. Digitalis (Appendix 17-2.
3. Carefully monitor all IV fluids and evaluation of overall hydration status.
4. Do not elevate the client's legs as this will rapidly increase the venous return and the circulating volume.

✦ *Goal: to provide psychological support and decrease anxiety.*

1. Approach client in a calm manner.
2. Explain procedures.
3. Administer sedatives.
4. Remain with client in acute respiratory distress.

✦ *Goal: to prevent recurrence of problem.*

1. Recognize early stages.
2. Maintain client in semi-Fowler's position.
3. Decrease levels of activity.
4. Extreme precaution in administration of fluids and transfusions.

Cancer of the Larynx

❑ **A malignancy of the vocal cords or some other part of the larynx. The majority of growths are primary site. If detected early, this type of cancer is curable by surgical resection of the lesion. (See Cancer, Chapter 8.)**

Assessment

1. Risk factors/etiology.
   a. More common in men 50 to 65 years old.
   b. History of tobacco smoking or chewing.
   c. Chronic laryngitis.
2. Clinical manifestations (may be asymptomatic).
   a. Voice changes, hoarseness.
   b. Persistent sore throat, difficulty swallowing.
   c. Dysphagia, feeling of foreign body in throat.
   d. Tendency to aspirate.
   e. Weight loss.
   f. Dyspnea is late.
3. Diagnostics
   a. Direct laryngoscopic examination.
   b. Biopsy of the lesion involved.
   c. CT scan and MRI.

Treatment

(Varies with the extent of the malignancy.)

1. Radiation—generally over several weeks; most successful when cancer is diagnosed early.
2. Chemotherapy—generally not effective in advanced situations..
3. Surgical intervention.
   a. Partial laryngectomy—preserves the normal airway and normal speech mechanism. If a tracheotomy is performed, it is removed after the risk of swelling and airway obstruction.
   b. Total laryngectomy—requires a permanent tracheotomy for breathing and an alternative method of speaking.
   c. If laryngectomy surgery is required, a gastrostomy tube may be inserted to maintain nutrition after surgery.
   d. Laser surgery may be used for small vocal cord tumors and be able to preserve a usable voice.

Complications.

1. Airway obstruction.
2. Hemorrhage.
3. Fistula formation.

Nursing Intervention

✦ *Goal: to prepare client for surgery.*

1. General preoperative preparation (Chapter 3).
2. Consult with surgeon as to the anticipated extent of the surgery.
3. Discuss with client the possibility of a temporary tracheotomy or if tracheotomy is anticipated to be permanent.
4. Encourage ventilation of feelings regarding a temporary or a permanent loss of voice postoperative.
5. If total laryngectomy is anticipated, schedule a visit from the speech pathologist or member of the laryngectomy club to reassure client of rehabilitation potential.
6. Establish a method of communication for immediate postoperative period.
7. Discuss nutritional considerations postoperatively.

✦ *Goal: to maintain patent airway postoperative laryngectomy.*

1. If tracheotomy is not performed, evaluate for hematoma and increasing edema of the incisional area precipitating respiratory distress (Figure 15-2).
2. Position in semi-Fowler's.
3. Humidified oxygen therapy.
4. Observe for signs and symptoms of hypoxia.
5. Avoid analgesics that depress respiration.
6. Promote good pulmonary hygiene.
7. If tracheostomy is present, suction as indicated (See Appendix 15-6).

✦ *Goal: to identify and control hemorrhage.*

1. Blood tinged sputum is expected for about 48 hours after tracheotomy.
2. Observe for pulsations of tracheostomy tube, it may be resting on the innominate artery.
3. Assess for hematoma or unilateral swelling.
4. Observe for mild bleeding, may occur prior to hemorrhage.

✦ *Goal: to promote nutrition postoperative laryngectomy.*

1. Method of nutritional intake depends on the extent of the surgical procedure.(See Appendix 18-9 for tube feedings.)
2. Gastrostomy tubes are frequently utilized until the suture line begins to heal.
3. Feedings may be started after initial edema has subsided.
4. Good oral hygiene, may need to suction oral cavity of client cannot swallow.
5. Treat nausea quickly to avoid vomiting.
6. Soft nonirritating foods when oral nutrition begins.
7. For a partial laryngectomy, the possibility of aspiration is a primary concern during the first few days after surgery.

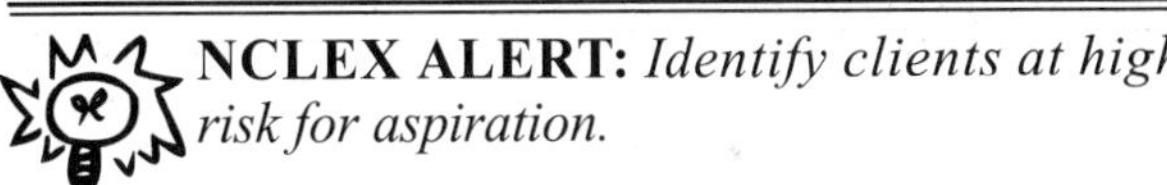
NCLEX ALERT: *Identify clients at high risk for aspiration.*

✦ *Goal: to identify resources for speech rehabilitation postoperative laryngectomy.*

1. If some of the vocal cord is left, client will have gradual improvement in voice; generally allowed to begin whispering two to three days postoperatively.
2. Follow-up visit from laryngectomy club member.
3. Arrange counseling with speech pathologist.
4. Identify different methods for speech management - esophageal speech, artificial larynx, etc.

Self Care

1. Encourage client to begin own suctioning and caring for the tracheostomy prior to leaving the hospital.
2. Assist the family in obtaining equipment for home use.
   a. System for humidification of air in home environment.
   b. Suction equipment necessary for tracheostomy care.

c. Equipment for care of the tracheostomy.
3. Precautions to take during showering.
4. Activities are encouraged.
5. Client should carry appropriate identification.

Cancer of the Lung

❑ **This is a tumor arising from within the lung. It may represent the primary site or may be a metastatic site from a primary lesion elsewhere. (See Cancer, Chapter 8.)**

Assessment

1. Risk factors.
   a. Smoking.
   b. Increased in males.
   c. Occupational exposure to and inhalation of irritants.
2. Clinical manifestations.
   a. Persistent chronic cough.
   b. Cough initially nonproductive, then becomes productive of purulent sputum.
   c. Hemoptysis.
   d. Recurring fever.
   e. Common sites of metastasis.
      (1) Liver.
      (2) Long bones.
      (3) Brain.
      (4) Vertebral column.
      (5) Lymph nodes - mediastinum,
   f. Pain is a late manifestation.
3. Diagnostics.
   a. Chest x-ray.
   b. Cytologic exam of the sputum.
   c. Bronchoscopy and biopsy.

Treatment

(Varies with extent of the malignancy.)

1. Radiation.
2. Surgery - treatment of choice early in condition..
   a. Lobectomy—removal of one lobe of the lung.
   b. Pneumonectomy—removal of the entire lung.
   c. Wedge and segmental resection - removal of a small area or a segment of the lung.
3. Chemotherapy.

Nursing Intervention

✦ *Goal: to prepare client for surgery.*

1. General preoperative preparations (Chapter 3).
2. Improve quality of ventilation prior to surgery.
   a. No smoking.
   b. Bronchodilator.
   c. Good pulmonary hygiene.
3. Discuss anticipated activities in the immediate postoperative period.
4. Encourage ventilation of feelings regarding diagnosis and impending surgery.
5. Establish baseline data for comparison postoperatively.
6. Orient client to the intensive care unit, if indicated.

✦ *Goal: to maintain patent airway and promote ventilation postoperative thoracotomy.*

1. Removal of secretions from tracheobronchial tree, either by coughing or suctioning.
2. Have client cough frequently and deep breathe.
3. Assessment of vital signs, correlate with sputum evaluation and auscultation of breath sounds.
4. Supplemental O_2 as indicated.
5. Control of pain so client can take deep breaths and cough.
6. Do not position the wedge resection or lobe resected client on the affected side for extended periods of time, this will hinder the expansion of the lung left on that side. If in stable condition, position in semi-Fowler's to promote optimum ventilation.

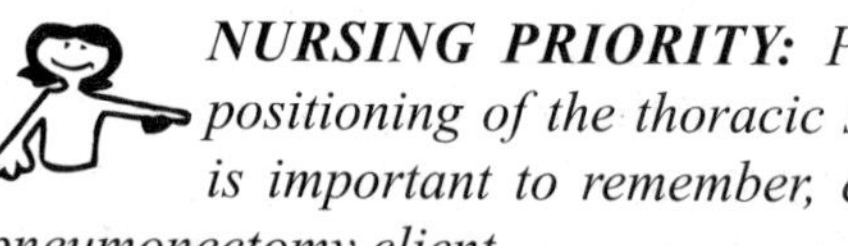

***NURSING PRIORITY:** Postoperative positioning of the thoracic surgery client is important to remember, especially the pneumonectomy client.*

7. If the pneumonectomy client experiences increased dyspnea, position them in semi-Fowler's. If positioned on the operative side, it may put increased tension on the suture line, if positioned on the unaffected side it will decrease lung expansion and inhibit ventilation.
8. Encourage ambulation as soon as possible.
9. Assess level of dyspnea at rest and with activity.
10. Maintain water-sealed drainage system (See Appendix 15-4. The pneumonectomy client will not have chest tubes, as no lung is left in the pleural cavity.)

✦ *Goal: to assess and support cardiac function postoperative thoracotomy.*

1. Monitor for dysrhythmias.
2. Assess adequacy of cardiac output.
3. Evaluate hourly urine output.
4. Administer fluids and transfusions with extreme caution; client is very conducive to development of pulmonary edema.

5. Evaluate fluid and electrolyte status.

✦ *Goal: to maintain normal range of motion and function of the affected shoulder postoperative thoracotomy.*

1. Skeletal exercises to increase abduction and mobility of the shoulders.
2. Encourage progressive exercises.

✦ *Goal: to assist client to understand measures to promote health postoperative thoracotomy.*

1. No more smoking; avoid respiratory irritants.
2. Decreased strength is common for approximately three weeks.
3. Continue activities and exercises.
4. Stop any activity that causes shortness of breath, chest pain, or undue fatigue.
5. Avoid lifting heavy objects until complete healing has occurred.
6. Return for follow-up care as indicated.

Study Questions—Respiratory System

1. First day postoperatively after a right lower lobe (RLL) lobectomy, the client deep breathes and coughs but has difficulty raising mucus. What indicates that the client is not adequately clearing secretions?

① Chest x-ray shows right-sided pleural fluid.
② A few scattered crackles on RLL auscultation.
③ PCO_2 increases from 35 to 45 mm Hg.
④ Decrease in forced vital capacity.

2. What nursing observation indicates that the cuff on an endotracheal tube is leaking?

① Rise in peak pressure on ventilator.
② Client is able to speak.
③ Increased swallowing efforts by client.
④ Increased crackles (rales) over left lung field.

3. The client with chronic obstructive pulmonary disease (COPD) is to be discharged home on continuous oxygen at 2 liters per minute via cannula. What information does the nurse provide to the client and his wife regarding the use of oxygen at home?

① Because of his need for oxygen, the client will have to limit activity at home.
② The use of oxygen will eliminate the client's shortness of breath.
③ Precautions are necessary because oxygen can spontaneously ignite and explode.
④ Oxygen will help to relieve the strain on the client's heart.

4. What symptoms would the nurse expect to observe in a 19-month-old client with a diagnosis of laryngotracheobronchitis?

① Predominant stridor on inspiration.
② Predominant expiratory wheeze.
③ High fever.
④ Slow respiratory rate.

5. The wife of a client with obstructive pulmonary disease (COPD) is worried about caring for her husband at home. Which statement by the nurse provides the most valid information?

① "You should avoid emotional situations that increase his shortness of breath."
② "Help your husband arrange activities so that he does as little walking as possible."
③ "Arrange a schedule so your husband does all necessary activities before noon; then he can rest during the afternoon and evening."
④ "Your husband will be more short of breath when he walks, but that will not hurt him."

6. Which statement correctly describes suctioning through an endotracheal tube?

① The catheter is inserted into the endotracheal tube; intermittent suction is applied until no further secretions are retrieved; the catheter is then withdrawn.
② The catheter is inserted through the nose and the upper airway is suctioned; the catheter is then removed from the upper airway and inserted into the endotracheal tube to suction the lower airway.
③ With suction applied, the catheter is inserted into the endotracheal tube; when resistance is met, the catheter is slowly withdrawn.
④ The catheter is inserted into the endotracheal tube to a depth of approximately 18 to 20 inches; suction is applied during withdrawal.

7. While a client's wife is visiting, she observes the client's chest tube bottle and begins to nervously question the nurse you regarding the amount of bloody drainage in the bottle. What is the best response by the nurse?

① "Your husband has been really sick; this must be a very difficult time, let's sit down and talk about it."
② "I have checked all of the equipment and it is working fine; you do not need to worry about it."
③ "The bottle contains approximately 300cc of normal saline; there is not as much blood in it as there appears to be."
④ "The chest tube is draining the secretions from his chest, it is important for him to deep breath frequently."

8. The nurse is caring for an infant experiencing respiratory distress and is being treated with CPAP (continuous positive airway pressure). The nurse is aware that for this treatment to be most effective the infant must be:

① Intubated and maintained on a controlled ventilation.
② Able to breath spontaneously.
③ Frequently stimulated to maintain respiratory rate.
④ Suctioned frequently to maintain alveolar ventilation.

9. The nurse is assessing a client with an endotracheal tube in place. What data confirms that the tube has migrated too far into the trachea?

① Decreased breath sounds over the left chest.
② There are increased rhonchi at the lung bases bilaterally.
③ Client is able to speak and there is excessive coughing.
④ Ventilator continues to alarm indicating decreased oxygen tension.

10. In which position does the nurse in the recovery room place a 6-year-old client following a tonsillectomy?

① Semi-Fowler's position, with the head turned to the side.
② Prone position, with the head of the bed slightly elevated.
③ On the back, with the head turned to the right side.
④ On the abdomen, with the head turned to the side.

11. The child's mother and father are both carriers of the cystic fibrosis gene, what is the genetic bases for the child to have cystic fibrosis?

① One out of every 4 offspring will have cystic fibrosis.
② The probability of producing an affected child is 25 percent with each pregnancy.
③ Since the mother and father are both positive for the gene, all of the children will be carriers.
④ Cystic fibrosis is inherited as a autosomal dominant trait and all children will be carriers.

12. The nurse understands that clamping a chest tube may cause what problem?

① Atmospheric pressure to enter the lung
② Tension pneumothorax
③ Bacterial infections in the pleural cavity.
④ Decrease in the rate and depth of respirations.

13. The nurse hears wheezing in the asthma client. What is the cause of this type of lung sound?

① Increased inspiratory pressure in the upper airways.
② Dilation of the respiratory bronchioles and increased mucus.
③ Movement of air through the narrowed airways.
④ Increased pulmonary compliance.

14. What is a finding on the nursing assessment that is associated with a diagnosis of pneumonia?

① Diminished breath sounds.
② Accessory use of thoracic muscles.
③ Hematemesis in the morning.
④ Dry hacking cough at night.

15. What is the procedure to non-invasively measure arterial oxygen levels?

① Pulse oximetry.
② Spriometry.
③ Blood gases.
④ Venogram.

16. Chronic obstructive pulmonary disease (COPD) clients are usually on low does oxygen via nasal cannula. The nurse understands that what problem may occur if the client receives too much oxygen?

① Hyperventilation.
② Tachypnea.
③ Hypoventilation or apnea.
④ Increased snoring.

17. A client has a diagnosis of right empyema. A thoracentesis procedure is to be done in the client's room. The nurse will place the client in what position for this procedure?

① Prone position with feet elevated.
② Sitting with upper torso over bedside table.
③ Lying on left side with right knee bent.
④ Semi-Fowler's with lower torso flat.

18. A client has thick pulmonary secretions. The nurse would anticipate which classification of medication to be ordered?

① Antihistamine.
② Expectorant.
③ Decongestant.
④ Bronchodilator.

19. A client has a history of atherosclerotic heart disease with a sustained increase in his blood pressure. What side effect may occur and is important to discuss with this client prior to his use of an over the counter decongestant?

① Urinary frequency and diuresis.
② Bradycardia and diarrhea.
③ Vasoconstriction and increased arterial pressure.
④ Headache and dysrhythmias

20. The nurse knows that immobility, estrogen therapy, and open reduction of a fractured femur all have the potential to cause what complication?

① Blood pressure fluctuation.
② Tachycardia and dysrhythmias.
③ Increased skin breakdown.
④ Pulmonary embolus.

21. Inflammation found in the bronchial tree of a client with acute bronchitis causes what problems?

① Increased temperature and headache
② Hyperventilation and bradycardia.
③ Sore throat with tachypnea.
④ Production of sputum and frequent cough.

22. A client complains of chest pain while breathing. The nurse hears a rubbing friction sound when auscultating the breath sounds. What is the nurses interpretation of this information?

① Bronchovesicular breath sounds are present.
② Client has angina with tactile fremitus.
③ A pleural friction rub is present.
④ Fluid is accumulating in the client's lungs.

23. What would the nurse expect to be present on the admission assessment of a client with chronic bronchitis?

① Peripheral edema, chest pain and hemoptysis.
② Dyspnea, productive cough, and wheezing.
③ Wheezing, dry cough, and peripheral edema.
④ Tachycardia, cyanosis, and non-productive cough.

24. The nurse is monitoring a client who is experiencing an acute asthma attack. What observations would indicate an improvement in the client's condition?

① Respiratory rate of 18 breaths per minute.
② Pulse oximetry of 88%.
③ Pulse rate of 110 beats per minute.
④ Productive cough with rapid breathing.

25. What complication might occur in a client who is experiencing an increasing problem with bronchospasm?

① Metabolic alkalosis.
② Hypertension.
③ Respiratory arrest.
④ Pneumonia.

26. For a chronic obstructive pulmonary client, what is the main risk factor that leads to a problem with pulmonary infection?

① Fluid imbalance with pitting edema.
② Pooling of respiratory secretions.
③ Decreased fluid intake and loss of body weight.
④ Decreased anterior-posterior diameter of his chest.

27. A client with active tuberculosis is admitted. The nurse would assess the client for what indications of an active disease process?

① Cough, low grade fever and night sweats.
② Tachycardia, oliguria, night sweats.
③ Upper body rash, night sweats, coughing.
④ Dyspnea, pleural edema, lack of appetite.

28. The nurse is checking a fellow employee's TB skin test. The employees forearm has a raised red area about 11mm in diameter after 72 hours. What is the best interpretation of this skin test?

① The skin reaction is negative.
② There is an allergy to the serum
③ Active tuberculosis is present.
④ Positive antibody response to TB bacillus.

29. An adult client is on 60% FIO_2, PO_2 is 58, and PCO_2 is 30mm HG. He is experiencing symptoms of tachypnea and tachycardia. The nurse would continue to closely assess the client for the development of what complication?

① Pneumonia.
② Chronic airflow limitation.
③ Cor pulmonale.
④ Acute respiratory distress syndrome.

Appendix 15-1: PULMONARY DIAGNOSTICS

X-RAYS:

CHEST X-RAY:
An X-ray of the lungs and chest wall; no specific pre- or post- care.

BRONCHOSCOPY:
Provides for direct visualization of larynx, trachea, bronchi; client is generally NPO for six hours prior to the exam; preoperative medication is given and the client's upper airway is anesthetized topically.
Nursing implications: after the exam, evaluate the client for return of gag reflex. Keep patient NPO until return of gag reflex. Bronchial washing or brushing may be done to obtain cells for cytology. Observe client for development of pneumothorax.

PULMONARY ANGIOGRAPHY:
Contrast material is injected into the pulmonary arteries and the angiography permits visualization of the pulmonary vasculature; definitive diagnosis for pulmonary emboli requires pulmonary angiography. May be sedated; exam is conducted in the X-ray department under fluoroscopic visualization.
Contraindications: (1) dye allergies, (2) unstable client, (3) uncooperative clients.
Complications: (1) cardiac dysrhythmias, (2) anaphylactic reaction to dye, (3) risk of death.

PATH-LAB STUDIES

SPUTUM STUDIES:
Best collected in the morning before the patient eats or drinks. Sputum should come from deep in the lungs.
Client should be instructed to rinse mouth out with water prior to collection, to decrease contamination.
Culture and Sensitivity (C & S) - obtained in order to determine presence of pathogenic bacteria; also determines to which antibiotic the specific organism is sensitive. Should be collected before anti-microbial therapy is started.
Acid-Fast Bacilli - sputum collection and analysis when tuberculosis is suspected.
Cytology - tumors in pulmonary system may slough cells into the sputum.

PULMONARY FUNCTION STUDIES:
Studies may be done for several reasons:(1) preoperative evaluation of pulmonary function; (2) evaluation of response to bronchodilator therapy; (3) differential diagnosis of pulmonary disease.
The client must be alert and cooperative; he/she should not be sedated. The client is taken to the pulmonary function laboratory and is asked to breathe into a cylinder from which a computer interprets and records data in specific values. Client should not smoke or use bronchodilating medications 6 hours prior to test.

PULSE OXIMETRY:
Measurement is made by placing a sensor on the finger or earlobe; a beam of light passes through the tissue and measures the amount of oxygen saturated hemoglobin. If probe is placed on the finger, remove any nail polish. Provides a method for continuously evaluating the oxygen saturation levels. It is non-invasive and there are no pre- or post- oximetry preparations. Readings may be incorrect if severe vasoconstriction has occurred or if PaO_2 is below 70%. Normal range is 95% or higher.

ARTERIAL BLOOD GAS STUDIES (ABGs): Measurement of the pH and partial pressures of dissolved gases (O_2, CO_2) of the arterial blood; requires approximately 3 cc of arterial blood, obtained through an arterial puncture. If client's O_2 concentration or ventilatory settings have been changed, or if a client has been suctioned, ABGs should not be drawn for at least 30 minutes (see Table 15-1 Normal ABG Values). Pressure should be maintained at the puncture site for a minimum of 5 minutes. The arterial blood sample should be tightly sealed and placed on ice.

THORACENTESIS:
Withdrawal of fluid from the pleural cavity; utilized for diagnostic as well as therapeutic purposes.
Nursing Implications:
1. Explain procedure to client.
2. Position client.
   a. Sitting on the side of the bed with the arms and head over the bedside table.
   b. If unable to assume sitting position, place on affected side with the head of the bed slightly elevated. Area containing fluid collection should be dependent.
   c. If client has a malignancy, cytotoxic drugs may be infused into the pleural space.
3. Support and reassure the client during the procedure.
4. After the procedure, position the client on his side with puncture side up, or in semi-Fowler's position, and monitor breath sounds.

Appendix 15-1: PULMONARY DIAGNOSTICS

MANTOUX SKIN TEST:
Does not determine if a client has active tuberculosis; a positive indicates that the client has been infected with the tubercle bacillus and has developed antibodies (sensitized). Purified protein derivative (PPD) is injected intradermally in the forearm. Results are read in 48-72 hours.

Nursing Implications:

1. Intradermal injection - a small needle (25 gauge) is used to inject 0.1 cc of purified protein derivative (PPD) under the skin. The needle is inserted bevel up; a raised area or "wheal" (6-10mm) will form under the skin.
2. The most common area for injection is the inside surface of the forearm.
3. Do not aspirate; do not massage area.
4. The client should be given specific directions to return, or plans should be made to read the test in 48 to 72 hours.
5. Interpretation: The area of induration is measured, not the area of erythema or inflammation.
   a. 5mm induration or more is positive in immunosuppresed clients, or people who have been recently exposed to active TB.
   b. 10mm induration is positive for people who are at increased risk of infection. This includes IV drug abusers, chronic medical conditions, children under 4 years, institutionalized people.
   c. 15mm induration is positive for people who do not meet any of the other criteria.
6. A chest X-ray, prophylactic medication and medical follow-up to determine if there is dormant TB, active TB, or the person was exposed and has an adequate immune response. It is also important to determine when and where the person came in contact with the TB bacillus.

NUCLEAR MEDICINE

LUNG SCAN: (V/Q Scan)
A procedure to determine defects in blood perfusion in the lung; particularly useful in the client suspected of having a pulmonary embolus or a ventilation/perfusion problem. For the perfusion component, a radioactive dye is injected and the specific uptake is recorded on X-ray film. For the ventilation portion, the patient breathes the tracer element through a face mask with a mouthpiece. Client not sedated or on dietary restrictions for the exam.

Appendix 15-2: RESPIRATORY MEDICATIONS

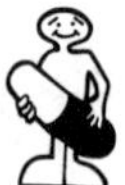

MEDICATIONS	SIDE EFFECTS	NURSING IMPLICATIONS

BRONCHODILATORS: Relax smooth muscle of the bronchi, promoting bronchodilation and reducing airway resistance. Also inhibits the release of histamine.

❖GENERAL NURSING IMPLICATIONS❖

— Metered Dose Inhalers (MDI) - hand-held pressurized devices that deliver a measured dose of drug with each "puff." When two "puffs" are needed, one minute should lapse between the two "puffs." A spacer may be used to increase the delivery of the medication.

—Dry Powder Inhalers (DPI) deliver more medication to lungs, does not require coordination as with MDI, one minute should lapse between "puffs".

— Bronchodilators - beta-$_2$ agonists and theophylline are given with caution in the cardiac client, since tachydysrhythmias and chest pain may occur.

— Aerosol delivery systems have less side effects and are more effective.

MEDICATIONS	SIDE EFFECTS	NURSING IMPLICATIONS
Epinephrine (**Adrenaline**): aerosol, SQ, IV	Headache Dizziness Hypertension Tremors Dysrhythmias	1. Do not use in clients with hypertension or dysrhythmias. 2. Primarily used to treat asthma attacks and anaphylactic reactions.
Theophylline (**Aminophylline**): PO, rectal, IV	Tachycardia Hypotension Nausea/vomiting Seizures	1. Theophylline blood levels should be drawn for long term use; therapeutic levels between 10-20 mcg/ml; above 20mcg/ml are toxic. 2. IV administration may cause rapid changes in vital signs. 3. Considered to be a third line drug for use with asthma.

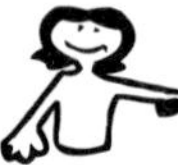

NURSING PRIORITY: *Monitor blood levels of medications.*

RAPID ACTING CONTROL

BETA$_2$ - AGONIST:

MEDICATIONS	SIDE EFFECTS	NURSING IMPLICATIONS
Albuterol (**Proventil, Ventolin**): MDI, DPI, PO Terbutaline (**Brethine**): aerosol, PO Pirbuterol (**Maxair**) MDI		1. Used for short term relief of acute reversible airway problems. 2. Not used on continuous basis in absence of symptoms. 3. Client teaching regarding proper use of MDI and DPI.

ANTI-CHOLINERGIC:

MEDICATIONS	SIDE EFFECTS	NURSING IMPLICATIONS
Ipratropium bromide (**Atrovent**) aerosol		1. Frequently used for COPD clients and severe asthmatics for treatment of acute airway problems. 2. Therapeutic effects begin within 30 seconds

LONG ACTING CONTROL

BETA$_2$-AGONIST:

MEDICATIONS	SIDE EFFECTS	NURSING IMPLICATIONS
Salmeterol (**Serevent**): DPI		1. Administered 2 times daily. 2. Not used for short-term relief, effects begin slowly and last for up to 12 hours.

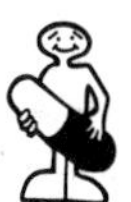

Appendix 15-2:
RESPIRATORY MEDICATIONS

MEDICATIONS	SIDE EFFECTS	NURSING IMPLICATIONS
LONG ACTING CONTROL		
CORTICOSTERIODS:		
Beclomethasone (**Beclovent**) MDI Triamcinolone acetonide (**Azmacort**) MDI	Oropharyngeal candidiasis, horseness	1. Works well with seasonal and exercise-induced asthma (EIA). 2. Prophylactic use decreases number and severity of attacks 3. May be used with beta-$_2$ agonist. 4. Gargle after each dose and use a spacer to decrease candidiasis.
NONSTERIODAL ANTIFLAMMATORY		
Cromolyn sodium (**Intal**) MDI Nedocromil sodium (**Tilade**)	Throat irritation, bad taste, cough	1. Prophylactic use decreases number and severity of attacks. 2. Prevents bronchoconstriction before exposure to known precipitant (e.g. exercise) 3. Administered via MDI - not for an acute attack.
LEUKOTRIENE MODIFIERS		
Montelukast (**Singular**) PO	Minimal side effects	1. Given to children over 6 years old. 2. Maximal effects develop within 24 hours.
Zafirlukast (**Accolate**) PO		1. Administer within 1 hour before or 2 hours after eating.

ANTITUBERCULAR: Broad-spectrum antibiotic specific to tubercle bacilli.

❖GENERAL NURSING IMPLICATIONS❖
— Client is not contagious when sputum culture is negative.
— Respiratory isolation when sputum is positive for bacilli.
— Treatment includes combination of medications for about 6 to 8 months.
— Monitor liver function studies for clients on combination therapy.
— Medications may be administered once daily or on a twice weekly schedule.
— Teach clients they should not stop taking the medications when they begin to feel better.
— Advise client to return to the doctor if he notices any yellowing of his skin or eyes, or begins to experience pain or swelling in joints, especially the big toe.

MEDICATIONS	SIDE EFFECTS	NURSING IMPLICATIONS
Isoniazid (**INH**): PO, IM	Peripheral neuritis Hypersensitivity Hepatotoxicity Gastric irritation	1. Administer with (pyridoxine) Vitamin B_6 to prevent peripheral neuritis. 2. Primary medication used in prophylactic treatment of tuberculosis.
Rifampin (**Rifadin**): PO	Peripheral neuropathy Hypersensitivity Gastric upset Hepatitis	1. Medication most commonly used with isoniazid. 2. May negate the effectiveness of birth control pills. 3. Body secretions may turn orange - urine, perspiration, tears.
Ethambutol (**EMG** or **Myambutol**): PO	Skin rash Gastric upset Peripheral neuritis Optic neuritis Increased uric acid levels	1. Frequently administered with rifampin and **INH**.
Pyrazinamide (**PZA Pyrazinamide**, **Fibrazid**): PO	Hepatotoxicity Increased uric acid levels	1. Should be taken concurrently with another antituberculosis agent.

Appendix 15-2: RESPIRATORY MEDICATIONS

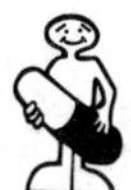

MEDICATIONS	SIDE EFFECTS	NURSING IMPLICATIONS
DECONGESTANTS: Produces decongestion by acting on sympathetic nerve endings to produce constriction of dilated arterioles.		
Ephedrine hydrochloride (**Bronkotabs, Tendral, Mini-Thins**): PO	Tremors Tachycardia Palpitations Nervousness Headache GI upset	1. Caution client regarding use of OTC medications (cough syrup, cold medications, allergy medications) as ephedrine is a common ingredient in all of these. 2. Cardiac and hypertensive clients should check with their physician prior to taking the medication. 3. May be abused by people seeking the increased CNS stimulation.
Phenylephrine hydrochloride (**Sinex, NEO-Synephrine, Rhinall, Sinarest Nasal**): PO, SQ, intra-nasal	Increased blood pressure Tachycardia Palpitations Trembling Light headedness	1. With intranasal preparations, rebound congestion may occur.
Phenylephrine (**Neo-Synephrine**): PO, nasal aerosol spray Pseudoephedrine: PO, nasal aerosol spray (**Sudafed**)	CNS stimulation, anxiety, insomnia	1. Will cause rebound congestion; caution clients to limit use of aerosol nasal sprays to 3 to 5 days. 2. Medications are frequently found in OTC combination decongestants.
ANTIHISTAMINE: Blocks histamine release at H_1 receptors.		
Diphenhydramine HCL (**Benadryl**): PO, IV, IM Clemastine (**Tavist**): PO Chlorpheniramine (**Chlortrimeton**): PO Loratadine (**Claritin**): PO Fexofenadine (**Allegra**): PO	Sedation Dysrhythmias Dry mouth	1. Used to treat mild allergic disorders. 2. Loratadine and terfenadine are non-sedating. 3. Antihistamines should not be taken during the third trimester of pregnancy. 4. May be found in numerous OTC combination medications. 5. Due to excessive drying effect, asthmatic clients should take medications only on recommendation of physician.
EXPECTORANT: Stimulates secretions. Reduces the viscosity of the mucus.		
Guaifenesin (**Robitussin**): PO	Nausea GI upset	1. Increase fluid intake for effectiveness.
ANTIVIRAL: Antiviral use for treatment of severe RSV in hospitalized children.		
Ribavirin (**Virazole**): aerosol	Anemia, increased respiratory problems	1. Should not be used with infants on mechanical ventilation. 2. Carefully monitor respiratory status of child. 3. Pregnant nurses should not have direct contact with medication.

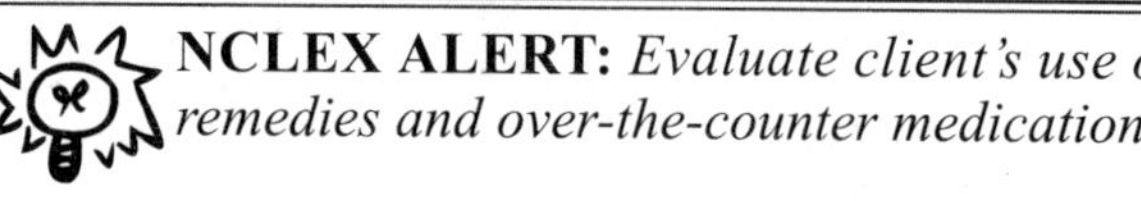

Appendix 15-3: SUDDEN AIRWAY OBSTRUCTION

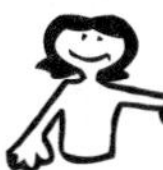

NURSING PRIORITY: *The procedure to remove airway obstruction is not effective in the child with epiglottitis or sudden airway obstruction due to inflammation of upper airways.*

✦ *GOAL: To identify respiratory obstruction.*

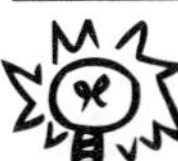

NCLEX ALERT: *If the adult client is coughing forcefully, do not interfere with attempts to cough and expel the foreign body. Do not administer any forceful blows to the back.*

1. If the victim can speak or cry, there is probably adequate air exchange.
2. If the victim cannot speak or cry but is conscious, proceed to implement abdominal thrusts to clear the obstructed airway.
3. If the victim is unconscious:
   a. Open the airway and evaluate breathing.
   b. If no evidence of breathing, attempt to ventilate via mouth to mouth or mouth to nose and mouth.
   c. If air does not enter the lungs, check for the patency of the airway and attempt to ventilate again.
   d. If still unable to ventilate, initiate procedure for relieving obstructed airway.

✦ *GOAL: To clear obstructed airway: Adult (conscious and unconscious).*

ADULT AND CHILD:

1. Conscious: Heimlich maneuver until obstruction is removed or victim becomes unconscious.
2. Unconscious: Evaluate airway and attempt to ventilate. If unable to ventilate, then proceed with steps for removal of foreign body.
   a. The rescuer kneels astride the victim's thighs; with the heel of the hand, apply forceful upward thrust to the abdomen well below the xiphoid and above the umbilicus.
   b. Administer 5 abdominal thrusts, return to the victim's head, evaluate the airway, attempt to ventilate. A blind sweep of the mouth may be done in adult with airway obstruction.
   c. If the above procedure does not relieve the airway, the steps for removal should be repeated until an open airway is established.
   d. Back blows are no longer recommended for relief of airway obstruction in the adult.

NCLEX ALERT: *The victim's airway must be cleared and ventilation established before continuing with further CPR efforts.*

✦ *GOAL: To clear obstructed airway: Infant (conscious and unconscious).*

1. Straddle the infant over the forearm with the head dependent.
2. Deliver 4 forceful back blows between the shoulder blades.
3. Supporting the head,, turn the infant back over and administer four chest thrusts (lower one-third of the sternum,, approximately one finger breadth below the nipple line).
4. Attempt to remove foreign body if it can be visualized.

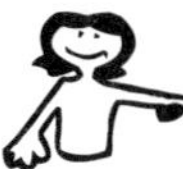

NURSING PRIORITY: *Do not do a blind sweep of the infant or child's mouth; the foreign body should be visualized before attempting to sweep the mouth.*

Appendix 15-4: WATER-SEALED CHEST DRAINAGE

PURPOSE:

1. To remove air and fluid from the pleural cavity.
2. To restore negative pressure in the pleural cavity and promote re-expansion of the lung.

PRINCIPLE OF WATER-SEALED CHEST DRAINAGE:

The water seal serves as a one-way valve; it prevents air, under atmospheric pressure, from re-entering the pleural cavity. On inspiration, air and fluid leave the pleural cavity via the chest tube; the water-seal keeps the air and fluid from re-entering. Both chest bottles and Pleur-Evac work on the same principle of water-sealed drainage systems.

NURSING PRIORITY: *There must be a water-seal between the client and the atmospheric pressure. In the bottle setup, the chest tube from the client must go under water before being exposed to the atmospheric pressure. In the Pleur-evac system, there is a water-sealed chamber between the client and the atmospheric pressure.*

EQUIPMENT:

Pleur-evac - a type of molded, plastic system that provides a three-chamber system. There is a waterseal chamber, a collection chamber and a suction control chamber. When suction is applied there should be a continuous, gentle bubbling in the suction control chamber.

One-bottle system - chest tube from client goes through underwater seal and drainage is accomplished by gravity. It is the simplest water-sealed system. Prior to the chest tube being connected, approximately 300 cc of normal saline is poured into the bottle. The chest tube is connected to the bottle opening that has a glass or plastic tube that extends approximately 2 cm under water. The amount of saline should be carefully marked on the bottle. The chest bottle serves both as the collection reservoir, and as the underwater seal. A positive pressure in the pleural space will force air and fluid out the chest tube; the air will bubble out, but the water-seal prevents air from being drawn back into the pleural cavity.

NURSING IMPLICATIONS:

Assessment
1. Evaluate character of respirations.
2. Evaluate for hypoxia.
3. Assess for symmetrical chest wall expansion.
4. Evaluate breath sounds bilaterally.
5. Palpate around insertion site for subcutaneous emphysema.

Intervention
1. Range of motion of the affected arm and shoulder.
2. Encourage coughing and deep breathing every two hours.
3. Encourage ambulation if appropriate.
4. Pain medications as indicated.
5. Low-or semi-Fowler's position.

Observe drainage system for proper functioning.
1. Water level in tubing from the client should fluctuate (tidal): rise on inspiration and fall on expiration.
2. Continuous bubbling should not occur in the fluid where water-seal is maintained; continuous bubbling indicates an air leak; continuous bubbling should occur only in the system that maintains a third chamber for suction control.
3. Initial bubbling may occur with coughing or with deep respiration as air is moved out of the pleural cavity.
4. Place a piece of tape on the outside of the drainage collection bottle to monitor amount of drainage. Be sure to indicate initial water added to bottle to establish water-seal.

Appendix 15-4: WATER-SEALED CHEST DRAINAGE

Maintain water-sealed system.

1. Keep all drainage equipment below level of client's chest.
2. Evaluate for dependent loops in the tubing; this increases the resistance to the drainage. All extra tubing should be coiled in the bed and flow in a straight line to the system.
3. Tape all connections.
4. Note characteristics and amount of drainage. Mark level on the drainage system PRN and every eight hours.
5. Vigorous "milking" or stripping chest tubes is controversial. Stripping or milking may be done when the chest tube becomes occluded with a clot, most often in the immediate postoperative time. Stripping should not be done routinely on all clients.
6. Change collection chamber when approximately half full. The increased volume in the collection chamber increases resistance to flow of drainage. It is institution policy whether the nurse can change the collection chamber.

Figure 15-3: Water Sealed Chest Drainage
Reprinted with permission: Phipps, WJ, Sands, JK, & Marek, JF (1999). *Medical Surgical Nursing: Concepts & Clinical Practice*, 6th ed. Philadelphia: Mosby, p.956

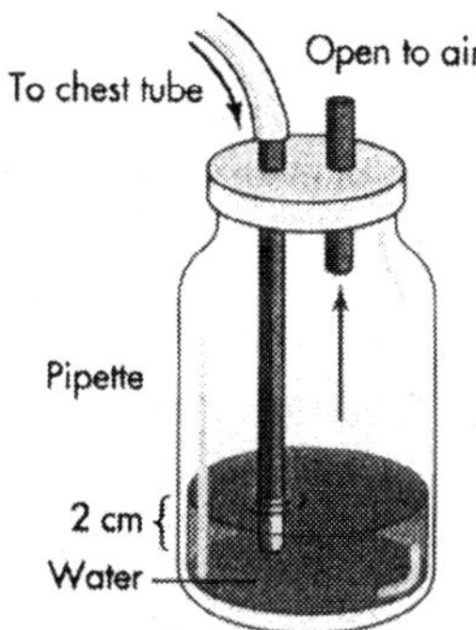

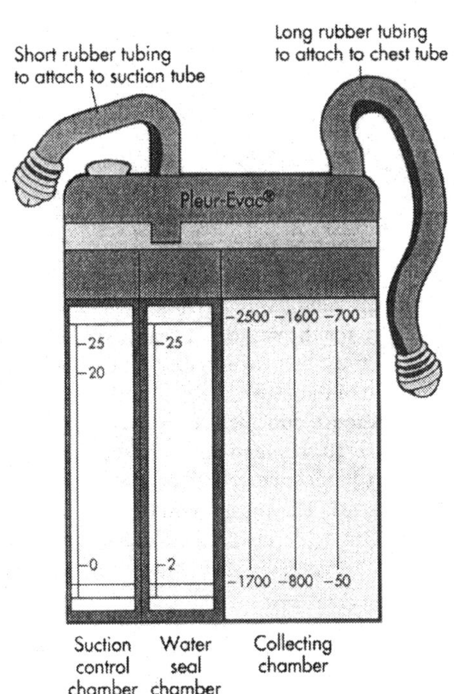

Appendix 15-4:
WATER-SEALED CHEST DRAINAGE

NCLEX ALERT: *Determine if chest drainage is functioning properly; adjust tubes to promote drainage; identify abvnormal chest tube drainage.*

Chest tube removal.

1. Criteria for removal of the tube:
   a. Minimum or no drainage.
   b. Fluctuations stop in the water-seal chamber.
   c. Chest X-ray reveals expanded lung.
   d. Client is breathing comfortably.
2. Procedure.
   a. Obtain equipment.
   b. Generally, the physician will want the client in a low-or semi-Fowler's position unless contraindicated.
   c. The physician will ask the client to exhale and hold it or to exhale and bear down. Either of these procedures will increase the intrathoracic pressure and prevent air from entering the pleural space.
   d. With the client holding his breath, the physician will quickly remove the tube and place an occlusive bandage over the area; client can then breathe normally.
   e. Assess the client's tolerance of the procedure; a chest X-ray should be done to determine that the lungs remain fully expanded.

Appendix 15-5:
ARTIFICIAL AIRWAYS

ENDOTRACHEAL INTUBATION:

Placement of an endotracheal (ET) tube through the mouth or nose into the trachea.

PURPOSE:

To provide an immediate airway; to maintain a patent airway; to facilitate removal of secretions to provide method for artificial ventilation.

Nursing Interventions:

1. Provide warm, humidified oxygen.
2. Establish method of communication since the client cannot speak; child cannot cry.
3. Maintain safety measures.
   a. Prevent client from removing tube inadvertently.
   b. Secure ET tube to the face.
   c. Child with an ET tube requires constant attendance.
4. As soon as tube is inserted and frequently afterwards assess symmetry of chest expansion and bilateral breath sounds. If tube slips farther into the trachea, it may pass into the right main stem bronchus, obliterating the left main-stem bronchus. Determine placement by checking breath sounds. After tube has been inserted, an Easy Cap can be placed over the end of the ET tube to determine oxygen saturation of exhaled air which will help to verify tube placement.
5. Cuff must remain inflated if client is on a volume ventilator or receiving IPPB treatments. If the client has adequate spontaneous respiration and is not on a ventilator, the cuff may be left deflated.
6. Provide oral hygiene; assess for pressure areas on the nose or the mouth.
7. Suction as indicated (see Appendix 15-6).

Appendix 15-5: ARTIFICIAL AIRWAYS

TRACHEOSTOMY:

A surgical opening into the trachea.

PURPOSE:
To maintain airway over an extended period of time; to facilitate removal of secretions.

Nursing Interventions:

1. Provide warm, humidified oxygen.
2. Establish method of communication, since client cannot speak; child is unable to cry.
3. Maintain safety measures.
   a. Secure tracheal tube to the client's neck.
   b. Prevent clothing or bed covers from occluding area of tracheal opening.
   c. Child with a tracheostomy requires continuous attendance.
4. Assess for symmetrical expansion of chest wall and bilateral breath sounds.
5. Maintain oral hygiene.
6. Inflate tracheostomy cuff during tube feedings or feedings by mouth.
7. Cuff must remain inflated if client is on a volume ventilator or receiving IPPB treatments. If the client has adequate spontaneous respiration, the cuff may be left deflated.
8. Suction as indicated (see Appendix 15-6).
9. The tracheal tube obturator should be taped to the head of the bed. If the tracheostomy tube is accidentally removed, the obturator is necessary for replacing the tube.
10. A fenestrated trach tube can be adapted so air will flow throughout normal passages; frequently used when client is beginning to be weaned from the ventilator. If client has respiratory difficulty when the inner cannula is removed, then immediately reinsert the cannula to provide tracheal airway. The tube can also be plugged so client can speak cough through normal airway. Make sure the cuff is deflated prior to plugging the tracheostomy.

NCLEX ALERT: *Provide tracheostomy care.*

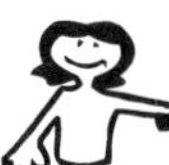

NURSING PRIORITY: *The cuff on a tracheostomy tube or on an ET tube is to facilitate the delivery of air to the lungs. The purpose of the cuff on either tube is not to maintain the tube position.*

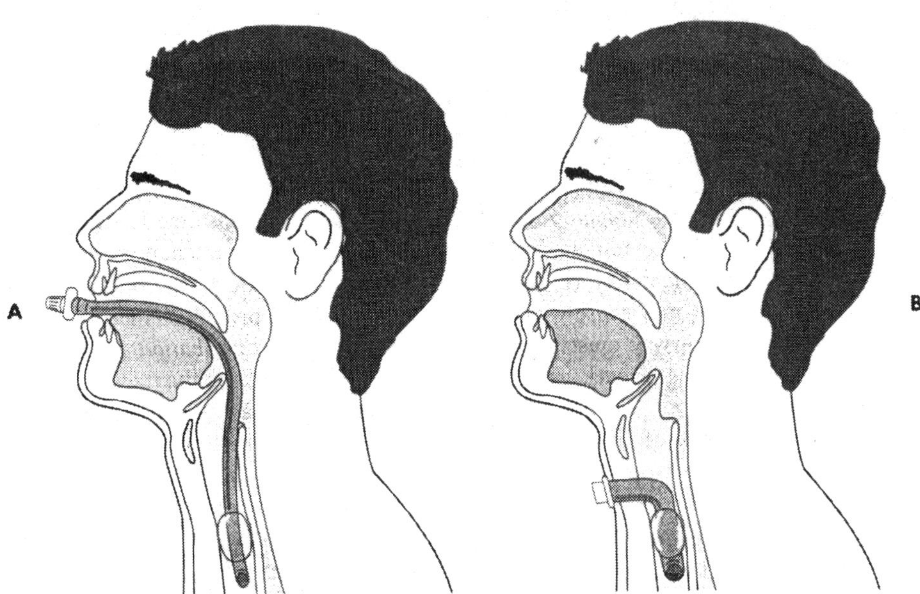

A, Position of endotracheal tube. **B,** Position of tracheostomy tube.

Figure 15-4: Position For Endotracheal/ Tracheostomy Tube.
Reprinted with permission: Phipps, WJ, Sands, JK, & Marek, JF (1999). *Medical Surgical Nursing: Concepts & Clinical Practice*, 6th ed. Philadelphia: Mosby, p.904

Appendix 15-6:
SUCTIONING THROUGH ARTIFICIAL AIRWAYS

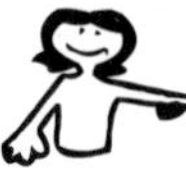

NURSING PRIORITY: *Suctioning the endotracheal tube or the tracheostomy is done to remove excess secretions and to maintain patent airway. The client should always be suctioned prior to deflating a cuff.*

1. Determine that the client needs to be suctioned.
   a. Auscultate lungs to detect presence of secretions.
   b. Observe client to see if he/she is experiencing immediate difficulty with removal of secretions.
2. Explain procedure if client is not familiar with it, or simply indicate to client that you are going to assist him/her with the removal of the secretions.
3. All equipment introduced into the trachea or the endotracheal tube should be sterile.
4. Prepare the equipment. Attach the suction catheter to the suction source while maintaining sterile glove and suction catheter.
5. If client is not in immediate danger of airway occlusion, hyperoxygenate with 100% O_2 for five to six minutes, or at least three hyperinflations.
6. Gently insert sterile catheter into the opening without suction being applied. Insert catheter to the point of slight resistance, then pull catheter back one to two centimeters.
7. Apply intermittent suction as you gently rotate the catheter on removal.
8. Each suctioning pass should not exceed 10 to 15 seconds in duration.
9. Reconnect client to oxygen source and evaluate if one suctioning episode was sufficient to remove secretions.
10. Hyperoxygenate client for 1-5 minutes after suctioning; assess vital signs and O_2 saturation, values should return to normal or to the previous levels prior to suctioning.
11. Avoid suctioning client prior to drawing arterial blood gases. Client should be allowed to stabilize for approximately 30 minutes prior to blood gases being drawn.
12. Monitor oximetry while suctioning, if oximetry does not come back to normal level immediately after suctioning, do not attempt to suction client again.

Complications of Suctioning:
1. Hypoxia -preoxygenate with high % of O_2 prior to and after suctioning.
2. Dysrhythmias -limit suctioning to 10-15 seconds, monitor rhythm during suctioning; if bradycardia develops, discontinue suctioning immediately .
3. Bronchospasm -try to time the suctioning with client's own cycle, insert tube during inspiration.
4. Airway trauma -maintain suction level below 120mm Hg.
5. Infection - use sterile technique; assess the color and quantity of sputum suctioned.
6. Atelectasis - use suction catheters that are approximately 1/3 or less of diameter of tube.

NCLEX ALERT: *Intervene to improve respiratory status, suction client's respiratory tract (oral, nasal, tracheostomy, and endotracheal tube).*

Appendix 15-7: OXYGEN

✦ *GOAL: The goal of oxygen therapy is to maintain an optimum level of oxygenation at the lowest effective level of FIO_2.*

METHODS OF ADMINISTRATION:
Oxygen is measured in liters per minute flow (LPM) — 2 to 8 LPM is the most commonly ordered range.

1. ***Low-flow systems*** - nasal cannula, standard mask, non-rebreather mask.
2. ***High-flow systems*** - Venturi mask, nebulizer mask, and volume ventilators. Oxygen is measured in fractions of inspired oxygen (FIO_2) in concentrations from 24% to 100% — 10 LPM is required to obtain accurate percentage flow.

HUMIDIFICATION:
1. Adds water vapor to inspired gas.
2. Prevents drying and irritation of respiratory membranes.
3. Loosens thick secretions, allowing them to be more easily removed.

INDICATIONS FOR OXYGEN ADMINISTRATION:
1. A decrease in oxygen in the arterial blood (hypoxemia).
2. An increase in the work of breathing.
3. Decrease the cardiac workload.

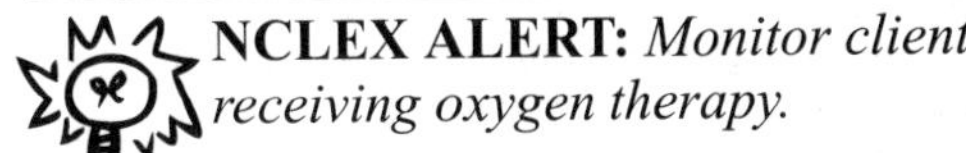

NCLEX ALERT: *Monitor client receiving oxygen therapy.*

OXYGEN SAFETY IN ADMINISTRATION:
1. Properly ground all electrical equipment.
2. Do not permit any smoking by anyone in the area.
3. Use water-base, not oil-base, lubricants.
4. Do not administer O_2 above 2-3 LPM to clients with chronic airway limitation (CAL).

OXYGEN TOXICITY:
A medically induced condition produced by inhalation of high concentrations of oxygen over a prolonged period of time. Toxicity is directly related to: concentration of oxygen, duration of therapy, degree of lung disease present.
1. Tracheal irritation and cough.
2. Dyspnea and increasing cough.
3. Decrease in vital capacity.
4. The PaO_2 continues to decrease, even with an increasing FIO_2.
5. Atelectasis.
6. Retrolental fibroplasia.

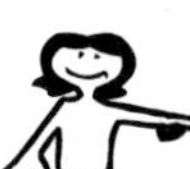

NURSING PRIORITY: *An arterial oxygen tension (PaO_2) of 150 mm Hg for four hours can cause retrolental fibroplasia in the neonate.*

Appendix 15-8: VENTILATORS

VOLUME-CYCLED VENTILATORS:

✦ Deliver air at a predetermined tidal volume. The machine delivers the volume of air within safe ranges of pressure. A pressure limit is set and an alarm will sound if the tidal volume cannot be delivered within the set pressure limits. The intrathoracic pressure is increased with the ventilator. This will decrease the venous blood return to the right side of the heart and subsequently decrease cardiac output.

Patterns Of Ventilation

1. **Assist** - the client initiates the cycle with inspiration.
2. **Controlled** -the machine controls rate and volume of the client's ventilatory cycle.
3. **Simulated intermittent mechanical ventilation (SIMV)** - delivers ventilation at inspiratory phase of client's spontaneous ventilation; may be used for weaning from ventilator.
4. **Positive end expiratory pressure (PEEP)** -maintains positive pressure at alveolar level at end expiration to facilitate the diffusion of oxygen. PEEP will increase the intrathoracic pressure, thus further decreasing the venous return.

Indications for use: acute respiratory failure (ARDS); clients unable to maintain patent airway; neuromuscular diseases causing respiratory failure.

5. **Continuous Positive Airway Pressure (CPAP)** -used to augment the functional residual capacity (FRC) during spontaneous breaths. Used to wean patients from ventilators and may be administered by face mask. Client or infant must have spontaneous respirations.

Nursing Implications:

NCLEX ALERT: *Identify changes in respiratory status and intervene to improve respiratory status.*

1. All alarms should be set and checked each shift.
2. An Ambu bag is placed in the client's room in case of mechanical failure of equipment.

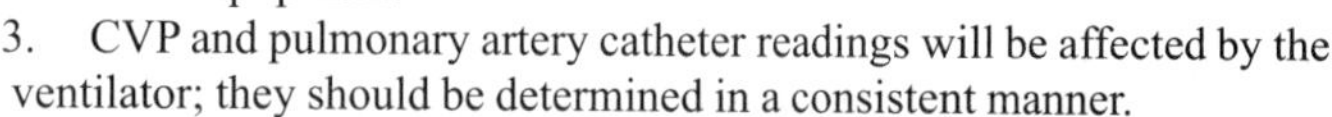

3. CVP and pulmonary artery catheter readings will be affected by the ventilator; they should be determined in a consistent manner.

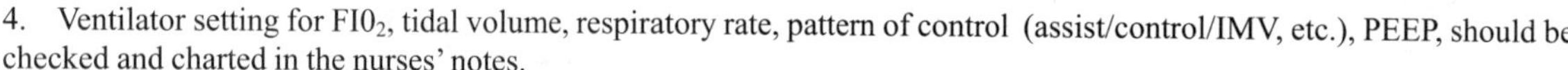

4. Ventilator setting for FIO_2, tidal volume, respiratory rate, pattern of control (assist/control/IMV, etc.), PEEP, should be checked and charted in the nurses' notes.
5. Assess client's tolerance of the ventilator; frequently, IV medications (Morphine, Pavulon, Valium) are utilized. If changes, weaning or removal of the ventilator are anticipated, do not medicate the client.
6. The client frequently experiences a high level of anxiety and fear. Explain equipment and alarms to the client and to the family. Maintain a calm, reassuring approach to the client.
7. When ventilator changes are made, carefully assess the client's response (pulse oximetry, vital signs).

Common Ventilator Alarms

1. High pressure alarm -occurs when tidal volume cannot be delivered at pressure limit.

Nursing Care: Increased secretions -suction; client biting tube -place oral airway; coughing and increased anxiety -administer sedative.

2. Low pressure alarm -occurs when the machine cannot deliver the tidal volume due to leak or break in the system.

Nursing Care: Disconnection - check all connections for break in system; client stops breathing on the SIMV mode -evaluate client tolerance; trach or ET tube cuff is leaking - check for air escaping around cuff, may need to replace trach tube if cuff is ruptured.

Weaning from Ventilators - may be done via SIMV, or T-piece on ET or trach with heated mist, or by pressure support ventilation from the ventilator. During weaning it is imperative the nurse maintain close observation for increasing dyspnea and hypoxia. If client becomes dyspneic, he should be returned to the ventilator at whatever parameters he was on and the doctor notified, anticipate ABGs to be drawn.

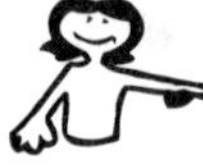

NURSING PRIORITY: *In case of problems with the ventilator, asses the client and if he is not being adequately ventilated, take him off the ventilator and maintain respirations via an ambu bag, and call for assistance.*

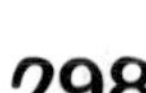

Appendix 15-9:
NURSING PROCEDURE ■ SPUTUM SPECIMEN COLLECTION ■

❑ Test analyzes sputum samples (material expectorated from client's lungs and bronchi during deep coughing) to diagnose respiratory disease, identify the cause of pulmonary infections, identify abnormal lung cells, and assist in managing pulmonary disease.

Key Points: Specimen Collection

- Encourage client to increase fluid intake the night before to assist in collecting specimen.
- Collect the specimen early in the morning, as bacteria is most concentrated at this time.
- No mouth wash prior to collection of specimen.
- Aerosal mist will assist to decrease thickness of sputum and increase effectiveness of coughing.
- Maintain strict asepsis and standard precautions in collecting and transporting specimen; utilize a sterile specimen collection container.
- Cytology specimens — obtain three morning specimens.
- Acid-fast bacillus — sputum collection over three consecutive days.
- Culture and sensitivity — initial specimen should be obtained before administering antibiotics.

Clinical Tips for Problem Solving

If client experiences pain while coughing,

Support painful area with roll pillows to minimize pain and discomfort.

Encourage client to take several deep breaths prior to beginning. This assists in triggering the cough reflex and areates the lungs.

If client is unable to obtain sputum specimen,

Attempt procedure early in the morning; when mucus production is greatest.

Notify physician to obtain orders for a bronchodilator or nebulization therapy.

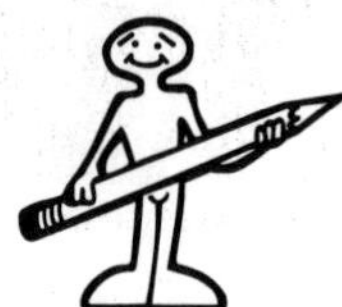

Notes

PHYSIOLOGY OF THE VASCULAR SYSTEM

Vessels

A. Arteries—primary function is to transport nutrients and oxygen to the cellular level.
   1. Elasticity allows for contraction and recoil in the cardiac cycle.
   2. Arterial vascular system is a high-pressure system with a rapid blood flow.

B. Capillaries—small microscopic vessels at the cellular level.
   1. Capillary bed is the area of circulation where the arterioles branch into capillaries and exchange between the circulating volume and the interstitial fluid occurs.
   2. Filtration, diffusion, and osmosis occur between the vascular compartment and the interstitial fluid compartment by means of the capillary bed.
   3. The interstitial fluid filters back through the capillary bed at the venous end through the venules, then into the larger venous vessels.

C. Veins—primary function of the veins is to return blood to the heart.
   1. Veins contain valves to prevent the back flow of blood and maintain direction of blood flow.
   2. Venous system is a low pressure system.

D. Circulatory systems.
   1. Systemic circulation—the flow of blood from the heart into the aorta through the arteries to the capillary bed where cellular nutrition and oxygenation occur.
   2. Pulmonary circulation—the flow of blood from the right ventricle through the pulmonary artery into the lungs, through the capillary beds of the lungs where the blood picks up oxygen and releases carbon dioxide and returns back into the left ventricle through the pulmonary veins.
   3. Hepatic-portal circulation—the flow of blood from the venous system of the stomach, intestines, spleen, and pancreas into the portal vein and through the liver for removal of foreign material; venous blood leaves the liver through the hepatic vein and into the vena cava for return to the heart.

E. Lymphatic system—primary function is to return fluid and protein to the blood from the interstitial fluid.
   1. Lymphatic system maintains homeostasis of the blood proteins, thereby maintaining blood volume.
   2. Changes in protein levels in the serum precipitate changes in the colloid osmotic pressure of the circulating volume.

Mechanics of Blood Flow

A. Blood flow is controlled by:
   1. The diameter of the vessel.
   2. The length of the vessel.
   3. The pressure at either end of the vessel.
   4. The viscosity of the blood.

B. Physiological control.
   1. Autoregulation—the ability of tissue to control its own blood flow.
      a. Lack of oxygen and accumulation of metabolic waste products initiate the autoregulatory system, which exerts changes in precapillary sphincters, thereby either increasing or decreasing blood supply.
      b. Autoregulatory system enables blood supply to vital organs (brain, kidney, heart) to remain relatively constant, even though blood pressure may fluctuate within normal ranges.
      c. Collateral circulation is part of autoregulatory mechanism for long-term control of blood flow; this mechanism is especially effective when obstruction to blood flow occurs gradually.
   2. Nervous system control.
      a. Parasympathetic nervous system.
         (1) Primary influence on blood flow is the regulation of the heart rate through the vagus nerve.
         (2) Baroreceptors are located in aortic arch and in carotid sinuses (carotid bodies) and are very sensitive to changes in pressure within vessel walls; increase in pressure causes stimulation of the vagus nerve, which in turn decreases the heart rate.
      b. Sympathetic nervous system.
         (1) Primary influence of sympathetic system is on arterioles for dilation and constriction of the vessels, in order to maintain peripheral resistance and vasomotor tone.
         (2) Peripheral resistance is resistance of arterioles to flow of blood.

(3) Dilation decreases peripheral resistance, thereby decreasing blood pressure; vasoconstriction increases peripheral resistance, thereby increasing blood pressure.

3. Normal components of serum influence blood pressure regulation.
   a. Angiotensin and vasopressin are vasoconstrictors.
   b. Histamine is a vasodilator.
   c. Epinephrine and norepinephrine.

Blood Pressure

A. Systolic blood pressure represents the ejection of the blood from the heart. The systolic pressure is determined primarily by the amount of blood ejected or the stroke volume (See Chapter 17).

B. Diastolic pressure represents the pressure remaining in the arteries at the end of systole. Diastolic pressure depends on the ability of the arteries to stretch and handle the blood flow.

C. Pulse pressure is the difference between the systolic and diastolic pressures.

D. Autonomic nervous system influence on blood pressure.
1. Parasympathetic system exerts control over blood pressure through stimulation of the vagus nerve.
2. Sympathetic nervous system controls blood pressure by:
   a. Maintaining peripheral resistance through constriction and dilation of the vessels.
   b. Increases heart rate and force of contraction.
   c. Causes constriction of the large veins which promotes an increase in venous return to the heart, thereby increasing cardiac output.

E. Renal influence on blood pressure.
1. Renin is an enzyme released by the kidney when there is a decrease in renal blood flow.
2. Renin breaks down to angiotensin II, which is a strong vasoconstrictor, and increases the blood pressure.
3. Activation of the renin-angiotensin system stimulates the adrenal cortex to increase secretion of aldosterone, thus precipitating sodium and water retention and increasing vascular volume.

F. The hypothalamus is stimulated to secrete vasopressin (ADH) when the blood pressure falls below normal; this increases the conservation of water, therefore increasing the blood pressure.

G. System assessment—see assessment of individual system involved.

DISORDERS OF THE VASCULAR SYSTEM

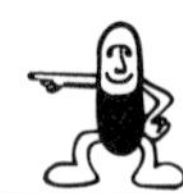

Arteriosclerosis

❑ **Arteriosclerosis is the most common disease of the arteries. The word means "hardening of the arteries."**

A. Atherosclerosis—most common classification of arteriosclerosis; characterized by stenosis and obstruction in the lumen of the vessel.
1. Lesions are found in the intima layer of the medium to large arteries.
2. Process is slow; generally no evidence of problems until a major artery is affected and there is severe decrease in blood supply to tissue supplied by artery involved.
3. Development of atherosclerosis. (Figure 16-1)
   a. Fibrous plaque and lipid irritation are progressive changes that occur within the arterial wall. The elevated plaques infiltrate the intima, or internal layer of the vessel, and precipitate varying degrees of obstruction in the arterial lumen. These changes begin in early adulthood and increase with age.
   b. In the final stage, there is development of a atherosclerotic lesion. The lesion increases in size and is associated with partial to complete obstruction of the lumen, resulting in severe ischemia or infarction of distal tissue.
4. Arteries commonly affected by atherosclerosis and the ensuing problems.
   a. Coronary arteries—myocardial infarction.
   b. Cerebrovascular arteries—cerebrovascular accident.
   c. Aorta —aortic aneurysm, peripheral occlusive disease.
   d. Renal artery
   e. Large peripheral arteries—peripheral occlusive disease.

Assessment

1. Modifiable risk factors.
   a. Diet high in saturated fats (cholesterol).
   b. Smoking.
   c. Obesity.
   d. Decreased activity.
   e. Stress.
2. Nonmodifiable risk factors.
   a. Familial tendencies.
   b. Age.

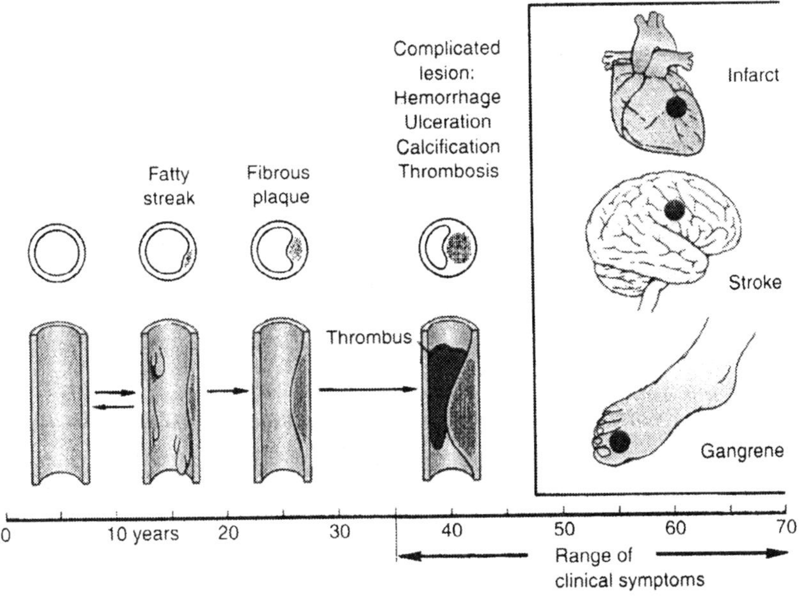

Fig 16-1: Schematic Concept of the Progression of Atherosclerosis.
Reprinted with permission: Smeltzer, SC, Bare, BG, (1999) *Brunner and Suddarth's Textbook of Medical Surgical Nursing,* 9th ed. Lippincott: Philadelphia, p. 689

3. Conditions accelerating atherosclerotic development.
   a. Diabetes mellitus.
   b. Hypertension.
4. Clinical manifestations—depend on artery involved.
5. Diagnostics (See Appendix 16-1).
   a. Clinical manifestation of specific area involved.
   b. Increased serum triglycerides, lipids, and cholesterol.

NCLEX ALERT: *Conduct cholesterol screening sessions, and adapt a diet to meet the special needs of a client.*

Treatment

1. Decrease cholesterol in diet (See Chapter 2)
2. Decrease risk factors (exercise, stop smoking, decrease weight, decrease stress).
3. Antihyperlipidemic medications (See Appendix 16-2).
4. Peripheral vasodilating medications.
5. Vascular surgery.
6. Sympathectomy.

Nursing Intervention

✦ *Goal: identify individuals at high risk (Table 16-1).*

1. Cholesterol 200 to 240 mg/dL - provide dietary information, recommend testing again in one year.
2. Cholesterol over 240 - low-fat diet and recommend further evaluation.

✦ *Goal: identify specific areas of involvement - see nursing intervention for specific areas.*

Chronic Arterial Occlusive Disease

❑ **Peripheral vascular disease (PVD) primarily involves narrowing and obstruction of the arteries of the extremities, especially the lower extremities. The atherosclerotic lesion causes chronic arterial obstruction, which leads progressively to decreased oxygen delivery to the tissue.**

A. Lesions are predominantly found in the lower aorta below the renal arteries, and extend through the popliteal area.
B. By the time symptoms occur, the artery is approximately 85 to 95 percent occluded.
C. The bifurcations at the renal, femoral, popliteal, and aortic iliac arteries are the most common sites affected.

Assessment

1. Risk factors (see also those for atherosclerosis).
   a. Generally occurs during the fifth or sixth decade of life.
   b. Familial tendency.
   c. Hypertension and diabetes accelerate the process.
2. Clinical manifestations.

Table 16-1: CHOLESTEROL AND LIPOPROTEIN LEVELS

Cholesterol (total)	120-200mg/dL
Low density lipoprotein (LDL)	<130mg/dL
High density lipoprotein (HDL)	>35mg/dL
Triglycerides	<200mg/dL

a. Intermittent claudication (ischemic pain on exercise).

b. Ischemic pain at rest (increasing severity).

c. Paresthesia of the feet.

d. Pallor when extremity is elevated.

e. Dependent rubor—dusky, purplish discoloration of extremity when in dependent position.

f. Decreased or absent peripheral pulses. (Figure 16-2)

(1) Pedal.

(2) Popliteal.

(3) Femoral.

g. Poor healing of injuries on the extremities.

h. Changes in the skin.

(1) Cool to touch.

(2) Shiny, fragile, poor turgor.

(3) Dry, scaly.

(4) Loss of hair on the lower leg.

i. Brittle, thick toenails.

j. Ulcerations and gangrene.

3. Diagnostics - (See Appendix 16-1).

a. Arteriogram.

b. Plethysmography and doppler assessment.

c. Exercise tolerance testing.

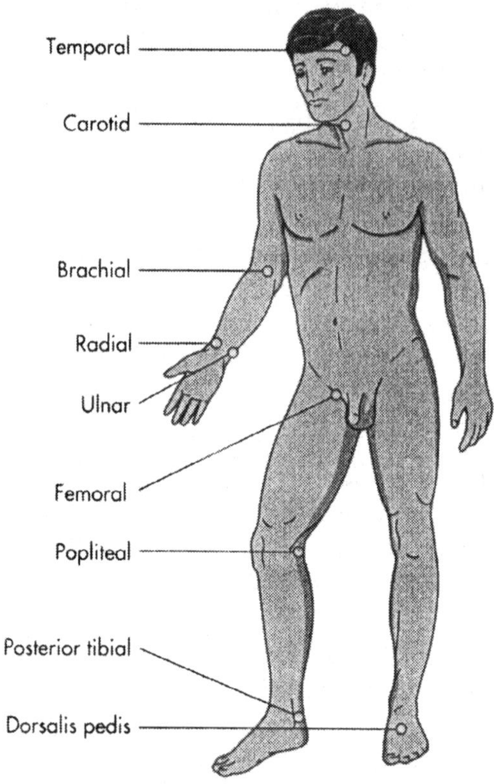

Figure 16-2: Body Sites for Peripheral Pulses.
Reprinted with permission: Phipps, WJ, Sands, JK, & Marek, JF (1999). *Medical Surgical Nursing: Concepts & Clinical Practice*, 6th ed. Philadelphia: Mosby, p. 619

Treatment

1. Medical.

a. Antiplatelet agents (aspirin, Persantin).

b. Stop smoking.

c. Decrease dietary cholesterol intake.

d. Exercise program as tolerated.

e. Fibrinolytic therapy (see Appendix 17-2).

f. Control diabetes and hypertension.

2. Surgical—procedures are done when intermittent claudication incapacitates the client, or when the circulation must be restored in order to salvage the limb.

a. Peripheral atherectomy - removal of plaque within the artery.

b. Bypass graft.

c. Intravascular stents.

3. Percutaneous transluminal angioplasty—utilization of a balloon catheter to compress the plaque against the arterial wall.

Nursing Intervention

✦ *Goal: to evaluate level of involvement of the extremity.*

1. Assess peripheral pulses; compare pulses of the lower extremities.

2. Evaluate skin on the affected extremity.

a. Color, warmth.

b. Capillary refill.

c. Condition of the skin and nail beds.

d. Presence of ulcers or lesions.

3. Assess tolerance to activity; determine at what point claudication occurs.

✦ *Goal: to prevent injury and infection.*

1. Avoid vigorous rubbing of the extremity.

2. Prevent skin breakdown at pressure sites—heel, ankle, knees; do not sit with legs crossed.

3. Heel covers and bed cradle to prevent pressure on the toes and heels.

4. Always wear shoes, avoid scratching feet.

✦ *Goal: to increase arterial supply and decrease venous congestion to the extremity.*

1. Encourage moderate exercise (i.e., walking).

a. Clients with cellulitis, leg ulcers or pain at rest should not exercise.

b. Explain to client the level of pain should be a guide to exercise, stop activity when pain occurs.

2. Active postural exercises (Buerger-Allen exercises).
3. Maintain constant warm temperature; do not use hot water bottles or heating pads.
4. Avoid pressure in the posterior popliteal area.
   a. Do not raise knee gatch on the bed without raising the foot of the bed to eliminate the pressure behind the knee.
   b. Avoid clothing that is tight and restricts circulation to the lower extremities (hose, girdles, etc.).
5. Stop smoking.

✦ *Goal: to provide preoperative care (See Chapter 3).*

✦ *Goal: to evaluate and promote circulation in affected extremity postoperative vascular surgery.*

1. Circulation checks initially every 15 minutes, then hourly, then routine. Assess for compartmental syndrome (Chapter 21) as well as graft thrombosis.
2. Encourage movement of the extremity as soon as client is awake.
3. Out of bed and ambulate as soon as indicated.
4. Do not raise the knee gatch of the bed.
5. Avoid flexion in the area of the graft (femoral or popliteal areas).
6. Monitor anticoagulation medications, maintain bleeding precautions.
7. Frequent assessment of graft area to determine adequacy of circulation and patency of graft.
8. Assess for development of dependent edema—common problem, client may require compression dressings or diuretic.

✦ *Goal: to understand measures to maintain health postoperative vascular surgery.*

1. Decrease weight if appropriate.
2. Avoid:
   a. Standing or sitting for prolonged periods of time.
   b. Constrictive clothing.
   c. Smoking.
3. Avoid trauma to the extremities.
4. Visually inspect extremities daily for:
   a. Discolored areas.
   b. Breaks in the skin.
   c. Infection.
5. Do not apply any type of direct heat to the legs.
6. Exercise daily as tolerated.
7. Daily wash, but do not soak, the feet; dry thoroughly.
8. Daily inspection and lubrication, do not use lotions on open lesions or sores.
9. Do not cut calluses or corns.
10. Proper care of toenails.

Self-Care

1. Determine client's activity level and work habits. Teach client methods to increase circulation during normal work day (do not cross legs, good chair, walking every hour if working at a desk, etc.).
2. Obtain a thermometer to test bath water, to prevent hot water burns.
3. Discuss clothing with client —good shoes, hose that do not constrict around the knee or ankle, socks that do not constrict or irritate the feet.

Raynaud's Syndrome

❑ **Raynaud's syndrome—intermittent episodic spasms of the arterioles of the extremities. Spasms are not necessarily correlated with other peripheral vascular problems.**

Assessment

1. Clinical manifestations.
   a. Increased incidence in females age 20 to 40.
   b. Symptoms are precipitated by:
      (1) Exposure to cold.
      (2) Emotional upset.
      (3) Nicotine and caffeine.
   c. Initially, there is pallor or cyanosis due to vasospasm; this causes numbness and tingling. As digits warm, there is redness, warmth, and throbbing as hyperemia occurs.
   d. Pulses may remain adequate.
   e. May progress to ulceration of the fingertips.
   f. Attacks are usually bilateral and intermittent.
   g. Obstructive disease may be associated with autoimmune disorders.

Treatment

1. No cure; treatment is based on symptoms.
2. Vasodilating medications.
3. Sympathectomy in severe situations.

Nursing Intervention

✦ *Goal: to assist client to understand disease implications and measures to decrease episodic attacks.*

1. Wear gloves when handling cold objects (refrigerator and freezer items).
2. Stop smoking.

3. Increase ability to cope with stress effectively.
4. Generally, there is no serious underlying disease problem.

Thromboangiitis Obliterans

❑ **A vasculitis of the small and medium size veins of the extremities. Also called Buerger's Disease.**

Assessment

1. Risk factors - primarily occurs in people who smoke.
2. Clinical manifestations.
   a. Intermittent claudication, rest pain in advances stages.
   b. Usually begins distally and spreads upward.
   c. Cyanosis and rubor of the extremity.
   d. Increased sensitivity to cold in the extremity.
   e. Edema of extremity.
   f. Peripheral pulses may be diminished or absent.
3. Diagnostics—based on clinical manifestations.
4. Complications: ulcerations and gangrene.

Treatment

No cure; treatment is based on symptoms; below-the-knee amputation may be done in extreme conditions.

Nursing Intervention

✦ *Goal: to evaluate level of involvement of the extremity and increase circulation to the extremity.*

1. Decrease or stop smoking.
2. Evaluate tolerance to activity.
3. Inspect feet for vascular changes.

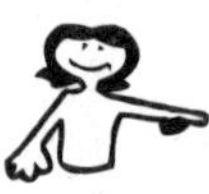

***NURSING PRIORITY:** The vascular problem has a direct relationship to cigarette smoking. In order for the condition to be controlled, the client must quit smoking.*

Aneurysm

❑ **A dilation or sac formed on the wall of an arterial vessel. The aneurysm may involve only one layer or all layers of the arterial wall.**

A. Types of aneurysms.
   1. Berry aneurysm (See Chapter 20).
      a. Occurs in intracranial arteries.
      b. Lesions are small and balloon-shaped.
      c. Problem occurs due to location and encroachment on brain tissue.
   2. Abdominal aortic aneurysm (AAA)—occurs primarily in the abdominal aorta below the renal arteries.
   3. Thoracic aortic aneurysm—located in the aorta in the thoracic area.

B. As the aneurysm enlarges there is an increasing risk of rupture.

C. Dissecting aneurysm.
   1. Characterized by bleeding between the layers of the vessel wall.
   2. With continual bleeding, dissection of the wall of the vessel occurs.
   3. Thoracic area is the most common site for dissection.

Box 16-1: Elderly Care Focus
Evaluation of Blood Pressure

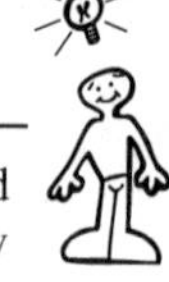

- If a client has been hypertensive for a long period of time, the client's "normal" blood pressure may need to be higher to maintain adequate blood flow and allow client to perform ADL.
- For clients over 65, high blood pressure may be defined as systolic over 160mm Hg and diastolic over 95mm Hg.
- Increased problems with orthostatic hypotension; teach client how to avoid.
- Obtain blood pressure standing, lying, and sitting. Make sure client has not had any nicotine or coffee for about an hour prior to taking blood pressure.
- Compliance problems occur when client has to take several medications for B/P, as well as cope with other chronic health problems.

Assessment

(Discussion is limited to aortic aneurysms; see Chapter 20 for nursing care of berry aneurysm).

1. Clinical manifestations—abdominal aortic aneurysm.
   a. May be asymptomatic.
   b. Back, flank, or abdominal pain.
   c. Epigastric discomfort.
   d. Pulsating abdominal mass may be palpable.
2. Clinical manifestations—thoracic aortic aneurysm.
   a. Generally asymptomatic.
   b. Client may complain of severe chest pain.
   c. Pressure on the esophagus may cause dysphagia.
   d. Pressure on the vena cava may cause edema.
   e. Dyspnea.
3. Clinical manifestations—dissecting aneurysms.
   a. Constant, intense pain.
   b. Drop in blood pressure rapidly leading to hemorrhagic shock.
   c. In AAA dissection, abdomen may remain soft.

4. Diagnostic (See Appendix 16-1).
   a. X-ray.
   b. Aortography.
   c. Sonography.
5. Complications—rupture, emboli, hemorrhage, and renal failure.

Treatment

Directed toward prevention of rupture; surgical resection of the aneurysm.

Nursing Intervention

✦ *Goal: to prepare client and family for anticipated surgery.*

1. Provide preoperative care (See Chapter 3).
2. Identify other chronic health problems.
3. Evaluate characteristic of pulses in the lower extremities and mark for evaluation postoperative.
4. Do not vigorously palpate the abdomen.
5. Evaluate for indications of dissection.
6. Keep blood pressure at lowest level for client tolerance.

✦ *Goal: to promote graft patency and circulation.*

1. General postoperative care. (See Chapter 3).
2. Maintain adequate blood pressure to facilitate filling of the graft.
3. Monitor for hemorrhage: assess increasing abdominal girth, back pain, indications of hypovolemia or shock.
4. Initially, hourly checks of peripheral circulation.
5. Evaluate urine output hourly.
6. Evaluate BUN and serum creatinine levels to assess renal function.

✦ *Goal: to maintain homeostasis and prevent infection.*

1. Monitor acid-base balance and promote pulmonary hygiene.
2. Maintain adequate body warmth in initial postoperative period.
3. Nasogastric suction in immediate postoperative period.
4. Evaluate status of GI system.
   a. Bowel sounds.
   b. Distention.
   c. Passage of flatus.
   d. Diarrhea.

Hypertension

❑ **Hypertension is a sustained increase in diastolic blood pressure.**

A. Classification.

1. Essential (primary, benign, idiopathic)—etiology unknown; accounts for approximately 85 to 95 percent of hypertensive clients.
2. Secondary—accounts for approximately 10 to 15 percent of hypertension cases; the sustained elevation is due to a secondary underlying health problem; most common type of hypertension in children.
   a. Increased secretion of catecholamines (pheochromocytoma).
   b. Increased release of renin (renal artery stenosis).
   c. Expansion of sodium and blood volume (Cushing's syndrome).
3. Malignant hypertension (hypertensive crisis)—a sustained increase in the diastolic pressure (140mm Hg) which is unresponsive to treatment and may be life-threatening.

Assessment

1. Risk factors in essential hypertension (See Table 16-1).
2. Clinical manifestations of essential hypertension, most often asymptomatic.

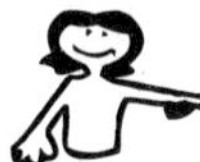

***NURSING PRIORITY:** B/P should be evaluated with the client lying, sitting and standing, as well as readings in both arms.*

   a. Sustained (two elevated pressures at least one week apart) average increase in systolic blood pressure at 140 mm Hg or higher and increase in diastolic blood pressure above 90 mm Hg.
   b. Headache, dizziness, palpitations.
   c. Epistaxis
   d. As vessel damage increases, symptoms are related to the area of the body affected.
      (1) Characterized by decreased blood supply to the heart, brain, kidneys, and retina.
      (2) There is progressive decrease in the function of these organs.
3. Clinical manifestations of malignant hypertension.
   a. Diastolic pressure above 140 mm Hg.
   b. Retinopathy, papilledema, renal failure.
   c. More critical in clients with previously compromised cardiovascular system.
   d. Blood pressure is unresponsive to medications.
4. Diagnostics.
   a. Sustained increase in diastolic pressure.
   b. Diagnostics to rule out problem of secondary hypertension.
5. Complications.

Table 16-2:
RISK FACTORS IN ESSENTIAL HYPERTENSION

NONMODIFIABLE FACTORS	
Age	Develops between 30 and 50 yr. of age. Peak incidence is 35 yr. of age.
Sex	Primarily affects men over 35 yr. and women over 45 yr.
Ethnic group	Blacks have twice the incidence of hypertension of whites.
Family history	Multifactorial genetic factors account for an estimated one-third of the cases of essential hypertension
MODIFIABLE FACTORS	
Obesity	Weight gain is associated with increased frequency of hypertension. High correlation of obesity and decreased physical activity with hypertension.
Stress	Stress results in increased sympathetic nervous system activity and increased peripheral resistance.
Cigarette smoking	Nicotine in cigarettes causes vasoconstriction and increased catecholamine release, resulting in increased heart rate.
Excess sodium intake	Relationship between high sodium intake and hypertension, especially in obese individuals.
Elevated serum lipids	Elevated levels of cholesterol and triglycerides are primary risk factors in atherosclerosis, which is a contributing factor to hypertension.

a. Coronary artery disease.

b. CHF—occurs when the left ventricle can no longer pump against the increased resistance to blood flow.

c. Cerebral vascular disease.

(1) Transient ischemic attacks (TIA).

(2) Cerebrovascular accident (CVA).

d. Nephrosclerosis—ischemia of the intrarenal vessels.

e. Retinopathy—ischemia of the arterioles in the retina.

f. Hypertensive crisis.

Treatment

1. Diet.

a. Sodium restriction.

b. Weight reduction, client should be within 10% of ideal body weight.

c. Decreased cholesterol and saturated fats.

Table 16-3:
STEP APPROACH TO DRUG THERAPY

Step 1:	Life style modifications. May begin on low dose of medication..
Step 2:	If blood pressure is not controlled, medication is increased or another medication is added.
Step 3:	If blood pressure is not controlled, a second medication may be substituted, or a third drug from another class is added.
Step 4:	If blood pressure is not controlled, a third or fourth drug is added and blood pressure is continued to be evaluated.

2. Regular exercise (avoid isometric exercises, i.e. weight lifting).
3. Antihypertensive medications (See Appendix 16-4 and Table 16-3).
4. Diuretics to decrease circulating volume (See Appendix 16-5).
5. Maintain optimal weight.
6. Avoid alcohol intake.
7. Decrease caffeine intake.
8. Stop smoking.
9. Assist client to cope effectively with stress.

Nursing Intervention

✦ *Goal: to identify the high-risk individual, and educate public regarding disease process.*

1. Encourage participation in community blood pressure screening programs.
2. Educate public regarding risk factors (Table 16-2).
3. Identify health promoting behavior for high-risk individuals.

a. Decrease weight.

b. Avoid smoking.

c. Control diabetes.

d. Decrease cholesterol intake.

e. Have regular blood pressure checkups.

✦ *Goal: to reduce blood pressure and assist client to maintain control.*

NCLEX ALERT: *Identify side effects, adverse effects/contraindications, client's understanding of medications.*

1. Assess response to medication regimen.

a. Antihypertensives (See Appendix 16-4).

b. Diuretics (See Appendix 16-5).

2. Evaluate blood pressure:

a. Client should be seated with arm at heart level.

b. No smoking or caffeine within past 30 minutes.
c. Use appropriate cuff size.
d. Two or more readings should be averaged.

3. Maintain low-sodium diet.
4. Assess changes in weight with regard to low sodium intake and diuretics.
5. When blood pressure is initially decreased, evaluate client's tolerance to decrease.
    a. Postural hypotension.
    b. Urinary output.
    c. Change in energy level.
    d. Changes in mental alertness.

Self-Care

1. Continue low-cholesterol, low-sodium diet. Assist client to identify easily prepared meals. Evaluate need for follow-up visit from the dietician.
2. Maintain optimum weight.
3. Maintain regular exercise.
4. Take prescribed medications.
    a. Take medication at regular times.
    b. Know the names and common side effects of the medications.

NCLEX ALERT: *Instruct client about self-administration of prescribed medications; evaluate client's compliance with prescribed therapy.*

5. Factors contributing to client's noncompliance with medications:
    a. Side effects of the medication.
    b. Cost of the medication.
    c. Poor relationship between client and health care providers.
6. Avoid hot baths, steam rooms, spas (increases vasodilating effect of medications).
7. Decrease problems of orthostatic hypotension.
    a. Get up slowly, sit at the bedside to regain equilibrium, then stand slowly.
    b. Wear elastic support hose.
    c. Lie or sit down when dizziness occurs.
    d. Do not stand or sit for prolonged periods of time.

NCLEX ALERT: *Teach health promotion information.*

8. Side effects of medication most often are temporary.
9. If sexual problems or impotence develop, contact physician. Do not stop taking medication.
10. Hypertensive medications need to be taken on a routine basis; if doses are missed, the client may experience rebound hypertension. Plan method for client to keep track of whether he has taken prescribed medications (daily pill box or marking on calendar, etc.).

Shock

❑ **Shock is a pathologic state that is characterized by inadequate blood flow and tissue perfusion.**

A. For adequate circulation to occur, all parts of the circulatory system must function effectively together.
    1. Vascular tone to maintain normal resistance of the vessels.
    2. Ability of the heart to maintain cardiac output.
    3. Adequate amount of total blood volume.

B. The initial problems precipitating shock and the specific treatment of the problems are very different; however, regardless of the precipitating cause of shock, the underlying problem is inadequate tissue perfusion.

C. Classification of shock (See Table 16-4).
    1. Hypovolemic shock.
    2. Cardiogenic shock.
    3. Distributive shock (vasogenic).

D. Body response to shock (See Table 16-5).

Assessment

Signs and symptoms of shock are essentially the same regardless of the precipitating cause.

1. Risk factors.
    a. Increased incidence in the very young and the very old.
    b. Increased incidence in clients with chronic progressive disease states.
    c. Trauma.
    d. Postoperative hemorrhage.
2. Clinical manifestations.
    a. The symptoms from shock are precipitated by a decrease in the mean arterial pressure (MAP -calculated as the diastolic pressure plus 1/3 of the difference between the systolic and diastolic pressures.) A decrease in MAP by 5-10mm Hg will stimulate compensatory mechanisms; there may also be a decrease in the pulse pressure.
    b. Initially, the only sign of impending shock may be tachycardia due to the ability of the body to adapt; body compensates by vasoconstriction

and increased cardiac rate, which will assist to maintain or even increase the blood pressure.

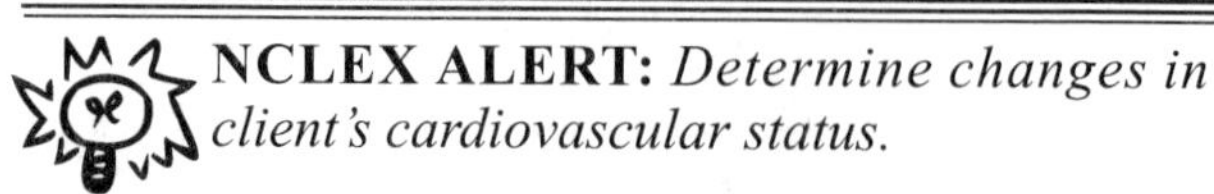

Table 16-4: CLASSIFICATION OF SHOCK

CLASSIFICATION	PATHOPHYSIOLOGY	CONDITIONS	TREATMENT AND CLINICAL IMPLICATIONS
HYPOVOLEMIC	Reduced venous return due to reduced blood volume; 15 percent to 25 percent reduction in volume.	Hemorrhage. Burns Severe fluid loss—dehydration.	1. Administer volume replacement—blood transfusion and volume expanders.
CARDIOGENIC	Heart is unable to effectively circulate the intravascular volume.	Dysrhythmias. MI. CHF.	1. Monitor EKG continuously. 2. Medications to increase cardiac output: digitalis and dopamine. 3. Evaluate CVP response to fluid therapy; easy to overload client. 4. Treat dysrhythmias.
DISTRIBUTIVE	Change occurs in the size of the vascular space without increase in circulating volume.		
Neurogenic →	Increased venous capacity due to a loss of peripheral vasomotor tone; cardiac function and blood volume may be normal.	Spinal cord injury, barbiturate OD, spinal anesthesia.	1. Administer vasoconstrictor medications as indicated. 2. Close record of intake to avoid circulatory overload. 3. Bradycardia may require atropine.
Septic → (toxic)	Dilation of blood vessels by humoral or vasoactive substances.	Overwhelming infection; generally gram-negative organism.	1. Evaluate for origin of infection. 2. Skin may remain warm. 3. Dopamine. 4. MAST suit.
Vasogenic → (anaphylactic)	Antigen - antibody reaction with release of histamine, causing vasodilation and fluid shift.	Transfusion reactions. Insect bites. Side effect of medications.	1. Maintain airway - problem with laryngeal edema. 2. Oxygen as indicated. 3. Epinephrine and **Benadryl**, IV. 4. MAST suit.
OBSTRUCTIVE	Physical impediment to the mainstream flow of blood.	Pericardial tamponade. Pulmonary embolism. Vena cava compression.	1. Will demonstrate increased CVP. 2. Treatment directed toward release of obstruction.

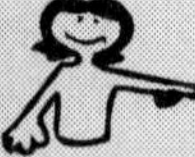

NURSING PRIORITY: *Shock is a dynamic condition. The client's status is constantly changing, either improving or deteriorating.*

Table 16-5: BODY RESPONSE TO SHOCK

A decrease in venous return, or failure of the heart to pump adequately, results in a decrease in cardiac output and a precipitating decrease in blood pressure.

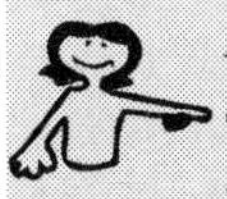

NURSING PRIORITY: As decreased cardiac output continues, the ability of the heart to pump progressively deteriorates, which eventually may lead to death.

The sympathetic nervous system is stimulated:

a. Facilitates vasoconstriction to shunt blood to vital organs (brain and heart).

b. Initiates tachycardia to increase cardiac output; tachycardia also occurs as the body attempts to meet circulatory demands.

Sequence of Events to Restore Blood Volume and Increase Blood Pressure

in blood flow to the kidney.

in activation renin-angiotensin.

release of aldosterone, ↑ in epinephrine and norepinephrine.

renal absorption.

in ADH secretion.

in water retention.

↑ in blood volume, which thus precipitates an increase in venous return to the heart.

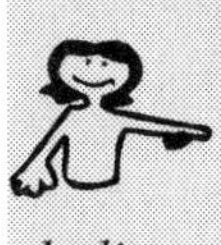

NURSING PRIORITY: Inadequate ventilation leads to hypoxia and to a decrease in myocardial functioning precipitating metabolic acidosis; metabolic acidosis then contributes further to tissue hypoxia.

c. Early (compensatory, non progressive): the body is able to compensate (vasoconstriction) with a blood pressure in low normal range and perfusion to vital organs.

(1) Oriented, may be restless, increased anxiety, apprehensive.

(2) Increase in pulse rate.

(3) Urine output may be slightly decreased, but within normal range.

(4) Cardiac output and MAP are maintained.

(5) Complaints of thirst and feeling cool.

d. Intermediate (progressive).

(1) Decreasing sensory perception.

(2) Cool, moist skin.

(3) Respirations become more rapid to increase oxygenation; may develop respiratory alkalosis.

(4) Skin color pale.

(5) Decrease in urine to oliguric levels.

(6) Tachycardia increases.

(7) 20mm Hg or greater decrease in MAP.

(8) Decrease in pulse pressure may occur before a decrease in bloodpressure.

e. Advanced (late).

(1) Progressively decreasing level of consciousness.

(2) Cool, moist skin.

(3) Cyanosis.

(4) Respirations become more labored; cellular hypoxia increases.

(5) Tachycardia to bradycardia.

(6) Anuria.

(7) Decrease in the bloodpressure.

(8) Development of metabolic acidosis.

3. Diagnostics—based on the clinical manifestations and history of underlying problems.

Treatment

Depends on the underlying problem.

1. Adequate fluid resuscitation.
2. Position to increase venous return but not compromise pulmonary status.
3. Medications to correct origin or to support cardiac output.
4. Oxygen therapy.

Nursing Intervention

✦ *Goal: to identify and correct cause of shock.*

✦ *Goal: to maintain adequate respiratory function.*

✦ *Goal: to maintain adequate circulation.*

1. Adequate blood volume—blood transfusions, positioning supine with legs elevated.
2. Adequate cardiac output—may be facilitated by intra-aortic balloon pump (IAPB).
3. Improve vascular tone.
   a. Medical anti-shock trousers or MAST are used to increase vascular resistance, and decrease vascular diameter by exerting external pressure on the blood vessels.
   b. Do not deflate until client is in situation for correction of the problem (i.e., surgery).
   c. Circulatory checks on extremities when MAST are in place.

NCLEX ALERT: *Implement measures to promote venous return (e.g., sequential compression devices, MAST trousers, anti-shock trousers, elastic stockings, etc.).*

✦ *Goal: to assess and support the cardiovascular and respiratory systems.*

1. Monitor blood pressure and MAP closely in response to administration of medications.

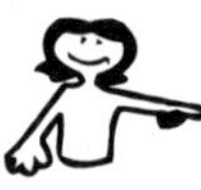

NURSING PRIORITY: *Decrease in blood pressure is a late sign of shock in young adults.*

---

2. Evaluate cardiac output in response to dysrhythmias.
3. Maintain bedrest.
4. Position supine with legs elevated and knees straight (modified Trendelenburg).
5. Maintain airway, evaluate rate and quality of respirations.
6. Evaluate ABGs for hypoxia and development of acidosis.
7. Provide supplemental oxygen.
8. Evaluate central venous pressure (See Appendix 17-5).
9. Maintain patent venous access for IV medications and fluid resuscitation, preferably a central line.
10. Foley catheter, hourly urine measurements.

✦ *Goal: to maintain homeostasis.*

1. Ongoing neuro status evaluations.
2. Maintain NPO; provide oral hygiene.

Table 16-6: NURSING MEASURES TO DECREASE VENOUS STASIS

✦ Encourage mobility; even standing at the bedside promotes venous tone.

✦ Elastic stockings:
—Hospitalized clients should wear them all the time.
—Removed for bath, but replaced prior to getting out of bed.
—Home clients generally wear them during the day, should be put on before getting out of bed; and removed when they go to bed.
—Do not allow stockings to bunch up behind the knee.
—Don't hang feet dependent when putting stockings on; elevate or put them parallel on the bed.

✦ Teach client to elevate legs for about 20 minutes every four or five hours.

✦ Avoid prolonged sitting; walk around every 1-2 hours.

✦ Don't cross legs when sitting

✦ Do not wear restrictive clothing.

✦ Maintain good fluid intake, avoid dehydration.

3. Evaluate for bowel sounds and distention due to visceral ischemia; insert nasogastric tube for distention.
4. Keep comfortably warm; do not allow chilling.
5. Do not administer medications PO, IM, or subcutaneous, due to decreased tissue perfusion.
6. Provide emotional support; continue to talk with client and describe procedures before they are done.
7. Avoid unnecessary nursing procedures.
8. Do not administer narcotics.

Venous Stasis Ulcers

❑ **Ulcers develop from increased venous tension and valve incompetence. This leads to venous stasis, poor venous return, edema and eventually ulceration.**

Assessment

1. Risk Factors:
   a. Venous hypertension
   b. Infection
   c. Diabetes
   d. Varicosities
2. Clinical Manifestations
   a. Stasis eczema is often the first indication.
   b. Sclerosis occurs due to long standing edema, leg becomes larger at the calf.
   c. Blistering and edema occurs.
   d. Ulcers exhibit a irregular margin.
   e. Appearance of wound varies from red granulation tissue to fibrinous tissue to necrosis.

f. Ulcer usually produces copious serous exudate.

3. Diagnostics: history and clinical manifestations.
4. Complicatons:
   a. Infection
   b. Delayed/poor healing.

Treatment

1. Measures to prevent venous stasis
   a. Compression, elevation of extremity.
   b. Topical wound care.
2. Removal of varicose veins.
3. Excision of ulcer with skin grafting.
4. Optimal skin care.

Nursing Intervention:

✦ *Goal: to prevent/treat venous stasis. (Table 16-6)*

1. Elastic stockings - applied before client gets out of bed, and removed before going to bed.
2. Compression devices -
   a. Compression boots - extremity may be covered with continuous compression bandage.
   b. Intermittent or sequential pneumatic compression devices - always check arterial circulation with any type of compression device.

NCLEX ALERT: *Implement measures: to promote venous return; to manage potential circulatory complications; to monitor wounds for signs and symptoms of infection.*

✦ *Goal: to prevent infection and promote healing.*

1. Keep area clean, may irrigate and cleanse noninfected wound with normal saline.
2. Hydrocolloid dressing over wound
3. Infected wounds will require daily wound care, as well as topical and/or systemic antibiotics.
4. Most often will maintain some type of compression over dressing.

✦ *Goal: to assist client/family to understand implications of condition and measures to maintain health.*

1. The majority of stasis ulcers will reoccur - teach clients measures to prevent venous stasis.
2. Wound care.
3. Measures to promote healing - decrease prolonged standing, good nutrition, weight control.

Varicose Veins

❑ **Varicose veins occur when veins in the lower trunk and extremities become congested and dilated because of the incompetent valves in the vessels, as well as loss of elasticity of the vessel wall.**

Assessment

1. Risk factors.
   a. Congenital weakness of the vessel walls.
   b. Obesity.
   c. Pregnancy.
2. Clinical manifestations.
   a. Dilated, tortuous subcutaneous veins.
   b. Cosmetic appearance of the vein is objectionable.
   c. Pressure or pain after prolonged standing.
   d. Pain is generally relieved by elevating the extremity.
3. Diagnostics—positive Trendelenburg test, clinical manifestations.

Treatment

1. Medical - prevent venous stasis. (Table 16-6)
2. Surgical.
   a. Scleropathy—injection of sclerosing agent into the affected vein.
   b. Surgical ligation of the veins; may be combined with vein stripping as well.

Nursing Intervention

✦ *Goal: to prevent development of complications*

1. Decrease venous stasis (Table 16-6)
2. Maintain firm pressure along the entire extremity (Jobst stockings, ace bandages, etc.).
3. Range of motion and active movement of extremities to promote venous return.

✦ *Goal: to assist client to understand implications of the condition and measures to maintain health.*

1. Avoid constrictive clothing.
2. Maintain good skin care of lower extremities.
3. Maintain weight control.
4. Avoid prolonged standing or sitting in the work environment.
5. Identify and avoid activities that increase venous pooling.
6. Wear support stockings.
7. Avoid constrictive clothing.

Thrombophlebitis

❑ **The formation of a thrombus that is associated with inflammation. Also called venous thrombosis or deep vein thrombosis—DVT.**

A. Thrombosis is the development of a clot in the vein; thrombophlebitis is the inflammation of the vein. Sometimes it is difficult to determine which problem occurred first.

B. Thrombus formation generally occurs as a result of:

1. Venous stasis.
2. Increased coagulability of the blood.
3. Damage to the endothelial wall of the vessel.

Assessment

1. Risk factors.
   a. Venous Stasis, (usually immobilization).
      (1) Surgery (hip surgery and open prostate surgery are high risk.)
      (2) Pregnancy.
      (3) Obesity.
   b. Hypercoagulability.
      (1) Malignancy.
      (2) Dehydration.
      (3) Blood dyscrasia.
      (4) Oral contraceptives.
   c. Vein wall trauma.

NCLEX ALERT: *Provide measures to prevent complications of immobility.*

2. Clinical manifestations.
   a. Superficial thrombophlebitis—area around the vein is tender to touch, reddened, and warm.
   b. Deep thrombosis.
      (1) Groin or calf tenderness.
      (2) Pain.
      (3) Warm, edematous area.
   c. Homan's sign—this is no longer considered an accurate indicator of thrombophlebitis.
   d. Unfortunately, the client is frequently asymptomatic.
3. Diagnostics (See Appendix 16-1).
   a. Phlebogram.
   b. Doppler ultrasound.
4. Complication—pulmonary emboli.

Treatment

1. Medical (primary method of treatment).
   a. Bedrest.
   b. Elevate extremity.
   c. Anticoagulant (See Appendix 16-3).
   d. Warm moist packs.
   e. Elastic stocking if edema is present after client is ambulatory.
   f. Elastic stocking on unaffected leg during period of bedrest.
2. Surgical intervention—done to prevent pulmonary emboli.
   a. Venous thrombectomy.
   b. Umbrella filter device in the vena cava.

Nursing Intervention

✦ *Goal: to prevent problem of thrombophlebitis.*

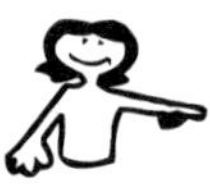

NURSING PRIORITY: *The most effective way to prevent the development of a pulmonary embolus is to prevent the development of DVT.*

1. Prophylactic measures for the surgical client (See Chapter 3).
2. Prevent complications of immobilization (See Chapter 3).
3. Prophylactic anticoagulation may be utilized in the high-risk client (hip and prostate surgery).
4. Nursing measures to promote venous return (see Table 16-6).

✦ *Goal: to decrease inflammatory response and prevent emboli formation.*

1. Bedrest with feet elevated.
2. Warm, moist soaks to dilate arteries and veins and to decrease lymphatic congestion.
3. Observe client for adverse reactions to anticoagulants (See Appendix 16-3).
4. Do not use pillow under the knees or elevate the knee gatch of the bed.
5. Monitor for development of pulmonary emboli (Chapter 15).
6. Utilization of pneumatic compression devices or sequential compression devices to facilitate venous return in immobilized clients.

Self-Care

1. Avoid oral contraceptives.
2. Stop smoking.
3. Teach methods to decrease venous stasis (Table 16-6).
4. Exercise regularly (especially walking).
5. Decrease weight if appropriate.
6. Decrease sodium in diet if edema is present.
7. Follow instructions regarding anticoagulation therapy at home.
8. Understand need for follow-up health care.⌘

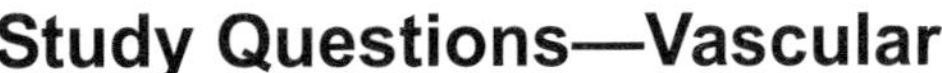

Study Questions—Vascular

1. On the initial assessment of a client with a CVP line, it is important for the nurse to establish the point from which the CVP should be measured. Where is this reference point?

① On the right side, mid-clavicular line where it intersects with the 5th intercostal space.
② Located mid-axillary at the level of the fifth intercostal space.
③ On the left midsternal border at the level of the 4th intercostal space.
④ On the anterior aspect of the thoracic cavity, left side at the 5th intercostal space

2. What is an important nursing action in order to safely administer Heparin?

① Check the prothrombin time (PT) and administer the medication if it is below 20 seconds.
② Utilize a 20 gauge, ½ inch needle, inject into the deltoid muscle and gently massage the area.
③ Dilute in 50cc D_5W and infuse by IVPB over 15 minutes, check the clotting time one half hour after infusion.
④ Utilize a 25 gauge, ½ inch needle, and inject the medication into the subcutaneous tissue of the abdomen.

3. A client with hypertension is concerned about her medications, and asks the nurse how long she is going to have to take all of these medications. What principle is the nurse's response based on?

① The client will be scheduled for an appointment in two months, the doctor will decrease her medications at that time.
② As soon as the blood pressure returns to normal levels, the client will be able to stop taking her medications.
③ In order to maintain stable control of the client's blood pressure, she will have to stay on the medications indefinitely.
④ The nurse cannot discuss the medications with client, she need's to talk to with the doctor.

4. The nurse is administering propranolol (*Inderal*) to a client who is being treated for hypertension. What is the desired client response to this medication?

① Vasodilation occurs, resulting in a decrease in the cardiac afterload.
② The cardiac rate is decreased, with a resulting decrease in the cardiac output.
③ A decrease in cardiac output and a rise in the arterial blood pressure.
④ Pericardial fluid is decreased, thus decreasing the cardiac workload.

5. The nurse is caring for a client who is six hours postpartum. What nursing actions decrease the incidence of postpartum thrombophlebitis?

① Encourage early ambulation and increased fluid intake.
② Bathroom privileges only and elevate the lower extremities.
③ Administer anticoagulants and evaluate the clotting factors.
④ Encourage her to breast-feed the infant as soon as possible.

6. A client diagnosed with peripheral vascular disease is being discharged. What risk factors are important for the nurse to discuss with the client?

① Orthostatic hypotension.
② Hypernatremia.
③ Smoking.
④ Hypoglycemia.

7. A major complication with the immobilized client is venous stasis. What is the most effective nursing intervention for this problem?

① Raise the foot of the bed for one hour then lower it to stimulate blood flow.
② Teach the client how to perform isotonic exercises while in bed.
③ Active range of motion of the upper body to stimulate cardiac output.
④ Assist the client to walk as soon and as often as possible.

8. A 48-year-old client has had her blood pressure evaluated weekly for one month. At the end of the month, the nurse averages out the weekly blood pressures at 150/96. The client is 20 pounds overweight and her cholesterol is 240mg/dL. What is important information for the nurse to include in the teaching plan for this client?

① Refer her to the doctor for further follow up and medications.
② Increase fiber in her diet and begin a daily 30 minute workout.
③ Decrease sodium intake and decrease the dietary calories from fat to 25-30% of total calories.
④ Reduce her cholesterol intake for one month and check her blood pressure three times a week.

9. Four hours post aortic-femoral bypass graft surgery, the nurse assesses the client and is unable to palpate pulses in the operative leg. The client complains of pain in the leg. What is the first nursing action?

① Massage the leg and apply warm towels.
② Elevate the leg and recheck the pulse.
③ Call the physician immediately.
④ Assist the client to ambulate.

10. The nurse is changing the sub-clavian dressing and IV tubing on a client with a central venous infusion line. What is included in this procedure?

① Scrubbing the client's chest with betadine and shave 6 inches around insertion site.
② Positioning the client with the head of the bed elevated and his head turned to the opposite side.
③ Increasing the IV infusion rate for 20 minutes to flush the line prior to changing it.
④ Putting the client on his back with the bed flat, have him hold his breath when the line is changed.

11. A client's blood pressure does not respond to increased IV fluids and his blood pressure continues to drop. The doctor orders an IV infusion of dopamine. What is one of the benefits of this medication in the treatment of shock?

① It increases the force of the myocardial contraction.
② There are fewer severe allergic reactions.
③ It causes rapid vasodilation of the vascular bed.
④ It supports renal perfusion by dilatation of the renal arteries.

12. The nurse is administering a fluid challenge to a client in hypovolemic shock. What nursing assessment data is most important in determining whether the client is responding favorably to the fluid replacement?

① Urine output increases from 25cc per hour to 40cc per hour.
② The systolic blood pressure increases from 80mmHg to 90mmHg.
③ The central venous pressure increases form 5cm to 7cm.
④ The PaO_2 increases to 90% on 60% oxygen.

13. The client returns to his room following a thoracotomy. What will the nursing assessment reveal if hypovolemia from excessive blood loss is present?

① A central venous pressure (CVP) of 5 cm of water, and urine output of 20cc per hour.
② Jugular vein distention with the head elevated 45°.
③ Chest tube drainage of 50 ml per hour in the first four hours.
④ Increased blood pressure and increased pulse pressure.

14. A hypertensive client asks the nurse what type of exercise she should do each day. What is the nurse's best response?

① Exercise for an hour, but only three times a week.
② Walk on the treadmill for 45 minutes every morning.
③ Begin walking, increase distance as you tolerate it.
④ Exercise only in the morning, stop when you get tired.

15. The nurse is preparing discharge teaching for a client with hypertension who is being treated with furosemide (*Lasix*) and clonidine (*Catapres*). The nurse would caution the client about which over-the-counter medications?

① Antihistamines.
② Acetaminophen.
③ Topical corticosteroid cream.
④ Decongestant cough preparations.

16. The nurse is titrating an IV infusion of sodium nitroprusside (*Nipride*). Fifteen minutes after starting the medication, the blood pressure goes from 190/120 to 120/90. What is a priority nursing action?

① Recheck the blood pressure and call the doctor.
② Decrease the rate and recheck the blood pressure in five minutes.
③ Stop the medication and keep the IV open with D5W.
④ Assess the client's tolerance of the current level of blood pressure.

17. The nurse is teaching a hypertensive client about his antihypertensive medications, furosemide (*Lasix*) and captopril (*Capoten*). What is important to include in this teaching?

① Stand up slowly to decrease problem with dizziness.
② Increase fluid intake due to increased loss of body fluids.
③ When you begin to feel better, the doctor will decrease your medications.
④ Stay out of the sunshine and make sure you have adequate sodium intake.

18. The nurse is preparing to administer spironolactone (*Aldactone*) to a client. After assessing the client, what data indicates the need to hold the medication?

① Potassium level of 5.8 mEq/L.
② Apical pulse rate of 58.
③ Blood pressure of 130/90.
④ Urine output 30cc per hour.

Answers and rationales to these questions are in the section at the end of the book entitled "Chapter Study Questions: Answers & Rationales."

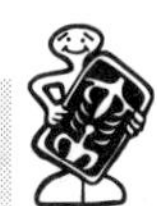

Appendix 16-1: VASCULAR DIAGNOSTICS

WHOLE BLOOD CLOTTING TIME	NORMAL VALUE	THERAPEUTIC VALUE	
SERUM STUDIES			
Activated Coagulation Time (ACT)	75-105 sec.	150-210 sec.	See Nursing Implications for clients on anticoagulant medications (Appendix 16-3). Range of values are dependent on reagents used in individual laboratories. Serum levels should be reported with the "control level" in order to evaluate results of study.
Prothrombin time (PT)	10-13 sec. range	1 to 2 ½ times normal	
Activated prothrombin time (aPTT)	Activated: 30 - 45 sec.	1 ½ to 2 ½ times normal	
International normalizing ratio (INR)	Mathematically calculated to maintain consistency.	2.0 to 3.5 (anticoagulation	

INVASIVE STUDIES

Study	Description	Nursing
Peripheral arteriography (angiography) Venography (phlebography)	Involves injection of a radiopaque dye into either the artery or the vein; x-rays are taken to identify atherosclerotic plaques, occlusions, traumatic injury or presence of aneurysms.	1. Explain procedures to client; mild sedative may be indicated; written consent required. 2. After procedure: a. Circulatory checks distal to the puncture site. b. Observe client for allergic reactions to the dye. c. Pressure dressings to puncture sites.

NONINVASIVE STUDIES

Doppler Ultrasonography—handheld doppler to detect flow of blood in peripheral arterial disease. Is not sensitive to early disease changes.

Computerized Tomography (CT) allows for visualization of the arterial wall and adjacent structures. Used for diagnosis of abdominal aortic aneurysm, graft occlusions.

Trendelenburg — Client lies supine with leg elevated and drains the veins, a tourniquet is applied at midthigh and the client is asked to stand. Veins normally fill from below or distally, a varicose vein will fill from above or proximally because of the incompetent valves. Do not leave tourniquet in place longer the 1 minute.

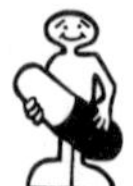

Appendix 16-2: ANTIHYPERLIPIDEMIC MEDICATIONS

MEDICATIONS	SIDE EFFECTS	NURSING IMPLICATIONS
ANTIHYPERLIPIDEMIC MEDICATIONS: Decreases LDL cholesterol, but preferably does not decrease the HDL cholesterol. First line of treatment for increased cholesterol is dietary therapy to reduce cholesterol intake.		
Cholestyramine (**Questran**): PO Colestipol (**Colestid**): PO	GI disturbances. Constipation.	1. Supplemental fat-soluble vitamins in long-term therapy. 2. Mix powder with several ounces of fluid for administration.
Nicotinic acid (**Niacin, Nicolar**): PO	Flushing. Hyperglycemia. Hyperuricemia. GI disturbances.	1. Used with caution in clients with gallbladder disease, diabetes and gout. 2. Flushing occurs in almost all clients; will diminish over several weeks.
Gemfibrozil (**Lopid**): PO	Rashes, GI disturbances, Hepatoxic	1. Should not be given to clients with pre-existing gall bladder disease.
Lovastatin (**Mevacor**): PO	Muscle breakdown	2. Will potentiate warfarin derivative anticoagulants (**Coumadin**).

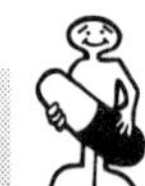

Appendix 16-3: ANTICOAGULANTS

MEDICATIONS	SIDE EFFECTS	NURSING IMPLICATIONS
ANTICOAGULANTS: Prolong coagulation by inactivation of clotting factors (heparin) and by decreasing synthesis of clotting factors (Coumadin).		
Heparin: IV, SQ	Hemorrhagic tendencies: hematuria, bleeding gums, frank hemorrhage.	1. Check the aPTT for normal levels vs therapeutic levels. 2. Protamine sulfate is the antidote. 3. Will not dissolve established clots. 4. May not be given PO. 5. Effective immediately after administration. 6. Anticoagulation effect is short. 7. Identify if heparin is being used to treat thromboembolic problem or as prophylaxis for thromboembolic problems.
Low Molecular Weight Heparin Enoxaparin (**Lovenox**) SQ Delteparin sodium (**Fragmin**) SQ		1. Use: prophylaxis for coagulation in high-risk clients (hip or knee replacement). 2. Dosage is not interchangeable with heparin. 3. Does not need as close control as regular heparin. 4. Leave the air loc in the prefilled syringe to prevent leakage.
Warfarin sodium (**Coumadin**): PO		1. Check the PT and INR to evaluate level of anticoagulation. 2. Vitamin K is the antidote. 3. Client teaching: —bleeding precautions (Table 14-2). —advise all health care providers of medication. —not recommended if pregnant or lactating.. —maintain routine checks on coagulation studies. 4. Utilized for long-term anticoagulation. 5. Check drug literature when administering with other medications; drug interactions are common. 6. Oral contraceptives may decrease effectiveness.

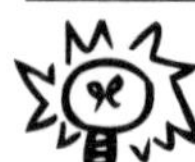

NCLEX ALERT: *The anticoagulant medications are consistently found on the examination.*

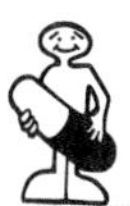

Appendix 16-4: ANTIHYPERTENSIVE MEDICATIONS

MEDICATIONS	SIDE EFFECTS	NURSING IMPLICATIONS

❖ GENERAL NURSING IMPLICATIONS ❖

— Advise client that postural hypotension may occur and how to decrease effects.
— Client should be instructed regarding sedation; hazardous activities should be avoided.
— Hypotension may be increased by hot weather, hot showers, hot tubs, and alcohol ingestion.
— Client should not abruptly discontinue medication or change dosage without consulting your health care provider.
— Encourage a low sodium diet and weight maintenance or reduction.
— Encourage to stop smoking.
— Have client report unpleasant side effects related to sexual dysfunction.
— Do not take over-the-counter cough medications or decongestants that contain pseudoephedrine, these medications cause an ↑ in blood pressure.

VASODILATORS: Acts directly on vascular smooth muscle to produce vasodilation.

MEDICATIONS	SIDE EFFECTS	NURSING IMPLICATIONS
Hydralazine HCl (**Apresoline**): PO, IM, IV	Tachycardia. Angina. Palpitations. Anorexia. Headache.	1. Advise client that postural hypotension may occur. 2. Medication may precipitate myocardial ischemia. 3. May be used in combination with other antihypertensive medications.
Nitroprusside (**Nipride**): IV	Nausea. Vomiting. Headache. Diaphoresis. Abdominal pain.	1. Used to treat hypertensive crisis, very rapid response. 2. Solution must be prepared immediately prior to use and protected from light during administration. 3. Administer via infusion pump to insure accurate flow rate. 4. Maintain continuous EKG and BP monitoring, preferably in a critical care setting.

CENTRALLY ACTING SYMPATHOLYTICS (ALPHA AGONISTS): Decreases sympathetic effect (norepinephrine) on BP and decreases sympathetic tone which leads to dilation of both arterioles and veins.

MEDICATIONS	SIDE EFFECTS	NURSING IMPLICATIONS
Clonidine (**Catapres**): PO, patch Methyldopa (**Aldomet**): PO, parenteral	Dry mouth & nasal mucosa, drowsiness, impotence, postural hypotension.	1. If withdrawn abruptly, may precipitate a hypertensive crisis. 2. More prolonged problems with postural hypotension and impotence.

ANGIOTENSIN-CONVERTING ENZYME INHIBITORS (ACE): Reduce peripheral vasculature resistance without increasing cardiac output, rate, or contractility; angiotension antagonist.

MEDICATIONS	SIDE EFFECTS	NURSING IMPLICATIONS
Captopril (**Capoten**): PO Enalapril (**Vasotec**): PO	Postural hypotension, GI distress, hyperkalmia, insomnia, potential aggravating nonproductive cough.	1. Instruct client to stay in bed for 3-4 hours after initial dose. 2. Monitor BP closely after the first dose for pronounced hypotension. 3. Monitor electrolytes; this medication causes retention of potassium. 4. Elderly client is at highest risk for postural hypotension.

BETA-ADRENERGIC BLOCKERS: See Appendix 17-2

CALCIUM CHANNEL BLOCKERS: See Appendix 17-2

Appendix 16-5: DIURETICS

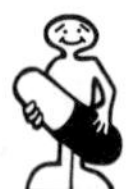

MEDICATIONS	SIDE EFFECTS	NURSING IMPLICATIONS

❖GENERAL NURSING IMPLICATIONS ❖

— Evaluate daily weights for fluid loss or gain.
— Maintain intake and output records.
— Monitor for hypokalemia.
— Advise client of foods that are potassium-rich.
— Administer medications in the morning.
— Teach clients how to decrease effects of postural hypotension.
— Monitor blood pressure response to diuretics.
— Interactions:
Digitalis action is increased in presence of hypokalemia.
Lithium levels may be increased in presence of hyponatremia.

LOOP DIURETICS: Block sodium and chloride reabsorption, which causes water and solutes to be retained in the nephron. Prevention of reabsorption of water back into the circulation causes an increase in excretion of the water, therefore diuresis.

MEDICATIONS	SIDE EFFECTS	NURSING IMPLICATIONS
Furosemide (**Lasix**): PO, IM, IV Ethacrynic acid (**Edecrin**): PO, IV Bumetanide (**Bumex**): PO	Dehydration, hypotension; excessive loss of potassium, sodium, chloride, hyperglycemia, hyperuricemia.	1. Strong diuretic that provides rapid diuresis. 2. Use with caution in elderly - CNS problems of confusion, headache.

THIAZIDE DIURETICS:

MEDICATIONS	SIDE EFFECTS	NURSING IMPLICATIONS
Chlorothiazide (**Diuril**): IV, PO Chlorthalidone (**Hygroton**): PO Hydrochlorothiazide (**Hydrodiuril, Esidrex**): PO	Dehydration, hypotension; excessive loss of potassium, sodium, chloride, hyperglycemia, hyperuricemia.	1. Frequently used as first line drug to control essential hypertension.

POTASSIUM-SPARING DIURETICS: Block the effect of aldosterone on the renal tubule.

MEDICATIONS	SIDE EFFECTS	NURSING IMPLICATIONS
Spironolactone (**Aldactone**): PO Triamterene (**Dyrenium**): PO	Menstrual irregularities, impotence, hypotension.	1. May be used in combination with other diuretics to reduce potassium loss. 2. Potassium-sparing effects may result in hyperkalemia. 3. Not used in clients in experiencing renal failure.

OSMOTIC DIURETIC: Increases osmotic pressure of the fluid in the renal tubule, thus preventing reabsorption of sodium and water

MEDICATIONS	SIDE EFFECTS	NURSING IMPLICATIONS
Mannitol (**Osmitrol**): IV	Pulmonary edema, CHF, tissue dehydration, nausea, vomiting.	1. Stop infusion if client begins to show symptoms of CHF, pulmonary edema. 2. Use an IV filter to prevent infusion of crystals.

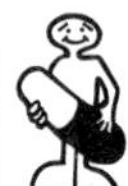

Appendix 16-6: MEDICATIONS USED FOR TREATMENT OF SHOCK

MEDICATIONS	SIDE EFFECTS	NURSING IMPLICATIONS

❖ GENERAL NURSING IMPLICATIONS ❖

— Most often limited to critical care settings; constant monitoring is required.
— Most often administered in diluted solution by IV drip.
— Careful, administered frequent observation and evaluation of blood pressure.
— Continuous EKG monitoring; observe client closely for cardiac dysrhythmias.
— Monitor urinary output every hour.
— Frequent and close monitoring of IV infusion site; leakage into tissue may cause tissue sloughing.
— Medications should not be administered to clients receiving MAO inhibitors or tricyclic antidepressants.

ADRENERGIC AGONIST / CATECHOLAMINE: Increases myocardial contractility, thereby improving cardiac output. Phentolamine (Regitine) is used to infiltrate tissue area if extravasation occurs.

MEDICATIONS	SIDE EFFECTS	NURSING IMPLICATIONS
Dopamine (**Intropin**)	Dysrhythmias (tachycardia), angina, hypertension, headaches.	1. Should not be used in clients with tachydysrhythmias or ventricular fibrillation. 2. If extravasation occurs, stop infusion immediately and infuse area with alpha-adrenergic antagonist. 3. In low doses, enhances renal blood flow.
Dobutamine (**Dobutrex**)	Tachycardia, dysrhythmias.	1. Positive inotropic effect: increased myocardial contractility, stroke volume, cardiac output. 2. Low doses will increase renal blood flow.
Amrinone (**Inocor**)		
Epinephrine hydrochloride (**Adrenalin**): IV	Tachydysrhythmias, angina.	1. Be sure to read label correctly and utilize correct strengths. 2. Observe for cardiac dysrhythmias. 3. Use in treatment of anaphylactic shock and cardiac arrest.
Norepinephrine (**Levophed**)		1. If extravasation occurs. The area needs to be infiltrated with alpha-adrenergic blocker Phentolamine (**Regitine**) 2. Monitor urine output carefully.

Appendix 16-7: VASCULAR ACCESS LINES

CENTRAL LINE - a line inserted into the venous system and progressed into the thoracic cavity with the end of the line in the superior vena cava or the right atrium.

NURSING IMPLICATIONS FOR CENTRAL LINE

—Most common insertion is percutaneous into the subclavian or jugular vein.
—A central line is necessary for a central venous pressure reading and for hyperalimentation solutions.
—Pulmonary artery catheters have a port at the level of the right atrium.
—When changing the tubing on straight central lines, position the client flat (if tolerated) and have him hold his breath and bear down when the line is opened. Immediately connect the new line and have the client breathe normally. Since the catheter goes into the thoracic cavity, it is subjected to changes in pressure, which increases the risk of air embolus.
—Maintain sterile technique when changing the dressing on the puncture site.

VASCULAR ACCESS DEVICES - long-term vascular lines for clients receiving IV therapy for 3 months or longer.-

Implanted ports (MediPort, Port-A-Cath)- port is implanted under the skin; activities are not restricted.

Tunneled ports (Hickman, Broviac)- requires surgical placement, has an external port. The distal tip of both catheters lies in the superior vena cava just above the right atrium. Not used to obtain CVP readings.

Peripherally inserted central catheter (PICC)- is placed in a peripheral vein, has an external port, area requires an occlusive dressing.

Triple or double lumen lines - a venous catheter that contains two or three separate ports and lines that are encased and inserted as one line; may be part of the vascular access devices (VAD). Since each line is separate, the infusing solutions do not mix.

NURSING IMPLICATIONS FOR VASCULAR ACCESS DEVICES:

Flushing - routine flushing may be required unless there is a continuous IV infusion. This should be done with normal saline or fibrinolytics. Type of solution, frequency, and volume depends on IV therapy and if blood was drawn from the line, as well as institution policy. Excessive force should never be used; syringes smaller then 10 cc should not be used because the smaller the syringe, the greater the pressure exerted.

Accessing - Gloves are worn and appropriate skin preparation done for implanted ports; external injection ports and connectors are cleansed prior to accessing.

Dressing Changes - Implanted sites require cleansing after exit, but do not require a dressing. External sites (PICCs and ports) require dressings, either gauze or transparent. Gauze dressings are changed every 48 hours; transparent dressings may not be changed for 5-7 days.

Changing lines - Clamping may be necessary during a tubing change to prevent air emboli; always use a flat or padded clamp to prevent damaging the line. If the line cannot be clamped, have the client hold his breath and bear down (Valsalva maneuver) during the line change.

PHYSIOLOGY OF THE CARDIAC SYSTEM

Structure of the Heart

A. The heart is located in the mediastinal space of the thoracic cavity.

B. The apex of the heart points downward and to the left; the apex comes in contact with the chest wall at about the fifth to sixth intercostal space. In the normal individual, the point of maximum impulse (PMI) may be palpated here; this is also the area to auscultate and evaluate the apical heart rate.

C. The heart is contained in a loose sac called the pericardium.
   1. Fibrous pericardium—the outer surface.
   2. Parietal layer—lines the fibrous pericardium.
   3. Epicardial (visceral layer)—vascular and is adherent to the heart.
   4. There is a potential space between the visceral and parietal layers of the pericardium. This area contains about 5-20cc of pericardial fluid to lubricate the sac and prevent friction from cardiac movement.

D. Myocardial wall.
   1. Epicardium—the outer surface.
   2. Myocardium—the middle layer of cardiac muscle.
   3. Endocardium—the lining of the inner surface of the cardiac chambers.

E. Cardiac chambers (Figure 17-1).
   1. Four chambers are located within the heart; these chambers represent two pumps.
   2. Both atria are the receiving chambers; both ventricles are the ejecting chambers.
   3. The right side of the heart has a thinner myocardium than the left side and is a low-pressure system.
   4. The left ventricle is composed of a thicker muscle, is a high-pressure system, and is capable of generating enough force to eject blood through the aortic valve and through the systemic circulation.

F. Cardiac valves—maintain the directional flow of blood through the heart chambers.
   1. Atrioventricular valves are controlled and supported by papillary muscle connected to the ventricular muscle, and chordae tendineae extending from papillary muscle to valve leaflets.
      a. Tricuspid valve lies between the right atrium and the right ventricle.
      b. Mitral valve lies between the left atrium and the left ventricle.
      c. Both valves prevent backflow of blood from the ventricles into the atria during systole.
   2. Semilunar valves (cusp valves) are controlled by the backward pressure of blood flow at the end of systole.
      a. Pulmonic valve—the outflow valve of the right ventricle into the pulmonary circulation.
      b. Aortic valve—the outflow valve of the left ventricle into the aorta.
      c. Both valves prevent the backflow of blood from the pulmonary artery and the aortic arch into the ventricle during diastole.

G. Direction of blood flow through the heart structure (See Figure 17-1).
   1. From the venous system, the blood enters the right atrium via the superior and inferior vena cavae; through the tricuspid valve into the right ventricle; ejected through the pulmonic valve into the pulmonary artery; to the lungs for oxygenation.
   2. Oxygenated blood returns to the left atrium via the pulmonary veins; through the mitral valve into the left ventricle; ejected through the aortic valve into the aortic arch; into the systemic circulation.
   3. The pulmonary artery is the only artery in the circulatory system to carry deoxygenated blood; the pulmonary vein is the only vein in the circulatory system to carry oxygenated blood.

Cardiac Function

A. Muscles are arranged in an interconnecting manner to allow for coordination of myocardial function. The sequential pattern of contraction and relaxation allows the cardiac muscle to function as a pump.

B. One complete cardiac cycle consists of contraction of the myocardium (systole) and subsequent relaxation of the myocardium (diastole).

C. The amount of blood ejected from the ventricle is the stroke volume.

D. Starling's law of the heart: the greater the cardiac muscles are stretched, the more forceful the contraction. If an increased amount of blood flows into the heart, then the heart will increase the force of contraction and eject a larger amount of blood.

E. Cardiac output (CO = SV x HR).
   1. The cardiac output can be determined by multiplying the stroke volume (SV) by the number of beats per minute (HR) (CO = SV x HR).

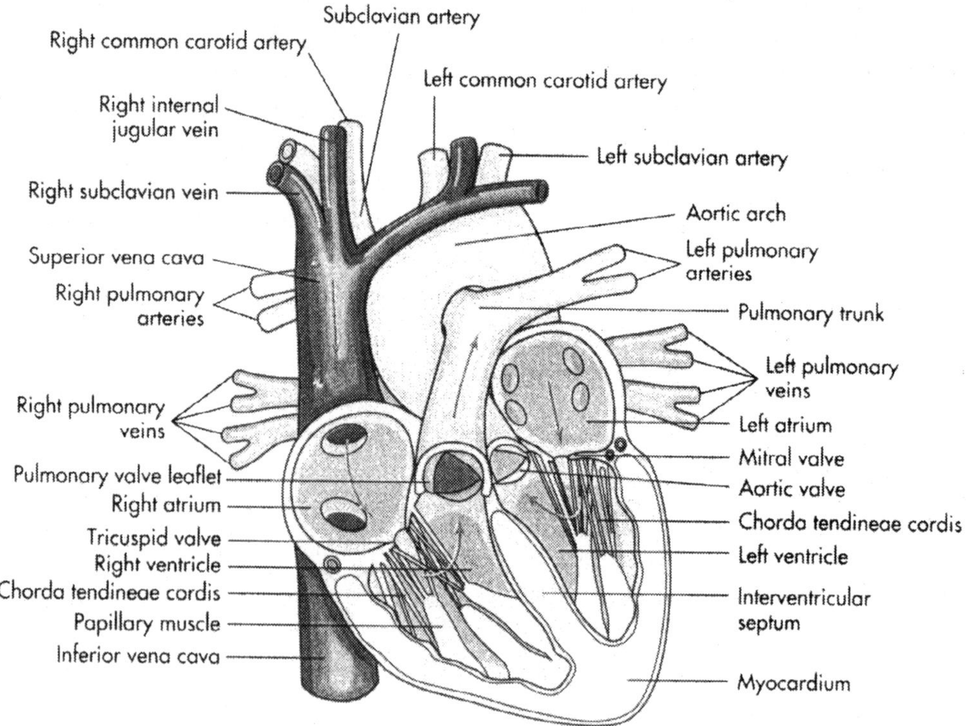

Figure 17-1: Circulation of Blood Through Chambers
Reprinted with permission: Phipps, WJ, Sands, JK, & Marek, JF (1999). *Medical Surgical Nursing: Concepts & Clinical Practice*, 6th ed. Philadelphia: Mosby, p. 604

2. The heart pumps approximately 5 liters of blood every minute.
3. The heart rate increases with exercise; therefore cardiac output increases.
4. The cardiac output will vary according to the amount of venous return.
5. Factors regulating stroke volume.
   a. Degree of stretch of the cardiac muscle prior to contraction (Starling's law); determined by the volume of blood in the ventricle at the end of diastole or diastolic filling.
   b. Contractility—ability of the myocardium to contract; contractility is increased by circulating catecholamines and medications such as digitalis.
   c. Preload—the filling of the ventricles at the end of diastole. The more the ventricles fill, the more the cardiac muscles are stretched, and the greater the force of the contraction during systole (Starling's law). If there is a decrease in the preload, then there is a decrease in contractility and in cardiac output.
   d. Afterload—the pressure in the aorta that the ventricles must overcome in order to pump blood into the systemic circulation. By decreasing the afterload, there is a decrease in the work load of the ventricles; this in turn will assist to increase the stroke volume and the cardiac output.

F. Innervation of the myocardium (autonomic nervous system).
   1. Parasympathetic (vagus nerve) stimulation.
      a. Slows rate of impulse generation at the S-A node.
      b. Slows transmission of the impulse through the A-V node.
      c. Atropine blocks vagal stimulation to the heart.
   2. Sympathetic stimulation.
      a. Increases heart rate.
      b. Increases force of contraction.

G. Factors that increase myocardial oxygen demands.
   1. Increased heart rate.
   2. Increased force of contractions.
   3. Increased afterload.

H. Cardiac compensatory mechanisms—when the normal compensatory mechanisms cannot maintain cardiac output to meet body needs, the client is in a state of cardiac decompensation.
   1. Acute.
      a. Sympathetic nervous system receptors initiate an increase in the release of epinephrine and norepinephrine to increase the cardiac rate and myocardial contractility.

b. Increased diastolic filling (preload) increases cardiac output by increasing the stretch of the myocardial muscle fibers; and therefore increasing the contractility (Starling's law). In a normal heart, this is the mechanism that functions when there is increased need in cardiac output, as in exercise. The increase in the stretch of the myocardial fibers and the increase in the contractile force also require an increase in oxygen consumption. If the myocardial fibers have a decreased oxygen supply and/or the demand on the myocardial muscle is over a prolonged period of time, decompensation will occur.

2. Chronic—ventricular hypertrophy increases cardiac output by increasing the size of the myocardial muscle. There is an increase in the diameter of the muscle fibers to further increase the contractility of the heart. This also increases the myocardial need for oxygen, and in the diseased myocardium the hypertrophy will eventually lead to a decompensated state.

Myocardial Blood Supply

A. Coronary arteries.
1. Originate at the coronary sinus just outside the aortic valve.
2. Provide the only source of oxygenated blood for the myocardium.
3. Arteries fill during diastole, requires a diastolic pressure of 60mmHg is required to adequately perfuse the coronary arteries.

B. Collateral circulation.
1. There are no direct connections between the large coronary arteries.
2. With gradual occlusion of large coronary vessels by ASHD, the smaller vessels increase in size and provide alternative blood flow.
3. Because of the development of collateral circulation, coronary artery disease may be well-advanced before the client experiences symptoms.

Conduction System

A. Controls the rate and rhythm of the heart.

B. Located in the myocardium are pathways for conduction of an electrical impulse which initiates contraction of the heart muscle.

C. Characteristics of cells in the conduction system.
1. Automaticity—the ability of certain conductive pathway cells to initiate an impulse spontaneously and consistently.
2. Excitability—the ability of a cell to respond to an impulse.
3. Conductivity—the ability of a cell to conduct an electrical impulse.
4. Refractoriness—the inability of a cell to respond to incoming stimuli.

D. Impulse generation.
1. Resting state—cell ready to receive an impulse.
2. Depolarization—flow of electrical current along cardiac membrane, initiating muscle contraction.
3. Repolarization—cells regain the electrical charge and are returned to a resting state.

E. Relationship of conducting pathways to the EKG.
1. P wave—indicative of the impulse generated from the S-A node; initiates atrial depolarization.
2. PR interval—delay of the impulse at the A-V node and bundle of His to promote ventricular filling.
3. QRS complex—passage of the impulse through the bundle of His, down the bundle branches, through the Purkinje fibers; depolarization of the ventricle occurs.
4. T wave—ventricular repolarization and return to the resting state.
5. S-T segment—above the base line in cardiac injury, and below the base line with ischemia.

System Assessment

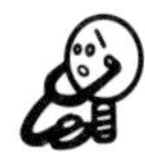

NCLEX ALERT: *Determine changes in client's cardiovascular status -this applies to assessment of clients in all areas and conditions.*

A. Health history.
1. Identify presence of risk factors for the development of arteriosclerotic disease.
2. Coping strategies.
3. Respiratory.
   a. History of difficulty breathing.
   b. Medications taken for respiratory problems.
   c. Determine normal activity level.
4. Circulation.
   a. History of chest discomfort (Table 17-1).
   b. History of edema, weight gain.
   c. History of syncope.
   d. Medications taken for the heart or for high blood pressure.

B. Physical assessment.
1. What is the general appearance of the client: any evidence of distress; what is the level of orientation and ability to think clearly?
2. Evaluate blood pressure.
   a. Pulse pressure—the difference between systolic and diastolic pressure.

b. Assess for postural hypotension—decrease in blood pressure when the client stands.

c. Take blood pressure sitting, standing, and lying if client is having problems with pressure changes. (see Chapter 16 for accurate blood pressure measurement)

d. Paradoxical blood pressure (paradoxical pulse)—a decrease in systolic BP of at least 10mmHg that occurs during inspiration.

3. Evaluate quality and rate of pulse; assess for dysrhythmias (see Appendix 17-3 for determining dysrhythmias).

a. Pulse deficit—the radial pulse rate is less than the apical pulse rate; occurs in atrial fibrillation.

b. Pulsus alternans—regular rhythm, but quality of pulse alternates with strong beats and weak beats.

c. Thready pulse—weak and rapid, difficult to count.

4. Assess quality and pattern of respirations and evidence of respiratory difficulty.

5. Auscultation of the heart.

a. Heart sounds heard during the cardiac cycle.

(1) S_1—closure of the mitral and tricuspid valves.

(2) S_2—closure of the aortic and pulmonic valves.

(3) S_3—represents rapid ventricular filling; normal in children and young adults, adults over 30-years-old may be indication of ventricular dysfunction.

(4) S_4—gallop sounds heard during atrial contraction are abnormal, may occur in tachycardia.

b. Presence of murmurs created by turbulent blood flow.

(1) Abnormal flow through diseased valves stenosis and insufficiency.

(2) Increased rate or velocity of blood flow.

(3) Flow of blood into a dilated chamber.

(4) Abnormal flow of blood between cardiac chambers (congenital heart disease).

c. Presence of a friction rub—rubbing and inflammation of the visceral and parietal layers of the pericardium. Pericardial friction rubs are heard throughout the respiratory cycle.

NCLEX ALERT: *Identify common abnormal heart sounds e.g. S3, S4.*

Table 17-1: ASSESSING CHEST PAIN

P	**PRECIPITATING FACTORS** May occur without precipitators Physical exertion Emotional stress Eating a large meal
Q	**QUALITY** Pressure Squeezing Heaviness Smothering Burning Severe pain Increases with movement
R	**REGION AND RADIATION** Substernal or retrosternal Spreads across the chest Radiates to the inside of either or both arms, the neck, jaw, back, upper abdomen
S	**SYMPTOMS AND SIGNS (ASSOCIATED WITH)** Diaphoresis, cold clammy skin Nausea, vomiting Dyspnea Orthopnea Syncope Apprehension Dysrhythmias Palpitations Auscultation of extra heart sounds Auscultation of crackles Weakness
T	**TIMING AND RESPONSE TO TREATMENT** Sudden onset Constant Duration > 30 minutes Not relieved with nitrates or rest Relief with narcotics

6. Evaluate adequacy of peripheral vascular circulation and for presence of peripheral edema.

7. Evaluate for presence of chest discomfort (Table 17-1).

a. Location.

b. Intensity of pain.

c. Precipitating causes.

DISORDERS OF THE CARDIAC SYSTEM

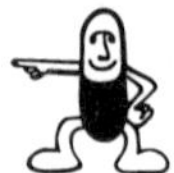

Angina Pectoris

❑ **Arteriosclerotic heart disease (*ASHD, coronary artery disease*) occurs as a result of the atherosclerotic process (Chapter 16) in the coronary arteries. The buildup of plaque or fatty material in the coronary artery causes a narrowing of the lumen of the artery and precipitates myocardial ischemia that causes chest pain.**

A. Pain (angina) occurs when oxygen demands of the heart muscle exceed the ability of the coronary arteries to deliver it.

B. Temporary ischemia does not cause permanent damage of the myocardium. Pain frequently subsides when the precipitating factor is removed.

C. Types of angina.

1. Chronic stable angina—predictable with level of stress or exertion, consistently responds well to medication; pain rarely occurs at rest.
2. Unstable angina (preinfarctional angina) pain may occur at rest; progressive in frequency of attacks; unpredictable, is not relieved with nitroglycerine sublingually.
3. Prinzmetal's (variant)—occurs at rest, may be due to coronary spasms.

Assessment

1. Risk factors/etiology.
   a. Arteriosclerotic heart disease (Table 17-2).
   b. Cardiac ischemia.
   c. Aortic valve disease (impedes filling of the coronary arteries).
   d. Increased cardiac demands.
      (1) Exercise.
      (2) Emotional stress.
      (3) Heavy meals.
      (4) Thyrotoxicosis.
      (5) Exposure to cold.
2. Clinical manifestations.
   a. Pain in varying levels of severity (Table 17-1).
   b. Pain most often is located retrosternal or just to the left of the sternum.
   c. Pain may radiate to neck, jaw, and shoulders.
   d. Client may describe pain as squeezing, choking, constricting, or as a vague feeling of pressure and indigestion.
   e. Frequently will deny seriousness of the pain.
   f. Most correlate with activity, ↑ cardiac demands.
   g. Pain is of short duration, generally about 5 minutes. May be longer if associated with anger or heavy meals.
   h. Accompanying symptoms may include: diaphoresis, increased anxiety, pallor, dyspnea.
3. Diagnostics (Appendix 17-1).
   a. Clinical manifestations.
   b. EKG.
   c. Stress test.

Table 17-2: RISK FACTORS IN ASHD

MODIFIABLE RISK FACTORS:
Elevated serum cholesterol levels
High blood pressure
Cigarette smoking
Sedentary life style
Obesity
Type A personality (high-pressure lifestyle, driving, competitive)
Diabetes mellitus

NON-MODIFIABLE RISK FACTORS:
Genetic predisposition
Positive family history of heart disease
Increasing age
Gender -occurs more often in men

NCLEX ALERT: *Teach health promotion information. Know the ASHD risk factors and be able to teach the client how to effectively reduce his risk factors.*

   d. Cardiac catheterization.

Treatment

1. Primary goal of treatment is to relieve pain and prevent future attacks.
2. Medication (Appendix 17-2).
   a. Vasodilators - nitroglycerin (Table 17-3).
   b. Beta-adrenergic blockers.
   c. Calcium-channel blockers.
   d. Antiplatelet medications (aspirin)
3. Surgical.
   a. Percutaneous transluminal angioplasty—a balloon is passed into the affected coronary artery to the area of obstruction. The balloon is inflated in an attempt to compress the atherosclerotic area and reestablish blood flow to the myocardium.
   b. Intracoronary stents—a tube placed in the coronary vessel to maintain patency.
   c. Cardiac revascularization (open heart surgery).
4. Restricted activity.
5. Supplemental oxygen.
6. Control of the modifiable risk factors. (Table 17-2)

Complications

1. Dysrhythmias (Appendix 17-3).
2. Myocardial infarction.

Nursing Intervention

✦ *Goal: to decrease pain and increase myocardial oxygenation.*

1. Assess characteristics of pain.

2. Evaluate vital signs.
3. Position client in reclining position with head elevated.
4. Begin supplemental O_2.
5. Administer medications.
   a. Nitroglycerin sublingual.
   b. Narcotic analgesics (morphine—IV in small increments until pain subsides).
   c. Aspirin
6. Maintain calm, reassuring atmosphere.

NURSING PRIORITY: *To relieve chest pain and to decrease cardiac damage resulting from an inadequate blood and oxygen supply to the myocardium, there must be an immediate reduction in the work load of the heart that results in a decrease in the oxygen consumption: rest, nitroglycerine, oxygen therapy.*

✦ *Goal: to evaluate characteristics of anginal pain and client's overall response.*
1. Does pain increase with breathing? (Anginal pain is generally not affected by breathing or changes of position.)
2. Assess activity tolerance or precipitating factor.
3. Assess characteristics of pain (Table 17-1).
   a. Length.
   b. Onset—gradual or sudden.
   c. Response of pain to nitroglycerin.
   d. Client's description of pain.
4. Evaluate response of pain to treatment or progression to more severe level.
5. Obtain a 12-lead EKG.
6. Assess respiratory status and response to pain.
7. Assess for presence of dysrhythmia and document as indicated.

✦ *Goal: to provide care postcardiac interventional procedures.*
1. Monitor for chest pain and hypotension; reocclusion is primary complication.
2. Frequent assessment of status of circulation distal to area of cannulation.
3. A sheath may be left in place; monitor area for bleeding, if it occurs put manual pressure on the area and notify the doctor.
4. Prevent flexion of affected extremity and maintain bedrest for 6-8 hours.
5. Avoid heavy lifting; may return to work in 1-2 weeks.
6. Notify the doctor of any bleeding at site and of chest pain or syncope.

Table 17-3: CLIENT EDUCATION FOR NITROGLYCERINE ADMINISTRATION

1. Keep in a tightly closed, dark glass container.
2. Carry supply at all times.
3. Fresh tablets should cause a slight burning under the tongue.
4. Purchase a new supply of medication every four to six months.
5. Take nitroglycerin prophylactically to avoid pain - sexual intercourse, exercise, walking, etc.
6. Take nitroglycerin when pain begins, and stop all activity.
7. If pain is not relieved in three to five minutes, take another nitroglycerin. Repeat procedure if still no relief.
8. If after taking a total of three nitroglycerin there is no pain relief, seek medical attention immediately.
9. Side effects of nitroglycerin are headache, dizziness, and flushing.

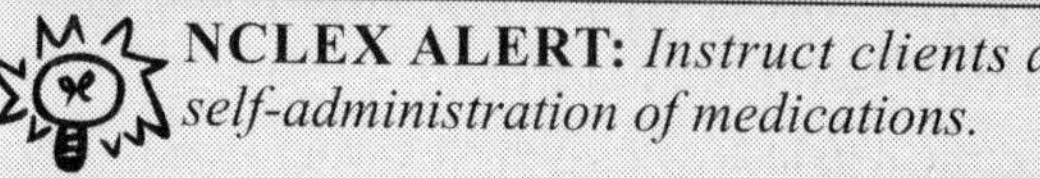
NCLEX ALERT: *Instruct clients about self-administration of medications.*

7. Assess ECG for evidence of ST segment changes.

Self Care
1. Education regarding ASHD.
   a. Will be able to identify personal risk factors and appropriate health practices to decrease risk factors.
   b. Will be able to identify factors precipitating pain.
2. Determine that client understands his medication regimen (Table 17-3).
3. Assess understanding of diet and exercise regime.
4. Assess understanding of seeking medical assistance if pain persists and is not relieved by medication.
5. Assist client to identify resources for counseling to decrease stress.

Myocardial Infarction

❑ **A *myocardial infarction* (MI, coronary occlusion, heart attack) is a total occlusion of a portion of a coronary artery. Following the occlusion, there is myocardial ischemia, injury or death.**

A. Infarction most often occurs in the area of the left ventricle.
B. The severity of the situation depends on the area of the heart involved, as well as the size of the infarction.
C. Healing process.
   1. In the first 24 hours, inflammatory process is well-established; leukocytes invade the area and cardiac enzymes are released from the damaged cells.
   2. 4 to 10 days—necrotic zone is well-defined.

3. 10 to 14 days—the formation of scar tissue foundation begins.

D. The presence of preestablished collateral circulation will assist in decreasing the size of the necrotic area.

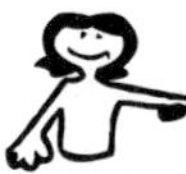

NURSING PRIORITY: *Danger of death from an MI is greatest during the first two hours.*

Assessment

1. Risk factors/etiology.
   a. ASHD.
   b. Sudden increase in exercise.
   c. Frequently no precipitating factors.
2. Clinical manifestations.
   a. Typical pain is severe, substernal, crushing, and unrelieved by nitroglycerin.
   b. Denial of the seriousness of the pain, frequently wait over 2 hours to seek assistance.
   c. Dyspnea.
   d. Nausea, vomiting, indigestion.
   e. Pale/dusky skin.
   f. Pain may radiate down arm or up the jaw.
   g. Onset is usually sudden.
   h. Diaphoresis.
   i. Extreme weakness.
   j. Decrease in blood pressure.
   k. Tachycardia.
   l. Syncope.
3. Diagnostics (Appendix 17-1).
   a. Serum laboratory studies.
      (1) Cardiac isoenzymes - CPK, Treponin are elevated.
      (2) Increase in WBC.
   b. Serial EKGs.
   c. Positron emission tomography.
   d. Radionuclide imaging.

Treatment

1. Supplemental oxygen.
2. IV line for medications.
3. Control dysrhythmias, especially tachycardia.
4. Medications (Appendix 17-2).
   a. Analgesics (morphine).
   b. Antidysrhythmic agents (lidocaine).
   c. Calcium blocking agents (verapamil).
   d. Anticoagulants (Appendix 16-2).
   e. Sedatives.
   f. Stool softeners.
5. Thrombolytic therapy (Appendix 17-2).
6. Pacemaker if conduction problems occur (Appendix 17-4).
7. Dietary restrictions.
8. Open heart surgery for myocardial revascularization.
9. PTCA—percutaneous transluminal coronary angiography or intra-coronary stents.

Complications

1. Cardiogenic shock.
2. Dysrhythmias (Appendix 17-3).
3. Congestive heart failure.

Nursing Intervention

✦ *Goal: to decrease pain and increase myocardial oxygenation (See related goal, Angina).*

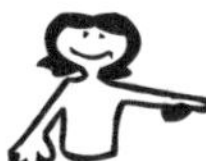

NURSING PRIORITY: *As long as chest pain persists, there is continuing cardiac ischemia.*

✦ *Goal: to evaluate characteristics of cardiac pain and client's overall response (See related goal, Angina).*

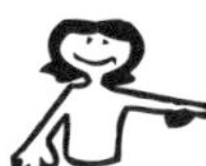

NURSING PRIORITY: *Decrease activity when client is tachycardic, with or without chest pain.*

✦ *Goal: to maintain homeostasis and decrease effects of MI.*

1. Cardiac monitor to identify serious dysrhythmia; document, treat, and report as indicated.
2. Frequent assessment for dyshyrthmias, murmurs, and presence of S_3, S_4.
3. Maintain IV access.
4. Maintain bedrest initially (1st 24 hours).
5. Frequent assessment of chest pain.
6. Evaluate urinary output and renal response.
7. Assess respiratory system for pulmonary congestion.
8. Evaluate peripheral circulation; assess for dependent edema.
9. NPO initially, then clear liquid; progress to light meals that are low in sodium and cholesterol.
10. Promote normal bowel pattern.
    a. Stool softeners.
    b. Bedside commode.

c. Caution against stimulation of the vagus nerve (Valsalva maneuver).

d. Increase fiber in diet.

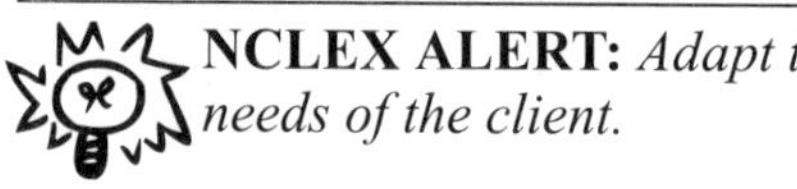

NCLEX ALERT: *Adapt the diet to special needs of the client.*

11. Decrease anxiety.
    a. Keep client informed regarding progress and immediate plan of care.
    b. Decrease sensory overload.
    c. Encourage verbalization of concerns and fears.
12. Monitor for changes in neurological status—confusion, disorientation, etc.
13. Monitor progressive activity.
    a. Early activities should not increase heart rate greater the 25% of resting rate.
    b. Assess heart rhythm, fatigue, and B/P after each activity.
    c. Resting tachycardia is a contraindication to activity.

NCLEX ALERT: *Determine changes in client's cardiovascular system. Monitor progress of cardiac client and evaluate tolerance to changes in activity.*

Self Care

1. Participate in organized cardiac rehabilitation program.
    a. Progressive monitored exercise.
    b. Dietary modifications.
    c. Stress management.
    d. Continued education regarding ASHD and decreasing personal risk factors.
2. Understand medication regimen.
3. Teach client how to take his pulse and check for rate and regularity.
4. Exercise in climate-controlled areas; teach client how to evaluate response to exercise (dyspnea, tachycardia, chest pain, etc).
5. Call the doctor for pain not controlled by nitroglycerine, significant changes in pulse rate, decreased tolerance to activity, syncope, increase in dyspnea.
6. Sexual intercourse generally can be resumed in 4-6 weeks post MI, or when the client can climb two flights of stairs without difficulty.
    a. Do not drink any alcohol prior to sexual activity.
    b. Take nitroglycerine prior to activity.
    c. Do not have sex after a heavy meal.
    d. Position for intercourse does not influence cardiac workload.

NCLEX ALERT: *Determine client's ability to perform self-care, whether the cardiac client understands his illness and if he can demonstrate knowledge of care.*

Congestive Heart Failure (CHF)

❑ **Congestive heart failure (cardiac decompensation, cardiac insufficiency, ventricular failure) is the inability of the heart to pump adequate amounts of blood into the systemic circulation in order to meet tissue metabolic demands; usually occurs secondary to dysrhythmias, acute myocardial infarction, or hypertension.**

Physiology of heart failure

A. Left-sided failure.
1. Results from failure of the left ventricle to maintain adequate cardiac output.
2. Blood backs up into the left atrium and into the pulmonary veins.
3. Increasing pressure in the pulmonary capillary bed causes lungs to become congested, resulting in impaired gas exchange.
4. Precipitating factors.
    a. MI (left ventricular infarct).
    b. Hypertension.
    c. Aortic and mitral value disease.
    d. Dysrhythmia.

B. Right-sided failure.
1. The right ventricle is unable to maintain adequate output.
2. Blood backs up into the systemic circulation and causes peripheral edema.
3. Precipitating factors.
    a. Left-sided heart failure.
    b. Chronic pulmonary hypertension.
    c. Right ventricular infarction.
    d. Excessive IV fluids.

C. Both sides of the heart are dependent on the other for adequate function.
1. Left-sided failure results in pulmonary congestion; this causes increase in pulmonary pressure, which puts increased workload on the right side of the heart and precipitates failure.

2. Although origin of problem may begin solely on one side, the majority of clinical situations involve failure on both sides.

D. High-output versus low-output failure.

1. High-output failure occurs when the body's needs for oxygen are excessively increased; the heart increases output, but is still unable to meet body needs (thyrotoxicosis and anemia).
2. Low-output failure occurs when the myocardium is so damaged that it cannot maintain adequate cardiac output; it is the failure of the heart as a pump.

E. Cardiac compensatory mechanisms will attempt to maintain the body requirements for cardiac output; when these mechanisms become ineffective, cardiac decompensation or failure will occur.

F. Edema development in right congestive heart failure.

1. With a decrease in the cardiac output, there is a decrease in tissue perfusion.
   a. A decrease in renal perfusion; the kidneys respond by stimulating the adrenal cortex to increase the secretion of aldosterone, thus increasing the retention of sodium and water.
   b. An increase in the secretion of ADH from the posterior pituitary gland, resulting in retention of sodium and water.
2. The above physiological responses increase the circulating fluid volume in an attempt to increase tissue perfusion.
3. With an increase in the venous pressure from the increased circulating volume, there is an increase in the capillary pressure and dependent, pitting edema occurs.

G. In children CHF occurs most often as the result of a structural problem of the heart. Ventricular function may not be impaired, but symptoms occur due to increased pulmonary artery pressure and pulmonary venous congestion.

Assessment

1. Risk factors/etiology.
   a. Myocardial disease.
   b. Valvular disease.
   c. Congenital heart disease.
   d. Fluid overload.
2. Clinical manifestations.(Table 17-4).
   a. Impaired cardiac function.
      (1) Tachycardia evaluated according to age level (see Table 15-2).
      (2) Cardiomegaly from dilatation and hypertrophy; PMI is displaced.
      (3) S_3 or S_4 (heart gallop) due to impaired ventricular function.
      (4) In infants, a failure to thrive and gain adequate weight.
      (5) Poor perfusion- cool extremities, weak pulses, poor capillary refill.
   b. Pulmonary congestion (left-sided failure).
      (1) Dyspnea, tachypnea.
      (2) Orthopnea.
      (3) Paroxysmal nocturnal dyspnea (PND) occurs while client is asleep.
      (4) Symptoms of respiratory distress and hypoxia (see Table 15-3).
      (5) Cough.
      (6) Congested breath sounds.
      (7) Feeding difficulties in infants, due to dyspnea.
      (8) Increase in PAP and PAWP (Appendix 17-5).
   c. Systemic congestion (right-sided failure).
      (1) Hepatomegaly—may be an early sign in children.
      (2) Peripheral pitting edema.
      (3) Dependent edema generalized in infants; evaluate by weight gain.
      (4) Ascites.
      (5) Increase in CVP (Appendix 17-5).

NCLEX ALERT: *Determine changes in client's cardiovascular status as related to his CHF.*

3. Diagnostics.
   a. Chest X-ray.
   b. EKG.
   c. Echocardiogram.

Treatment

1. Treatment of the underlying problem.
2. Prevention.
   a. Prophylactic antibiotics in rheumatic heart disease prior to medical procedures.
   b. Effective early treatment of hypertension.
   c. Early treatment of dysrhythmia.
3. Oxygen.
4. Bedrest.
5. Medications (Appendix 17-2).

a. Cardiac glycosides.

b. Diuretics.

c. Potassium.

d. Vasodilators (decrease the afterload).

e. Aspirin.

6. Decreased sodium diet in adults, sodium not as severely restricted in infants and children.
7. Fluid restrictions, adults and older children. Infant seldom need fluid restriction because of difficulty feeding.

Complications

1. Pulmonary edema.
2. Cardiogenic shock.
3. Dysrhythmias.

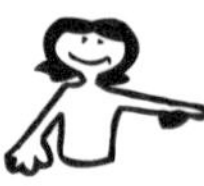

***NURSING PRIORITY:** The goals for therapeutic intervention in clients with congestive failure are:*

** Improve cardiac output—digitalis and oxygen.*

** Decrease the afterload—decrease activity, administer vasodilator.*

** Decrease the preload—diuretics, decrease sodium and fluid intake, place client in semi-Fowler's position.*

Nursing Intervention

✦ *Goal: to decrease cardiac demands and improve cardiac function.*

1. Assess vital signs and compare with other physical assessment data.
2. Limit physical activity.
3. Maintain normal body temperature; avoid chilling.
4. Provide supplemental oxygen.
5. Provide uninterrupted sleep when possible.
6. Minimize crying in children and infants.
7. Chilling increases oxygen consumption, especially in infants.
8. Decrease stress and anxiety; encourage parents to remain with child.

✦ *Goal: to decrease circulating volume.*

NCLEX ALERT: *Check for interactions among client's drugs, foods and fluids. For clients receiving digitalis and diuretics, it is very important to monitor the serum potassium level. A severe decrease in the serum potassium may affect cardiac rhythm, and may precipitate digitalis toxicity.*

Table 17-4: ASSESSMENT FINDINGS OF CONGESTIVE HEART FAILURE

RIGHT-SIDED (Systemic symptoms)
Neck vein distention
Generalized edema (anasarca)
Dependent pitting edema
Nausea, vomiting
Anorexia
Altered GI function
Weight gain
Ascites
Decreased urinary output
Liver engorgement
Electrolyte imbalances
Dysrhythmias
Elevated CVP
LEFT-SIDED (Pulmonary symptoms)
Dusky skin and nail beds
Chest pain
Tachycardia
Decreased systolic BP
Ventricular ectopics
S_3 and S_4
Shift of the PMI to the left
Irritability, restlessness
Decreased cardiac output
Increased PAWP
Wheezing crackles
Dyspnea
Productive cough

1. Assess breath sounds, distended neck veins, peripheral edema.
2. Decreased sodium diet and fluid restriction.
3. Evaluate fluid retention by accurate daily weight (5 pounds = 2 liters of fluid).
4. Accurate intake and output.

✦ *Goal: to reduce respiratory distress.*

1. Position.

a. Adult in Fowler's or in an armchair.

b. Infants and small children may breathe better side-lying with the knees drawn up to the chest.

c. Infants may be placed in an infant seat.

d. Make sure diapers are loosely pinned and safety restraints do not hinder maximum expansion of the chest.

e. Do not elevate client's legs as this increases venous return.

f. Hold infant upright over the shoulder with knees flexed (knee chest position).

2. Administer oxygen, oxygen hood for infants, cannula for adults and older children..
3. Evaluate breath sounds and presence of hypoxia.
4. Do not allow infants to cry for extend periods.

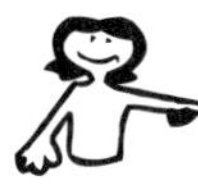

NURSING PRIORITY: Infants: if cyanosis decreases with crying the problem is usually pulmonary; if cyanosis increases with crying the problem is usually cardiac.

✦ *Goal: to monitor for development of hypoxia (Chapter 15).*

✦ *Goal: to maintain nutrition.*

1. Provide small, frequent feedings; allow client adequate time, every 3 hours is good schedule for infants.
2. Infants may need to be gavaged, due to increased work of sucking.
3. Infants generally not on fluid restriction, due to decreased intake from dyspnea.
4. Do not prop the bottle; burp the infant frequently.

Rheumatic Heart Disease

❑ **An inflammatory disease primarily affecting connective tissue, especially cardiac valves.**

A. Usually preceded by a group A beta hemolytic *streptococcal* infection.

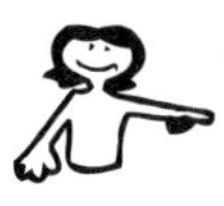

NURSING PRIORITY: Prevention and adequate treatment of streptococcal infections prevents the development of rheumatic fever.

1. Tissue damage believed to be related to an autoimmune process.
2. Antibodies produced in response to streptococcal infection react with connective tissue (cardiac tissue, joints).

B. Myocardial involvement characterized by inflammation of the endocardium, pericardium, and myocardium.

1. Endocarditis produces scarring of the cardiac valves.
2. Mitral and aortic valves are most commonly affected, either by valvular stenosis or valvular insufficiency.

Assessment

1. Risk factors/etiology - previous infection by *beta hemolytic streptococcus*.
2. Clinical manifestations—symptoms vary; no specific symptom or sign is diagnostic of rheumatic fever. Criteria for the diagnosis requires a combination of symptoms to be present.
   a. Carditis
   b. Migratory polyarthritis.
   c. Chorea.
   d. Erythema marginatum.
   e. Subcutaneous nodules

Treatment

1. Adequate treatment of streptococcal infection.
2. Bedrest until tachycardia subsides.
3. Salicylates to control inflammatory process.
4. Prophylactic treatment.
   a. Initiated after acute therapy.
   b. Monthly administration of IM penicillin over extended period of time.
   c. Administration of prophylactic penicillin before and after medical procedures which increase risk factor of infection (GU procedures, dental work, etc.).

Complications

Severe valvular damage precipitates the development of congestive heart failure and may require open heart surgery for replacement of diseased valve.

Nursing Intervention

(Child is generally cared for in the home environment).

✦ *Goal: to assist parents and family to provide home environment conducive to healing and recovery.*

1. Decrease activity; bedrest if pulse rate is increased or if febrile.
2. Friends may visit for short periods; child is not contagious.
3. Maintain adequate nutrition.
   a. May be anorexic during the febrile phase.
   b. Soft or liquid foods as tolerated.
   c. Assist child with feeding if choreic movements are severe.
   d. Maintain adequate hydration.
4. Administer analgesics for arthralgia.
5. Reassure child that chorea and joint involvement is only temporary and there will be no residual damage.

✦ *Goal: to assist parents to understand need for long-term prophylactic antibiotic therapy.*

1. Importance of preventing recurring infections.
2. Include child in planning, especially when numerous injections are involved.
3. Importance of prophylactic therapy prior to invasive medical procedures.
4. Continued medical follow-up for the development of valvular problems as child grows.

Endocarditis (Bacterial, Infective)

❑ **Endocarditis is an infection of the valves and inner lining of the heart.**

A. Organisms tend to grow on the endocardium in an area of increased turbulence of blood flow, or in areas of previous cardiac damage (rheumatic heart disease, congenital malformations).

B. Bacteria may enter from any site of localized infection.

C. Organism grows on the endocardium and produces a characteristic lesion consisting of vegetation, fibrin deposits, collagen; the lesion then may invade adjacent valves.

D. Lesion is fragile and may break off and embolize elsewhere.

Assessment

1. Risk factors/etiology.
   a. Most often bacterial (streptococcal) but may be fungal or viral.
   b. History of pre-existing heart condition.
   c. History of recent invasive procedures: minor surgery, dental procedures, procedures involving the urinary tract.
2. Clinical manifestations.
   a. Symptoms of systemic infection.
   b. Murmur develops or changes occur in previous murmurs.
   c. Symptoms secondary to emboli (left sided endocarditis).
      (1) Spleen—splenomegaly, upper left quadrant pain.
      (2) Kidney—flank pain, hematuria.
      (3) Brain—hemiplegia, decreased level of consciousness.
      (4) Pulmonary—dyspnea, chest pain, hemoptysis.
      (5) Peripheral manifestations—splinter hemorrhages in nail bed, changes in retina.
   d. Hematological symptoms.
      (1) Anemia.
      (2) Petechiae (common).
3. Diagnostics.
   a. History to identify site of entry.
   b. EKG changes.
   c. Blood cultures.

Treatment

1. IV antibiotic therapy for 4-6 weeks. (Appendix 6-10).
2. Bedrest if high fever or if evidence of cardiac damage.
3. Prophylactic antibiotics for 3-5 years, especially in children with history of rheumatic fever or congenital anomalies.
4. Surgical intervention for severe valvular damage.

Complications

1. Congestive heart failure.
2. General systemic emboli.

Nursing Intervention

✦ *Goal: to assist parents to understand need for long-term prophylactic therapy. (See related Goal, rheumatic fever).*

✦ *Goal: to maintain homeostasis and prevent complications.*

1. IV antibiotic medications.
2. Assess activity tolerance, restricted activities until:
   a. Temperature is normal.
   b. Resting pulse is below 100.
   c. EKG is stable.
3. Evaluate for complications of emboli and congestive heart failure.

Self Care

1. Teach family how to administer IV antibiotics.
2. Progressive activity to gradually increase tolerance.
3. Client/family understand need for continued antibiotics.
4. Report temperature elevations, fever, chills, anorexia, weight loss, and increased fatigue.

Pericarditis

❑ **Pericarditis is an inflammation of the pericardium.**

A. Acute pericarditis—may be dry or may cause excessive fluid accumulation in the pericardial space.

B. Chronic pericarditis—fibrous thickening of the visceral and parietal pericardium; thickening inhibits cardiac filling during diastole.

Assessment

1. Risk factors/etiology.
   a. Acute.
      (1) Infection.
      (2) Myocardial injury.
      (3) Hypersensitivity (collagen diseases, SLE, drug reactions).
      (4) Metabolic disorders (uremia, myxedema).
2. Clinical manifestations.

a. Acute.

(1) Precordial pain.

(2) Pericardial friction rub caused by myocardium rubbing against inflamed pericardium.

(3) Pain increases with respirations, sitting may relieve pain.

b. Chronic—symptoms are characteristic of gradually occurring CHF; chest pain is not a prominent symptom.

3. Diagnostics (acute and chronic).

a. EKG changes.

b. Increased sedimentation rate.

c. History of precipitating causes.

Complications

1. Cardiac tamponade.
2. Pericardial effusion.

Treatment

1. Acute.
   a. Treat underlying problem.
   b. Bedrest.
   c. Anti-inflammatory medications.
   d. If pleural effusion and tamponade occur, then pericardiocentesis (aspiration of fluid from the pericardial sac).

Nursing Intervention

✦ *Goal: to maintain homeostasis and promote comfort.*

1. Assess characteristics of pain; administer appropriate analgesics.
2. Upright position, with client leaning forward, may relieve the pain.
3. Decrease anxiety, as client often associates problem with an MI; assist client to distinguish the difference.
4. Observe for symptoms of cardiac tamponade.
   a. Pulsus paradoxus - precipitous decrease in systolic blood pressure on inspiration.
   b. CVP increased, presence of JVD.
   c. Heart sounds are muffled or distant.
   d. Narrowing pulse pressure.
5. In clients with chronic pericarditis, evaluate for symptoms of CHF and initiate appropriate nursing intervention.

Cardiac Valve Disorders

A. Etiology of valve disease.

1. Congenital heart disease.
2. Rheumatic heart disease.
3. Bacterial endocarditis.
4. Ischemia secondary to ASHD.

B. Mitral valve is most commonly involved, followed by the aortic valve.

C. Valvular stenosis—a narrowing of the valve opening and progressive obstruction to blood flow; increase in workload of the cardiac chamber pumping through the stenosed valve.

D. Valvular insufficiency (incompetency, regurgitation)—impaired closure of the valve allows blood to flow back into the cardiac chamber, thereby increasing the workload of the heart.

Disorders of the Mitral Valve

A. Stenosis—increases workload on the left atrium as it attempts to force blood through the narrow valve.

B. Mitral insufficiency (regurgitation) —with each cardiac contraction, the left ventricle forces blood back into the left atrium.

C. With both conditions, the left atrium dilates and hypertrophies due to an increase in workload. This causes an increase in pulmonary pressure and the subsequent development of CHF.

Assessment

1. Risk factors - associated with history of rheumatic fever and endocarditis.
2. Clinical manifestations.
   a. Exertional dyspnea, orthopnea.
   b. Progressive fatigue due to decrease in cardiac output.
   c. Narrow pulse pressure.
   d. Cardiac murmur (diastolic).
   e. Systemic embolization.
   f. Palpitations.
   g. Developing CHF.
   h. Atrial fibrillation.
3. Diagnostics.
   a. Echocardiogram.
   b. Cardiac catheterization (Appendix 17-1).

Treatment

1. Prevention of CHF.
   a. Digitalis (Appendix 17-6).
   b. Diuretics.
   c. Beta blockers to decrease cardiac rate.
2. Prophylactic anticoagulation to prevent embolus formation.
3. Prophylactic antibiotics.

4. Open heart surgery for valve replacement when there is evidence of progressive cardiac failure.

Nursing Intervention

✦ *Goal: to prevent development of rheumatic heart disease and provide prophylactic treatment to individuals with history of rheumatic heart disease.*

✦ *Goal: to identify early development of congestive heart failure.*

***NURSING PRIORITY:** The primary care for the client with cardiac valve disease is to maintain homeostasis and prevent the development of CHF. The client should be advised to avoid excessive fatigue and should be assessed according to the level of activity tolerance.*

Disorders of Aortic Valve

A. Aortic stenosis—increased (afterload) work of the left ventricle as it attempts to propel blood through the narrowed valve.

B. Aortic insufficiency—increased (afterload) work of the left ventricle as blood leaks back into the left ventricle after contraction.

C. With both conditions, the left ventricle dilates and hypertrophies due to increased pressure and this will precipitate left ventricular failure.

Assessment

1. Clinical manifestations.
   a. Syncope and vertigo.
   b. Angina (condition interferes with coronary artery filling).
   c. Dysrhythmia.
   d. Systolic murmur.
   e. Dyspnea. and increasing fatigue.
   f. Congestive heart failure.
   g. Widened pulse pressure with aortic insufficiency, decreased in aortic stenosis.
2. Diagnostics (same as mitral valve disease).

Treatment

(Same as mitral valve disease).

Nursing Intervention

(Same as mitral valve disease).

Cardiovascular Disease in Pregnancy

❑ **Rheumatic heart disease, congenital heart defects and mitral valve prolapse account for the greatest incidence of cardiac disease in pregnancy.**

A. Normal physiological alterations of pregnancy that increase cardiovascular stress.
   1. Increase in oxygen requirements.
   2. Increase in cardiac output.
   3. Increase in plasma volume.
   4. Weight gain.
   5. Hemodynamic changes during delivery.

B. As normal pregnancy advances, cardiovascular system is unable to maintain adequate output to meet increasing demands. Classification of the severity of cardiac disease in pregnancy is presented in Table 17-5.

C. Increased incidence of prematurity and low birth weight is indicative of the inability of the heart to meet the demands of the growing fetus.

Assessment

Clinical manifestations indicative of cardiac decompensation are those of impending CHF.

1. Frequent cough, progressive dyspnea.
2. Progressive general edema.
3. Syncope with exertion.
4. Excessive fatigue for level of activity.
5. Dysrhythmia.
6. Congested breath sounds.
7. Cardiac decompensation increases with length of gestation; 28 to 32 weeks has highest incidence of CHF.

Treatment

1. Management of the pregnant client.
   a. Good nutritional intake; iron supplement, may require decrease in calories to avoid excessive weight gain.
   b. Limited physical activity.
   c. Sodium and fluids may be limited but not severely restricted.
   d. Diuretics and digitalis only if cardiac disease is severe.
   e. May be hospitalized at 28 to 32 weeks due to impending CHF.
   f. If coagulation problems occur, heparin is utilized because it does not cross the placenta.
   g. Prophylactic penicillin to prevent infection (endocarditis).
2. Management of the client during intrapartum.
   a. Outlet forceps may be used to shorten labor.
   b. Regional anesthesia generally utilized for delivery.
   c. Supplemental oxygen.

3. Management of the client during postpartum -treated symptomatically according to status of cardiovascular system; the postpartum period is a time of increased risk for CHF in the mother.

Nursing Intervention

✦ *Goal: to assist client to maintain homeostasis during pregnancy.*

1. Written information regarding nutritional needs.
2. Nursing assessment to identify early symptoms of CHF.
3. Frequent rest periods; activity may be severely restricted the last trimester.

***NURSING PRIORITY:** One of the most effective means of decreasing the cardiac workload is to decrease activity; therefore, the pregnant client needs to avoid excessive fatigue to prevent or decrease cardiac decompensation.*

4. Decrease stress by keeping client informed of progress.

✦ *Goal: to assist client to maintain homeostasis during intrapartum.*

1. Close observation of pulmonary function during labor.
2. Evaluate information from continuous fetal and maternal monitoring.
3. Discourage pushing during labor to prevent Valsalva maneuver and increase cardiac stress.
4. Position on left lateral side with head and shoulders elevated.
5. Prepare for vaginal delivery.
6. Provide pain relief as indicated.
   a. Pain increases cardiac work.
   b. Evaluate effects of analgesia on fetus.

✦ *Goal: to maintain homeostasis in postpartal period.*

1. Assessment of pulmonary and cardiac adaptation to changes in hemodynamics.
2. Maintain semi-Fowler's position or left lateral position with the head elevated.
3. Gradual progression of activities (depending on cardiac status) as indicated by:
   a. Pulse rate.
   b. Respiratory status.
   c. Activity tolerance.
4. Progressive ambulation as soon as possible, to prevent venous thrombosis.
5. Assist mother and family to prepare for discharge.

CONGENITAL HEART DISEASE

Table 17-5: CLASSIFICATION OF CARDIOVASCULAR DISEASE

Class I	Physical activity is not limited; no discomfort from normal activity. No anginal pain.
Class II	Physical activity is slightly limited; comfortable at rest, normal activity precipitates fatigue, dyspnea and anginal pain.
Class III	Physical activity is markedly decreased; less than normal activity precipitates excessive fatigue, dyspnea and anginal pain.
Class IV	Physical activity is severely restricted, as symptoms of cardiac insufficiency are present at rest.

Source: Criteria Committee, New York Heart Assoc.

A. Clinical manifestations depend on the severity of the defect and the adequacy of pulmonary blood flow.

B. Normal pressure in the right side of the heart is lower than the left side; blood will flow from an area of high pressure to an area of low pressure.

C. Acyanotic defects are not immediately incompatible with life, because blood flows through the defect from the left side of the heart to the right. No deoxygenated blood flows into the left ventricle; considered a left-to-right shunt.

D. Cyanotic defects initially may be incompatible with life. Specific defects precipitate a pressure change, so blood is shunted from the right to the left side of the heart and deoxygenated blood enters the left ventricle; considered a right-to-left shunt.

E. Severe acyanotic defects that are not corrected may progress to a cyanotic shunt. In the acyanotic, left-to-right shunt, there is an increase in the pulmonary vascular resistance due to thickening of the pulmonary vasculature. As the resistance in the pulmonary circulation increases, there is a subsequent increase in the pressure in the right ventricle. The increased pressure in the right ventricle may reverse the left-to-right, acyanotic shunt, to a right-to-left, cyanotic shunt.

F. Physical consequences of congenital defects.
   1. Retarded physical growth.
      a. Failure to gain weight, often due to poor nutrition.
      b. Tachycardia and tachypnea precipitate increase in caloric requirements.
   2. Excessive fatigue, especially during feedings.
   3. Frequent upper respiratory infections.
   4. Dyspnea.
   5. Tachycardia.
   6. Tachypnea.

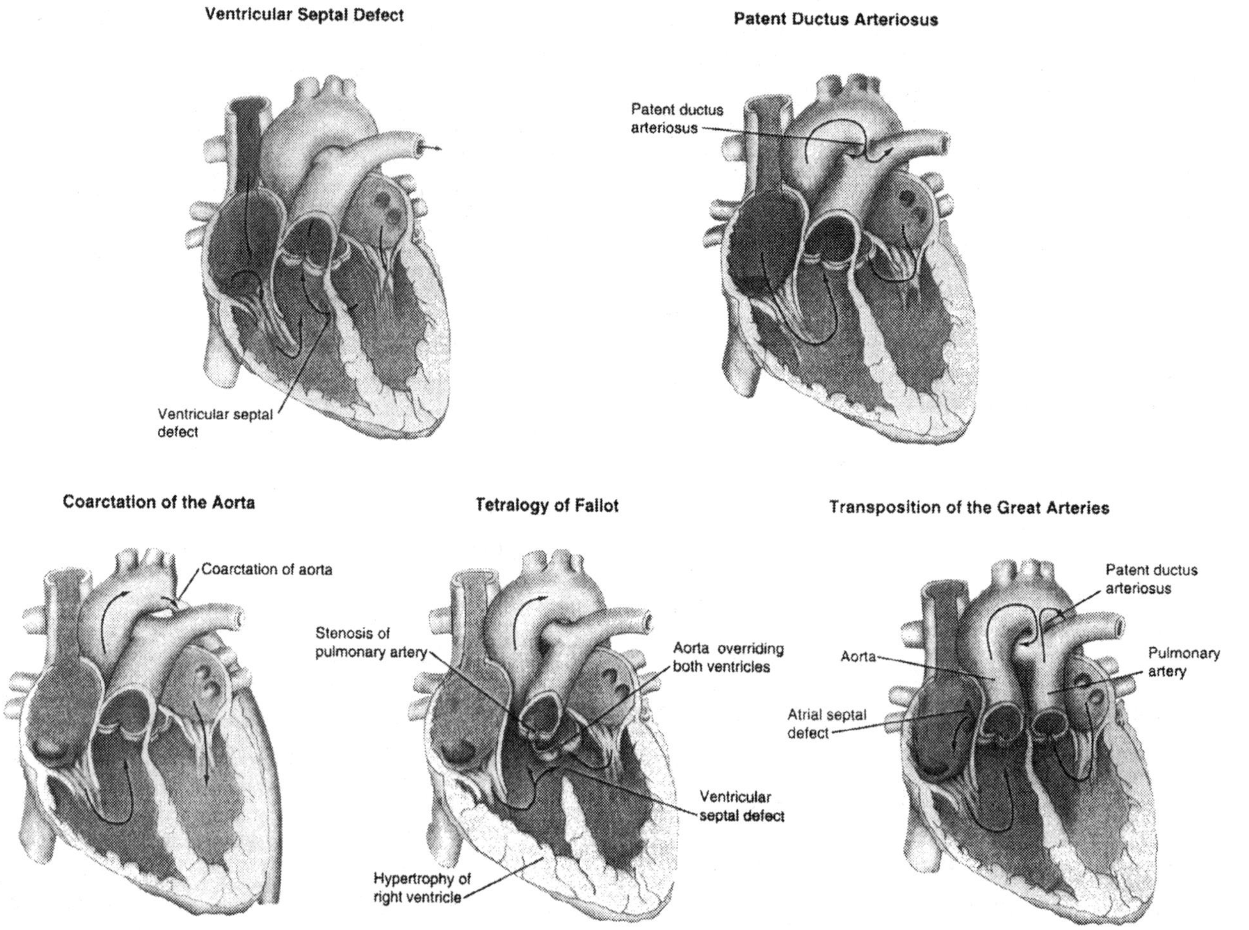

Figure 17-2: Congenital Heart Defects
Reprinted with permission: Gorrie, T., McKinney, E., & Murray, S., (1998) *Foundations of Maternal-Newborn Nursing,* 2nd ed, Philadelphia: W.B. Saunders, p 874.

7. Cyanotic defects.
   a. Cyanosis (cyanotic defect).
   b. Clubbing (cyanotic defect).
   c. Squatting (cyanotic defect); older children will "squat" in order to shunt blood into the pulmonary circulation. By squatting, the venous return from the lower extremities is reduced, and there is an increase in the systemic resistance. The decrease in the preload from the venous system, and the increase in the afterload on the arterial side, will cause pressure changes in the heart that will decrease the right-to-left shunt. The changes in pressure increase the amount of blood pumped into the pulmonary vasculature. This decreases the right-to-left shunt and increases the oxygenation of circulating blood.
   d. Hypercyanotic spells - most often in children 2mo-1year old, sudden acute cyanosis, may be associated with period of increased agitation.

G. Diagnostics (Appendix 17-1).
   1. Cardiac catheterization.
   2. Chest X-ray.
   3. Echocardiogram.
   4. Predisposing maternal history.
   5. Clinical manifestations.

Acyanotic Congenital Defects

A. Ventricular septal defect (VSD) (Figure 17-2)—abnormal opening between the right and left ventricles; majority close spontaneously in one to three years.
   1. Clinical manifestations.
      a. Loud systolic murmur.
      b. Overloading of the right ventricle and an increase in pulmonary blood flow will precipitate CHF.

B. Atrial septal defect (ASD) (Figure 17-2)—abnormal opening between the atria; often due to failure of foramen ovale to close; may be asymptomatic.

1. Clinical manifestations.
   a. Diastolic murmur.
   b. Right atrial and ventricular hypertrophy.
   c. CHF usually does not occur.

C. Patent ductus arteriosus (PDA) (Figure 17-2)—failure of the ductus arteriosus to close at birth.

1. Clinical manifestations.
   a. Systolic or continuous (machinery) murmur.
   b. Bounding pulses.
   c. Left atrial dilatation, and left ventricle hypertrophy.
   d. CHF may result if left ventricle cannot handle volume overload.
2. Treatment.
   a. Surgical ligation of the vessel; recommended for all children due to an increase in bacterial endocarditis in later years.
   b. Pharmacologic treatment may be done with indomethacin. This NSAID medication changes the oxygen concentration of the tissue and enhances tissue changes that close the defect.

D. Coarctation of the aorta (Figure 17-2)—a narrowing of the aorta; specific symptoms depend on the location of the coarctation in relation to arteries coming off the aortic arch.

1. Clinical manifestations.
   a. Marked differences in blood pressure in the upper and lower extremities; area proximal to the defect has a high pressure and a bounding pulse.
      (1) Epistaxis.
      (2) Headaches.
      (3) Bounding radial and temporal pulses.
      (4) Dizziness and fainting.
   b. Area distal to defect has decreased blood pressure and weaker pulse.
      (1) Lower extremities are cooler, mottling is present.
      (2) Weak peripheral and femoral pulse.

Cyanotic Heart Defects

A. Tetralogy of Fallot (Figure 17-2).

1. Consists of four defects.
   a. Ventricular septal defect.
   b. Pulmonic stenosis.
   c. Overriding aorta.
   d. Right ventricle hypertrophy.
2. The pulmonic stenosis causes the blood to shunt through the VSD (right-to-left cyanotic shunt). The degree of cyanosis relates to the level of severity of the pulmonic stenosis.
3. May not demonstrate cyanosis at birth due to a patent ductus arteriosus.
4. Clinical manifestations.
   a. Polycythemia to compensate for chronic hypoxia.
   b. Hypercyanotic spells ("tet" spells - caused by increase in right-to-left shunt).
      (1) Acute cyanosis.
      (2) Irritability and pallor.
      (3) Tachypnea.
      (4) Flaccidity and possible loss of consciousness.
   c. Posturing or squatting in the older child.
   d. Does not develop CHF because overload of right ventricle flows into the aorta and the left ventricle; therefore, pulmonary congestion does not occur.
5. Treatment.
   a. Depending on severity of shunt, repair may be done in infancy or delayed until later years; usually done between 18 to 36 months.
   b. Palliative surgery (Blalock-Taussig procedure) to increase pulmonary blood flow may be necessary to sustain life. More extensive surgery will be done later.
6. Complications—even with repair, child may experience residual VSD, pulmonary insufficiency, and conduction disturbances, especially problems with heart block.

B. Transposition of the great vessels (Figure 17-2).

1. Condition where the pulmonary artery arises from the left ventricle, and the aorta arises from the right ventricle.
2. Incompatible with life unless another defect (ASD or PDA) exists for mixing of oxygenated and deoxygenated blood.
3. Clinical manifestations—severity depends on adequacy of an associated communicating defect.
   a. May be severely cyanotic at birth.
   b. If septal defect is large or PDA is present, cyanosis occurs with crying and feeding.
   c. Problems of CHF occur if a child has a large VSD due to increase in pulmonary blood flow.
4. Treatment.
   a. Palliative surgery to create or increase the atrial septal defect, decrease pulmonary vascular resistance and prevent CHF.

b. Complete repair is generally done before one year of age.

C. Truncus arteriosus (Figure 17-2)—an inadequate separation of the aortic and pulmonary vessels, resulting in a common trunk for aortic and pulmonary blood flow; a VSD exists where the common vessel enters the ventricle.

1. Clinical manifestations.

a. May have minimal cyanosis at birth.

b. A few weeks after birth there is marked evidence of CHF.

c. Harsh systolic murmur.

2. Treatment.

a. The level of pulmonary vascular disease will influence the type of repair that is necessary.

b. Repair is done as soon as possible to prevent the development of CHF and growth retardation.

Nursing Intervention

(Primarily directed toward the infant who has a serious defect requiring home care prior to corrective surgery).

✦ *Goal: to evaluate infant's response to cardiac defect.*

1. Evaluate infant's Apgar score at birth.
2. Evaluate adequacy of weight gain.
3. Assess feeding problems.
   a. Poor sucking reflex.
   b. Poor coordination of sucking, swallowing, breathing.
   c. Fatigues easily during feeding.
4. Frequency of upper respiratory infections.
5. Cyanosis at rest or precipitated by activity.
6. Presence and quality of pulses in extremities.
7. Bacterial endocarditis is a primary concern prior to and after correction of congenital defect.

✦ *Goal: to assist parents in adjusting to diagnosis.*

1. Allow family to grieve over loss of perfect infant.
2. Evaluate parents' level of understanding of the child's problem.
3. Foster early parent-infant attachment; encourage touching, holding, and general physical contact.
4. Assist the family to develop relationship which fosters optimum growth and development of all family members. (See Chapter 3 for psychosocial aspect of chronically ill children.)

NCLEX ALERT: *Provide emotional support to family, assist family members to manage care of a client with a chronic illness.*

✦ *Goal: to detect, prevent, and treat CHF.*

✦ *Goal: to provide appropriate nursing interventions for the client undergoing open heart surgery for repair of defect.*

Cardiac Surgery

A. Types of procedures.

1. Open heart surgery is performed with the utilization of the cardiopulmonary bypass machine. This machine allows for full visualization of the heart while maintaining perfusion and oxygenation.
2. Closed heart surgery is performed without the utilization of the bypass machine. The most common closed heart procedure is the mitral commissurotomy.

Nursing Intervention

(For pre- and postoperative care see Chapter 3).

✦ *Goal: to prepare the client psychologically and physiologically for surgery.*

1. Evaluate client's history for other chronic health problems.
2. Establish baseline data for postoperative comparison.
3. Appropriate preoperative teaching according to age level; frequently includes a visit to the intensive care unit (parents should accompany the child on the visit).
4. Discussion of immediate postoperative nursing care and anticipated nursing procedures.
5. Correct metabolic imbalances.
6. Establish and maintain adequate hydration.
7. Anticipate adjustments in medication schedule prior to surgery.
   a. Digitalis dosage is usually decreased.
   b. Diuretics may be discontinued 48 hours prior to surgery.
   c. Long-acting insulin will be changed to regular insulin.
   d. Antihypertensive medication dosage may be modified.
8. Alleviate all possible sources of infection.

✦ *Goal: to evaluate and promote cardiovascular function postoperatively.*

1. Maintain adequate blood pressure.
2. Evaluate for dysrhythmia; document and treat accordingly (Appendix 17-3).

3. Maintain client in semi-Fowler's position.
4. Evaluate fluid and electrolyte balance.
   a. Record daily weight and compare with previous weight.
   b. Assess for hypokalemia and hyperkalemia.
   c. Assess for adequate hemoglobin and hematocrit.
   d. Evaluate hemodynamic levels for adequate volume (Appendix 17-5).
   e. Hourly urine output to evaluate adequacy of renal perfusion.
   f. IV fluids as indicated.
5. Observe for hemorrhage - most often identified by increase in chest drainage.
6. Evaluate adequacy of peripheral circulation.
7. Mediastinal chest tubes are frequently placed in the pericardial sac to prevent tamponade. These tubes are cared for in the same manner as pulmonary chest tubes.
8. Bedside hemodynamic monitoring as indicated (Appendix 17-5).

✦ *Goal: to evaluate and promote respiratory function.*

1. Volume ventilators via an ET tube may be utilized for approximately 12-24 hours postoperatively. Generally, children are extubated sooner than adults.
2. Maintain water-sealed drainage for mediastinal/chest tubes (Appendix 15-4).
3. Pulmonary hygiene via ET tube.
4. Promote good respiratory hygiene after extubation.
5. Evaluate ABGs for adequate oxygenation as well as acid-base balance.
6. Encourage activity as soon as possible. Client should be out of bed the first postoperative day.
7. Monitor pulse oximetry levels.

✦ *Goal: to evaluate neurological status for complications postoperatively.*

1. Recovery from anesthesia within appropriate time frame.
2. Able to move all extremities equally.
3. Appropriate response to verbal command.
4. Evaluate neuro signs.

✦ *Goal: to prevent complications of immobility (Chapter 3) postoperatively.*

✦ *Goal: to decrease anxiety and promote comfort postoperatively.*

1. Frequent orientation to surroundings.
2. Careful explanation of all procedures.
3. Prevent sensory overload.
4. Promote uninterrupted sleep.
5. Administer pain medications as appropriate.

Common complications after cardiac surgery.

1. Dysrhythmia (Appendix 17-3).
   a. Premature ventricular contractions.
   b. Ventricular tachycardia.
   c. Atrial dysrhythmias are common with mitral valve replacement.
   d. Conduction blocks.
2. Hypovolemia.
   a. Low cardiac output may be due to hypovolemia.
   b. Frequently, vasoconstriction is present immediately after surgery. Vasodilation occurs as client's body temperature increases and precipitates hypovolemia.
   c. Evaluate hemodynamic parameters for adequacy of cardiac output.
   d. Observe client closely for response to fluid replacement, as fluid overload occurs very rapidly, especially in children.
3. Emboli.
   a. Pulmonary emboli.
   b. Arterial emboli.
      (1) Occur most frequently following valvular surgery.
      (2) May be on prophylactic anticoagulants.
      (3) Evaluate neurological system for evidence of cerebral emboli.
4. Cardiac tamponade.
   a. Pressure on the heart caused by a collection of fluid in pericardial sac.
   b. Pressure prevents adequate filling of ventricles, thereby decreasing cardiac output.
   c. Pulsus paradoxus—precipitous decrease in systolic blood pressure on inspiration; diagnostic for tamponade.
   d. CVP is frequently increased, blood pressure is decreased.
   e. Heart sounds are frequently described as distant.
   f. A decrease in drainage may occur in the mediastinal tubes.
   g. Treatment involves re-establishing patency of mediastinal tube, pericardialcentesis, or surgical exploration of bleeding areas.
5. Psychosis (most common in adults).
   a. Characteristics.

(1) Inappropriate verbal response.
(2) Disorientation to time and place.
(3) Vision and auditory hallucinations.
(4) Paranoid delusions.

b. Prevention of psychosis.
(1) Maintain orientation to time and place.
(2) Maintain continuity in nursing staff.
(3) Carefully explain all procedures.
(4) Encourage ventilation of feelings.⌘

Study Questions—Cardiac System

1. The nurse is preparing a client for a cardiac catheterization. What is the best explanation regarding the purpose of a cardiac catheterization with coronary angiography?

① Evaluate the exercise tolerance.
② Study the conduction system.
③ Evaluate coronary artery blood flow.
④ Measure the pumping capacity of the heart.

2. The nurse is caring for a client with cor pulmonale. What nursing assessment information correlates with an increase in venous pressure ?

① Jugular vein distention with client sitting at a 45° degree angle.
② Crackling sounds over the lower lobes with client in an upright position.
③ Bradycardia, restlessness, and an increase in respiratory rate.
④ Jugular vein distention with the client supine and the head of the bed flat.

3. The nurse is administering nitroglycerine IV to relieve chest pain. What is the therapeutic action of this medication?

① Increase diuresis and glomerular filtration which results in decreased venous return.
② Increase the force of contraction of the myocardium, thereby increasing oxygen delivery.
③ Produce an immediate analgesic effect and relieve the chest pain.
④ Increase the coronary blood supply and decrease the afterload.

4. In discharge planning for the client with congestive heart failure, the nurse discusses the importance of adequate rest. What information is most important?

① A warm, quiet room is necessary.
② Bedrest promotes venous return.
③ A hospital bed is necessary.
④ Bedrest decreases cardiac work load.

5. The nurse is assessing a client who is being stabilized from a myocardial infarction. What finding on the nursing assessment would indicate inadequate renal perfusion?

① Decreasing serum BUN level.
② Specific gravity of less than 1.010.
③ Urine output of less than 30 ml per hour.
④ Low urine osmolarity and creatinine clearance.

6. The nurse applies a Nitro-Dur patch on a postoperative cardiac client. What nursing observation indicates that a Nitro-Dur patch is achieving the desired effect?

① Chest pain is relieved by nitroglycerin.
② Performs activities of daily living without chest pain.
③ Able to control pain with frequent changes of patch.
④ Tolerates minimal activity without pain.

7. The nurse is evaluating a client's progress. What information would be indicative of a cardiac compensatory mechanism?

① Ventricular dilation, hypertrophy, and tachycardia.
② Hepatomegaly, splenomegaly, and cardiac hypertrophy.
③ Headache, drowsiness, and confusion.
④ Bradycardia, restlessness, and hyperventilation.

8. During the night, a client diagnosed with an acute myocardial infarction is found to be restless and diaphoretic. What is the best nursing action?

① Check his temperature and determine his serum blood glucose level.
② Turn the alarms low and decrease the number of times you interrupt sleep.
③ Check the monitor to determine his cardiac rhythm and evaluate vital signs.
④ Call the physician to obtain an order for sedation.

9. Which statement by the client indicates that he understands how to take the nitroglycerin sublingual?

① "If I have a chest pain, I'll immediately stop what I am doing, sit down and take the medication."
② "I'll chew the tablet then let it dissolve in my mouth."

③ "I'll take only one dose. If the pain doesn't stop, I'll call the doctor."

④ "If I have chest pain, I'll call the doctor and put two tablets under my tongue."

10. The nurse is providing preoperative care for a cardiac surgery client. During this preoperative preparation what is an important nursing action?

① Perform a thorough nursing assessment to provide an accurate baseline for evaluation postoperatively.

② Discuss with the client the steps of myocardial cellular metabolism and the anticipated surgical response.

③ Provide preoperative education regarding the mechanics of the cardiopulmonary bypass machine.

④ Discuss with the client and family the anticipated amount of postoperative chest tube drainage.

11. An elderly client is taking Digitalis .025mg bid and *Lasix* 40mg daily for her congestive heart failure. She is complaining of increased lethargy and nausea over the past two days, however she is still able to take her medication. Her blood pressure is 150/98, pulse is 110 and irregular, respirations are 18. What laboratory information is most important for the nurse to evaluate?

① Hemoglobin, hematocrit, and white blood cell count.

② Arterial blood gases and acid base balance.

③ Blood urea nitrogen (BUN) and serum creatinine.

④ Serum electrolytes, particularly potassium.

12. A client is in first degree block. What is a nursing measure to assess the status of this dysrhythmia?

① Count the radial pulse for one full minute.

② Determine the cardiac rate at the PMI.

③ Evaluate an EKG or monitor strip.

④ Hourly pulse checks and correlate with blood pressure.

13. A cardiac client is on a monitor and the nurse observes ventricular tachycardia at a rate of 160 beats per minute. The client is awake and coherent. What is the first nursing action?

① Immediately defibrillate.

② Administer lidocaine IV push.

③ Begin cardio-pulmonary resuscitation.

④ Start oxygen at 6L/minute.

14. A client is admitted for evaluation of his permanent pacemaker. What data would the nurse identify as confirming that the pacemaker is not working correctly?

① Pulse rate of 96, regular rate, and rhythm.

② Irregular pulse rate with premature ventricular beats.

③ Monitor shows atrial premature beats.

④ Pulse rate of 48 with premature ventricular beats.

15. The nurse is assessing a cardiac client's apical pulse. Where is the stethoscope placed to correctly auscultate this pulse?

① To the left of the sternal border in the middle of the sternum.

② Second intercostal space at the mid-clavicular line.

③ At the third intercostal space, just left of the sternal border.

④ Left mid clavicular line at the level of the fifth intercostal space.

16. A cardiac client's vital signs are: 110/78, pulse of 52, and respiratory rate is 18. Atropine (atropine sulfate) is administered IV push. What nursing assessment indicates a therapeutic response to the medication?

① Pulse rate increases to 70.

② Systolic blood pressure increased by 20mmHg.

③ Dilation of the pupils.

④ Decreased oral secretions.

17. The nurse is taking the history from a client with congestive heart failure (CHF) secondary to hypertension. The nurse identifies what data as supportive of the client's medical diagnosis?

① Dyspnea after walking one block.

② Weight loss of 15 pounds over last 3 months.

③ Lower extremity edema in the evenings.

④ Dizziness and fainting when getting up too quickly.

18. A client is admitted with mitral valve disease and left ventricular dysfunction. What is the most reliable test to determine the cardiac status?

① Electrocardiogram.

② Stress test.

③ Cardiac catheterization.

④ Echocardiogram.

19. What would be the home care goal for a client who has bacterial endocarditis?

① To begin exercise regime as soon as possible.

② To monitor urinary output.

③ To continue antibiotic therapy.

④ To decrease activity until pulse stabilizes.

20. What is the primary pathophysiological reason for performing coronary artery bypass surgery?

① Decrease oxygen overload to the cardiac muscle.
② Increase oxygen supply to the heart muscle.
③ Reduce plaque buildup in the carotid artery.
④ Reduce overall contractility of the heart muscle.

21. A client has left-sided heart failure and the nurse notes he has symptoms of dyspnea and orthopnea. What is the most immediate short-term goal?

① Continue heparin therapy for peripheral edema.
② Assess the stressors in the client's home life.
③ Check urinary output for kidney perfusion.
④ Decrease venous return to the heart.

22. A client is being discharge with sublingual nitroglycerin tablets. What is important to teach him?

① Keep the nitroglycerin in a breathable container.
② Keep the nitroglycerin in a clear container.
③ Take two nitroglycerin tablets together for severe chest pain.
④ Take a nitroglycerin at the first onset of chest pain.

23. The congestive heart failure (CHF) client has digoxin ordered. In evaluating the therapeutic effectiveness of the drug, what would the nurse expects to find?

① Decreased cardiac workload and heart rate.
② Increased cardiac workload and output.
③ Diaphoresis with decreased output.
④ Increased heart rate with increased respirations.

24. A client has heart failure. What is the expected physiological response of the body when edema is reduced?

① Increased real body weight.
② Increased rales across all lung fields.
③ Increased respiratory rate.
④ Increased urinary output.

25. A nurse notices jugular vein distention in her cardiac client when his head is elevated 45°. What condition will the nurse further assess for in this client?

① Dehydration.
② Left-sided heart failure.
③ Congestive heart failure.
④ Cardiovascular accident.

Answers and rationales to these questions are in the section at the end of the book entitled "Chapter Study Questions: Answers & Rationales."

Appendix 17-1: CARDIAC DIAGNOSTICS

SERUM LABORATORY STUDIES:

Cardiac Enzymes:

Enzymes are drawn to evaluate myocardial damage and to identify myocardial infarction.
Lactate dehydrogenase (LDH) -isoenzymes LDH_1 specific for cardiac damage - 14-26% of total LDH.
Increases 24-48 hours after MI, peaks in 48-72 hours.

Creatinine Phosphokinase - 5-35 ug/ml
CPK isoenzymes: M—associated with muscle, B—associated with the brain. Elevation in the isoenzyme MB may indicate damage to the myocardial muscle if the value of the MB is over 5% of the total CPK.
CPK-MB increases within 3-6 hours after an MI, peaks in 12 - 24 hours (sometimes peaks at levels 6 times the normal value), returns to normal in 3 - 4 days. Normal is 0-6% of total CPK
Troponin level is elevated within 4-6 hours after an MI, it peaks within 10-24 hours. Normal is .0 to 3.1ng/ml.

Nursing Implications:
1. Enzymes must be drawn on admission and obtained in a serial manner thereafter. There is a characteristic pattern to the increases and decreases of the enzymes in the client with a myocardial infarction.
2. The larger the infarction, the larger the enzyme response.
3. The increased levels of Treponin and CPK are the most significant. With the rapid rise and subsequent decrease in CPK, the pattern may be missed.
4. IM injections, medications, other disease entities, and tissue injury will affect enzyme changes; however, isoenzymes help discriminate myocardial tissue damage from other tissue injury.

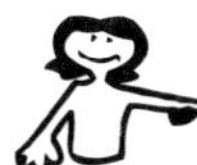

***NURSING PRIORITY:** For CPK greater than 120 IU/L, assess the client for symptoms of an acute MI. Serum levels may be checked every 6 - 8 hours during the acute phase of an MI.*

C-reactive Protein:

Identification of the protein that is synthesized by the liver and is not normally present in the blood except when there is tissue trauma. The protein attaches to the bacteria as part of the immune response. The response to the test assists to evaluate severity and course of inflammatory conditions. May be used to help differentiate between viral and bacterial infections - protein level does not increase with viral infections.
Normal -trace elements are present; any other titer level is significant.
Nursing Implications -Client is NPO for 6-8 hours prior to test being drawn.

Serum Electrolytes: (EKG changes with potassium levels).
Hyperkalemia - (1) Tall, peaked T wave, (2) Widening of the QRS, (3) Ventricular fibrillation.
Hypokalemia -(1) PVCs, (2) Ventricular tachycardia, (3) Ventricular fibrillation.

Erythrocyte Sedimentation Rate:

Used as a gauge for evaluating progression of inflammatory conditions; inflammatory process precipitates a rapid settling of the red cells.
Normal values vary greatly, depending on the laboratory method utilized.

NONINVASIVE DIAGNOSTICS:

Electrocardiogram (EKG, ECG):

A graphic representation of the electrical activity of the heart, generally conducted utilizing a twelve-lead format. Test to identify conduction in rhythm disorders and the occurrence of ischemia, injury or death of myocardial tissue.

Holter Monitor:

Client is connected to a small portable EKG unit with recorder which records the client's heart activity for approximately 24 hours. The client is supposed to keep a log of activity, pain, palpitations. Client should not remove leads, but is encouraged to maintain normal activity. The client should not shower or bathe while the monitor is in place. He should not remove the leads at any time. The recording is analyzed and compared to the client's activity log.

Appendix 17-1:
CARDIAC DIAGNOSTICS

Exercise Stress Test:
This test involves the client exercising, usually on a treadmill which increases with speed and incline to increase the heart rate. EKG leads are attached to the client and the response of the heart to exercise is evaluated.
Nursing Implications:
1. Appropriate pretest preparation, establish baseline vital signs, and cardiac rhythm..
2. Client should:
   a. Avoid smoking and eating immediately prior to test.
   b. Avoid stimulants, eating, and extreme temperature changes immediately after test.
3. Cardiac monitoring constantly during test, blood pressure is monitored periodically.
4. Reasons for terminating an exercise stress test: chest pain, greatly increased heart rate, EKG changes - significant ST segment depression.
5. If any of the above changes occur, the test is terminated and is said to be a positive stress test.

Echocardiogram:
An ultrasound procedure to evaluate function, structure and valvular function of the heart. These sound waves are displayed on a graph and interpreted.

Transeophageal echocardiography - provides a higher quality picture than regular echocardiogram. The throat is anesthetized and an esophageal scope is inserted.
Nursing implications:
1. NPO for 8 hours prior to test.
2. Check for gag reflex prior to resuming PO fluids.

INVASIVE DIAGNOSTICS:

Cardiac Catheterization:
This is an invasive procedure where a catheter is passed through an artery or vein into the heart. Cardiac catheterization will provide data regarding status of the coronary arteries, as well as cardiac muscle function, valvular functions, and left ventricular function (ejection fraction).

Nursing Implications:
1. Pretest preparation.
   a. NPO six hours before test.
   b. Check for dye allergy, especially iodine and shellfish.
   c. Record quality of distal pulses for comparison post-test.
   d. Record height and weight (may be used to determine amount of dye to use).
   e. Appropriate client education (lying still on hard table, flushed feeling when dye is injected, etc.).
2. Post-test.
   a. Evaluate catheterization site for hematoma formation.
   b. Evaluate circulatory status (pulses distal to catheterization site, color, sensation of the extremity.)
   c. Assess for dysrhythmias.
   d. Avoid flexion, keep extremity straight for 6-8 hours.
   e. Keep head of bed elevated at 15° or less.
   f. Fluids will be encouraged to flush the dye out of the body (dye is hyperosmolar and can lead to fluid volume overload).

Positron Emission Tomography:
Provides information regarding the perfusion and the metabolism of an area of the heart. The procedure takes about 2-3 hours and a radioactive dye is injected IV followed by glucose.

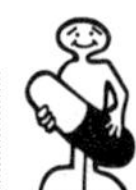

Appendix 17-2:
CARDIAC MEDICATIONS

MEDICATIONS	SIDE EFFECTS	NURSING IMPLICATIONS
NITRATES: Increase blood supply to the heart by dilating the coronary arteries; cardiac workload is reduced due to decrease in venous return because of peripheral vasodilation.		
Isosorbide dinitrate (**Isordil, Sorbide**): PO Nitroglycerin (**NTG, Nitrostat**): sublingual Nitroglycerin (**Nitro-BID, Nitrol**): topical	Headaches (will diminish with therapy), postural hypotension, syncope, blurred vision, dry mouth, reflex tachycardia.	1. Advise client that alcohol will potentiate postural hypotension. 2. Educate client regarding self-medication. (Table 17-3). 3. Report to physician continuous headaches, blurred vision, or dry mouth. 4. Topical application is used for sustained protection against anginal attacks. 5. Avoid skin contact with topical form; remove all previous applications when applying topical form. 6. Purpose of transdermal is to prevent chest pain and allow client to maintain ADL's.
CALCIUM CHANNEL BLOCKERS: Blockade of calcium channel receptors in the heart causes decreased cardiac contractility and a decreased rate of sinus and A-V node conduction.		
Diltiazem (**Cardizem**) PO, IV Nifedipine (**Procardia**): PO Verapamil (**Calan, Isoptin**): IV, PO	Constipation, exacerbation of CHF, hypotension, bradycardia, peripheral edema.	1. ***Uses:*** chronic stable angina, hypertension, and supraventricular dysrhythmias. 2. Nifedipine is less likely to exacerbate pre-existing cardiac conditions; is not effective in treating dysrhythmias. 3. Intensifies cardiosuppressant effects of beta blocker medications.
BETA-ADRENERGIC BLOCKING AGENTS: Blockade of $beta_1$ receptors in the heart causes: decreased heart rate, decreased force of contraction, and decreased rate of A-V conduction.		
Nadolol (**Corgard**): PO Propranolol (**Inderal**): PO, IV Metoprolol (**Lopressor**) PO, IV Timolol (**Blocadren**) PO Atenolol (**Tenormin**)	Bradycardia, CHF, hypotension, depression, lethargy and fatigue.	1. Evaluate client for precipitation of and/or increase of CHF, or dysrhythmia involving heart block. 2. May increase effectiveness of calcium channel blockers. 3. Teach clients how to decrease effects of postural hypotension 4. Teach clients not to stop taking medication when they feel better. 5. Bradycardia is common adverse effect. 6. Check pulse prior to administering. 7. If diabetic, monitor blood glucose levels, hypoglycemic symptoms may be blocked. 8. ***Uses:*** angina, hypertension, and cardiac dysrhythmias.

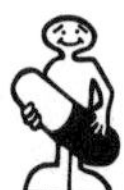

Appendix 17-2:
CARDIAC MEDICATIONS, *Continued*

MEDICATIONS	SIDE EFFECTS	NURSING IMPLICATIONS
ANTIDYSRHYTHMIC MEDICATIONS: Decrease cardiac excitability, delay cardiac conduction either in the atrium or ventricle. Atropine is cardiac stimulant for bradycardia.		
❖**GENERAL NURSING IMPLICATIONS**❖ — Assess client for changes in cardiac rhythm and impact on cardiac output. — Evaluate effect of medication on dysrhythmia and resulting effects on cardiac output. — Client should be on bedrest and cardiac monitor for IV administration. — Have atropine available for cardiac depression resulting in symptomatic bradycardia. — All cardiac depressant medications are contraindicated in clients with sinus node or A-V node blocks. — Digitalis will enhance cardiac depressant effects. — Closely monitor for dysrhythmias that are precipitated by the treatment. —See Appendix17-3, Cardiac Dysrhythmias.		
Quinidine sulfate (**Quinidine Sulfate, Quinidex**): PO	Vertigo, nausea, vomiting and diarrhea; progressive AV block, cinchonism-tinnitus, visual problems, headache	1. ***Uses:*** supraventricular dysrhythmias and to convert client to sinus rhythm. 2. Medication is not recommended to be administered parenterally.
Disopyramide (**Norpace**): PO	Anticholinergic - urinary retention, dry mouth, constipation, bradycardia, hypotension.	1. High incidence of urinary retention. 2. Contraindicated for use in clients with CHF. 3. ***Use:*** ventricular dysrhythmias.
Lidocaine hydrochloride (**Xylocaine**): IV	Drowsiness, confusion, seizures, severe depression of cardiac conduction.	1. ***Use:*** ventricular dysrhythmias.
Tocainide (**Tonocard**) PO	GI disturbances especially nausea, tremors, possible pulmonary fibrosis.	1. ***Use:*** to prevent/control ventricular dysrhythmias.
Mexiletine (**Mexitil**) PO	GI Disturbances- N/V, diarrhea; CNS disturbances -tremor, dizziness.	1. ***Use:*** to prevent/control ventricular dysrhythmias.
Amiodarone hydrochloride (**Cardarone**) PO, IV	GI disturbance, pulmonary toxicity.	1. ***Use:*** Treatment of ventricular fibrillation and tachycardia that are refractory to other treatment. 2. Hypotension occurs in majority of clients; keep clients on bedrest during treatment.
Procainamide (**Pronestyl**): PO, IV	Systemic lupus erythematosus-like syndrome, blood dyscrasias, hypotension, prolonged QT interval.	1. ***Use:*** short and long term control of ventricular and supraventricular dysrhythmias. 2. If joint pain and inflammation occur, client should contact physician.
Propranolol Hydrochloride (**Inderal**):PO, IV	(See previous discussion of beta adrenergic blockers)	
Atropine sulfate: IV, PO, SQ, IM	Dry mouth. Blurred vision. Dilated pupils. Tachycardia	1. ***Use***: block cardiac stimulation, primarily for bradycardias that are hemodynamically significant, or PVCs related to slow heart rate. 2. Assess client's cardiac output in response to the bradycardic episode.

Appendix 17-2:
CARDIAC MEDICATIONS, *Continued*

MEDICATIONS	SIDE EFFECTS	NURSING IMPLICATIONS
FIBRINOLYTIC MEDICATIONS: Bind to fibrin in a thrombus and initiate fibrinolysis to break up a clot. Convert the circulating plasminogen to plasmin to begin fibrinolysis; are not clot specific.		
❖ **GENERAL NURSING IMPLICATIONS** ❖ — Therapy should begin as soon as the myocardial infarction is diagnosed, or when there is history of prolonged angina. — Bleeding precautions (Table 9-1). — Streptokinase should be administered with an IV filter.		
Streptokinase (**Streptase, Kabikinase**) IV Alteplase (**tPA, Activase**) IV Reteplase (**Retavase**) IV	Bleeding and hypotension.	1. Obtain base vital signs and coagulation studies. Must be infused via IV pump and client monitored every 15 minutes. 2. Must be administered as soon as possible after symptoms begin to occur. 3. ***Use***: MI, PE, DVT, contraindicated in clients with active bleeding.
CARDIAC GLYCOSIDES (Digitalis): Increase myocardial contractility and cardiac output; decrease conduction of impulses through the A-V node.		
❖**GENERAL NURSING IMPLICATIONS** ❖ —Take the apical pulse for a full minute; if the rate is below 60 in an adult, below 90 in a child, hold the medication and notify the physician. —Evaluate for tachycardia, bradycardia, and irregular pulse. If there is significant change in rate and rhythm, hold the medication and notify the physician. —Evaluate serum potassium levels and response to diuretics, hypokalemia potentiates action of digitalis. —Gastrointestinal symptoms are frequently the first indication of digitalis toxicity. —Teach client not to increase or double dose for missed doses. —Quinidine and verapamil both increase plasma levels of digitalis. —To achieve maximum results rapidly, a loading dose is administered, then reduced to a maintenance dose. —Digibind is a digitalis antagonist, may be used for digitalis toxicity, watch for decreased potassium levels and client response to decreased digitalis levels.		
Digoxin (**Lanoxin**): PO, IV	Anorexia, nausea, vomiting, visual disturbances, fatigue, drug induced dysrhythmias.	1. Therapeutic plasma levels of digoxin are 0.5-2.0 ng/ml. 2. First sign of toxicity is usually GI symptoms. 3. ***Uses:*** supraventricular tachycardia, CHF.
Digitoxin (**Crystodigen**): PO		1. Effects of medication last much longer than digoxin, more difficult to adjust.

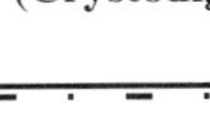
GERIATRIC PRIORITY: *Elderly clients are more sensitive to digitalis and are more likely to experience digitalis toxicity.*

NCLEX ALERT: *Monitor blood levels of medications.*

Appendix 17-3: CARDIAC DYSRHYTHMIAS

❑ **A *dysrhythmia* (arrhythmia) is defined as an interruption in the normal conduction of the heart, either in the rate or the rhythm.**

CHARACTERISTICS OF NORMAL SINUS RHYTHM:

Rate - 60 to 100
Rhythm - regular
P waves - present, precede each QRS
P-R interval - .12 to .20 seconds
QRS - present and under .10 second

Dysrhythmias may be classified according to rate, either bradycardia or tachycardia. They are also classified according to their origin - atrial or ventricular. Ventricular dysrhythmias are more life-threatening than atrial dysrhythmias. (See Table of Common Dysrhythmias.)

Nursing Implications:

1. Evaluate client's tolerance of the dysrhythmia.
2. Maintain adequate cardiac output.
3. Convert abnormal rhythm to normal sinus rhythm.
4. Prevent complications.

INTERPRETATION OF ELECTROCARDIOGRAM:

1. Determine the heart rate. Count the "P" waves in a six second strip to determine the atrial rate, and the "R" or "Q" waves to determine the ventricular rate.
2. Are the QRS complexes occurring at regular intervals?
3. Are "P" waves present for each QRS complex?
4. Measure the "P-R" interval.
5. Measure the "QRS" interval.
6. Identify the "T" wave and "S-T" segment.
7. Correlate findings with characteristics of normal sinus rhythm.

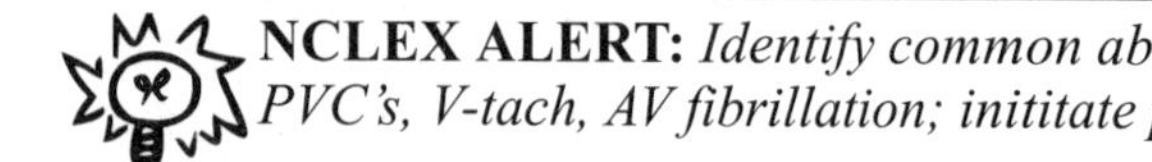

NCLEX ALERT: *Identify common abnormalities on client's cardiac monitor (sinus tachycardia, PVC's, V-tach, AV fibrillation; inititate protocol to manage cardiac dysrhythmias.*

Figure 17-3: Normal QRS Complex

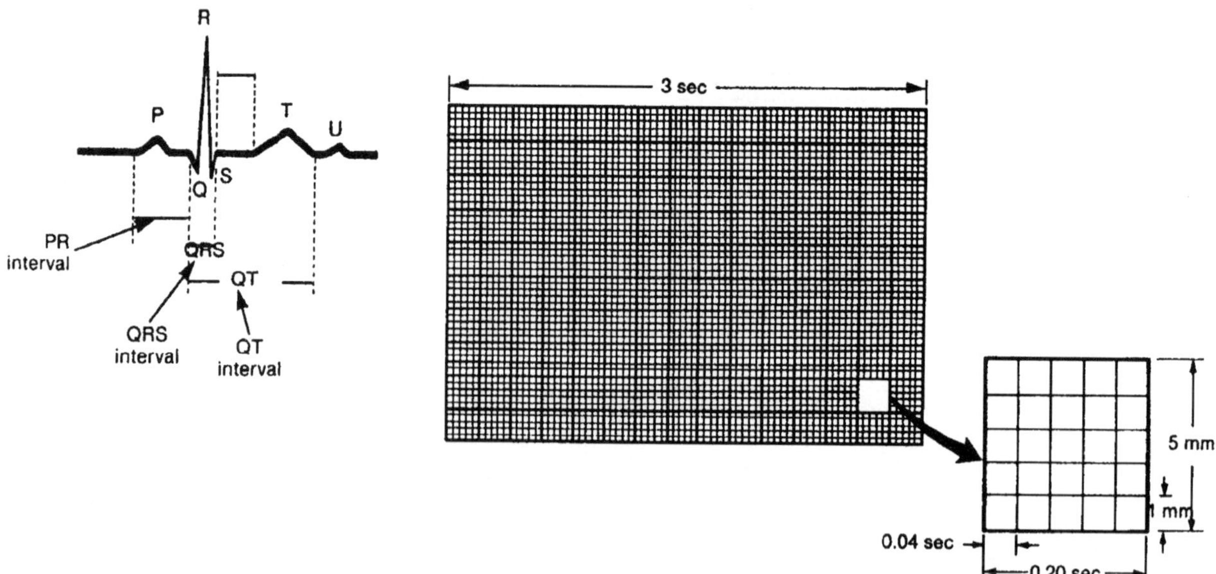

Appendix 17-3: TABLE OF COMMON DYSRHYTHMIAS

RHYTHM	CHARACTERISTICS	INTERVENTIONS/IMPLICATIONS
SINUS BRADYCARDIA	Sinus rhythm below a rate of 60.	Assess client for tolerance of the rate. If hypotension or decreasing LOC occur, the rhythm is treated. ***Treatment:*** atropine.
ATRIAL FIBRILLATION	Grossly irregular rate; cannot identify P waves or P-R interval on the EKG. Controlled rate 60 to 100. Uncontrolled rate 140 to 180.	Evaluate client for systemic emboli from clots that tend to form in the fibrillating atrium; a decrease in cardiac output will occur with the tachycardia; maintain bedrest until rate is controlled. Pulse deficit may occur. ***Treatment:*** digitalis, quinidine, verapamil, cardioversion.
ATRIOVENTRICULAR BLOCK		
First degree block	Prolonged P-R interval; all P waves are followed by a QRS complex.	May be due to digitalis toxicity or electrolyte imbalance; also seen in myocardial ischemia; identify and treat the underlying cause. Must have an EKG tracing to identify.
Third degree or complete block	No correlation between atrial impulses and ventricular response. Rate: atrial rate 80 to 90, with ventricular rate around 30.	May occur after an MI; symptoms depend on client's tolerance to the rhythm; very unstable and frequently leads to cardiac standstill. ***Treatment:*** atropine, pacemaker.
PREMATURE VENTRICULAR CONTRACTIONS	A premature ectopic beat; occurs within a basic rhythm; is of ventricular origin; no P waves; wide, bizarre QRS complex.	Indicative of ventricular irritability, considered to be significant and should be treated if they: 1. Occur in excess of six beats per minute. 2. Occur in a consecutive manner, or pairs. 3. Occur on a T wave of a preceding complex. ***Treatment:*** Oxygen, lidocaine, procainamide, bretylium ; PVCs frequently precede ventricular tachycardia.
VENTRICULAR TACHYCARDIA	Looks like a row of PVCs in configuration, wide and bizarre; very rapid rate of 125 to 200.	Severe decrease in cardiac output; potentially life-threatening situation. ***Treatment:*** lidocaine, procainamide, bretylium
VENTRICULAR FIBRILLATION	Very rapid, disorganized rate; cannot identify QRS complexes; erratic conduction.	If client is unconscious there is no cardiac output, initiate a code and begin CPR. ***Treatment:*** defibrillation, epinephrine, lidocaine, bretylium, procainamide.
ASYSTOLE	No electrical activity. "Straight line".	No cardiac output. Initiate CPR. ***Treatment:*** external pacemaker, epinephrine, atropine.

Appendix 17-4: PACEMAKERS

Temporary - an external generator is utilized; a catheter is inserted in the antecubital vein and lodged in the right ventricle; utilized only in the hospitalized client; used in emergency situations and in severe cases of bradycardia involving low cardiac output, as in conditions of cardiac block. Since pacing wires are on the outside of the body the client is at a high risk for electrical and electro-magnetic interference.
Permanent - an internal generator is inserted into soft tissue of upper chest or abdomen and electrodes are positioned according to the pacing mode; procedure planned and conducted under fluoroscopy and optimal conditions; used in persistent chronic heart block or sustained bradycardia.

Pacing Modes
Fixed rate - Fires constantly without regard to the client's own heart beats. Is used when there is no electrical activity in the heart (asystole).
Demand - the heart is stimulated to beat when the client's pulse rate falls below a set value or rate (majority of the pacemakers have a set rate between 60-72, if client's pulse rate falls below the set value, the pacemaker will be initiated); utilized in both temporary and permanent pacing. The pacemaker "senses" the initiation of a beat and the following conduction. If a normal cardiac beat is initiated and conducted, the pacemaker does not initiate an impulse.
Atrioventricular - The ventricle is sensed, and the atrium is paced. If the ventricle does not depolarize, then it is also paced.
Universal atrioventricular - both the atrial and ventricular circuits sense and pace in the respective chambers. This most closely resembles the normal conduction system.

Pacemaker Failure - an ECG must be available to verify pacemaker failure.
Failure to sense -the pacemaker does not sense the client's own heartbeats. This is dangerous as the pacer impulse may be discharged during a critical time in the cardiac cycle.
Failure to pace -A malfunction in the pacemaker generator, or it may be due to dislodgment of the leads.
Failure to capture - May occur with a low battery or poor connection. The pacemaker is discharging the impulse, however there is not a responding cardiac contraction.

Client Education:

1. Advise the client of the set rate of his pacemaker; teach him to take his pulse every day and record on calendar. Notify the physician if the pulse is lower than the set rate.
2. Avoid constrictive clothing that puts pressure on or irritates the site; report any signs of infection.
3. Safe environment - avoid areas of high voltage, magnetic force fields, large running motors.
4, Wear a medical alert identification, and advise all health care professionals regarding the pacemaker.
5. Avoid activity that requires vigorous movement of arms and shoulders.
6. Client's pulse rate should not drop below the preset rate; if this occurs, the pacemaker is not functioning properly and it needs to be reported.
7. Follow-up care and monitoring of pacemaker is important; pacemaker may need to be reprogrammed.

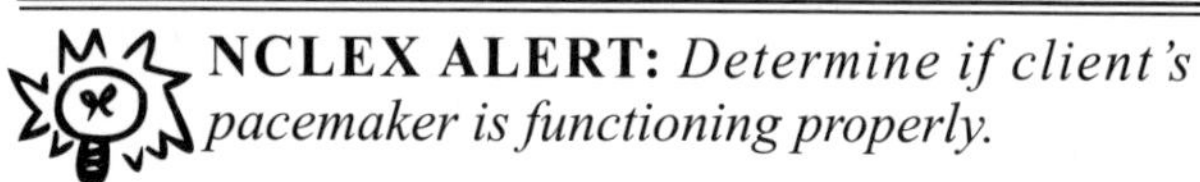

Appendix 17-5: BEDSIDE HEMODYNAMIC MONITORING

CENTRAL VENOUS PRESSURE MONITORING (CVP):

❑ **CVP is an indication of the pressure within the right atrium or within the large veins in the thoracic cavity. An IV catheter is placed in the superior vena cava or in the right atrium via the subclavian vein or jugular vein. A CVP reading may also be obtained from a the proximal lumen of the pulmonary artery catheter.**

Interpretation of Pressure Readings:
Normal response may range from 2 to 12 mm of H_2O pressure. CVP is a dynamic measurement; it must be correlated with client's overall clinical status for correct interpretation.

CVP reading is influenced by:
1. Venous return to the heart (venous tone and vascular volume).
2. Intrathoracic pressure.
3. Function of the left heart.
4. Coughing or straining will increase CVP.

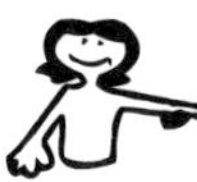

NURSING PRIORITY: *The CVP is an index of the ability of the right side of the heart to handle venous return.*

NURSING PRIORITY: *Rising CVP may indicate hypervolemia or poor cardiac contractility. Decreasing CVP may indicate state of hypovolemia or vasodilation.*

Nursing Considerations:
1. Each CVP reading should be measured from the same zero level point (level of the right atrium or the phlebostatic axis). The zero level on the manometer, or the transducer should be placed at this level to obtain the reading. Client should be supine to obtain the measurements; head may be slightly elevated, but the position should be consistent for all measurements.
2. If the CVP catheter is patent in the thoracic cavity, fluid in the manometer, or the digital readout will fluctuate with respirations or changes in thoracic pressure when the reading is obtained.
3. Patency of the CVP line is maintained via IV infusion drip.
4. Catheter should be stabilized on the skin at the insertion site and an occlusive sterile dressing applied.

Complications:
Air emboli and infections.

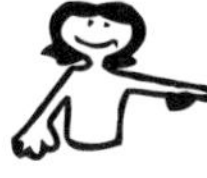

NURSING PRIORITY: *To obtain hemodynamic measurements, the zero point of the transducer must be at the level of the right atrium, which is the midaxillary line at the fourth or fifth intercostal space.*

Appendix 17-5:
BEDSIDE HEMODYNAMIC MONITORING, *Continued*

PULMONARY ARTERY PRESSURE MONITORING (SWAN-GANZ)

❑ **A multi-lumen catheter is inserted and advanced through the right atrium and right ventricle into the pulmonary artery. The flow of blood carries the catheter into the pulmonary artery. Heparinized saline is infused under pressure to maintain the patency of the line.**

Interpretation of Pressure Readings:

(Pressure readings are obtained via a transducer; for readings to be accurate, the zero level of the transducer must be at the level of the right atrium.)

Right Atrial Pressure (RA): normal 2 -12 mm/Hg; is a direct measurement of the pressure in the right atrium.

Pulmonary artery pressure (PAP): normal is 15-25/8-10 mm Hg, with a mean pressure around 15 mmHg. Mean PAP is increased in clients with chronic pulmonary diseases and in CHF.

Pulmonary capillary wedge pressure (PAWP or PCWP): normal is 8 to 13 mm Hg. It is determined as a mean pressure and is obtained by inflating or wedging a small balloon on the catheter tip in a distal branch of the pulmonary artery. The wedge pressure is indicative of pressure in the left cardiac chambers and reflects the function of the left atrium and ventricle.

Nursing Considerations:

1. Maintain patency of line via a heparinized flush solution administered under pressure.
2. The transducer should be at the level of the right atrium to ensure accurate measurements.
3. Catheter should be secured to the skin and covered with an occlusive dressing. Each time the PCWP is evaluated, it is imperative that the balloon or the wedge be deflated in order to prevent pulmonary infarction.

Complications:

Infections, pulmonary artery rupture, pulmonary infarction, air emboli.

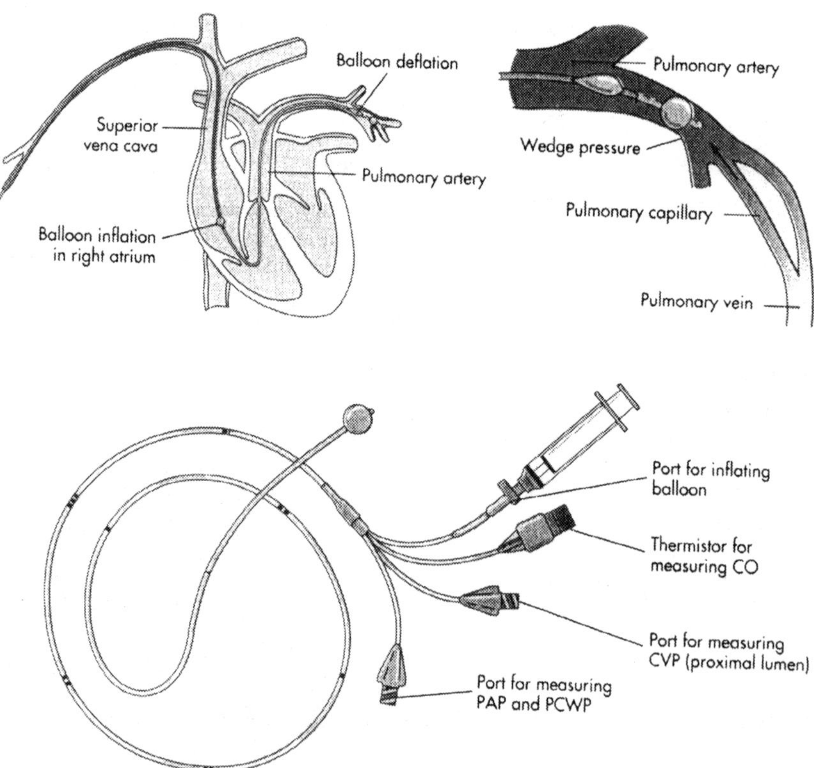

Figure 17-4: Four Lumen Thermodilution Pulmonary Artery Catheter

Reprinted with permission: Phipps, WJ, Sands, JK, & Marek, JF (1999). *Medical Surgical Nursing: Concepts & Clinical Practice*, 6th ed. Philadelphia: Mosby, p. 634

Appendix 17-6: CARDIOPULMONARY RESUSCITATION (CPR)

❑ **The American Heart Association has established standards for cardiopulmonary resuscitation. For further delineation of the procedure, consult the American Heart Association Cardiopulmonary Resuscitation Guidelines. The American Heart Association defines a child as 1 year to approximately 8 years and infant as birth to one year. Basic cardiac life support involves the ABCs of CPR - Airway, Breathing, and Circulation.**

1. **Airway.**
   - Identify that victim is unconscious.
   - Activate the EMS system or code blue protocol.
   - Place client in position to open airway.
   - Open the airway: head tilt, chin lift.
   - Determine if victim is breathing (Look, listen, and feel for breaths).
   - If victim is breathing, place in recovery position.
   - If victim is not breathing, initiate rescue breathing.
2. **Breathing.**
   - Maintain the open airway.
   - Pinch nostrils closed.
   - Give 2 full breaths utilizing mouth-to-mouth technique (mouth-to-nose and mouth may be utilized in small children and infants).
3. **Check the pulse.** After giving two full breaths, check the pulse. On the adult and child, check the carotid; on the infant, check the pulse on the inside of the upper arm midway between the elbow and shoulder. If the pulse is present, continue rescue breathing.
   Adult: 1 breath every 5 seconds or 12 per minute.
   Child and Infant: 1 breath every 3 seconds or 20 per minute.
   If pulse is absent, begin external cardiac compressions.

NURSING PRIORITY: *Do not check the pulse prior to establishing ventilation. An open airway and rescue breathing must be established before continuing any further in the CPR sequence.*
PEDIATRIC PRIORITY: *Be careful not to hyperextend the infant's head, it may block the airway. Don't pinch the nose shut on an infant, cover the nose with your mouth. Breathe slowly, just enough to make the chest rise.*

4. **External cardiac compression.**
   - Place the victim on a firm surface. If the client is in the bed, put a cardiac board behind the victim. DO NOT attempt to remove the victim from the bed.
   - Locate the lower half of the sternum in the adult and the child. For the adult, place one hand over the lower sternum; place the other hand on top of the previous hand. For a child, utilize the heel of one hand. For an infant, locate the nipple line; the area for compression is one finger's width below the line; use two fingers for compression.
   - Depress the sternum 1 ½ to 2 inches in the adult; children depress 1 to 1 ½ inches; infants depress ½ to 1 inch.
   - Compression and relaxation should be of equal duration.

   Adult:
   One rescuer and two rescuers - 15 compressions (keep rate sustained at minimal of 100 per minute) to 2 ventilations.
   Infant and Child:
   One rescuer - 5 compressions (maintain rate greater than 100 per minute) to 1 ventilation.
   Infant - one man only
   Child may be one may or two man, but rate and compressions remain same
5. **Do not interrupt CPR for more than 5 seconds.**
6. **Termination of CPR: The nonphysician individual should continue resuscitation efforts until one of the following occurs:**
   - Spontaneous circulation and ventilation have been restored.
   - Resuscitation efforts are transferred to another equally responsible person who continues the resuscitation procedure.
   - A physician, or physician-directed person, assumes responsibility for resuscitation procedure.
   - The victim is transferred to an emergency medical service (i.e., paramedics and ambulance).
   - The rescuer is exhausted and unable to continue resuscitation.

NCLEX ALERT: *Perform cardiopulmonary resuscitation.*

Appendix 17-7:
DEFIBRILLATION

❑ Defibrillation - Depolarization of the electrical impulses in the heart to allow the heart's own intrinsic pacemaker to regain control of cardiac rhythm.

Unsynchronized cardioversion (defibrillation) — depolarization of cardiac cells in an emergency situation with a life threatening dysrhythmia.

1. Always begin CPR if client is pulse-less and unconscious; do not wait for a defibrillator.
2. Make sure everyone is clear of the bed and the client is not laying in fluids.
3. Defibrillation is usually started at 200j and progresses to a higher energy level (300-360) if necessary.
4. Document rhythm after defibrillation.
5. Remain with client and closely assess for adequacy and stability of cardiac output and cardiac rhythm.
6. Make sure everyone is clear from touching the bed or client

Synchronized cardioversion — depolarization of cardiac cells to allow the sinus node to regain control of cardiac rhythm.

1. An elective, planned procedure.
2. Requires client teaching and informed consent.
3. Document rhythm prior to cardioversion and immediately afterwards.
4. The defibrillator is set (synchronized) to deliver the electrical discharge during the QRS complex, this prevents the discharge from occurring on the T-wave.
5. Remain with client and closely assess for adequacy and stability of cardiac output and cardiac rhythm.

Implantable cardioverter defibrillators (ICD)

1. Used in clients who have survived one or more episodes of sudden death from ventricular dysrhythmias, or from refractory ventricular dysrhythmias not associated with an MI.
2. Implantable device can also be used as a pacemaker.
3. Inserted in a subcutaneous pocket in the subclavicular or abdominal area.
4. Client should avoid contact sports, increase activity gradually, carry ICD identification information.
5. Client should avoid working over large motors, and move away from devices of dizziness occurs.
6. Common response to device is anxiety and fear.
7. Assess for fluid hazards - IV fluids and urine may conduct voltage.

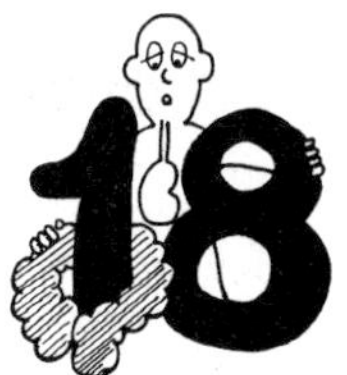

PHYSIOLOGY OF THE GASTROINTESTINAL (GI) SYSTEM

Ingestion, Digestion, Absorption, and Elimination Process

A. Ingestion—intake of food.
   1. Swallowing (deglutition) completes the process of ingestion.
   2. Intake of food is influenced by appetite center located in hypothalamus.
   3. Appetite stimulated by an empty stomach, decrease in body temperature, hypoglycemia, habit, and the sight, smell, and taste of food.
   4. Appetite inhibited by stomach distention, illness with fever, hyperglycemia, nausea or vomiting, and some drugs (e.g. amphetamines).

B. Digestion—physical and chemical breakdown of food.
   1. Involves chemical, mechanical, and hormonal activity.
   2. Ptyalin, an enzyme, acts on food in the mouth and begins starch digestion.
   3. Food moves through the esophagus by peristalsis to the stomach.
   4. Digestion of proteins occurs in the stomach.
   5. Stomach acts as a reservoir for food.
   6. Length of time food remains in stomach depends on type of food, gastric motility, and psychologic factors; average time 3 to 4 hrs.
   7. Carbohydrates leave stomach the fastest; proteins and fats leave the slowest.
   8. pH is acidic in stomach, which promotes the enzyme in gastric juice, pepsin, to break down proteins into protease and peptones.
   9. Lipase acts to split fats.
   10. Chyme (food mixed with gastric secretion) moves through the pylorus to the small intestine.
   11. Hormones are released into the bloodstream. Secretion stimulates pancreas to secrete an alkaline fluid. Cholecystokinin and pancreozymin (CCK-PZ) are produced and released by the duodenal mucosa, which stimulates contraction of the gall bladder and relaxation of the sphincter of Oddi.
   12. Bile is released from gallbladder and fats are emulsified.

C. Absorption—transfer of food products into circulation.
   1. Occurs in small intestine which has numerous villi to increase absorptive surface area.
   2. Simple sugars (from carbohydrates), fatty acids (from fats), and amino acids (from proteins), water, electrolytes, and vitamins are absorbed.

D. Elimination—excretion of waste products.
   1. Large intestine, absorbs water and electrolytes, and forms feces.
   2. Serves as a reservoir for fecal mass until defecation occurs.

System Assessment

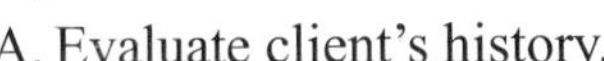

A. Evaluate client's history.
   1. Changes in bowel habits.
   2. Changes in dietary habits.
   3. Weight loss or gain.
   4. Pain.
   5. Nausea and vomiting.
      a. Associated with pain.
      b. Precipitating factors.
   6. Presence or problems with flatulence.

B. Assess vital signs in client's overall status.

C. Assess for presence and characteristics of pain.

D. Assess client's mouth.
   1. Presence of adequate saliva.
   2. Overall condition of teeth.
   3. Overall condition of tongue.
   4. Presence of the gag reflex.

E. Evaluate the abdomen (client should be lying flat).
   1. Divide the abdomen into four quadrants and describe findings according to the quadrants (Figure 18-1).
   2. Evaluate the general contour of the abdomen.
   3. Evaluate for presence of surgical or trauma scars or ostomies.
   4. Assess for presence of and characteristics of bowel sounds.

NCLEX ALERT: *Assessment: To determine characteristics of bowel sounds; note characteristics of bowel sounds.*

      a. Normally soft, gurgles should be heard every 5-15 seconds.

b. Loud, high pitched sounds may be heard when a client is hungry or has gastroenteritis.

c. Borborygmi - loud, gurgling bowel sounds; may precede diarrhea.

d. Hypoactive bowel sounds are at rate of one every minute or longer.

5. Palpate the abdomen; begin with nontender areas first.

a. Is it soft to palpation?

b. Presence of distention.

c. Presence of masses.

F. Assess rectal area.

G. Evaluate elimination patterns and effects of aging on GI tract (Box 18-1).

H. Evaluate dietary pattern and fluid intake.

I. Assess stool specimen.

1. Color.

2. Consistency.

3. Odor.

4. Presence of blood or mucus.

DISORDERS OF THE GASTROINTESTINAL SYSTEM

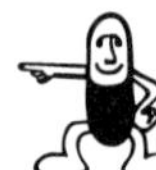

Nausea and Vomiting

❑ **Nausea is an unpleasant feeling that vomiting is imminent. Vomiting is an involuntary act in which the stomach contracts and forcefully expels gastric contents.**

A. Loss of fluid and electrolytes is the primary consequence of repeated vomiting; the very young and the elderly are more susceptible to complications of fluid imbalances.

B. Prolonged vomiting will precipitate a metabolic problem.

1. Metabolic alkalosis is associated with prolonged vomiting and loss of hydrochloric acid.

2. Metabolic acidosis occurs with *severe* prolonged vomiting of contents of the small intestine resulting in loss of bicarbonate.

Assessment

1. Precipitating Causes.

a. Pathogenic—related to a disease process.

(1) Intestinal obstruction.

(2) Peptic ulcer disease

(3) Increased intracranial pressure.

(4) Ingestion of toxic substances (food poisoning).

(5) Vertigo.

b. Iatrogenic—resulting from a disease treatment.

(1) Chemotherapy/radiation.

(2) Medications.

(3) Postoperative.

c. Psychogenic.

(1) Psychosis/neurosis.

(2) Reaction to psychological trauma.

d. Pregnancy.

NCLEX ALERT: *Monitor client's hydration status; modify client's care based on results of diagnostic tests..*

2. Assessment.

a. Identify precipitating cause.

b. Assess frequency of vomiting, amount of vomiting, and contents of vomitus.

c. Hematemesis—presence of blood in vomitus.

(1) Bright red blood is indicative of hemorrhage.

(2) Coffee-ground material is indicative of blood retained in the stomach; the digestive process has broken down the hemoglobin.

d. Projectile vomiting—vomiting not preceded by nausea and expelled with excessive force.

e. Presence of fecal odor and bile in vomitus indicates a back flow of intestinal contents into stomach.

3. Diagnostics—clinical manifestations.

Treatment

1. Eliminate the precipitating cause.

2. Antiemetics (See Appendix 18-2).

3. Parenteral replacement of fluid if loss is excessive.

Nursing Intervention

✦ *Goal: to prevent recurrence of nausea and vomiting, and ensuing complications.*

1. Prophylactic antiemetics for clients with a tendency toward vomiting.

2. Prompt removal of unpleasant odors, used emesis basin, used equipment and soiled linens.

3. Good oral hygiene.

4. Position conscious client on side or in semi-Fowler's position; position unconscious client on the side with head of bed slightly elevated, to promote drainage of oral cavity.

Figure 18-1: Organs of the Gastrointestinal System
Reprinted with permission: Phipps, WJ, Sands, JK, & Marek, JF (1999). *Medical Surgical Nursing: Concepts & Clinical Practice*, 6th ed. Philadelphia: Mosby, p. 1236

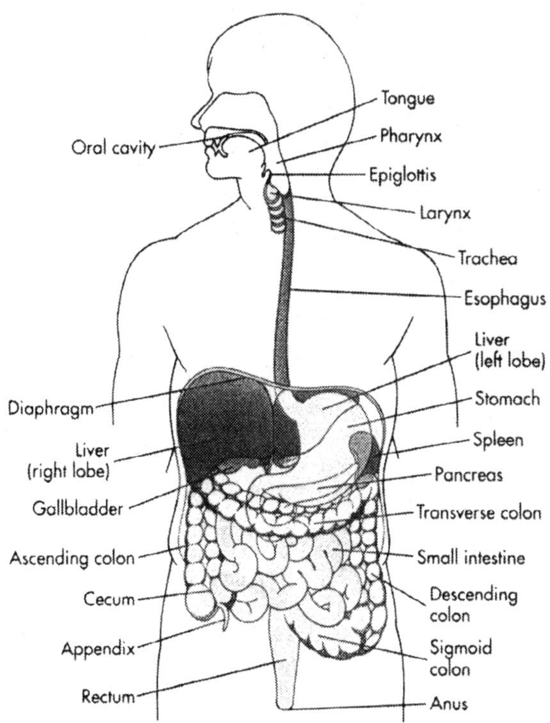

5. Withhold PO food and fluid initially after vomiting; begin oral intake slowly with clear liquids.
6. Assess for bowel sounds on postoperative clients; do not begin PO fluids until bowel sounds are present.
7. Support abdominal incisions during prolonged vomiting.

✦ *Goal: to relieve nausea and vomiting.*
1. Administer antiemetics as indicated.
2. Evaluate precipitating causes; relieve if possible.
3. Use gastric decompression with a nasogastric tube if indicated.

✦ *Goal: to assess client's response to prolonged vomiting.*
1. Fluid and electrolyte status.
2. Continued presence of gastric distention.
3. Overall vital sign changes.
4. Intake and output.
5. Assess for adequate hydration.
6. Evaluate weight loss.

Constipation

❑ **Constipation exists when the interval between bowel movements is longer than normal for the individual and the stool is dry and hard.**

Box Test 18-1: Elderly Care Focus
Changes in GI System Related to Aging.

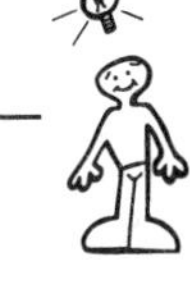

- Decreased hydrochloric acid and decreased absorption of vitamins; encourage frequent small feedings that are high in vitamins.
- Decreased peristalsis and decreased sensation to defecate; encourage diet high in fiber and minimum of 1500 of fluid daily, encourage physical activity
- Decreased lipase from pancreas to aid in fat digestion; encourage smaller meals since diarrhea may be caused by increased fat intake.
- Decreased liver activity with decreased production of enzymes for drug metabolism, tendency toward accumulation of medications instruct clients not to double up on their medications, especially cardiac medications.

Assessment

1. Precipitating causes.
   a. Inadequate bulk in the diet.
   b. Inadequate fluid intake.
   c. Immobilization.
   d. Ignoring the urge to defecate.
   e. Diseases of the colon and rectum.
   f. Side effects of medications.
2. Clinical manifestations.
   a. Abdominal distention.
   b. Decrease in the amount of stool.
   c. Dry, hard stool.
   d. Straining to pass the stool.
3. Diagnostics—clinical manifestations.

Treatment

1. Change dietary intake—increase bulk and fluids.
2. Bulk laxatives or enemas for occasional constipation problem(Appendix 18-3).
3. Instruct to maintain normal bowel schedule and do not ignore urge to defecate.
4. Discourage long-term use of laxatives and enemas.

Nursing Intervention

✦ *Goal: to identify client at risk of developing problems and institute preventive measures (Box 18-2).*

✦ *Goal: to implement treatment measures for fecal impaction removal.*
1. Considered an impaction if no BM for 3 days or passage of small amounts of semisoft or liquid stool.
2. Very young and very old most susceptible for problems with impaction.
3. Steps in removing:

a. Manually check for presence with nonsterile, lubricated gloved finger.

b. Gently, attempt to break up impaction.

c. Follow with suppository, enema, or laxative as ordered by physician.

d. Emphasis is on *prevention* of impaction.

NCLEX ALERT: *Evaluate client's use of home remedies and OTC drugs. Assess what the client is using for constipation; frequently, the geriatric client is using harsh laxatives.*

Diarrhea

❑ **Rapid movement of intestinal contents through the small bowel.**

1. Significant increase in number of stools.
2. Decrease in the consistency of the stool, with an increase in fluid content.
3. Infants and elderly are most susceptible to complications of diarrhea.
4. Complications of severe diarrhea.
   a. Dehydration resulting in hypovolemia.
   b. Metabolic acidosis.

Assessment

1. Precipitating causes.
   a. Intestinal inflammation and infections.
   b. Food and drug intolerance, tube feedings.
   c. Food poisoning.
   d. Bowel disorders.
   e. Malabsorption problems.
   f. Parasitic infections.
   g. Rotavirus is the most common pathogen in young children - contact precautions.
   h. Psychological factors.
2. Clinical manifestations.
   a. Frequent, watery bowel movements.
   b. Stools may contain undigested food, mucus, pus, or blood.
   c. Frequently foul-smelling.
   d. Abdominal cramping, distention, and vomiting frequently occur with diarrhea.
   e. Weight loss.
   f. Hyperactive bowel sounds.
   g. May precipitate dehydration, hypovolemia, hypokalemia, and shock.
3. Diagnostics.
   a. Clinical manifestations.
   b. Stool culture.
   c. X-rays of the GI tract.

Treatment

1. Treat the underlying problem.
2. Decrease activity and irritation of the GI tract by decreasing intake.
3. Parenteral replacement of fluid and electrolytes if diarrhea is severe.
4. Administer antidiarrheal medications (See Appendix 18-4).

Nursing Intervention

✦ *Goal: to decrease diarrhea and prevent complications.*

1. Identify precipitating causes and eliminate if possible.
2. Decrease food intake; more soft, nonirritating food.
3. Oral rehydrating solutions (Pedialyte, Rehydrate, Infalyte) and progress fluids and diet as tolerated.
4. Administer medications as indicated.
5. Maintain good hygiene in the rectal area to prevent skin excoriation.
6. Decrease activity.

✦ *Goal: to evaluate client's response to diarrhea.*

1. Evaluate changes in vital signs correlating with fluid loss.
2. Evaluate electrolyte changes and urine specific gravity.
3. Intake and output, daily weight if diarrhea is progressive.
4. Assess changes in abdominal distention and cramping.
5. Ongoing evaluation of characteristics of diarrhea.

✦ *Goal: to prevent spread of diarrhea.*

1. Good hand washing techniques.
2. Contact based precautions.
   a. Proper disposal of diapers and soiled linens close to bedside.
   b. Instruct family regarding hand washing techniques.
   c. Keep bedpans, soiled linens, diapers away from clean areas.

Rotavirus

❑ **Most common pathogen in young children hospitilized for diarrhea.**

A. Affects all age groups and is most common in cool weather.

B. Incubation period is 1-3 days.

C. Important source of nosocomial infections in hospital.

D. Is frequently associated with an upper respiratory infection.

Assessment.

1. Clinical manifestations.
   a. Abrupt onset.
   b. Nausea/vomiting and abdominal pain.
   c. Persistent foul smelling, explosive, diarrhea.
   d. Fever last approximately 48 huors.
2. Diagnostics.
   a. History regarding onset and duration.
   b. Laboratory electrolytes to determine status of hydration.

Nursing Intervention.

✦ *Goal: to maintain fluid and electrolyte balance (see nursing interventions for client with diarrhea)*

1. Fluid and electrolyte replacement, initially oral rehydration therapy with solutions to replace electrolytes (oral rehydration solutions)
2. Monitor IV fluids in situations of severe diarrhea.
3. Antidiarrheal medications (Appendix 18-4), monitor stools, child is at increased risk for developing a paralytic ileus.
4. Strict monitoring of hydration status.
5. May begin food as soon as child can tolerate, generally soft, easily digestible food, but does not have to be clear liquids.

✦ *Goal: to decrease infection and prevent spread.*

1. Contact precautions in hospital
2. Instruct parents regarding importance of handwashing, and how to care for infant/child at home.
3. Maintain "clean" and "dirty" areas in the room.
4. Antibiotics are most often not indicated because of the risk of developing pseudo-membranous colitis.

Gastroesophageal Reflux Disease (GERD)

❑ **Condition is caused by the backward flow of gastrointestinal contents into the esophagus (esophageal reflux). Reflux is often associated with a *hiatal hernia;* the herniation of the upper portion of the stomach through the diaphragm into the thoracic cavity.**

A. Esophageal reflux occurs and the esophagus is exposed to acid.

B. The acid breaks down the esophageal mucosa and an inflammatory response is initiated.

Box 18-2: Elderly Care Focus:
Preventing Fecal Impaction

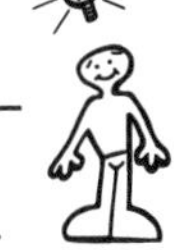

- Increase intake of high-fiber foods - raw vegetables, whole grain breads and cereals, fresh fruits.
- Increase fluid intake - water and juice.
- Maintain regular activity - daily walking in immediate area.
- Discourage use of laxatives and enemas - client becomes dependent on them.
- Encourage use of bulk-forming products to provide increased fiber (methylcellulose, psyllium).
- Encourage bowel movement at same time each day.
- Try to position client on bedside commode rather than on a bedpan.
- If client is experiencing diarrhea, check to see if stool is oozing around an impaction.

Assessment

1. Risk factors.
   a. Increase in gastric volume or intra-abdominal pressure.
   b. Sphincter tone of the lower esophagus (LES) is decreased.
   c. Increased occurrence of reflux from nicotine, high-fat foods, caffeine.
   d. Hiatal hernia.
2. Clinical manifestations.
   a. Reflux esophagitis (heartburn, dyspepsia).
   b. Increased pain after meals; may be relieved by antacids.
   c. Activities that increase intra-abdominal pressure increase esophageal discomfort.
   d. Pain may radiate to back and neck.
   e. Regurgitation not associated with belching or nausea.
3. Diagnostics - 24-hour pH monitoring, esophageal manometry, esophagoscopy.

Treatment

1. Medical
   a. Diet therapy - decrease fatty foods; small frequent meals.
   b. Medications- histamine receptor antagonist, antacids, gastrointestinal stimulants. (Appendix 18-5).
2. Surgical - surgical correction of the hernia.

Nursing Intervention

✦ *Goal: to decrease esophageal reflux.*

1. Drink adequate fluids at meals to increase food passage; avoid carbonated beverages.
2. Avoid temperature extremes in foods.

3. Avoid drinking fluids 3 hours prior to bedtime.
4. Elevate the head of the bed on 6-8 inch blocks.
5. Lose weight to decrease abdominal pressure gradient.
6. Avoid tobacco, alcohol, NSAIDs, salicylates.
7. Decrease intake of highly seasoned foods
8. Frequent small meals to prevent gastric dilation.
9. Avoid any food which precipitates discomfort (fats, caffeine, chocolate, nicotine will decrease esophageal sphincter tone).
10. Do not lie down after eating.

✦ *Goal: perform preoperative nursing interventions prior to surgery.*

✦ *Goal: provide postoperative nursing care.*

1. If surgical thoracic approach, the client will have chest tube postoperatively.
2. Client should continue same dietary restrictions postoperatively.

Gastritis

❑ **This condition is an inflammation of the gastric mucosa.**

A. Acute gastritis is generally self-limiting with no residual damage.

B. Chronic gastritis is due to repeated irritation of the gastric mucosa caused by a breakdown of normal protective mucosal barrier.

Assessment

1. Risk factors/etiology.
   a. Often due to dietary indiscretion (gastric irritants - coffee, aspirin, alcohol, etc.).
   b. Alcohol intake (especially chronic).
   c. Contaminated foods (*Staphylococcus* or *Salmonella* organisms).
   d. Medications causing gastric irritation (aspirin, corticosteroids, chemotherapy)
2. Clinical manifestations.
   a. Epigastric tenderness.
   b. Nausea, vomiting.
   c. Anorexia.
   d. Chronic gastritis.
      (1) May precipitate pernicious anemia.
      (2) May be secondary to uremia.
      (3) Peptic ulcer disease
   e. Smoking aggravates condition.
3. Diagnostics.
   a. Endoscopic examination of the gastric mucosa with biopsy.
   b. Stool examination for occult blood.
   c. Gastric analysis.

Treatment

1. Medical management.
   a. Eliminate cause.
   b. Antiemetics, antacids.
2. Surgical intervention if medical treatment fails or hemorrhage occurs.

Nursing Intervention

✦ *Goal: to decrease gastric irritation.*

1. May be NPO initially, with IV fluid and electrolyte replacement.
2. Administer antiemetics, antacids.
3. Bed rest.
4. Begin clear liquids when symptoms subside.

✦ *Goal: to assist client to identify and avoid precipitating causes.*

Gastroenteritis

❑ **This is an inflammatory process involving the mucosa of the stomach and the small bowel.**

Assessment

1. Risk factors/etiology.
   a. *Salmonella*—fecal oral transmission by direct contact or via contaminated food.
   b. Staphylococcal—transmission via foods that were handled by contaminated carrier.
   c. Dysentery *E-coli,* and *Shigella.*
2. Clinical manifestations.
   a. Abdominal cramping.
   b. Vomiting and diarrhea.
   c. Fever.
   d. Dehydration with excessive loss of fluid.
3. Diagnostics—identify causative agent.

Treatment

Appropriate medication for causative agents.

Nursing Management

✦ *Goal: to maintain hydration and electrolyte balance, and to prevent spread of disease.*

1. NPO until vomiting ceases.
2. Examine anal area for irritation, apply moisture barrier.
3. IV fluid replacement if severe dehydration occurs.
4. Begin clear liquids gradually after vomiting ceases.
5. Contact based precautions.

✦ *Goal: to provide symptomatic nursing care for diarrhea, nausea, and vomiting (See general intestinal disorders).*

Peptic Ulcer Disease (PUD)

❑ **PUD is ulceration of the gastric mucosa as a result of the digestive action of hydrochloric acid and pepsin.**

A. Types of peptic ulcers.
   1. Duodenal (most common).
   2. Gastric.
   3. Stress-induced ulcers, drug-induced ulcers.

A. Histamine release occurs with the erosion of the gastric mucosa in both duodenal and gastric ulcers. This stimulates further secretion of gastric acid and formation of mucosal edema. The continued erosion will eventually damage the blood vessels, leading to hemorrhage or to erosion through gastric mucosa.

B. Characteristics
   1. Factors contributing to development.
      a. Presence of *Helicobacter pylori.*
      b. Medications that alter gastric mucosa and secretions.
      c. Increased physical stress (trauma, postoperative).
      d. Psychosocial stress (duodenal ulcers).
      e. Smoking, alcohol.
   2. Clinical manifestations.
      a. Pain
         (1) Gastric ulcer - mid-epigastric, variable, may be worse with food.
         (2) Duodenal ulcer - right epigastric area, occurs 2 to 4 hours after meals, relieved by food and antacids.
      b. Weight gain with duodenal ulcer loss with gastric ulcer.
      c. Nausea and vomiting.
      d. Bleeding when ulcer erodes through a vessel.

Diagnostics

(All types)
   1. X-ray of upper GI system.
   2. Esophagogastroduodenoscopy (EGD).

Treatment

   1. Medications (Appendix 18-5)
      a. Antacids.
      b. Histamine receptor antagonist.
      c. Anticholinergic medications for duodenal ulcers.
      d. Prostaglandin analogs and acid pump inhibitors.
      e. Medications for to *H. pylori* bacteria.
         (1) Metronidazole (**Flagyl**).
         (2) Omeprazole (**Prilosec**).
         (3) Clarithromycin (**Biaxin**).
   2. Life style modifications.
      a. Avoid foods that cause discomfort.
      b. Decrease smoking.
      c. Decrease activity and psychological stress.
   3. Surgical interventions (indicated in complications).
      a. Vagotomy—decreases acid-secreting stimulus to gastric cells.
      b. Pyloroplasty—widens the pyloric valve to enhance gastric emptying; may be done in association with vagotomy.
      c. Gastric resection —acute obstruction, hemorrhage, perforation, chronic recurring ulcers.

Complications

   1. Hemorrhage.
      a. Hematemesis, melena, or both.
      b. Hypovolemic shock (See Chapter 16).

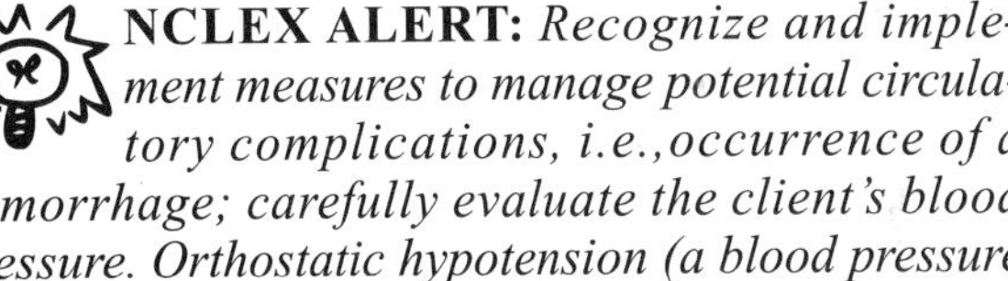

NCLEX ALERT: *Recognize and implement measures to manage potential circulatory complications, i.e., occurrence of a hemorrhage; carefully evaluate the client's blood pressure. Orthostatic hypotension (a blood pressure decrease of 10 mm Hg or more) may be indicative of hypovolemia.*

   2. Perforation of ulcer into the peritoneal cavity.
      a. Sudden, severe, diffuse, upper abdominal pain.
      b. Abdominal muscles contract as abdomen becomes rigid.
      c. Bowel sounds absent.
      d. Respirations become shallow and rapid.
      e. Severity of peritonitis is proportional to size of perforation and amount of gastric spillage.
   3. Gastric obstruction.
      a. Clients with a long history of ulcer disease.
      b. Progression of pain from epigastric to generalized upper abdominal pain.
      c. Increasing abdominal discomfort.
      d. Relief may be obtained by vomiting.
      e. Increased bowel sounds.

NCLEX ALERT: *Teach client methods to prevent complications associated with diagnosis.*

Nursing Intervention

✦ *Goal: to promote health in clients with PUD.*

1. Identify factors in lifestyle contributing to development of ulcer.
2. Identify factors which precipitate pain and discomfort.
3. Do not take over-the-counter medications, especially aspirin compounds and NSAIDs.
4. Identify stress factors in lifestyle. Counseling may be indicated to help client improve ability to cope with stress.

NCLEX ALERT: *Evaluate use of home remedies and OTC drugs. The PUD client may have been using antacids for a prolonged time.*

✦ *Goal: to relieve pain and promote healing.*

1. Dietary modifications.
   a. Encourage small, frequent meals.
   b. Nonstimulating, bland foods are generally tolerated better during healing of acute episodes.
   c. Assist client to identify specific dietary habits which accelerate or precipitate pain.
   d. Promote good nutritional habits.
2. Identify characteristics of pain and activities that increase/decrease pain.

✦ *Goal: to assess for complications of gastric obstruction (see discussion of obstruction in this unit).*

✦ *Goal: to assess for complications of hemorrhage.*

1. Assess for symptoms indicating hemorrhage.
   a. Evaluate hemoglobin and hematocrit levels.
   b. Assess for distention, increase in pain, and tenderness.
   c. Correlate vital signs with changes in client's overall condition.
   d. Assess stools and nasogastric drainage for presence of blood.
2. If hemorrhage occurs:
   a. Establish peripheral infusion line, preferably with large gauge needle for blood infusion.
   b. Insert indwelling urinary catheter to monitor urinary output.
   c. Insert nasogastric tube for removal of gastric contents and maintain gastric suction.
   d. May implement iced saline lavage.
   e. Prepare to administer whole blood transfusion (Appendix 14-3) and IV fluids.
3. Position client supine with legs slightly elevated.
4. Begin oxygen.
5. Initiate preoperative preparation (See Chapter 3).

Table 18-1: DUMPING SYNDROME

❑ **Condition occurs when a large bolus of gastric chyme and hypertonic fluid enter the intestine.**

✦ *Goal: to assess for symptoms of condition.*

Weakness, dizziness, tachycardia.
Epigastric fullness and abdominal cramping.
Diaphoresis.
Generally occurs within 15 to 30 minutes after eating.
Condition is usually self-limiting and resolves in about 6 -12 months.

✦ *Goal: to prevent dumping syndrome.*

- Decrease amount of food eaten at one meal.
- Decrease carbohydrates, decrease salt intake, increase proteins and fats as tolerated.
- No added fluid with meal or for one hour following meal.
- Position client in semi recumbent position during meals; client should lie down on the left side for 20 to 30 minutes after meals to delay stomach emptying.
- Manifestations usually occur within 5-30 minutes after eating.
- Hypoglycemia may occur 2-3 hours after eating, caused by rapid entry of high carbohydrates into jejunum.

NCLEX ALERT: *Implement measures to improve client's nutritional intake. Prevent the dumping syndrome and/or care for client experiencing the dumping syndrome.*

✦ *Goal: to assess for complications of perforation and peritonitis(see discussion of peritonitis in this unit).*

✦ *Goal: to assist client to return to homeostasis postoperative gastric resection.*

1. General postoperative care as indicated (See Chapter 3).
2. Maintain nasogastric suction until peristalsis returns (Appendix 18- 7).

NCLEX ALERT: *Monitor/maintain gastrointestinal drainage. Distention and obstruction of the nasogastric tube is a common problem in this client.*

3. After removal of nasogastric tube, assess for:
   a. Increasing abdominal distention.
   b. Nausea, vomiting.
   c. Changes in bowel sounds.
4. No PO fluids until client is able to tolerate removal of nasogastric tube.
5. Begin PO fluids slowly—clear liquids, then progress to bland, soft diet.
6. Based on client's condition, total parenteral nutrition may be necessary to maintain adequate nutrition.
7. Encourage ambulation to promote peristalsis.

✦ *Goal: to identify dumping syndrome (see Table 18-1).*

✦ *Goal: to prevent the development of pernicious anemia postoperative total gastric resection: (Vitamin B_{12} deficiency, Chapter 14).*

Appendicitis

❑ **Appendicitis is an inflammation of the appendix and is the most common reason for abdominal surgery during childhood.**

A. Obstruction of the blind sac of the appendix precipitates inflammation, ulceration, and necrosis.

B. Problems arise when the necrotic area ruptures, spilling intestinal contents into the peritoneal cavity, causing peritonitis.

Assessment

1. Risk factors/etiology.
   a. Rare in children under two years old.
   b. Peak incidence in 20-30 year-old.
2. Clinical manifestations.
   a. Begins with vague abdominal pain.
   b. Pain becomes more persistent and consistent; more intense at McBurney's point (right lower quadrant).
   c. Pain may be characterized as rebound pain or tenderness.
   d. Anorexia, nausea, vomiting.
   e. Low-grade fever.
   f. Client assumes a characteristic position of side-lying with the knees flexed.
   g. Sudden relief from pain may be indicative of ruptured appendix.
3. Diagnostics.
   a. Clinical manifestations.
   b. Leukocytosis.
4. Complications—peritonitis.

Treatment

1. Appendectomy.
2. More extensive abdominal surgery must be done if appendix has ruptured (abdominal laparotomy).

Nursing Intervention

✦ *Goal: to assess clinical manifestations and to prepare for surgery as indicated.*

1. Careful nursing assessment for clinical manifestations.
2. Maintain child/client NPO until otherwise indicated.
3. Maintain bed rest in position of comfort.

NCLEX ALERT: *Determine need for administration of PRN pain medications. Do not give narcotics for pain control prior to confirming a diagnosis of appendicitis, as they mask signs if the appendix ruptures.*

4. Do not apply heat to the abdomen; cold applications may provide some relief or comfort.
5. Do not administer enemas.
6. Avoid unnecessary palpation of abdomen.

NCLEX ALERT: *Determine if client is prepared for surgery or procedures. Appendicitis is a very common problem; know how to care for client during diagnostic phase.*

✦ *Goal: to maintain homeostasis and healing postoperative appendectomy (See Chapter 3).*

✦ *Goal: to prevent abdominal distention and assess bowel function postoperative abdominal laparotomy.*

1. Remain NPO.
2. Gastric decompression by nasogastric tube; maintain patency and suction.
3. Monitor abdomen for distention.
4. Assess peristaltic activity.
5. Evaluate and record character of bowel movement.

✦ *Goal: to decrease infection and promote healing postoperative abdominal laparotomy.*

1. Position client in semi-Fowler's to localize infection, prevent spread of infection or development of subdiaphragmatic abscess.
2. Antibiotics are usually administered via IV infusion, monitor response to antibiotics as well as status of IV infusion site.

3. Monitor vital signs frequently (2 to 4 hours) and evaluate for infectious process.
4. Provide appropriate wound care; evaluate drainage from abdominal Penrose drains and incisional area.

NCLEX ALERT: *Promote progress of wound healing: the abdominal laparotomy client frequently has drains and a large incision.*

✦ *Goal: to maintain adequate hydration and nutrition, and promote comfort postoperative abdominal laparotomy.*

1. Maintain adequate hydration via IV infusion.
2. Evaluate tolerance to PO liquids when nasogastric tube is removed.
3. Begin clear liquids PO when peristalsis returns.
4. Progress diet as tolerated.
5. Administer analgesics as indicated.

NCLEX ALERT: *Identify infection; peritonitis is common postoperatively from a ruptured appendix.*

Peritonitis

❑ **Peritonitis is a generalized inflammatory process of the peritoneum.**

A. Intestinal motility is decreased and fluid accumulates as a result of the inability of the intestine to reabsorb fluid.

B. Fluid will leak into the peritoneal cavity, precipitating fluid, electrolyte and protein loss as well as fluid depletion.

Assessment

1. Risk factors/etiology.
   a. Chemical peritonitis results from gastric ulcer perforation or a ruptured ectopic pregnancy.
   b. Bacterial peritonitis results from traumatic injury (abdominal trauma, ruptured appendix).
   c. Chemical peritonitis is rapidly followed by bacterial peritonitis.

NCLEX ALERT: *Monitor status of postoperative client; identify infection. Peritonitis is a potential complication any time the abdomen is entered, either from trauma or from surgery.*

2. Clinical manifestations.
   a. Presence of precipitating cause.
   b. Pain over involved area; rebound tenderness.
   c. Abdominal distention.
   d. Abdominal muscle rigidity ("board-like" abdomen).
   e. Fever.
   f. Anorexia, nausea, vomiting.
   g. Increased pulse, decreased blood pressure, shallow respirations.
   h. Decreased or absent bowel sounds.
   i. Hypovolemia, dehydration.
   j. Shallow respirations in attempt to avoid pain.
3. Diagnostics.
   a. CBC — ↑ WBC.
   b. X-ray of abdomen.
   c. Paracentesis, to evaluate abdominal fluid.
   d. History.

Treatment

1. Identify and treat precipitating cause (may require surgical intervention).
2. Antibiotics.
3. IV fluids.
4. Decrease abdominal distention.

Nursing Intervention

✦ *Goal: to maintain fluid and electrolyte balance and reduce gastric distention.*

1. Maintain nasogastric suction.
2. Maintain IV fluid replacement: usually normal saline or lactated Ringer's solution.
3. Administer potassium supplements with caution due to possible complication of poor renal function.
4. Evaluate peristalsis and return of bowel function.
5. Maintain intake and output records.
6. Assess for problems of dehydration and hypovolemia.
7. Encourage activities to facilitate return of bowel function.
   a. Encourage ambulation.
   b. Attempt to decrease analgesics and maintain adequate pain control.
   c. Maintain adequate hydration.

✦ *Goal: to reduce infectious process.*

1. Administer antibiotics via IV infusion; assess client's tolerance of antibiotics and status of infusion site.
2. Evaluate vital signs and correlate with progress of infectious process.

3. Maintain semi-Fowler's position to enhance respirations as well as to localize drainage and prevent subdiaphragmatic abscess.

Diverticulosis

❑ **The condition in which an individual has multiple diverticuli is known as *diverticulosis*.**

❑ **Meckel's diverticulum is a congenital anomaly that is characterized by an outpouching or diverticulum of the ileum.**

A. Diverticulum—dilatation or out pouching of a weakened area in the intestinal wall.

B. Diverticulitis—inflammation of the diverticulum.

Assessment

1. Risk factors/etiology.
   a. Increased incidence in clients over 45 years old.
   b. Diverticulitis—bacterial invasion and an inflammatory reaction.
      (1) May be due to constipation and low-fiber diet.
      (2) Indigestible fibers (corn, seeds, etc.) will precipitate diverticulitis.
   c. The edema that accompanies the inflammation results in increased swelling and bowel irritation.
2. Clinical manifestations.
   a. Diverticulum, including Meckel's, is usually asymptomatic; symptoms vary with degree of inflammation.
   b. Intermittent left lower quadrant tenderness, abdominal cramping.
   c. Inflammatory changes may precipitate perforation or abscess formation.
   d. Diverticulitis.
      (1) Fever.
      (2) Left lower quadrant pain, usually accompanied by nausea and vomiting.
      (3) Abdominal distention.
      (4) Frequently constipated.
      (5) May progress to intestinal obstruction.
3. Diagnostics.
   a. Stool examination for occult blood.
   b. Barium enema.
   c. Colonoscopy.

Treatment

1. Medical management of uncomplicated diverticulum.
   a. High-residue diet.

Table 18-2: UNDIAGNOSED ABDOMINAL PAIN

✦ **DO NOT:**
Give anything by mouth.
Put any heat on the abdomen.
Give an enema.
Give strong narcotics.
Give a laxative.

✦ **DO:**
Put on bed rest.
Place in a position of comfort.
Assess hydration.
Assess abdominal status: distention, bowel sounds, passage of stool or flatus, generalized or local pain.

   b. Bulk laxatives, stool softeners.
   c. Anticholinergic medications (Appendix 18-5).
   d. Enemas are avoided.
2. Treatment for acute diverticulitis.
   a. Antibiotics.
   b. NPO.
   c. IV fluids.
   d. Possible surgery and colon resection if obstruction or perforation occur.
   e. Analgesics—frequently meperidine (**Demerol**) is given.

Nursing Intervention

✦ *Goal: to assist client to understand dietary implications and maintain prescribed therapy to prevent exacerbations.*

1. Understand high-fiber diet.
2. Avoid indigestible roughage such as nuts, popcorn, raw celery, corn, seeds.
3. Maintain high-fluid intake.
4. Avoid large meals.
5. Avoid alcohol.
6. Weight reduction if indicated.
7. Avoid activities which increase intra-abdominal pressure (straining at stool, bending, lifting, tight restrictive clothing).

NCLEX ALERT: *Adapt the diet to the special needs of the client; determine client's ability to perform self-care.*

✦ *Goal: to decrease colon activity in client with diverticulitis.*

1. Maintain NPO.
2. Bed rest.
3. Adequate hydration via parenteral fluids.
4. As attack subsides, introduce PO fluids gradually.

Self-Care

1. High-fiber diet that is low in undigestible fibers.

2. If client has any abdominal distress, then all fiber should be avoided until tenderness resolves.
3. Report fevers, consistent abdominal pain, and dark, tarry stools.

Crohn's Disease

❑ **Crohn's disease is a type of inflammatory bowel disease. It is most often a chronic, nonspecific, inflammatory disease of the gastrointestinal tract.**

A. Most commonly affects the small bowel, especially in the area of the terminal ileum. Lesions may also arise in the cecum and ascending colon.

B. Edema, inflammation, fibrosis occur involving all layers of the bowel wall.

C. Inflammatory process occurs in patchy segments, separated by normal tissue.

D. Client may experience periods of complete remission that alternate with exacerbations.

Assessment

1. Risk factors/etiology.
   a. May begin in adolescence; peak incidence occurs between ages 20 and 40 years.
   b. Familial tendencies.
2. Clinical manifestations.
   a. Abdominal pain.
   b. Diarrhea; may become more severe with emotional upset or poorly tolerated foods.
   c. Steatorrhea due to inefficient bile salt resorption.
   d. Nausea and vomiting.
   e. Abdominal tenderness, fistulas and abscesses.
   f. Nutritional deficits.
   g. As disease progresses:
      (1) Weight loss.
      (2) Dehydration.
      (3) Electrolyte imbalance.
      (4) Anemia.
3. Diagnostics.
   a. Stool analysis to rule out bacterial or parasitic infection.
   b. Barium enema (the pretest procedures may be modified for this client; always check with the physician).
   c. Colonoscopy.

Complications

1. Perirectal and intra-abdominal fistulas and abscesses.
2. Inflammation of the intestine, leading to perforation and generalized peritonitis.
3. Nutritional deficiencies.

Treatment

1. Dietary modifications—bland, easily digested foods to promote absorption in small intestine. Encourage client to eat small servings several times a day.
2. Medications.
   a. Corticosteroids to reduce the inflammation.
   b. Sulfasalazine (an antimicrobial agent) to control diarrhea.
   c. Immunosuppressive agents in long-term management of chronic problems.
   d. Antidiarrheal medications.
   e. Anticholinergics.
3. Surgical intervention if fistulas, perforation, bleeding, or intestinal obstruction occur.

Nursing Intervention

✦ *Goal (acute): to decrease inflammatory response and promote healing.*

1. Evaluate and maintain adequate hydration status.
2. NPO to decrease bowel activity; fluids are introduced gradually.
3. IV fluids; may require parenteral hyperalimentation.
4. Evaluate electrolyte status.
5. Good skin hygiene around anal area to prevent excoriation due to diarrhea.
6. Antidiarrheal agents.
7. If fistulas form, the client is most often malnourished; may require total parenteral nutrition (TPN).
8. Assess characteristics in patterns of stool.

Self-Care

1. Dietary modifications—teach client to eat small, frequent meals that are high in protein and calories.
2. Medication regimen—precautions regarding steroids or immunosuppressive medications.
3. Symptoms of reoccurrence of the problem; when to call the physician.
   a. Continued diarrhea and weight loss.
   b. Chills, fever, malaise.
4. Dressings and wound care if fistula is present.
5. Identify appropriate measures to decrease stress in lifestyle.

Ulcerative Colitis

❑ **Ulcerative colitis is an inflammation and ulceration of the colon and rectum, it is more common than Crohn's disease.**

A. Area of inflammation is diffuse involving mucosa and submucosa of the intestinal wall; inflammatory process progresses to scar formation.

B. Problem frequently begins in the rectum and spreads in a continuous manner up the colon; seldom is the small intestine involved.

C. Mucosa develops ulcerated areas and can precipitate hemorrhage.

D. Condition has periods of exacerbations and remissions; frequently is associated with psychological factors and stress.

E. May have exacerbations of acute symptoms or, as disease progresses becomes chronic.

Assessment

1. Risk factors/etiology.
   a. May occur at any age; peaks at ages 15-40 years.
   b. Increased incidence in Jewish population.
   c. Familial tendencies.
   d. Increased incidence in females.
   e. Psychophysiological characteristics.
2. Clinical manifestations.
   a. Diarrhea, frequently bloody, may have 20 or more stools per day.
   b. Abdominal pain, rebound tenderness.
   c. Fever.
   d. Rapid depletion of fluid and electrolytes during exacerbation.
   e. Anorexia, weight loss
   f. Anemia.
3. Diagnostics.
   a. Colonoscopy.
   b. Barium enema.
   c. Stool studies.

Complications

1. Obstruction, perforation, abscess, fistulas.
2. Increased incidence for development of colon cancer.

Treatment

1. Moderate to mild disease.
   a. Anti-inflammatory medications (corticosteriods).
   b. Vitamin replacement.
   c. Antidiarrheal medications (Appendix 18-4).
   d. Antimicrobials (sulfasalazine).
   e. Diet decreased in roughage, no milk or milk products, high protein, high calorie.
2. Severe or acute disease.
   a. NPO.
   b. IV fluid replacement.
   c. Anti-inflammatory medications.
3. If condition does not respond to medical management or if complications occur, colon resection and ileostomy (Appendix 18-12) may be done.

Nursing Intervention

Nursing goals and activities are essentially the same as for the client with regional enteritis (Crohn's disease).

Intestinal Obstruction

❑ **Interference with normal peristalsis and impairment to forward flow of intestinal contents is known as *intestinal obstruction*.**

A. Types of obstruction.
   1. Mechanical obstruction.
      a. Strangulated hernia.
      b. Intussusception of the bowel (common in infants and small children).
      c. Volvulus—twisting of the bowel.
      d. Tumors—cancer (most frequent cause of obstruction in the elderly).
      e. Adhesions.
   2. Neurogenic—interference with nerve supply in the intestine.
      a. Paralytic ileus or adynamic ileus occurring from abdominal surgery or inflammatory process.
   3. Vascular obstruction—interference with the blood supply to the bowel.
      a. Infarction of superior mesenteric artery.
      b. Bowel obstructions related to intestinal ischemia may occur very rapidly and be life-threatening.

B. Regardless of the precipitating cause, the ensuing problems are a result of the obstructive process.

C. The higher the obstruction in the intestine, the more rapid symptoms occur.

D. Fluid, gas, and intestinal contents accumulate proximal to the obstruction. This causes distention proximal to the obstruction and bowel collapse distal to the obstruction.

E. As fluid accumulation increases, so does pressure against the bowel. This precipitates extravasation of fluids and electrolytes into the peritoneal cavity. Increased pressure may cause the bowel to rupture.

F. The location of the obstruction determines the extent of fluid and electrolyte imbalance and acid-base imbalance.

1. Dehydration and electrolyte imbalance do not occur rapidly if obstruction is in the large intestine.
2. If obstruction is located high in the intestine, dehydration occurs rapidly due to the inability of the intestine to reabsorb fluids.
3. If persistent vomiting is a problem, the client will develop metabolic alkalosis; if contents of the small intestine are lost via vomiting, metabolic acidosis will occur.

Assessment

1. Risk factors/etiology—identify type of obstruction and precipitating cause.
2. Clinical manifestations.
   a. Vomiting occurs early and is more severe if obstruction is high; may not occur if obstruction is below the ileum.
   b. Abdominal distention.
   c. Bowel sounds initially may be hyperactive proximal to the obstruction and decreased or absent distal to the obstruction; eventually, all bowel sounds will be absent.
   d. Colicky-type abdominal pain.

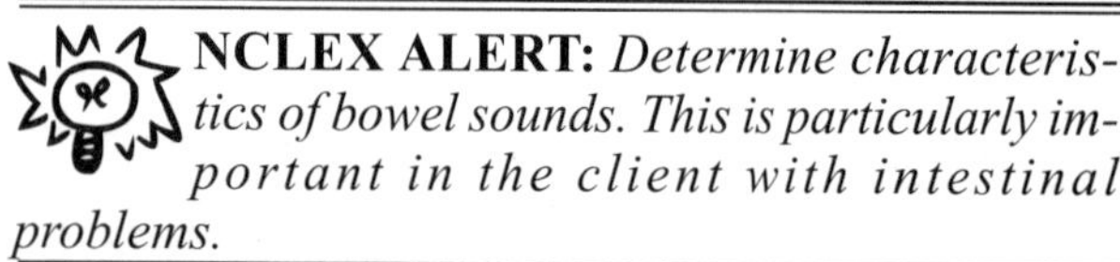

NCLEX ALERT: *Determine characteristics of bowel sounds. This is particularly important in the client with intestinal problems.*

3. Diagnostics.
   a. X-ray of the abdomen.
   b. Evaluation of history of abdominal problems.
   c. Leukocytosis.
   d. Barium enema.
4. Complications—peritonitis.

Treatment

1. Mechanical and vascular intestinal obstructions are generally treated surgically; ileostomy or colostomy may be necessary.
2. Treatment of neurogenic obstruction consists of intestinal intubation and decompression (Appendix 18-9).
3. Maintain fluid and electrolyte balance and adequate nutrition.

Nursing Intervention

✦ *Goal: to prepare client for diagnostic evaluation and to maintain ongoing nursing assessment for pertinent data (Appendix 18-1).*

✦ *Goal: to decrease gastric distention, maintain hydration and electrolyte balance.*

1. Client is kept NPO.
2. Maintain nasogastric suction, or intestinal suction (Appendix 18-8).
3. Maintain IV fluid replacement: most often normal saline or lactated Ringer's solution.
4. Administer potassium supplements with caution due to complications of decreased renal function.
5. Evaluate peristalsis and return of bowel function.
6. Maintain accurate intake and output records.
7. Assess for problems of dehydration and hypovolemia.
8. Measure abdominal girth to determine if distention is increasing.
9. Encourage activities to facilitate return of bowel function.
   a. Encourage physical activity as tolerated.
   b. Attempt to decrease amount of medication required for effective pain control.
   c. Maintain hydration.

✦ *Goal: to provide appropriate preoperative preparation when surgery is indicated (See Chapter 3).*

✦ *Goal: to maintain homeostasis and promote healing postoperative abdominal laparotomy (See Chapter 3).*

✦ *Goal: to maintain fluid and electrolyte balance and prevent gastric distention postoperatively. (See Preoperative Goal above).*

✦ *Goal: to decrease infection and promote healing postoperatively.*

1. Antibiotics are administered via IV infusion. Monitor client's response to antibiotics, as well as status of IV infusion site.
2. Monitor vital signs frequently and evaluate for presence or escalation of infectious process.
3. Provide wound care. Evaluate drainage and healing from abdominal Penrose or Jackson-Pratt drains as well as from abdominal incisional area.

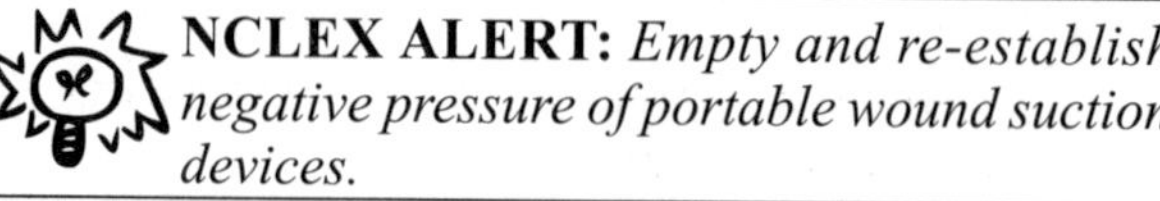

NCLEX ALERT: *Empty and re-establish negative pressure of portable wound suction devices.*

✦ *Goal: to reestablish normal nutrition, and promote comfort postoperative abdominal laparotomy.*

1. Evaluate tolerance of liquids when nasogastric tube is removed.
2. Begin clear liquids initially and continue to evaluate presence of peristalsis.
3. Progress diet as tolerated.
4. Administer analgesics as indicated.
5. Promote psychological comfort.
   a. Respond promptly to requests.
   b. Carefully explain procedures.
   c. Encourage questions and ventilation of feelings regarding status of illness.

Hernias

❑ **A hernia is a protrusion of the intestine through an abnormal opening or weakened area of the abdominal wall.**

A. Types.
   1. Inguinal—a weakness where the spermatic cord in men and the round ligament in women passes through the abdominal wall in the groin area; more common in men.
   2. Femoral—protrusion of the intestine through the femoral ring; more common in women.
   3. Umbilical—occurs most often in children when the umbilical opening fails to close adequately; occurs in adults in an area where the rectus muscle is weak.
   4. Incisional—weakness in the abdominal wall due to a previous incision.
   5. Classification.
      a. Reducible—hernia may be replaced into the abdominal cavity by manual manipulation.
      b. Incarcerated—hernia may not be replaced back into the abdominal cavity.
      c. Strangulated—blood supply and intestinal flow in the herniated area are obstructed; strangulated hernia leads to intestinal obstruction.

Assessment

1. Clinical manifestations.
   a. Hernia protrudes over the involved area when the client stands or strains.
   b. Severe pain occurs if hernia becomes strangulated.
   c. Strangulated hernia occurs with symptoms of intestinal obstruction.
2. Diagnostics.
   a. History.
   b. Clinical manifestations.

Treatment

1. General elective surgery to prevent complications of strangulation (herniorrhaphy).
2. Strangulated hernia involves resection of the involved bowel.

Nursing Intervention

✦ *Goal: to prepare client for surgery if indicated (See Chapter 3).*

✦ *Goal: to maintain homeostasis and promote healing postoperative herniorrhaphy.*

1. General postoperative nursing care (See Chapter 3).
2. Repair of an indirect inguinal hernia: assess male clients for development of scrotal edema.
3. Encourage deep breathing and turning.
4. If coughing occurs, teach client how to splint the incision.
5. Restrain from heavy lifting for approximately 6 to 8 weeks postoperative.

Intussusception

❑ **The telescoping of one portion of the intestine into another, which may result in an intestinal obstruction. The common site is the ileocecal valve.**

Assessment

1. Risk factors/etiology.
   a. Incidence of problem increases in clients with cystic fibrosis or celiac disease.
   b. Most common cause of intestinal obstruction in children from ages 3 months to 5 years.
   c. More common in males.
2. Clinical manifestations.
   a. Child is healthy with sudden occurrence of acute abdominal pain.
   b. Pain may be episodic characterized by periods of absence of pain.
   c. Vomiting occurs initially.
   d. Child may pass one normal stool, then as condition deteriorates, he may pass a stool described as "currant jelly" (a mixture of blood and mucus).
   e. Abdominal tenderness and distention.
   f. A "sausage-shaped" mass may be palpated in the abdomen.
3. Diagnostics - radiographic studies to determine free air in the abdomen prior to a barium enema.

Treatment

1. Initial treatment may consist of a water soluble contrast and air pressure to reduce intussusception.
2. Barium enema may also be used for reduction as well as confirming the problem. BE does have increased risk of peritonitis if there is a perforation.

Nursing Intervention

✦ *Goal: to assist in diagnostic evaluation and maintain ongoing nursing assessment for pertinent data.*

1. Careful assessment of client's physical and behavioral symptoms.
2. Maintain NPO and assess for electrolyte imbalance.
3. Nasogastric suctioning may be necessary.
4. Monitor all stools; passage of normal stool may indicate reduction of the intussusception.
5. A barium enema would be contraindicated if there is air in the abdomen, high fever, vomiting, and/or signs of peritonitis.
6. Prepare child for barium enema as though surgery will follow - NPO, nasogastric tube, IV fluids.

✦ *Goal: to provide preoperative preparation of client or child and parents if surgery is indicated (See Chapter 3).*

✦ *Goal: to maintain homeostasis and promote healing postoperative surgery (See Chapter 3).*

✦ *Goal: (See nursing interventions postoperative intestinal obstruction)*

Pyloric Stenosis

❑ **The obstruction of the pyloric sphincter by hypertrophy and hyperplasia of the circular muscle of the pylorus.**

Assessment

1. Risk factors/etiology.
   a. Occurs most often in first born, full-term infants.
   b. More common in male infants.
   c. Seen more frequently in white infants.
2. Clinical manifestations.
   a. Onset of vomiting may be gradual, occurring in first few weeks, or may develop forceful, projectile vomiting from four to six weeks of age.
   b. Emesis is not bile stained.
   c. Vomiting occurs shortly after feeding.
   d. Infant is hungry and nurses well.
   e. Infant does not appear to be in pain or acute distress.
   f. Weight loss if untreated.
   g. Stools decrease in number and in size.
   h. Dehydration as condition progresses; hypochloremia, and hypokalemia as vomiting continues.
   i. Upper abdomen is distended and an "olive-shaped" mass may be palpated in the right epigastric area.
3. Diagnostics.
   a. Palpation of abdominal mass.
   b. Prolonged vomiting
   c. X-ray studies of the upper GI tract.
   d. Treatment—surgical release of the pyloric muscle (pyloromyotomy).

Nursing Intervention

✦ *Goal: to restore and maintain hydration and electrolyte balance; initiate appropriate preoperative nursing activities.*

1. If infant is being fed PO:
   a. Feed slowly with infant in upright position.
   b. Frequent bubbling during feeding to prevent gastric distention.
   c. After feeding, position infant slightly on the right side in high-Fowler's or in an infant seat.
   d. Minimal handling after feeding.
2. Monitor vital signs and for signs of peritonitis.
3. Assess hydration status and electrolyte balance.
4. If child is dehydrated, may be placed NPO with continuous IV infusion.
5. Accurate intake and output records—complete description of all vomitus and stools.
6. Monitor electrolyte balance closely, especially serum calcium, sodium and potassium levels.
7. Gastric decompression and suction may be utilized preoperatively; maintain patency of tube and record drainage.
8. Preoperative teaching for parents.

✦ *Goal: to maintain adequate hydration and promote healing postoperative pyloromyotomy.*

1. Postoperative vomiting in the first 24 to 48 hours is not uncommon.
2. Assess infant's response to surgery.
3. Continue to monitor infant in the same manner as in the preoperative period.
4. Feedings are initiated early; bottle-fed infant may begin with clear liquids, then diluted formula; gradually increase length of time nursing for breast- fed infant.
5. Continue feedings in the same manner as preoperatively.

6. Monitor infant's response to feedings.
7. Encourage parents to visit and be involved in child's care.

✦ *Goal: to assist parents to provide appropriate home care postoperative pyloromyotomy.*

1. No residual problems are anticipated after surgery.
2. Instruct parents regarding care of the incisional area.

Oral Cancer

A. May occur in any area of the mouth; frequently curable if discovered early.

B. Sites of oral cancer.
1. Lips.
2. Tongue.
3. Salivary gland.
4. Floor of the mouth.

C. Types of oral cancer.
1. Basal cell carcinoma—occurs primarily on the lips; results from excessive exposure to sunlight.
2. Squamous cell carcinoma—occurs on the lower lip and the tongue; associated with alcohol intake and tobacco use.

Assessment

1. Risk factors/etiology.
   a. Smoking.
   b. Continuous oral irritation due to poor dental hygiene.
   c. Chewing tobacco.
2. Clinical manifestations.
   a. Leukoplakia—whitish patch on oral mucosa or tongue (premalignant lesion).
   b. Oral lesions tend to be fixed and hard; may ulcerate.
   c. Pain and dysphagia are late symptoms.
3. Diagnostics—biopsy of suspected lesion.

Treatment

1. Surgery.
   a. Surgical resection.
   b. Reconstructive surgery.
2. Radiation—radioactive seeds may be implanted into the affected area. (See Chapter 8)
3. Chemotherapy.

Nursing Intervention

✦ *Goal: to prevent oral cancer*

1. Avoid chemical, physical or thermal trauma to the mouth.
2. Good oral hygiene, brushing and flossing.
3. Prevent constant irritation in the mouth, repair dentures or other dental problems.
4. See a doctor for any oral lesion that does not heal in 2-3 weeks.

✦ *Goal: to prepare client for surgery.*

1. General preoperative care (See Chapter 3).
2. Discuss with physician the anticipated extent of surgery; reinforce information with client.
3. Emphasis on good oral hygiene.
4. If reconstructive surgery is anticipated, encourage ventilation of feelings regarding anticipated changes in body image.

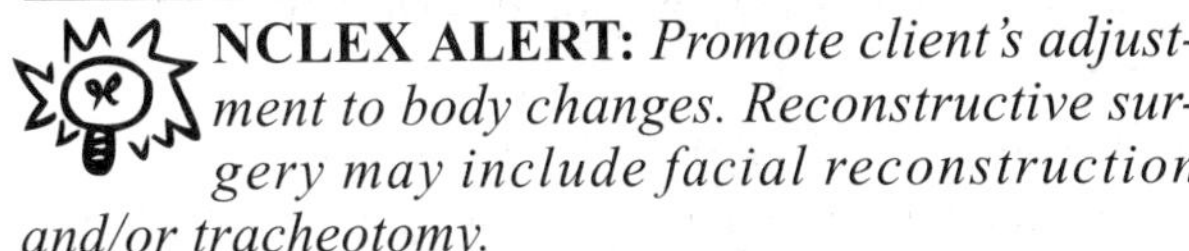

NCLEX ALERT: *Promote client's adjustment to body changes. Reconstructive surgery may include facial reconstruction and/or tracheotomy.*

✦ *Goal: to maintain patent airway postoperatively.*

1. Immediate postoperative position: should be supine with head turned or client positioned on side; when client is awake, elevate head of bed slightly to promote venous and lymphatic drainage.
2. Evaluate swelling around suture areas.
3. Evaluate ability of client to handle oral secretions.
4. Respiratory assessment to identify problems of hypoxia.
5. Occasionally the client may have a tracheostomy (depends on the extent of surgery).
6. Good pulmonary hygiene.

✦ *Goal: to maintain oral hygiene and prevent injury and infection postoperatively.*

1. Type of oral hygiene is indicated by the extent of the procedure.
   a. Mouth irrigations.
   b. Soothing mouth rinses (cool normal saline or non-irritating antiseptic solutions).
   c. If dentures are present, clean mouth well before replacing.
   d. Oral hygiene before and after PO intake.
2. Avoid using stiff toothbrushes and metal-tip suction catheters.

✦ *Goal: to maintain nutrition postoperatively.*

1. Monitor return of bowel sounds before beginning tube feedings or PO intake.
2. May be necessary to maintain nutrition by parenteral hyperalimentation (Appendix 18-7).
3. Oral intake.

a. Liquid, soft, nonirritating foods.

b. No extremes in temperature of food.

c. Small, frequent feedings.

d. Provide privacy and do not rush during meals.

Self- Care

1. Assist client to identify community resources for individual problems in rehabilitation.

   a. Speech therapist.

   b. Dietician.

   c. Counseling.

   d. Home health care agency if appropriate.

2. Assist client to decrease or stop smoking.

3. Assist client to maintain good oral hygiene, dressing care, and take medications.

4. Teach client to identify symptoms of complications and to notify physician.

Cancer of the Stomach

❑ **Cancer may occur in any portion of the stomach. The majority of the lesions are in the pyloric area.**

A. Metastasis generally occurs by direct extension of the malignant growth into adjacent organs and structures (esophagus, spleen, pancreas, etc.).

B. Due to the ability of the stomach to accommodate the growing tumor, symptoms may not be evident until metastasis has occurred.

Assessment

1. Risk factors/etiology.

   a. Increased incidence in men.

   b. Peak incidence at 50 to 70 years of age.

   c. Familial tendencies.

   d. Increased incidence in presence of other chronic gastric problems.

2. Clinical manifestations.

   a. Early symptoms.

      (1) Progressive loss of appetite; indigestion.

      (2) Continuous GI discomfort.

   b. Later symptoms.

      (1) Weight loss.

      (2) Enlarged lymph nodes in supraclavicular chain.

      (3) Traces of occult blood in stools, anemia.

   c. Presence of a palpable mass in the stomach; ascites or bone pain from metastasis may be first symptom.

3. Diagnostics.

   a. Gastroscopy and biopsy.

   b. Upper GI series.

Treatment

No successful treatment other than removal of tumor. The gastric tumor is usually not diagnosed until the advanced stages.

Nursing Intervention

See nursing intervention for gastric resection.

Cancer of the Colon and Rectum

❑ **This type of cancer is the most prevalent internal cancer in the United States.**

A. Most common sites.

   1. Sigmoid colon.

   2. Rectum.

   3. Cecum and ascending colon.

B. 50% of malignant tumors are in the rectum, 20-30% are in the sigmoid and descending colon.

Assessment

1. Risk factors/etiology.

   a. Peak incidence occurs after age 40.

   b. May be associated with ulcerative colitis.

   c. High-fat, low-residue diet.

   d. Family history of colon cancer.

2. Clinical manifestations.

   a. Symptoms are vague early in disease state.

   b. Change in bowel habits - constipation and diarrhea.

   c. Change in shape of stool (pencil- or ribbon-shaped, as in sigmoid or rectal cancer).

   d. Weakness and fatigue.

   e. Pain is a late symptom.

   f. Rectal bleeding.

   g. Bowel obstruction.

3. Diagnostics.

   a. Sigmoid and colonoscopy.

   b. Rectal examination.

   c. Hemoccult stool test.

Treatment

1. Colon resection—may have resection without a colostomy or may have an extensive abdominal-perineal resection which includes formation of a permanent colostomy.

2. Radiation therapy.

3. Chemotherapy.

Nursing Intervention

✦ *Goal: to provide information to high risk clients.*

1. High fiber, low fat diet.
2. Digital rectal exams yearly after age 40.
3. Guaiac and colonoscopy after age 50.
4. Aspirin (81mg) daily to decrease risk.

✦ *Goal: to provide preoperative care.*

1. Determine extent of surgery anticipated - does not always have a colostomy.
2. Bowel preparation— low-residue diet, cathartics 24 hours prior to surgery, begin prophylactic antibiotics.
3. Enemas to cleanse bowel evening prior to surgery.
4. If colostomy is to be done, discuss implications and identify appropriate area on abdomen for stoma. (Appendix 18-12).
5. Prepare client for change in body image.

✦ *Goal: to provide appropriate wound care postoperative abdominal-perineal resection.*

1. Client will have three incisional areas:
   a. Abdominal incision.
   b. Incisional area for colostomy.
   c. Perineal incision.

NCLEX ALERT: *Identifying factors interfering with wound healing, and identifying infection are areas that could be easily tested on the care of this client.*

2. Perineal wound may be closed with a Penrose drain inserted, or may be left open to heal by secondary intention.
   a. Irrigate the perineal wound.
   b. Warm sitz bath to promote debridement and increase circulation to the area.
3. Rectal incision frequently packed after surgery, irrigations and dressing changes will begin after packing is removed.
4. Abdominal wound and perineal wound need frequent dressing changes due to profuse drainage postoperatively.
5. Healing of the perineal wound may take several months.
6. Position client on his side.
7. Assess status of stoma and healing (Appendix 18-12).

✦ *Goal: to maintain homeostasis and promote healing postoperative abdominal perineal resection, or colon resection. (See Chapter 3).*

1. Infections, hemorrhage, wound disruption, thrombophlebitis, and stomal problems are the most common complications.
2. Assist client to begin to become independent with colostomy care early in recovery period (See appendix 18-12).

Self-Care

1. Recovery period is long; assist client and family to identify community resources.
2. Assist client and family to identify resources and obtain equipment for colostomy care (Appendix 18-12).
3. Return for frequent medical checkups.
4. Identify community resources for client - home health visits, social services, etc.

Celiac Disease

❑ **Also known as sprue, gluten-induced enteropathy, and malabsorption syndrome. This disease is an inborn error in metabolism of rye, wheat, barley and oat products.**

A. Symptomatology generally begins within 1 year to 5 years of age.
B. Severe malnutrition results from a loss of nutrients via the stool.

Assessment

1. Etiology—congenital defect in metabolism.
2. Clinical manifestations.
   a. Symptomatology begins when child has increased intake of gluten type foods -cereals, breads, pastas, etc.
   b. Watery, pale diarrhea.
   c. Vomiting, anorexia.
   d. Poor weight gain, failure to thrive.
   e. Constipation, vomiting, and abdominal pain may be the initial presenting signs/systems.
   f. Abdominal distention.
3. Diagnostics.
   a. Stool analysis.
   b. Jejunal biopsy.

Treatment

Primarily dietary management; gluten-free diet (See Chapter 3).

Nursing Intervention

✦ *Goal: to assist parents to understand diet therapy and promote optimal nutrition intake.*

1. Written information regarding a gluten-free diet; corn and rice may be substituted for grains in diet.

2. Diet should be high-calorie, high-protein, low-fat.
3. Teach parents how to read food labels for grain content.
4. Important to discuss with parents and older children necessity of maintaining a lifelong gluten-restricted diet; problems may occur in teenagers who relax their diet and experience an exacerbation of the disease state.
5. Lack of adherence to dietary restrictions may precipitate growth retardation, anemia, and bone deformities.

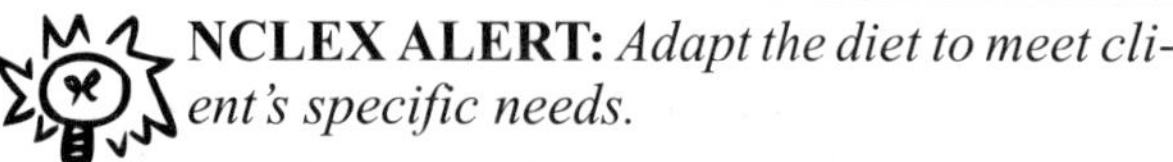
NCLEX ALERT: *Adapt the diet to meet client's specific needs.*

Hirschsprung's Disease

❑ **Hirschsprung's disease (congenital aganglionic megacolon) is characterized by a congenital absence of innervation in a segment of the colon wall.**

A. May precipitate a neurogenic bowel obstruction, cause of 25% of neonatal intestinal obstructions.

B. Most common site is the rectosigmoid colon; colon proximal to the area dilates (i.e., megacolon).

Assessment

1. Risk factors/etiology—congenital, may be associated with Down syndrome.
2. Clinical manifestations.
   a. Varies according to age and amount of colon involved.
   b. Inadequate or absent peristalsis.
   c. Newborn.
      (1) Failure to pass meconium with in 24-48 hours after birth.
      (2) Vomiting.
      (3) Abdominal distention.
      (4) Reluctance to take fluids.
   d. Older infant.
      (1) Failure to thrive.
      (2) Abdominal distention.
      (3) Persistent constipation, impactions.
3. Diagnostics.
   a. Rectal biopsy.
   b. Barium enema.

Treatment

Surgical correction usually involves creation of a temporary colostomy, then a pull-through of the colon to a point near the rectum. After the reanastomosis has healed, the temporary colostomy is closed.

Nursing Intervention

✦ *Goal: to promote normal attachment and prepare infant and parents for surgery:*

1. Allow parents to ventilate feelings regarding congenital defect of infant.
2. Foster infant-parent attachment.
3. General preoperative preparation of the infant; neonate does not require any bowel preparation.
4. Careful explanation of colostomy to parents.

✦ *Goal: see nursing intervention postoperative abdominal surgery for intestinal obstruction.*

✦ *Goal: to assist parents to understand and provide appropriate home care for the child postoperative colostomy.*

1. Colostomy is most often temporary.
2. Parents should be actively involved in colostomy care prior to discharge.

Hemorrhoids

❑ **Dilated varicose veins of the anus and rectum are called *hemorrhoids.***

Assessment

1. Risk factors/etiology.- caused by conditions which increase anorectal pressure.
   a. Pregnancy.
   b. Prolonged constipation.
   c. Prolonged standing or sitting.
   d. Portal hypertension.
2. Clinical manifestations.
   a. Internal hemorrhoids occur above the intestinal sphincter; become constricted, and are painful.
   b. External hemorrhoids occur below or outside external sphincter; appear as protrusions at the anus.
   c. Thrombosed hemorrhoid—a blood clot in a hemorrhoid that causes inflammation and pain.
   d. Rectal bleeding during defecation.
3. Diagnostics—rectal examination.

Treatment

1. Ointments to shrink mucous membranes.
2. Stool softeners.
3. Sitz bath.
4. Excision of the hemorrhoid - cryosurgery, laser removal, internal ligation.

Nursing Intervention

✦ *Goal: to provide appropriate information to assist client to manage problem at home.*

1. Avoid prolonged standing or sitting.
2. Sitz bath to decrease discomfort.
3. Over-the-counter ointments to decrease discomfort.
4. Ice pack, followed by a hot sitz bath, if severe discomfort occurs.
5. Avoid constipation and straining at stool.

Self-Care

1. Encourage bulk laxatives to promote soft stool for first bowel movement.
2. Rectal pain may be severe; analgesics, local moist heat, as appropriate.
3. Review preventive techniques; weight loss and decrease problems with constipation.⌘

Study Questions—Gastrointestinal System

1. On the third day postoperative gastric resection, the client's nasogastric tube is draining bile-colored liquid containing coffee ground material. What is the best nursing action?

① Continue to monitor the amount of drainage and correlate it with any change in vital signs.

② Reposition the nasogastric tube and irrigate the tube with normal saline.

③ Call the physician and discuss the possibility that the client is bleeding.

④ Irrigate the nasogastric tube with iced saline and attach the tube to gravity drainage.

2. The nurse is providing preoperative care for a client who will have a gastric resection. What will the preoperative teaching include?

① A nasogastric tube will be in place several days after surgery.

② The client will be started on a low residue, bland diet about 2 days after the surgery.

③ Explain the anticipated prognosis and implications that he may have a malignancy.

④ A Foley catheter will be in place for one week after surgery.

3. The nurse is planning care for the client scheduled for gastroduodenoscopy and a barium swallow. What will the nursing care plan include?

① Anticipating the client will receive a low residue diet in the evening and then be NPO 6 to 12 hours prior to the test.

② Discussing with the client the nasogastric tube and the importance of gastric drainage for 24 hours posttest.

③ Explaining to the client that he will be NPO for 24 hours after the test to make sure his stomach can tolerate food.

④ Discussing the general anesthesia and explain that he will wake up in the recovery room.

4. In preparing a pediatric client for an appendectomy, the nurse would question which doctor's orders?

① Penicillin 600,000u IVPB, now.

② Obtain signed consent form from parents.

③ Administer enemas until clear.

④ 500cc Ringer's Lactate at 50cc per hour.

5. What are the best nursing actions to promote comfort prior to surgery in a client with appendicitis?

① Ambulate to increase the passage of flatus to decrease distention prior to surgery.

② Position on side, legs flexed to the abdomen with the head slightly elevated.

③ Position on left side, apply a warm K-Pad to the abdomen.

④ Administer **Demerol** and allow to assume the position of comfort.

6. A client returns to his room from surgery after having a colon resection. He complains of feeling cold, what is the best nursing action?

① Apply a heating pad to the client's back for warmth.

② Recognize that this is a symptom of shock and notify the physician.

③ Realize that the client is bleeding internally and call the physician.

④ Apply several blankets to maintain the body temperature at a normal level.

7. In planning discharge teaching for the postop gastrectomy client, the nurse includes what information regarding dumping syndrome?

① The syndrome will be a permanent problem and the client should eat 5 to 6 small meals per day.

② The client should decrease the amount of fluid consumed with the meal and for one hour after the meal.

③ The client should increase the amount of complex carbohydrates and fiber in his diet.

④ Activity will decrease the problem, it should be scheduled about one hour after meals.

8. The nurse is assessing a child with a tentative diagnosis of appendicitis. The nursing assessment is most likely to reveal what characteristics concerning the pain?

① Rebound tenderness in the right lower quadrant, associated with decreased bowel sounds and vomiting.

② Gnawing pain, radiating through to the lower back, with severe abdominal distention.

③ Sharp pain with severe gastric distention, frequently associated with hemoptysis.

④ Pain on light palpation in mid-epigastric area, chronic low grade fever and diarrhea.

9. What is the priority nursing action for the post-operative client complaining of nausea in the recovery room after gastric resection?

① Evaluate the nasogastric tube for patency.

② Call the physician for an antiemetic order.

③ Place client in semi-Fowler's position so he will not aspirate.

④ Medicate the client with a narcotic analgesic.

10. The nurse knows that a conclusive diagnosis of pyloric stenosis will be made by what test?

① A flat plate of the abdomen.

② A colonoscopy.

③ An altered electrolyte balance.

④ An upper gastrointestinal series.

11. A client is admitted with duodenal ulcers. What will the nurse anticipate the history to include?

① Recent weight loss.

② Increasing indigestion after meals. Awakening with pain at night.

③ Awakening with pain at night.

④ Episodes of vomiting.

12. A client returns to the floor after surgical creation of a continent ileostomy (Kock's). What will the care of this ileostomy include?

① Placing a catheter in the stoma for drainage.

② Irrigating it with normal saline after 24 hours.

③ Attaching an ostomy bag with careful checking for watertight seal.

④ Assessing for skin excoriation and increased drainage due to location of stoma.

13. The nurse is conducting discharge dietary teaching for a client with diverticulosis and is recovering from an acute episode of diverticulitis. The nurse would determine that the client understood his dietary teaching by which client statement?

① "I will need to increase my intake of protein and complex carbohydrates to increase healing."

② "Peanuts, fruits, and vegetables with seeds can cause problems and I should avoid them."

③ "I will not put any added salt on my food and I will decrease foods that are a saturated fat.

④ "Milk and milk products can cause a lactose intolerance, if this occurs I need to decrease my intake of these products."

14. The nurse is caring for a client who has a bleeding duodenal ulcer. The nurse identifies what assessment data as indicative of a gastric perforation?

① Increasing abdominal distention and tight abdomen.

② Decreasing hemoglobin and hematocrit with bloody stools.

③ Diarrhea with increased bowel sounds and hypovolemia.

④ Decreasing blood pressure with tachycardia and disorientation.

Answers and rationales to these questions are in the section at the end of the book entitled "Chapter Study Questions: Answers & Rationales."

Appendix 18-1: GASTROINTESTINAL SYSTEM DIAGNOSTICS

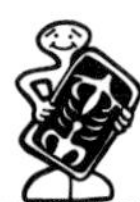

X-RAY

UPPER GASTROINTESTINAL SERIES OR BARIUM SWALLOW:
X-ray examination utilizing barium as a contrast material; used to diagnose structural abnormalities and problems of the esophagus and stomach.

Nursing implications:
1. Explain procedure to client.
2. Maintain client NPO 8 to 12 hours prior to procedure.
3. After examination promote normal excretion of barium to prevent impaction.
4. Stool should return to normal color within 72 hours.

LOWER GASTROINTESTINAL SERIES OR BARIUM ENEMA:
X-ray examination of the colon using barium as a contrast medium; barium is administered rectally.

Nursing implications:
1. Maintain client NPO for 8 hours prior to test or give clear liquids the morning of the examination.
2. Colon must be free of stool; laxatives and enemas are administered the evening prior to test; enemas may also be given the morning of the procedure.
3. Explain to client that he/she may experience cramping and feel urge to defecate during the procedure.
4. After the procedure, increase fluids and administer a laxative to assist in expelling the barium.

ENDOSCOPY

ESOPHAGOSCOPY, GASTROSCOPY:
The direct visualization of the esophagus, stomach, and duodenum via a flexible, fiberoptic, lighted scope; inflammation, ulcerations, tumors, and esophageal varices may be observed.

Nursing implications prior to procedure:
1. Maintain client NPO for 6 to 8 hours prior to procedure.
2. May give preoperative medication for relaxation and to decrease secretions.
3. Explain to client that local anesthesia will be utilized to anesthetize the throat prior to insertion of the scope.
4. Assess client's mouth for dentures and removable bridges.

Nursing implications after the procedure:
1. Maintain client NPO until the gag reflex returns.
2. Use throat lozenges or warm saline gargles for relief of sore throat.
3. Position client on his side to prevent aspiration until gag/cough reflex returns.
4. Observe for signs of perforation - bleeding, fever, dysphagia, substernal or epigastric pain.

PROCTOSIGMOIDOSCOPY:
Direct visualization of the distal sigmoid colon and rectum.
Nursing implications prior to procedure:
1. Colon and rectal area must be free of stool prior to the examination; clear liquid diet prior to test, enemas the evening before and possibly the morning of the procedure.
2. Explain to client the knee-chest position and the need to take a deep breath during the insertion of the scope; client will feel urge to defecate as scope is passed.
3. Sedatives are administered prior to test.

Nursing implications post procedure:
1. Observe for rectal bleeding and signs of perforation following the test.
2. Assist client to upright position - observe for orthostatic hypotension.
3. Warm sitz bath will assist to relieve any anal discomfort.

COLONOSCOPY:
Examination of the colon using a flexible, fiberoptic scope.
Nursing implications:
1. Bowel preparation.
2. Client preparation regarding conscious sedation (See Chapter 3).
3. Assessment of abdomen for pain and bleeding post procedure.

Appendix 18-1: GASTROINTESTINAL SYSTEM DIAGNOSTICS

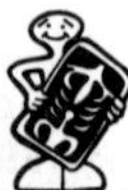

ANALYSIS OF SPECIMENS

PARACENTESIS - Peritoneal Tap and Lavage
Procedure - a catheter or trocar is inserted into the peritoneal cavity, most often just below the umbilicus.

Purpose:
1. To determine effect of blunt abdominal trauma.
2. Investigate presence of ascites.
3. Identify cause of acute abdominal problems, i.e. perforation.

- To determine intra-abdominal bleeding after a blunt trauma to the abdomen, the solution (normal saline) is rapidly infused into the peritoneal cavity. The fluid is aspirated or allowed to drain by gravity. Normal fluid should return clear with a slight yellow cast. If a positive tap is obtained, the client may have abdominal injuries that require surgery.
- If client has abdominal fluid from ascites or other abdominal pathology, a specimen of the fluid is obtained without instilling fluid.

Nursing Implications:
1. Nasogastric tube may be used to maintain gastric decompression during procedure.
2. Have the client void prior to procedure.
3. Maintain sterile field for puncture, drainage procedure.

Complications:
1. Perforation of bowel -peritonitis.
2. Introduction of air into abdominal cavity; client may complain of right referred shoulder pain from air under the diaphragm.
3. If client had a full bladder at the time of insertion of the trocar, there could be bladder perforation and peritonitis.

STOOL EXAMINATION:
Stool is examined for form, consistency, and to see if it contains mucus, blood, pus, parasites, or fat. Stool will be examined for presence of occult blood.

Nursing implications:
1. Collect stool in sterile container if examining for pathological organisms.
2. Client may be on a specific type of diet prior to test being done.
3. A fresh, warm stool is required for evaluation of pathogenic organisms.
4. Collect the stool sample from various areas of the stool.
5. Guaiac testing for occult blood is positive when the paper turns blue.

Appendix 18-2:
ANTIEMETICS

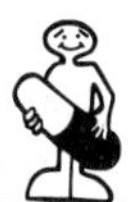

MEDICATIONS	SIDE EFFECTS	NURSING IMPLICATIONS
PHENOTHIAZINE DERIVATIVES: Depresses the chemoreceptor trigger zone and vomiting center.		
Chlorpromazine hydrochloride (**Thorazine**): PO, suppository, IM Promethazine (**Phenergan**): PO, IM, suppository Prochlorperazine (**Compazine**): PO, suppository, IM Thiethylperazine maleate (**Torecan**): PO, suppository, IM	Central nervous system depression, drowsiness, photosensitivity.	1. Sub-q injection may cause tissue irritation and necrosis. 2. Use with caution in pediatrics; do not administer **Thorazine** to infants under six months, **Compazine** to children under 20 pounds or under two years old, or **Torecan** to children under 12. 3. **Thorazine** should be used only in situations of severe nausea or vomiting.
ANTIHISTAMINES: Depresses the chemoreceptor trigger zone.		
Hydroxyzine (**Atarax, Vistaril**): PO, IM Dimenhydrinate (**Dramamine, Marmine**): PO, suppository, IM	Sedation; anticholinergic effects -blurred vision, dry mouth, difficulty in urination and constipation; paradoxical excitation may occur in children.	1. Caution client regarding sedation - should avoid activities that require mental alertness. 2. Administer early in order to prevent vomiting. 3. Use with caution in clients with glaucoma and asthma. 4. Sub-q injection may cause tissue irritation and necrosis.
GI STIMULANT: Stimulates motility of upper GI tract		
Metoclopramide (**Reglan**): PO, IM, IV	Restlessness, drowsiness, fatigue	1. Used to decrease problems with esophageal reflux. 2. Use with caution when increase in GI motility may be dangerous (intestinal perforation, obstruction).

Appendix 18-3:
LAXATIVES

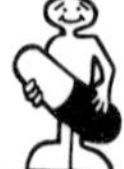

MEDICATIONS	SIDE EFFECTS	NURSING IMPLICATIONS
❖ GENERAL NURSING IMPLICATIONS ❖ — Laxatives should be avoided in clients who have nausea, vomiting and/or undiagnosed abdominal pain and cramping, or any indications of appendicitis. — Dietary fiber should be taken for prevention of and in first line of treatment for constipation. — Daily intake of fluids should be increased. — Constipation is determined by stool firmness and frequency. — Increasing activity will increase peristalsis and decrease constipation. — Narcotic analgesics and anticholinergics will cause constipation. — A laxative should be used only briefly and in the smallest amount necessary. — Use with caution during pregnancy.		
BULK LAXATIVES: Stimulate peristalsis and passage of soft stool.		
Methylcellulose (**Citrocel**) Psyllium (**Metamucil, Perdiem**) Fibercon Bran	Esophageal irritation, impaction, abdominal fullness, flatulence.	1. Not immediately effective; 12 to 24 hours before effects are apparent. 2. Use with caution in clients with difficulty swallowing. 3. Administer with full glass of fluid to prevent problems with irritation and impaction. 4. Fibercon is a tablet form, others are powder form to be mixed with fluids.
STOOL SOFTENERS OR SURFACTANTS: Decrease surface tension allowing water to penetrate feces		
Ducusate Potassium (**Colace**) *Combination with stimulant:* Docusate Calcium (**Surfak**) Ducusate sodium (**Dialose Plus**)	Occasional mild abdominal cramping.	1. Do not use concurrently with mineral oil. 2. Not recommended for children under 6 years old.
STIMULANT OR CONTACT LAXATIVES: Stimulate and irritates the large intestine to promote peristalsis and defecation.		
Bisacodyl (**Dulcolax**): suppository, PO Phenolphthalein (**Modane, Ex-Lax**): PO Senna concentrate (**Senokot**): PO, suppository	Diarrhea, abdominal cramping.	
BOWEL EVACUANT: Non-absorbable osmotic agents that pulls fluid into the bowel.		
Polyethylene glycol (**GoLytely, Colyte**) Magnesium Citrate		1. Primary use is in preparing the bowel for examination. 2. Client should fast 4-5 hours prior to administration. 3. Food (except clear liquids) is contraindicated within 2 hours of medication. 4. GoLYTELY involves large amount of fluid for client to drink (4L); provide 8-10 ounces chilled at a time to increase client consumption and taste. 5. Best if consumed over 3-4 hours. 6. Evacuates cause frequently bowel movements, advise client to plan accordingly.

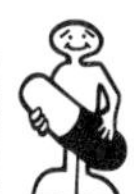

Appendix 18-4:
ANTIDIARRHEAL AGENTS

MEDICATIONS	SIDE EFFECTS	NURSING IMPLICATIONS
OPIOIDS: Suppress peristalsis, facilitating water and electrolyte reabsorption.		
Paregoric: PO Diphenoxylate HCL + Atropine (**Lomotil**): PO	Nausea, vomiting, paralytic ilius, abdominal cramping.	1. Interacts with MAO inhibitors. 2. Not recommended during pregnancy 3. Encourage increased fluids. 4. Avoid activities that require mental alertness.
ABSORBENTS AND EMULSIONS: Soothing effects and absorb toxic substances.		
Attapulgite (**Donnagel**) PO: Loperamide HCL (**Immodium**): PO	May precipitate an impaction	1. May interfere with absorption of PO medications. 2. Should not be given to clients with fever > 101°. 3. Do not give in presence of bloody diarrhea

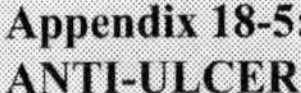

Appendix 18-5:
ANTI-ULCER

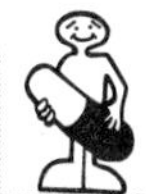

MEDICATIONS	SIDE EFFECTS	NURSING IMPLICATIONS
ANTACID: An alkaline substance that will neutralize gastric acid secretions; non-systemic.		
Aluminum Hydroxide (**Amphojel**)	Constipation. Phosphorus depletion with chronic utilization.	1. Avoid administration within 1 to 2 hours of other oral medications. Medications should be taken frequently, before and after meals and at bedtime. 2. Instruct clients to take medication even if they do not experience discomfort. 3. Clients on low-sodium diets should evaluate sodium content of various antacids. 4. Administer with caution to the cardiac client, as GI symptoms may be indicative of cardiac problems.
Aluminum hydroxide and magnesium salt combinations (**Gelusil, Maalox, Gaviscon**)	Constipation or diarrhea. Hypercalcemia. Renal calculi.	
Sodium preparation: Sodium bicarbonate, (**Rolaids, TUMS**): PO	Rebound acid production. Alkalosis.	1. Discourage use of sodium bicarbonate, due to occurrence of metabolic alkalosis.
HISTAMINE H_2 RECEPTOR ANTAGONISTS: Reduces volume and concentration of gastric acid secretion.		
Cimetidine (**Tagamet**): PO, IV, IM	Rash, confusion, lethargy, diarrhea, dysrhythmias	1. Take with or after meals. 2. May be used prophylactically or for treatment of PUD. 3. Do not take with PO antacids.
Ranitidine (**Zantac**): PO, IM, IV	Headache, GI discomfort, jaundice, hepatitis	1. Use with caution in clients with liver and renal disorders. 2. Do not take with aspirin products. 3. Wait 1 hour after administration of antacids.
Niaztidine (**Axid**): PO	Anemia, dizziness	
Famotidine (**Pepsid**) PO, IV	Headache, dizziness, constipation, diarrhea	1. Used with caution in clients with renal or hepatic problems. 2. Dosing may be done with meals or without regard to meal time. 3. Caution clients to avoid aspirin and other NSAIDs.

Appendix 18-5: ANTI-ULCER

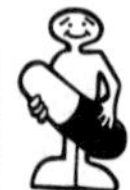

MEDICATIONS	SIDE EFFECTS	NURSING IMPLICATIONS
PROTON PUMP INHIBITORS: Inhibit the enzyme that produces gastric acid.		
Omeprazole (**Prilosec**): PO Lansoprazole (**Prevacid**): PO	Headache, diarrhea, dizziness	1. Administer before meals. 2. Do not crush, chew or open capsules 3. Sprinkle granules of **Prevacid** over food; do not chew granules.
CYTOPROCTECTANT: Binds to diseased tissue provides a protective barrier to acid.		
Sucralfate (**Carafate**): PO	Constipation, GI discomfort.	1. Avoid antacids. 2. Use: prevention and treatment of duodenal ulcers. 3. May impede the absorption of medications that require an acid medium.
PROSTAGLANDIN ANALOGUE: Suppresses gastric acid secretion, increases protective mucus and mucosal blood flow.		
Misoprostol (**Cytotec**)	GI problems, headache.	1. Contraindicated in pregnancy. 2. Indicated for prevention of NSAID-induced ulcers.
ANTICHOLINERGICS (antispasmodics): Inhibit secretion of gastric acids.		
Dicyclomine hydrochloride (**Bentyl**): PO Hyoscyamine (**Levsin**): PO Propantheline (**Pro-Banthine**): PO, IM	Drowsiness, dry mouth, urinary retention, blurred vision, constipation, orthostatic hypotension	1. Use with caution in clients with glaucoma. 2. Evaluate for anticholinergic side effects. 3. Do not administer at same time as antacids.

Appendix 18-6: INTESTINAL ANTIBIOTICS

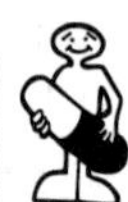

MEDICATIONS	ACTION	SIDE EFFECTS	NURSING IMPLICATIONS
Kanamycin sulfate (**Kantrex**): PO Neomycin sulfate (**Mycifradin Sulfate**): PO	Decrease bacteria in the GI tract; utilized to sterilize bowel prior to surgery.	(See Chapter 6)	(See Nursing Implications, Aminoglycosides in Chapter 6).
Paromomycin (**Humatin**): PO	Used to treat diarrhea caused by *E. Coli*, amebicidal.	Vomiting and diarrhea	1. Administer with meals. 2. Administer with caution in clients with ulcerative bowel disease.

Appendix 18-7: HYPERALIMENTATION

DEFINITION

A method for providing nutrients that support body growth as well as maintain body systems; indications for hyperalimentation are:

1. Inadequate protein intake to support tissue healing.
2. Conditions that interfere with the process of nutrition: ingestion, digestion, absorption.

✦ *Goal: to maintain client in positive nitrogen balance and promote healing.*

Routes of Administration

1. **Peripheral** - partial parenteral nutrition (PPN) (fat emulsions, dextrose solutions below 20%) is administered via a large peripheral vein when nutritional support is indicated for short period of time.
2. **Central** - total parenteral nutrition (TPN): a parenteral line (PICC, Hickman, Broviac, central line) is inserted via the jugular or subclavian vein and threaded into the vena cava; utilized for nutritional support in the client who requires in excess of 2500 calories per day for an extended period of time. Solutions utilized are hypertonic and require rapid dilution.

Nursing Implications:

1. Solution should be mixed by a pharmacist under a laminar flow hood and sterile environment.
2. Orders are written daily, based on the current electrolyte and protein status; always check the doctor's order for correct fluid for the day.
3. Solution may be refrigerated for up to 24 hours, but solution should be at room temperature before administering.
4. Maintain constant flow rate; if solution is behind, than determine how much and divide that amount over about 24 hours and gradually increase rate to level of previous infusion order. Do not randomly speed up the infusion to "catch up" ; an infusion pump is required.
5. Monitor serum blood glucose on a regular basis; some institutions require glucose testing every 4-6 hours.
6. Infusion is initiated and discontinued on a gradual basis to allow the pancreas to compensate for increased glucose intake.
7. Use IV tubing with filters.
8. Assess client for weight gain and tissue healing.
9. Clients allergic to eggs should not receive any lipid solutions.

Maintenance

1. Solution and administration equipment is changed every 24 hours.
2. Sterile occlusive dressing should be utilized at the catheter site. It should be changed at least every 48 hours, utilizing sterile technique.
3. Do not mix any medications or blood components with the hyperalimentation solution.
4. Do not draw blood or measure CVP from hyperalimentation line.
5. Maintain record of daily weight, blood glucose, and intake and output.
6. Check client's IV site for signs of infection.

Complications:

1. Infections, septicemia.
2. Fluid volume overload.
3. Electrolyte imbalances.
4. Serum glucose fluctuations - both hyper-and hypoglycemia.
5. Air embolus from central line (see Appendix 16-7 for care of central line).

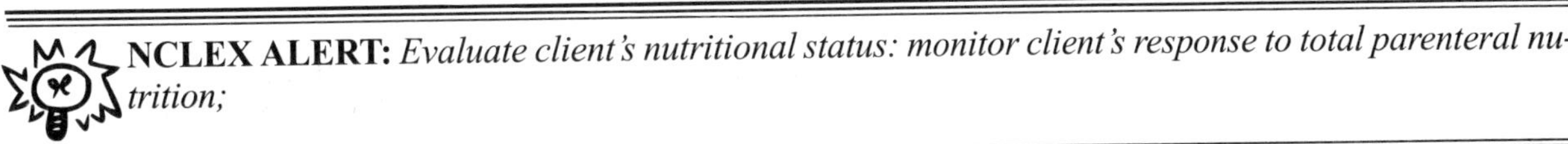

NCLEX ALERT: *Evaluate client's nutritional status: monitor client's response to total parenteral nutrition;*

COMPLICATIONS

1. Hyperglycemia - usually caused by too rapid an infusion of solution.
2. Hyperosmolar coma - caused by failure to recognize original hyperglycemia; treatment consists of insulin and IV fluid to correct water deficit.
3. Septicemia - strong glucose solutions provide good medium for bacteria; strict aseptic techniques in dressing changes and fluid preparation.
4. Air embolus (central line) - increased tendency to occur during insertion of central catheter line and during dressing changes; place in Trendelenburg position during insertion and during dressing changes.

Appendix 18-8:
NURSING PROCEDURE ■ NASOGASTRIC AND INTESTINAL TUBES ■

NASOGASTRIC TUBES:

1. **Levin Tube** - single lumen.
   a. Suctioning gastric contents.
   b. Administering tube feedings.
2. **Salem Sump Tube** - double lumen (smaller blue lumen vents the tube and prevents suction on the gastric mucosa, maintains intermittent suction regardless of suction source.).
   a. Suctioning gastric contents.
   b. Maintaining gastric decompression.

✓ **Key Points:**

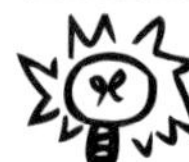

NCLEX ALERT: *Insert feeding/nasogastric tubes, and determine if characteristics of nasogastric drainage are with normal limits.*

- Prior to insertion, position the client in high-Fowler's position if possible.
- Use a water-soluble lubricant to facilitate insertion.
- Measure the tube from the tip of the client's nose to the earlobe and from the nose to the xiphoid process to determine the approximate amount of tube to insert to reach the stomach.
- Flex the client's head slightly forward; this will decrease the chance of entry into the trachea.
- Insert the tube through the nose into the nasopharyngeal area; ask the client to swallow, and as the swallow occurs, progress the tube past the area of the trachea and into the esophagus and stomach. Withdraw tube immediately if client experiences respiratory distress.
- Secure the tube to the nose; do not allow the tube to exert pressure on the upper inner portion of the nares.
- Validating placement of tube.
  a. Aspirate gastric contents via a syringe attached to the end of the tube.
  b. Measure pH of aspirated fluid. (pH of gastric secretions is 0-4.0)
  c. Place the stethoscope over the gastric area and inject a small amount of air through the nasogastric tube. A characteristic sound of air entering the stomach from the tube should be heard.
- Characteristics of nasogastric drainage
  a. Normally is greenish -yellow, with strands of mucus.
  b. Coffee-ground drainage – old blood that has been broken down in the stomach.
  c. Bright red blood – bleeding from the esophagus, the stomach or swallowed from the lungs.
  d. Foul-smelling (fecal odor) -occurs with reverse peristalsis in bowel obstruction; increase in amount of drainage with obstruction.

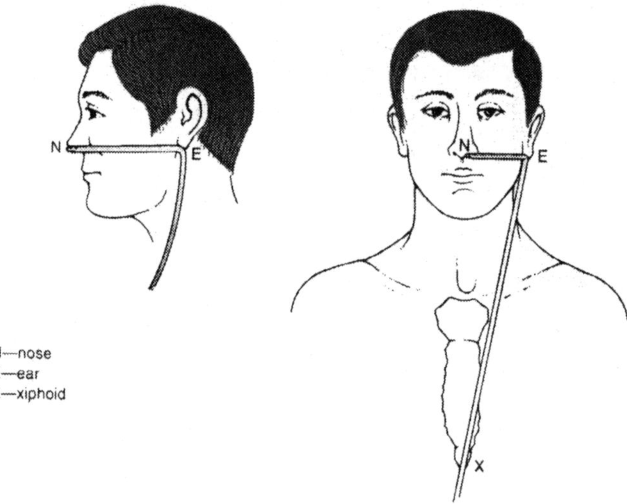

Figure 18-2: Gastrointestinal Intubation
Reprinted with permission: Smeltzer, SC, Bare, BG, *Brunner and Suddarth's Textbook of Medical Surgical Nursing,* 9th ed. Lippencott: Philadelphia, p 835

Appendix 18-8:
NURSING PROCEDURE ■ NASOGASTRIC AND INTESTINAL TUBES ■

Clinical Tips for Problem Solving

- **Abdominal distention** - check for patency and adequacy of drainage, determine position of tube, assess presence of bowel sounds, position in semi-Fowler's and observe for respiratory compromise from distention.
- **Nausea and vomiting around tube** - validate position of tube with air, then irrigate with small amount of normal saline; tube may not be far enough into stomach, try repositioning. If tube patency cannot be established, tube may need to be replaced.
- **Inadequate or minimal drainage** - validate placement and patency; tube may be in too far and is past pyloric valve, or not in far enough and is in the upper portion of the stomach. Reassess length of tube insertion and characteristics of drainage.

NCLEX ALERT: *ALWAYS check the placement of a gastric tube prior to injecting or irrigating it; placement should be checked each shift, do not adjust or irrigate the naso gastric tube on a client after a gastric resection.*

INTESTINAL TUBES:

1. Provide intestinal decompression proximal to a bowel obstruction. Prevent/decrease intestinal distention.
2. Placement Of a tube containing a mercury weight and allowing normal peristalsis to propel tube through the stomach into the intestine to the point of obstruction where decompression will occur.

TYPES:

1. **Cantor and Harris Tubes.**
   a. Approximately 6 to 10 feet long.
   b. Simple lumen.
   c. Mercury placed in rubber bag prior to tube insertion.
2. **Miller-Abbot Tube.**
   a. Approximately 10 feet long.
   b. Double lumen.
   c. One lumen utilized for aspiration of intestinal contents.
   d. Second lumen utilized to instill mercury into the rubber bag after the tube has been inserted into the stomach.

Nursing Implications:

1. Maintain client on strict NPO.
2. Initial insertion usually done by physician and progression of the tube may be monitored via an X-ray.
3. After the tube has been placed in the stomach, position the client on the right side to facilitate passage through the pyloric valve.
4. Advance the tube 2 to 4 inches at regular intervals as indicated by the physician.
5. Encourage activity, to facilitate movement of the tube through the intestine.
6. Evaluate the type of gastric secretions being aspirated.
7. Do not tape or secure the tube until it has reached the desired position.
8. Tubes may be attached to suction and left in place for several days.
9. Offer the client frequent oral hygiene, if possible offer hard candy or gum to reduce thirst.
10. Removal of the tube depends on the relief of the intestinal obstruction.
    a. May be removed by gradual pulling back (4-6 inches per hour) and eventual removal via the nose or mouth.
    b. May be allowed to progress through the intestines and expelled via the rectum.

Appendix 18-9: NURSING PROCEDURE ■ TUBE FEEDING ■

SHORT TERM TYPES

1. **Nasogastric**: Provides alternative means of ingesting nutrients for clients.
2. **Nasoenteric Tube (Dobhoff Tube)**: A weighted tube of soft material that is placed in the small intestine to decrease chance of regurgitation. In the Dobhoff tube, placement may be evaluated by placing the stethoscope more to the right of the mid-epigastric area. Fluoroscopy or X-ray will validate the position of the tube.

LONG-TERM TYPES

1. **Percutaneous Endoscopic Gastrostomy (PEG)**: A tube is inserted percutaneously into the stomach; local anesthesia and sedation is used for tube placement.
2. **Percutaneous Endoscopic Jejunostomy (PEJ)**: A tube is inserted percutaneously into the jejunum.
3. **Gastrostomy:** A surgical opening is made into the stomach and a gastrostomy tube is positioned with sutures.

✓ **Key Point: Methods of administering a tube feeding**

- Continuous—controlled with a feeding pump. Decreases nausea and diarrhea.
- Intermittent—prescribed amount of fluid infuses over specific time. For example 350 cc is given over 30 minutes.
- Bolus—a prescribed amount of feeding is drawn into a syringe or poured through a funnel and allowed to infuse by gravity flow. The least preferred method.
- Cyclic—involves feeding infused via a pump for a part of a day, usually 12 to 16 hours. This method may be used for weaning from feedings.

Clinical Tips for Problem Solving

- Position client on right side in high-Fowler's position for intermittent or bolus feeding.
- Aspirate contents of stomach to determine residual. If residual is over 100 cc, or equal to 1/2 of the amount of the next feeding, it may be necessary to withhold feeding until residual diminishes.
- Return aspirated contents to stomach to prevent electrolyte imbalance.
- When administering bolus, hold tube feeding container no more than *18 inches above client's abdomen*. Used for short- term feeding.
- Do not force solution through the tube with pressure or a syringe.
- Flush the tube with 30 to 50 cc of water:
  (a) Following tube feeding
  (b) Every 4 hours for continuous feeding
  (c) Before and after each medication administration.
- When the PEG or PEJ tubes are placed, note the length of tube protruding from the abdomen. This tube should be routinely checked to determine if the tube is migrating from the original insertion point.
- Avoid diarrhea:
  (a) Slow rate of infusion.
  (b) Keep equipment clean to avoid bacterial contamination.
  (c) Check for fecal impaction; diarrhea may be flowing around impaction.
  (d) Identify clients with medical conditions that would precipitate diarrhea.
- For continuous feeding (intermittent or bolus), change feeding reservoir every 24 hours.

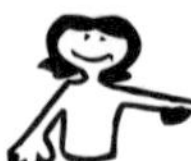

***NURSING PRIORITY:** If in doubt of a tube's placement or position, stop or hold the feeding and obtain an X-ray confirmation of location.*

NCLEX ALERT: *Change rate and amount of tube feeding based on client's response.*

Appendix 18-10: NURSING PROCEDURE ENEMAS

TYPES OF ENEMAS

CLEANSING: Stimulate peristalsis through irritation of colon and rectum and by distention.

Soap Suds: Mild soap solutions stimulate and irritate intestinal mucosa. Dilute 5 ml of castile soap in 1000 ml of water.

Tap Water: Give with caution to infants or to adults with altered cardiac and renal reserve.

Saline: For normal saline enemas, use a smaller volume of solution.

Prepackaged disposable enema (Fleet): Approximately 125 cc, tip is pre-lubricated and does not require further preparation.

✓ **Key Points: Administering an Enema**

- Fill water container with 750 to 1000 cc of lukewarm solution, (500 cc or less for children, 250 cc or less for an infant), 99°F to 102°F. Solutions that are too hot or too cold, or solutions that are instilled too quickly, can cause cramping and damage to rectal tissues.
- Allow solution to run through the tubing so that air is removed.
- Place client on left side in Sims' position.
- Lubricate the tip of the tubing with water-soluble lubricant.
- Gently insert tubing into client's rectum (3 to 4 inches for adult, 1 inch for infants, 2 to 3 inches for children), past the external and internal sphincters.
- Raise the water container no more than 12 to 18 inches above the client.
- Allow solution to flow slowly. If the flow is slow, the client will experience fewer cramps. The client will also be able to tolerate and retain a greater volume of solution.
- After you have instilled the solution, instruct client to hold solution for 10 to 15 minutes.
- Oil retention: enemas should be retained at least 1 hour. Cleansing enemas are retained 10 to 15 minutes.

Clinical Tips for Problem Solving

If client expels solution prematurely: —

- Place client in supine position with knees flexed.
- Slow the water flow and continue with the enema.

If enema returns are not clear prior to surgery or diagnostic testing:: —

- Repeat enema. If, after three enemas, returns are still not clear, notify physician.

If client complains of abdominal cramping during instillation of fluid: —

- Slow the infusion rate by lowering the fluid bag.
- If cramping does not subside, then discontinue the enema.

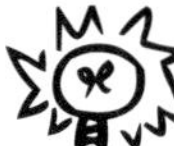

NCLEX ALERT: *Administer an enema. Pay attention to safety and comfort factors regarding amount of fluid, height of container, and distance of inserting enema tubing into rectum.*

Appendix 18-11:
NURSING PROCEDURE ■ STOOL SPECIMEN ■

TYPES OF STOOL

- Narrow, ribbon-like stool → spastic or irritable bowel, or obstruction.
- Diarrhea → spastic bowel, viral infection.
- Blood and mucus, soft stool → bacterial infection.
- Mixed blood or pus → colitis.
- Yellow or green stool → severe, prolonged diarrhea.
- Black stool → GI bleeding or intake of iron supplements.
- Tan, clay-colored, or white stool → liver or gallbladder problems.
- Red stool → colon or rectal bleeding; some medications and foods can may also cause a red coloration.
- Fatty stool, pasty or greasy → intestinal malabsorption, pancreatic disease.

✓ **Key Points: Collecting the Specimen**

- Always wear gloves during procedure.
- Use clean bedpan or bedside commode to collect stool; do not use stool that has been in contact with toilet bowl water or urine.
- Collect stool specimen in a clean, dry container. If stool is to be evaluated for organisms, use a sterile container. Use a tongue blade to obtain specimens from several areas of the stool and place in the stool collection container.
- The client collecting a stool specimen for occult blood needs to follow directions regarding diet restrictions (no red meat, beets, or foods that may cause the stool to turn red or lead to a false-positive).
  Take the specimen to the laboratory. Do not allow it to remain on the unit.

NCLEX ALERT: *Obtain specimen from clients for laboratory tests.*

Appendix 18-12:
NURSING PROCEDURE ■ CARE OF THE CLIENT WITH AN OSTOMY ■

TYPES OF OSTOMY

COLOSTOMY—opening of the colon through the abdominal wall; stool is generally semisoft and bowel control may be achieved.

ILEOSTOMY—opening of the ileum through the abdominal wall; stool drainage is liquid and excoriating; drainage is frequently continuous; therefore, difficult to establish bowel control. Fluid and electrolyte imbalance is a common complication.

Kock's ileostomy - may be referred to as a "continent" ileostomy; an internal reservoir for stool is surgically formed. Decreases problem of skin care due to frequent irritation of stoma by drainage. Primary complications are leakage at the stoma site and peritonitis.

✦ *Goals:*

1. Maintain physiological and psychological equilibrium.
2. Assist client to maintain total care of colostomy or ileostomy prior to discharge.

Preoperative Care:
1. Preoperative education: actively involve family and client; encourage questions concerning the procedure.
2. Client frequently on a low-residue diet prior to surgery to decrease intestinal contents.
3. Placement of stoma evaluated and site selected with client standing. Avoid skin creases and folds, selecting site that does not interfere with clothing.

✓ **Key Points: Postoperative Nursing Implications - Initial Care**

- Measure the stoma and select an appropriately sized appliance. Stoma will shrink postoperatively, which necessitates changes in size of the appliance.
- Appliance should fit easily around the stoma and protect the skin.
- Keep the skin around the stoma clean, dry, and free of intestinal juices. Prevent contamination of the abdominal incision.
- Change the skin appliance only when it begins to leak or becomes dislodged.

✓ **Key Points: Irrigation**

- Do not irrigate an ileostomy or maintain regular irrigations in child with colostomy.
- Irrigate colostomy at same time each day, to assist in establishing a normal pattern of elimination.
- Involve client in care as early as possible.
- In adults, irrigate with 500 to 1,000 cc warm tap water.

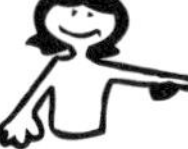

***NURSING PRIORITY:** Do not:*
(1) force catheter into the stoma.
(2) insert the catheter over four inches.
(3) use more than 1,000 cc of irrigation fluid.
(4) irrigate more than once a day.
(5) irrigate in the presence of diarrhea.

- Place the client in a sitting position for irrigation, preferably in the bathroom with the irrigation sleeve in the toilet.
- Elevate the solution container approximately 12 to 18 inches and allow solution to flow in gently. If cramping occurs, lower fluid or clamp the tubing.
- Allow 25 to 45 minutes for return flow. Client may want to walk around before the return starts.
- Encourage client to participate in care of his or her own colostomy. Have client perform return demonstration of colostomy irrigation prior to leaving the hospital.
- Assist the client to control odors - diet and odor-control tablets.
  Kock's ileostomy -is drained when client experiences fullness. May have a magnetic ring implanted into stoma and a magnetic cap on the outside. The reservoir is drained using a catheter.

Appendix 18-12:
NURSING PROCEDURE ■ CARE OF THE CLIENT WITH AN OSTOMY ■

Clinical Tips for Problem Solving

If water does not flow easily into colostomy stoma:

- Change angle or position of catheter slightly.
- Check for kinks in tubing from container.
- Check height of irrigating container.
- Encourage client to change positions, relax, and take a few deep breaths.

If client experiences cramping, nausea, or dizziness during irrigation:

- Stop flow of water, leaving catheter in place.
- Do not resume until cramping has passed.
- Check water temperature and height of water bag; if water is too hot or flows too rapidly, it can cause dizziness.

If client has no return of stool or water from irrigation:

- Be sure to apply drainable pouch, solution may drain as client moves around.
- Have client increase fluid intake; he may be dehydrated.
- Repeat irrigation next day.

If diarrhea occurs:

- Do not irrigate colostomy.
- Check client's medications; sometimes they may cause diarrhea.
- If diarrhea is excessive and/or prolonged, notify physician.

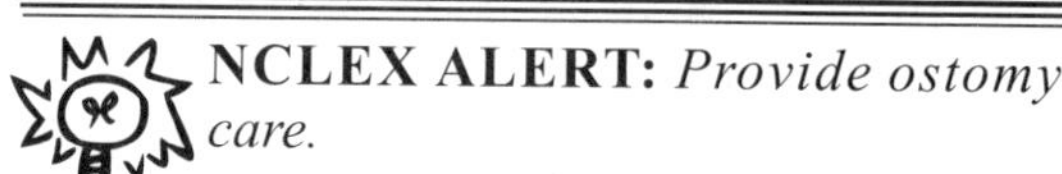

NCLEX ALERT: *Provide ostomy care.*

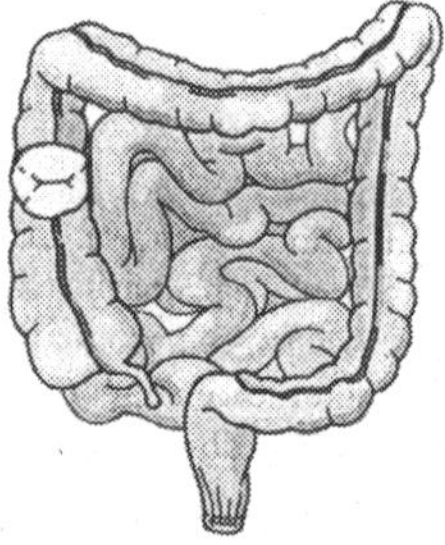

The **ascending colostomy** is done for right-sided tumors.

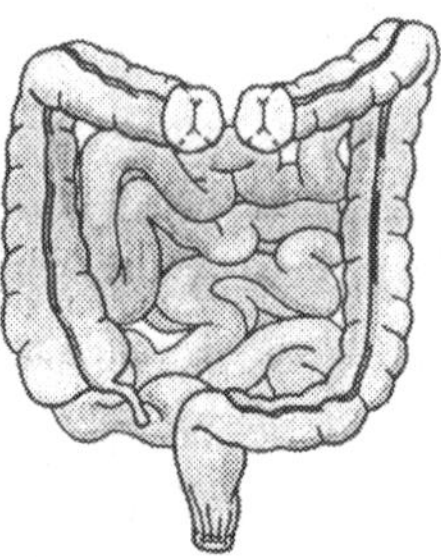

The **transverse (double-barreled) colostomy** is often used in such emergencies as intestinal obstruction or perforation because it can be created quickly. There are two stomas. The proximal one, closest to the small intestine, drains feces. The distal stoma drains mucus. Usually temporary.

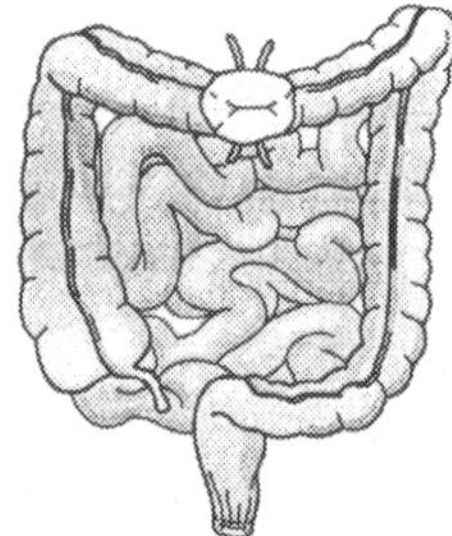

The **transverse loop colostomy** has two openings in the transverse colon, but one stoma. Usually temporary.

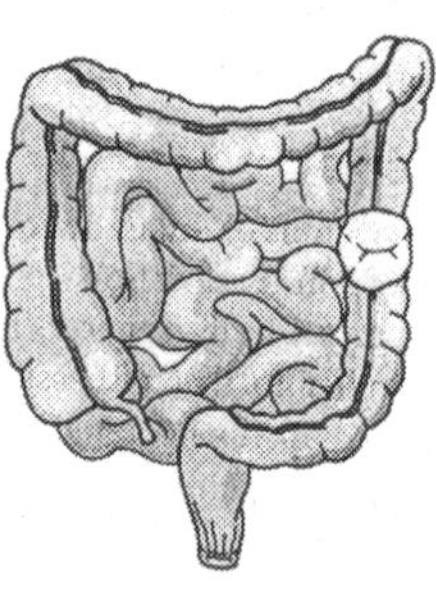

Descending colostomy

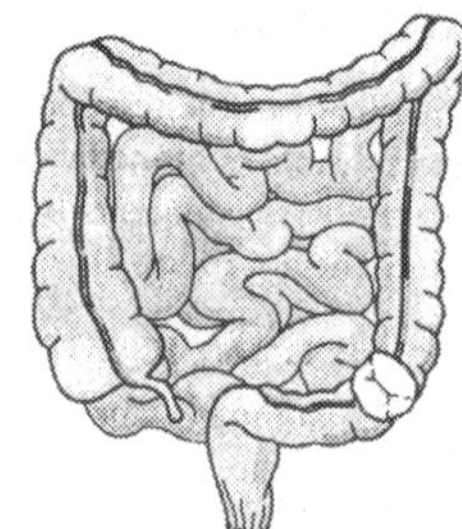

Sigmoid colostomy

Figure 18-3: Types of Ostomies

Reprinted with permission: Phipps, WJ, Sands, JK, & Marek, JF (1999). *Medical Surgical Nursing: Concepts & Clinical Practice*, 6th ed. Philadelphia: Mosby, p. 1336

HEPATIC AND BILIARY SYSTEM

PHYSIOLOGY OF THE HEPATIC AND BILIARY SYSTEM

Organs of the Hepatic and Biliary System

A. Liver.
1. Located in the upper right portion of the abdominal cavity just under the diaphragm; vascular organ; protected by the rib cage.
2. Blood flow into the liver is from two sources.
   a. Portal vein carries venous blood from the stomach, intestines, pancreas, and spleen into the liver. The venous blood is rich in nutrients absorbed from the GI system.
   b. The hepatic artery provides oxygenated blood to the liver.
   c. The portal vein and hepatic artery enter the liver via a common vessel and flow through the liver tissue; blood then leaves the liver via the hepatic vein and empties into the inferior vena cava.
3. Due to pressure differences in the hepatic and portal veins, the liver may normally store 200 to 400 cc of blood.
4. The liver produces approximately 600 to 1200 cc of bile daily.
   a. Bile drains from the liver via the common bile duct.
   b. Common bile duct enters the duodenum, either in close proximity to, or in conjunction with, the pancreatic duct.
5. The liver is susceptible to many pathologic processes. It can sustain 90 percent damage with loss of tissue and still remain functional.

B. Gallbladder.
1. A muscular, elastic sac located on the under- surface of the liver.
2. The cystic duct from the gallbladder joins the common bile duct from the liver.
3. Gallbladder is capable of storing 20 to 50 cc of bile. When food enters the duodenum, the gallbladder contracts; the sphincter of Oddi, which controls the release of bile, relaxes and bile enters the intestine via the common duct.
4. When the sphincter of Oddi closes, bile flows back into the gallbladder for storage.
5. The primary function of the gallbladder is concentration and storage of bile.

Functions of the Liver

A. Synthesis of absorbed nutrients.
1. Serum glucose regulation.
   a. Glucose from carbohydrate metabolism is converted to glycogen, which is stored in the liver and released according to body demands.
   b. Gluconeogenesis refers to the ability of the liver to produce glucose from non-carbohydrate sources, such as amino acids and the glycerol portion of fats. This process is initiated when the body requirements for glucose are in excess of the stored glycogen in the liver.
2. Lipid (fat) metabolism.
   a. Preliminary breakdown of fatty acids as a source of body energy.
   b. When glucose availability for metabolism is limited, fatty acids may be broken down for production of energy. This results in formation of ketone bodies.
   c. Utilization of fatty acids for production of cholesterol, lipoprotein, and phospholipid.
3. Protein metabolism.
   a. Synthesis of plasma proteins.
   b. Deaminization—breakdown of amino acids for energy or for conversion to glucose or to fat.
   c. Synthesis of nonessential amino acids.
   d. Ammonia is a by-product of protein metabolism. It is converted to urea by the liver and excreted by the kidney.

B. Synthesis of prothrombin for normal clotting mechanisms. Vitamin K is necessary for adequate prothrombin production.

C. Vitamin and mineral storage.
1. Produces and stores vitamins A and D.
2. Vitamin B_{12} and iron are stored in the liver.

D. Drug metabolism—barbiturates, amphetamines, and alcohol are metabolized by the liver.

E. Production of bile and bile salts.
1. Bile is continuously formed in the liver.
2. Bile salts are produced in the liver; cholesterol is necessary constituent of bile salts.
3. Bile and bile salts emulsify fat for digestion and absorption in the intestine.
4. Bilirubin, a bile pigment, is excreted by the liver.
   a. The spleen removes and breaks down the hemoglobin in the worn out red cells. This results in the production of bilirubin.
   b. Bilirubin is carried from the spleen to the liver for excretion.

c. Bilirubin is conjugated in the liver (made water-soluble) and secreted into the bile.

(1) A small amount of unconjugated bilirubin (indirect) is released into the circulation and is not water-soluble.

(2) Conjugated bilirubin (direct) has been processed through the liver to form a water-soluble substance.

(3) Conjugated bilirubin is secreted into the bile and flows into the small intestine for fat digestion.

(4) Conjugated bilirubin is converted into urobilinogen in the large intestine and is reabsorbed and returned to the liver or excreted in feces. Normally, only a small amount of urobilinogen is excreted in the urine.

System Assessment

A. History.

1. History of liver, gallbladder, or jaundice problems.
2. History of bleeding problems.
3. History of reproductive problems.
4. Medication intake.
5. Recent association with anyone with jaundice.
6. Alcohol consumption.

B. Physical assessment.

1. Inspection.

a. Skin.

(1) Presence of vascular angiomas, skin lesions, or petechiae.

(2) Hydration status.

(3) Color of the skin (jaundiced).

(4) Presence of peripheral edema.

b. Abdomen.

(1) Evidence of jaundice.

(2) Contour of the abdomen.

(3) Presence of visible abdominal wall veins.

2. Palpation of the abdomen.

a. Pain, tenderness.

b. Presence of distention.

c. Hepatomegaly.

d. Splenomegaly.

C. Nutritional assessment.

1. Weight gain or loss.
2. Dietary intake.
3. Problems of anorexia, nausea and vomiting.

Pathophysiology of Jaundice

A. Jaundice may begin so gradually that it is not noticed immediately.

B. The increased levels of bilirubin cause a yellowish discoloration of the skin. It may be first observed as a yellow color in the sclera of the eye. Serum bilirubin levels must exceed 2mg/dL for jaundice to occur. The yellow discoloration is due to deposits of bilirubin in the skin and body tissue.

C. Types of jaundice.

1. Hemolytic jaundice.

a. Occurs with an increase in the breakdown of red blood cells, which produces an increase in the amount of unconjugated bilirubin in the blood.

b. The liver cannot handle the level of increase in unconjugated bilirubin. The bilirubin is not water-soluble; therefore, it cannot be excreted. Unconjugated bilirubin is lipid-soluble and is capable of entering nerve cells and causing brain damage.

c. The increased production of urobilinogen will increase the amount of bilirubin excreted in the urine and feces.

d. Causes of hemolytic jaundice.

(1) Blood transfusion reactions.

(2) Sickle cell crisis.

(3) Hemolytic anemias.

(4) Hemolytic disease of the newborn.

2. Hepatocellular jaundice.

a. Results from the inability of the liver to clear normal amounts of bilirubin from the blood.

b. Increase in serum levels of unconjugated and conjugated bilirubin.

c. Causes of hepatocellular jaundice.

(1) Hepatitis.

(2) Cirrhosis.

(3) Hepatic cancer.

3. Obstructive jaundice.

a. Results from an impediment to bile flow through the liver and the biliary system.

b. The obstruction may be within the liver, or it may be outside the liver.

c. Causes of obstructive jaundice.

(1) Hepatitis.

(2) Liver tumors.

(3) Cirrhosis.

(4) Obstruction of the common bile duct by a stone.

DISORDERS OF THE HEPATIC SYSTEM

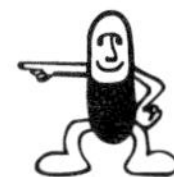

Hepatitis

❑ **Widespread inflammation of the liver tissue is called *hepatitis*.**

A. Types of hepatitis (Table 19-1).

1. Hepatitis A (HAV, infectious hepatitis).
   a. Mode of transmission.
      (1) Carriers are most contagious just prior to onset of symptoms (jaundice).
      (2) The route of infection is predominately fecal-oral.
      (3) Transmission via sexual contacts as well as percutaneous transmission is possible, but are not primary methods of transmission.
      (4) Virus is present in feces for 7-10 days prior to person becoming ill.
   b. Primarily a disease of children because of mode of transmission and day care centers.
   c. Mortality is low, there is an increase in fatalities in the geriatric population.
   d. Administration of immune serum globulin (IgG) to exposed individuals increases the immune resistance and or decreases the severity of the illness (passive immunization).
2. Hepatitis B (HBV, serum hepatitis).
   a. Mode of transmission.
      (1) Percutaneous inoculation with contaminated needles or instruments is primary mode.
      (2) Non-percutaneous transmission, contact with body fluids containing hepatitis B surface antigen (sexual contact).
      (3) Infants of mothers with HBV may contract the disease in utero, at birth, or postnatal.
      (4) Infected asymptomatic carrier.
   b. Identification of the hepatitis B surface antigen (HB_sAg, Australian antigen).
      (1) Identification of antigen in potential blood donors has significantly decreased transmission via blood transfusions.
      (2) Antigen is present in blood, vaginal secretions, menstrual fluid, semen, saliva, and respiratory secretions (see Table 19-1).
   c. Administration of hepatitis B immunoglobulin (HBIG) will provide some temporary immunity.
   d. HBV vaccine should be administered to everyone as a standard immunization. (See Table 2-1)
3. Hepatitis C (non-A non-B)—transmission is very similar to HBV, multiple causative agents; percutaneous inoculation (IV drug abusers), blood transfusions, and there is an increased incidence in crowded living conditions.
4. Toxic and drug-induced hepatitis.

B. The inflammatory process causes hepatic cell degeneration and necrosis. Hepatitis A is generally self-limiting, with liver regeneration and complete recovery. Hepatitis B and C are more serious and can progress to total destruction of the liver.

NCLEX ALERT: *Teach health promotion information, follow infection control guidelines/protocols. Prevention of transmission in the hospital as well as teaching the importance of personal hygiene in preventing the transmission of hepatitis virus.*

Assessment

(Regardless of the type, the clinical picture is similar.)

1. Risk factors/etiology.
   a. Hepatitis A.
      (1) Common in young children and young adults.
      (2) Increased incidence in crowded living conditions and areas of poor hygiene.
      (3) Infected food handlers may be the source of infection.
      (4) May be transmitted from contaminated water, or milk products, or shellfish from contaminated waters.
      (5) Primary route of transmission is fecal-oral.
   b. Hepatitis B.
      (1) Contact with serum of an infected individual.
      (2) Blood transfusions.
      (3) Virus is transmitted in body fluids such as saliva and semen.
      (4) Affects all ages.
2. Clinical manifestations - all clients experience inflammation of the liver tissue and exhibit similar symptoms.
   a. Anicteric phase
      (1) Anorexia, nausea.
      (2) Upper right quadrant discomfort.
      (3) Malaise, headache.
      (4) Low-grade fever.
      (5) Hepatomegaly.

Table 19-1: HEPATITIS

HEPATITIS A (HAV)	HEPATITIS B (HBV)	HEPATITIS C (HCV)
Transmission modes:		
Poor personal hygiene Oral-anal sexual practices Contaminated food, water, and shellfish (commonly spread by infected food handlers)	Blood and blood products Skin or mucous membrane break by inoculation (needle sticks, cuts, ear piercing, tattooing, or contaminated drug paraphernalia) Sexual contact Hepatitis D is very similar to HBV	Blood and blood products Sexual contact Close contact, IV drug use Closely associated with HBV
Incubation period:		
2 to 6 weeks (average: 4 weeks); also the most contagious period	6 weeks to 6 months (average: 12 weeks) Contagious as long as serum marker (surface antigen) appears	6-7 weeks
High-Risk Individuals:		
Household contacts Sexual contacts Institutions, day care centers, schools	Household contacts Sexual contacts Dental, laboratory, and medical personnel Multiple blood transfusion recipients IV drug users	Multiple blood transfusion recipients Sexual contacts IV drug users

NCLEX ALERT: *Follow infection control guidelines; standard precautions include blood and body fluids.*

b. Icteric phase (jaundiced).

(1) Dark urine due to increased excretion of bilirubin.

(2) Pruritus.

(3) Stools light and clay-colored.

(4) Liver remains enlarged and tender.

c. Posticteric phase (after jaundice).

(1) Malaise.

(2) Easily fatigued.

(3) Hepatomegaly remains for several weeks.

d. Anicteric hepatitis (absence of jaundice).

(1) Frequently occurs in children.

(2) Many clients with hepatitis A, and hepatitis (non-A, non-B) may not show clinical jaundice.

(3) Unexplained fever.

(4) General GI disturbances.

(5) Anorexia and malaise.

e. Onset of hepatitis A is more acute; symptoms are generally less severe.

f. Onset of hepatitis B is more insidious; symptoms are more severe.

3. Diagnostics (Appendix 19-1).

a. Increased alanine aminotransferase (ALT) aspartate amino-transferase (AST), serum bilirubin.

b. Presence of HB_sAg in serum of hepatitis B client.

Treatment

1. No specific medications.
2. Encourage good nutrition, no specific dietary modifications, client will probably not tolerate a high-fat diet.
3. Decreased activity.

Complications

1. Chronic, active hepatitis.
2. Fulminant hepatitis—severe, acute case of hepatitis.
3. Permanent destruction of liver cells, leading to cirrhosis.
4. Total destruction of the liver.

Nursing Intervention

✦ *Goal: to control and prevent hepatitis.*

1. Understand characteristics of transmission and preventive measures for hepatitis A.

a. Good personal hygiene, especially hand washing.

b. Participate in community activities for health education, (i.e., environmental sanitation, food preparation, etc.).

c. Identification of individuals at an increased risk of exposure includes household, intimate sexual, and institutional contacts with the active disease.

d. Administer immune serum globulin (IgG) within two weeks of exposure.

e. Implement standard precautions.

f. Client should abstain from sexual activities during periods of communicability.

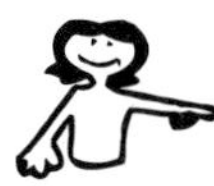

GERIATRIC PRIORITY: Elderly clients are at higher risk for liver damage and for complications of hepatitis.

2. Understand characteristics of transmission and preventive measures for hepatitis B.

   a. Identification of individuals at increased risk of exposure; includes oral or percutaneous contact with HB_sAg positive fluid, or sexual contact within four weeks of jaundice.

   b. Administration of hepatitis B vaccine.

3. Maintain strict contract based standard precautions in hospitalized client with questionable diagnosis of hepatitis (Appendix 6-10).

✦ *Goal: to promote healing and regeneration of liver tissue.*

1. Bed rest with bathroom privileges initially; progressive activity according to liver function tests.

2. Promote psychological and emotional rest.

   a. Strict bed rest may increase anxiety.

   b. Frequently, young adults are very concerned about body image; encourage verbalization and emphasize temporary nature of symptoms.

   c. Maintain communication and frequent contact.

3. Promote nutritional intake.

   a. Anorexia and decreased taste for food potentiate the problem.

   b. Small frequent feedings of favorite foods, good oral hygiene, and food served in a pleasant atmosphere.

4. Encourage increased fluid intake.

Self-Care

1. There is a continued need for adequate rest and nutrition until liver function tests are normal.

2. Avoid alcohol and OTC medications, especially those containing acetaminophen and phenothiazine.

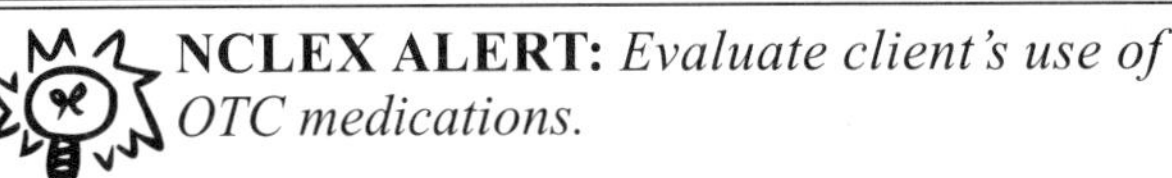

NCLEX ALERT: *Evaluate client's use of OTC medications.*

3. Clients with hepatitis B should avoid intimate and sexual contact until the presence of antibodies to the HB_sAg are present and the client is no longer contagious.

4. If possible, client should have his own bathroom.

5. Client and family must understand importance of personal hygiene and good hand washing.

6. Client should not donate blood.

Hepatic Cirrhosis

❑ **This is a chronic, progressive disease of the liver characterized by degeneration and destruction of liver cells.**

A. Liver regeneration is disorganized and results in the formation of scar tissue, which in time will exceed the amount of normal liver tissue.

B. Types of cirrhosis.

   1. Laennec's—associated with alcohol abuse; with excessive alcohol intake, there is wide spread inflammation and destruction of liver cells, which results in widespread scar formation.

   2. Postnecrotic—can follow hepatitis or exposure to hepatotoxin.

   3. Biliary—diffuse fibrosis and scarring, due to chronic biliary obstruction and infection.

   4. Cardiac — increase in venous pressure associated with long-term right-sided heart failure.

C. Complications of cirrhosis.

   1. Portal hypertension.

      a. Structural changes in the liver result in obstruction to normal hepatic blood flow, which causes increased pressure in the portal circulation.

      b. Collateral circulation develops as the body attempts to reduce the increased portal pressure. Common areas for collateral channels are:

         (1) Lower esophagus at the area of the gastric vein.

         (2) Anterior abdominal wall.

         (3) Parietal peritoneum.

         (4) Rectum.

      c. Esophageal varices form from collateral vessels in the lower esophagus.

      d. Splenomegaly occurs from the increase of congestion in the splenic bed; may lead to leukopenia and thrombocytopenia.

      e. Caput medusae—dilated veins around the umbilical area.

2. Peripheral edema and ascites.
   a. Edema results from:
      (1) Impaired liver synthesis of protein resulting in decreased colloid osmotic pressure (hypoalbuminemia).
      (2) Portal hypertension, malnutrition.
   b. Ascites—accumulation of serous fluid in the peritoneal cavity.
      (1) With increased pressure in the liver, excessive protein and water leak out of the liver into the abdomen.
      (2) The presence of hypoalbuminemia results in decreased colloid osmotic pressure, which facilitates movement of fluid and protein into the abdominal cavity.
      (3) Hyperaldosteronism causes increased amounts of sodium and water to be retained.
3. Hepatic encephalopathy (coma) results from the inability of the liver to detoxify ammonia.
   a. Ammonia is a byproduct of protein metabolism.
   b. Large quantities of ammonia remain in the systemic circulation and cross the blood-brain barrier, producing toxic neurological effects.

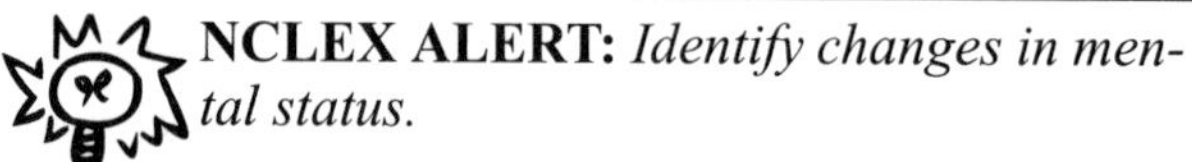

NCLEX ALERT: *Identify changes in mental status.*

Assessment

1. Risk factors/etiology.
   a. Excessive, prolonged alcohol consumption.
   b. Nutritional deficiencies.
   c. Frequently, a combination of alcohol and nutritional deficiency.
   d. Predisposing chronic hepatic and biliary infections.
2. Clinical manifestations.
   a. GI disturbances—anorexia, indigestion, change in bowel habits.
   b. Changes in the skin.
      (1) Jaundice (hepatocellular and biliary).
      (2) Spider angiomas on the face, neck and shoulders.
      (3) Palmar erythema—reddened areas in the palm that blanch with pressure.
   c. Blood disorders.
   d. Anemia.
   e. Thrombocytopenia.
   f. Coagulation disorders.
   g. Changes in sexual characteristics: gynecomastia, impotence in males; amenorrhea, vaginal bleeding in females.
   h. Peripheral neuropathy—probably due to inadequate intake of vitamin B complex.
   i. Hepatomegaly, splenomegaly.
   j. Portal hypertension.
      (1) Esophageal varices which bleed easily.
      (2) Hemorrhoids.
      (3) Collateral veins visible on abdominal wall.
      (4) Development of edema and ascites.
      (5) Edema generally occurs in feet, ankle and presacral area.
      (6) Severe abdominal distention and weight gain with ascites.
      (7) Presence of fluid waves in the abdomen.
   k. Portal-systemic encephalopathy.
      (1) Changes in mental responsiveness.
      (2) Level of concentration—ask client to repeat a series of numbers; if he has encephalopathy he will be unable to repeat a 4- to 6-digit sequence.
      (3) Memory—determine his ability to recall recent events (yesterday or past week) and remote events (last year).
      (4) Apraxia—deterioration in writing and drawing; ask him to write his name or draw a figure.
      (5) Asterixis—ask him to hold his hands out in front of him and dorsiflex his hands at the wrist and extend his fingers; a flapping of the hands occurs will occur.
3. Diagnostics.
   a. Elevated aspartate aminotransferase (AST) and alanine aminotransferase (ALT).
   b. Decrease in total protein, hypoalbuminemia.
   c. Prolonged prothrombin time.
   d. Altered bilirubin metabolism.

Treatment

1. Cirrhosis.
   a. Rest.
   b. Dietary modification—increase calories and carbohydrates; protein and fat as tolerated.
   c. Vitamin supplement, especially vitamin B complex.
   d. Abstinence from alcohol.
2. Ascites.

a. Salt-poor albumin via IV infusion.
b. Sodium restriction in dietary intake.
c. Fluid restriction in severe ascites.
d. Diuretics.
e. Paracentesis.
f. Peritoneal venous shunt (LeVeen shunt)—a surgical procedure for reinfusion of ascitic fluid.
g. Surgical procedures to decrease portal hypertension by shunting portal blood flow.

3. Esophageal varices.
   a. Surgical procedures to decrease portal hypertension by shunting portal blood flow.
   b. Mechanical compression of bleeding varices via esophageal gastric balloon tamponade (Sengstaken-Blakemore tube, Figure 19-1).
   c. Blood transfusions to restore volume from bleeding varices (preferably fresh whole blood).
   d. Administration of vasopressin (**Pitressin**) IV directly into mesenteric artery to control bleeding.
   e. Injection sclerotherapy—injection of a sclerosing agent directly into esophageal varices. Bleeding may recur since there has been no reduction in portal hypertension.
4. Decrease portal systemic encephalopathy
   a. Restriction of dietary protein intake.
   b. Decreases the normal flora in the intestines to reduce bacterial activity on protein (**Neomycin**).
   c. Lactulose—produces an acidic environment in the intestine and thereby decreases bacterial activity.
   d. Control of GI hemorrhage to decrease protein available in the intestine.

Nursing Intervention

✦ *Goal: to promote health in the cirrhotic client.*

1. Proper diet—increased protein as tolerated, adequate carbohydrates.
2. Adequate rest.
3. Avoid potential hepatotoxic over-the-counter drugs.
4. Avoid aspirin and acetaminophen.
5. Abstinence from alcohol.
6. Attention and care should be given the alcoholic client without being judgmental or moralizing.
7. Client should understand symptoms indicative of complications and when to seek medical advice.
8. Regular medical checkups.

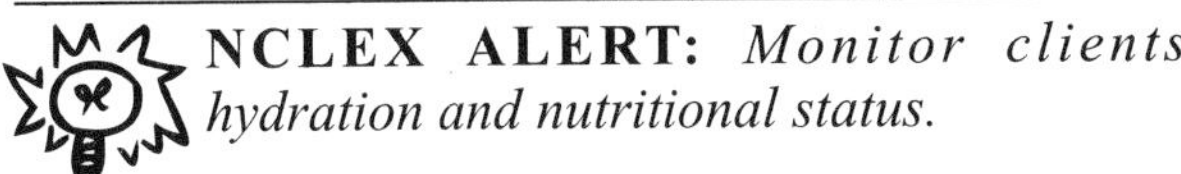

NCLEX ALERT: *Monitor clients hydration and nutritional status.*

✦ *Goal: to maintain homeostasis and promote liver function.*

1. Rest and activity schedule based on clinical manifestations and lab data.
2. Measures to prevent complications of immobility (See Chapter 3).
3. Assist client to maintain self-esteem.
   a. Maintain positive, accepting atmosphere in the delivery of care.
   b. Encourage ventilation of feelings regarding disease.
4. Assist in ADLs as necessary to prevent undue fatigue.
5. Promote nutritional intake.
   a. Good oral hygiene.
   b. Between-meal nourishment.
   c. Provide food preferences when possible.
   d. Antiemetic prior to meals if necessary.
   e. Iron and vitamin supplements, especially vitamin B complex.
   f. Nasogastric or parenteral feeding if unable to maintain adequate intake.
6. Decrease discomfort of pruritus secondary to jaundice.
7. Good skin care to prevent breakdown.
8. Evaluate serum electrolytes, especially potassium, due to diuretics to decrease ascites and edema.
9. Monitor temperature closely due to increased susceptibility to infection.
10. Assess for bleeding tendencies and prevent trauma to the mucous membrane.
11. Measure abdominal girth to determine if it is increasing from ascitic fluid.(Figure 19-1)

✦ *Goal: if esophageal varices are present, decrease risk of active bleeding.*

1. Soft, nonirritating foods.
2. Discourage straining at stool.
3. Decrease esophageal reflux.
4. No salicylate compounds (aspirin).
5. Evaluate for active bleeding.
   a. Monitor vital signs.
   b. Assess for melena.
   c. Assess for hematemesis.

✦ *Goal: to decrease bleeding from esophageal varices .*

1. Gastric lavage with iced saline.
2. Assess and prevent complications associated with of sclerotherapy.
   a. The client is sedated and the throat is anesthetized prior to the procedure.
   b. Via an endoscopy, the physician injects the sclerosing agent into the varices.
   c. Bleeding from the varices should stop within minutes.
   d. Client may experience chest discomfort for 2 to 3 days; administer an analgesic.
   e. Esophageal perforation and ulceration are complications associated with treatment; observe client for development of severe chest pain.
   f. Observe for return of active bleeding.

✦ *Goal: to decrease esophageal bleeding with a esophageal tamponade balloon.*

1. Constant observation is required while the balloons are inflated.
2. The client is *absolutely* NPO, provide frequent oral and nasal hygiene.
3. Constant tension/traction is applied to maintain the pressure against the esophageal sphincter by the gastric balloon. The gastric balloon is *not* to be deflated while tension is present and the esophageal balloon is inflated.
4. Keep the head of the bed elevated, to decrease gastric regurgitation and nausea.
5. Keep scissors at the bedside in case the esophageal balloon moves into the oropharynx area and causes obstruction of trachea. If this should occur, the lumen to the esophageal balloon should be cut to immediately deflate the balloon and relieve the obstruction.

✦ *Goal: to assess for and prevent complications associated with ascites.*

1. Decrease sodium intake.
2. Diuretics, potassium supplements.
3. Daily measurements of abdominal girth.
4. Maintain semi-Fowler's position, to decrease pressure on the diaphragm.
5. Assess daily weight.

✦ *Goal: to assess for and prevent complications of hepatic encephalopathy.*

1. Frequent assessment of responsiveness.
2. Assess for sensory and motor abnormalities (asterixis).
3. Decrease production of ammonia.
   a. Decrease protein in diet.
   b. Increase carbohydrates and fluids.
   c. Decrease activity, since ammonia is by-product of metabolism.
   d. GI bleeding will increase ammonia levels due to breakdown of red blood cells.
4. Prompt treatment of hypokalemia.

✦ *Goal: to provide appropriate pre-and postoperative care if surgical procedure is indicated (See Chapter 3).*

1. An anastomoses of the high pressure portal system to the low pressure systemic venous system to create a shunt to decrease portal hypertension (portosystemic shunt), thereby decreasing problems with esophageal varices and ascites.
2. Client at increased risk for postoperative complications.
   (1) Hemorrhage.
   (2) Electrolyte imbalance.
   (3) Seizures.
   (4) Delirium tremens.
3. Surgical procedures do not alter course of progressive hepatic disease.

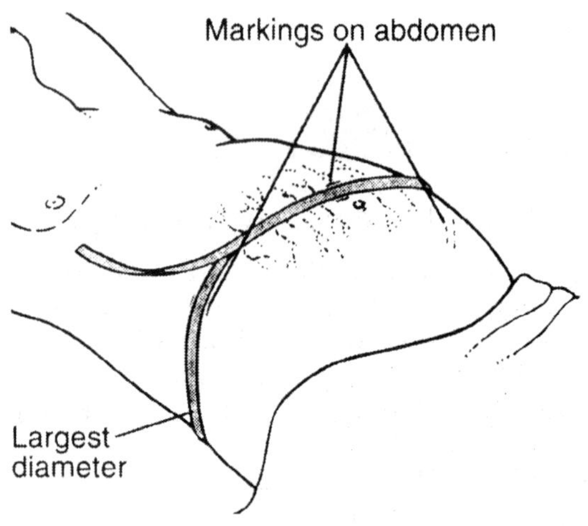

Figure 19-1: Mearsuring Abdominal Girth
With the client supine, the nurse brings the tape measure around the client and takes a measurement at the largest diameter of the abdomen. Before removing the tape, the nurse marks the client's abdomen along the sides of the tape on the client's flanks (sides) and midline to ensure that later measurements are taken in a consistent manner.
Reprinted with permission: Ignatavicius, D., Workman, L., Mishler, M. (1995). *Medical Surgical Nursing: A Nursing Process Approach,* p. 1671.

Cancer of the Liver

❑ **Primary cancer of the liver is rare. Metastatic cancer is more common.**

A. Liver is common site for metastasises, due to increased rate of blood flow and capillary network.

B. Metastasises are found in liver in approximately one-half of all late-stage cancer victims.

C. Prognosis is poor.

Assessment

1. Risk factors/etiology—malignancy elsewhere in the body.
2. Clinical manifestations.
   a. Anorexia, weight loss.
   b. Fatigue, anemia.
   c. Right upper quadrant pain.
   d. Ascites and jaundice.
3. Diagnostics.
   a. Liver scan and biopsy.
   b. Hepatic arteriogram.

Treatment

Primarily palliative.

1. Surgical excision of tumor if it is localized.
2. Chemotherapy—very poor response.

Nursing Intervention

Focused on maintaining comfort; nursing care is the same as for the advanced cirrhotic client.

DISORDERS OF THE BILIARY TRACT

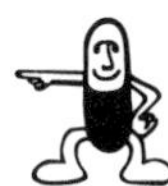

Cholelithiasis and Cholecystitis

❑ **Cholelithiasis is the presence of stones in the gallbladder; this is the most common form of biliary disease. Cholecystitis is an inflammation of the gallbladder, which is frequently associated with stones; this condition may be acute or chronic.**

Assessment

1. Risk factors/etiology.
   a. Cholelithiasis.
      (1) Supersaturation of bile with cholesterol causes precipitate to occur.
      (2) Conditions upsetting cholesterol and bile balance are infection and disturbances of cholesterol metabolism.
      (3) Increased incidence in females, especially during pregnancy.
      (4) Increased incidence after age 40.

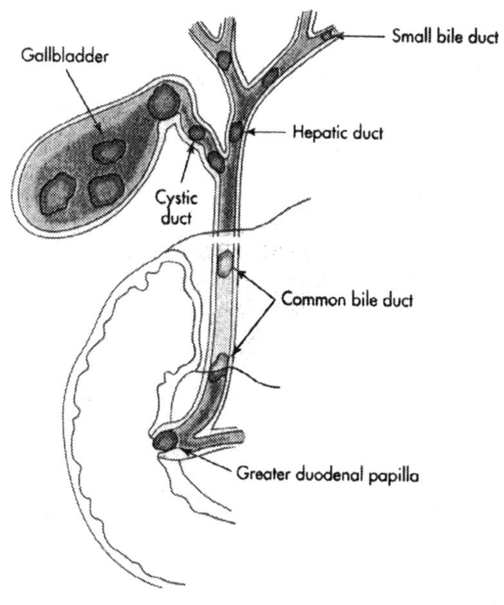

Figure 19-2: Common Sites of Gallstones
Reprinted with permission: Phipps, WJ, Sands, JK, & Marek, JF (1999). *Medical Surgical Nursing: Concepts & Clinical Practice*, 6th ed. Philadelphia: Mosby, p. 1374

      (5) Obesity.
   b. Cholecystitis.
      (1) Associated with stones.
      (2) *E.coli* is common bacteria involved.
      (3) May also be associated with neoplasms, anesthesia, adhesions.
2. Clinical manifestations.
   a. Cholelithiasis—severity of symptoms depend on the mobility of the stone and whether or not obstruction occurs.
      (1) Epigastric distress.
      (2) Feeling of fullness.
      (3) Abdominal distention.
      (4) Vague pain in the right upper quadrant after eating meals high in fat.
   b. Obstruction of cystic ducts by stones precipitating biliary colic.
      (1) Severe abdominal pain radiating to the back and shoulder.
      (2) Nausea, vomiting, tachycardia, diaphoresis.
      (3) Pain occurs several hours after eating a heavy meal.
      (4) Jaundice may occur with obstruction of bile flow.

(5) Urine may become very dark and stools clay-colored.

c. Cholecystitis.

(1) Abdominal guarding, rigidity and rebound tenderness.

(2) Fever.

(3) Pain aggravated by deep breathing.

(4) May present suddenly with severe pain.

3. Diagnostics (Appendix 19-1).

a. Oral cholecystogram.

b. IV cholangiography.

c. Biliary ultrasonography.

d. Increase in direct and indirect bilirubin.

Treatment

1. Cholecystectomy for cholelithiasis—surgical removal of the stones.

2. Cholecystitis.

a. Anticholinergics to decrease secretions and promote relaxation of the gallbladder.

b. Analgesics—usually meperidine (**Demerol**); morphine can cause a spasm in the sphincter of Oddi, causing increase in pain.

c. Antibiotics.

d. Atropine and propantheline (**Pro-Banthine**) will relieve spasm and decrease pain.

3. Laparoscopic cholecystectomy.

a. 3 small incisions are made.

b. Decreases risk to client.

c. Client may be admitted on a 23-hour basis.

d. Early ambulation and decreased pain.

4. Decrease dietary fat intake.

Nursing Intervention

✦ *Goal: to decrease attack of pain and inflammatory response.*

1. Low-fat liquid diet during acute attack.

2. Low-fat solids added as tolerated.

3. IV fluids and gastric decompression if nausea and vomiting are severe.

4. Antibiotics and analgesics.

5. Assess for indications of infection.

✦ *Goal: if surgery is indicated, to provide appropriate preoperative nursing care (See Chapter 3).*

✦ *Goal: to maintain homeostasis and prevent complications postoperative cholecystectomy.*

1. General postoperative care for clients having abdominal surgery (See Chapter 3).

2. Evaluate tolerance to diet and progress diet gradually to low-fat solids.

3. Penrose drain may be in place; client will frequently have large amounts of serosanguineous drainage; change dressing as indicated.

4. T-tube may be utilized to maintain patency of bile duct and bile drainage until edema subsides.

a. Maintain tube to gravity drainage.

b. Observe amount and color of bile drainage.

c. Do not irrigate or clamp tube.

d. Observe for bile drainage around the tube.

e. Observe and record drainage.

f. Postoperatively, drainage usually around 500 cc per day for several days postoperative; gradually, drainage will decrease and the doctor will remove the tube.

5. Monitor urine and stool for changes in color.

✦ *Goal: to assist client to understand implications of disease process and measures to maintain health postoperative cholecystectomy.*

1. Dietary teaching regarding low-fat diet.

2. Weight reduction if appropriate.

3. Avoid heavy lifting.

4. Understand symptoms indicating bile obstruction (i.e., stool and urine changes), and advise physician accordingly.⌘

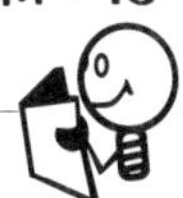

Study Questions—Hepatic/Biliary System

1. The postcholecystectomy client has a T-tube in place after surgery. What is the purpose of the T-tube in the care of this client?

① Remove bile leaking from the incision.
② Provide a means of wound irrigation.
③ Drain bile from the common bile duct.
④ Prevent rupture of the inflamed gall bladder.

2. Which position is best for the client postoperative abdominal cholecystectomy?

① Side lying, to prevent aspiration.
② Semi-Fowler's position, to facilitate breathing.
③ Supine, to decrease strain on the incision line.
④ Prone, to reduce nausea.

3. An obese 44-year-old woman with a history of chronic cholecystitis is to receive vitamin K preoperatively. What is the purpose of this medication?

① Increase the digestion and utilization of fats.
② Support the immune system and promote healing.
③ Aid in the emptying of the bile from the gallbladder.
④ Facilitate coagulation activities of the blood.

4. A client 3 days post cholecystectomy has a T-tube that has stopped draining. What is the best nursing action?

① Flush the tube with 5cc normal saline.
② Reposition the patient.
③ Continue to monitor.
④ Assess for tube placement.

5. What client statement would indicate to the nurse the client understands the discharge teaching regarding his cirrhosis?.

① "I will decrease vitamin B intake."
② "I need to continue **Thorazine** nightly."
③ "I will weigh every day in the A.M."
④ "I can eat my regular diet".

6. The nurse is caring for a client with chronic hepatitis B (HBV). What will the teaching plan for this client include?

① Avoid sexual activity.
② Report any clay colored stools.
③ Eat a high protein diet.
④ Perform daily urine bilirubin checks.

7. The client returns to his room post liver biopsy, the nurse positions the client on his left side and assesses for bleeding. What is a priority nursing assessment?

① Assess vital signs.
② Monitor for shock.
③ Check pretest PT and PTT values.
④ Determine adequacy of urinary output.

8. A client with portal hypertension and ascites has had a paracentesis to relieve respiratory compromise. What medication will the nurse anticipate the client will receive?

① $D_{10}W$.
② Meperidine (**Demerol**)
③ IV Albumin.
④ Furosemide (**Lasix**).

9. The nurse is making a home visit to a client with hepatitis A (HAV). Prior to assessing the client, the nurse will gather the equipment and perform what action next?

① Wipe the bedside table with alcohol preps.
② Place the supplies on the bedside table.
③ Place paper towels on the bedside table.
④ Put on a gown and gloves.

10. While talking with a client diagnosed with end stage liver disease, the nurse noticed the client is unable to stay awake and seems to fall asleep in the middle of his sentence. The nurse recognizes these symptoms to be indicative of what condition?

① Hyperglycemia.
② Increased bile production.
③ Increased blood ammonia levels.
④ Hypocalcemia.

Answers and rationales to these questions are in the section at the end of the book entitled "Chapter Study Questions: Answers & Rationales."

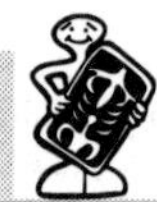

Appendix 19-1: DIAGNOSTICS OF THE HEPATIC AND BILIARY SYSTEM

LABORATORY TESTS	NORMAL	NURSING IMPLICATIONS
SERUM LABORATORY TESTS		
BILIRUBIN		
Direct Indirect Total	0.1 to 0.4 mg/dL 0.2 to 0.8 mg/dL 0.3 to 1.3 mg/dL	A rise in the serum level of bilirubin will occur if there is excessive destruction of red blood cells or if the liver is unable to excrete normal amounts of bilirubin.
BROMSULPHALEIN EXCRETION (BSP TEST)	Less than 5 percent retention 45 min after injection	Retention is increased in liver cell damage or decreased liver blood flow. Client is NPO prior to the test. Dye is injected and sample is drawn in 45 minutes. Observe client for reaction to dye.
PROTEIN STUDIES		
Total serum protein Serum albumin Serum globulin	6.0 to 8.2 gm/dL 3.5 to 5.5 gm/dL 2.0 to 3.5 mg/dL	Proteins are responsible for maintaining the colloid oncotic pressure in the serum. Synthesis of protein and normal serum protein levels are affected by various liver impairments.
PROTHROMBIN TIME	11 to 13 seconds	Prothrombin time may be prolonged in liver disease. Evaluates vitamin K deficiency.
SERUM ENZYMES		
Lactic dehydrogenase (LDH)	70-200 IU/L	Elevated in liver damage.
Aspartate aminotransferase (AST) Alanine aminotransferase (ALT),	10 to 26 units 10 to 35 units	
Serum alkaline phosphatase (ALP)	Depends on method utilized	Primary source of alkaline phosphatase in the body is from the bone and liver. Abnormally high readings may be associated with either liver or bone disease and must be correlated with presenting clinical symptoms.
SERUM BLOOD AMMONIA	15-45ug/dL	Increasing blood ammonia is indicative of the inability of the liver to convert ammonia to urea.
HEPATITIS ANTIGENS AND ANTIBODIES	Negative for antigens	Antigens indicate hepatitis. Antibodies indicate exposure, current disease, or immunization of Hepatitis B.
BIOPSY		
LIVER BIOPSY Needle aspiration of liver tissue.		1. Client NPO for 6 hours prior to procedure. 2. Blood coagulation studies should be available on the chart prior to biopsy procedure. 3. Immediately prior to needle insertion have client take a deep breath, exhale completely and hold breath. This immobilizes the chest wall and decreases the risk of penetration of the diaphragm with the needle. 4. Bed rest for 24 hours. Client may be positioned on the right side, to apply pressure and decrease risk of hemorrhage. 5. Assess for complications of pneumothorax and hemorrhage immediately after biopsy - assess for right upper abdominal pain or referred shoulder pain; observe for development of bile peritonitis. 6. Vital signs should be evaluated hourly for 8 to 12 hours.

NCLEX ALERT: *Monitor status of client after a procedure -position the client on his/her right side with a pillow under the costal margin to facilitate compression of the liver.*

Appendix 19-1: DIAGNOSTICS OF THE HEPATIC AND BILIARY SYSTEM

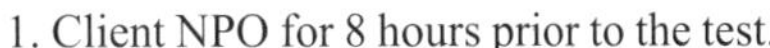

X-RAY

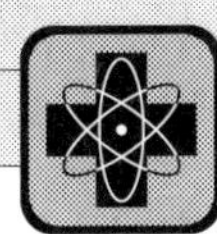

CHOLANGIOGRAPHY
IV injection of radiopaque dye to visualize the biliary duct system.

1. Client NPO for 8 hours prior to the test.
2. Assess for sensitivity to iodine.
3. Evaluate for iodine reaction after the test.
4. Drink large amounts of fluid after test to increased excretion of dye.

ORAL CHOLECYSTOGRAM (GALLBLADDER SERIES)
X-ray visualization of the gallbladder to determine the gallbladder's ability to concentrate and store the dye ingested and the patency of the biliary duct system.

1. Assess client for sensitivity to iodine.
2. Administer radiopaque dye PO evening prior to examination: six tablets, one given every 5 minutes. Client is NPO after dye ingestion.
3. Evaluate for side effects of the dye.
4. Client may be given a fatty meal before or during the x-ray procedure. This depends on the type of diet, type of radiopaque contrast media being used and what particular function is being assessed (e.g., emptying of gallbladder, contraction of gallbladder, etc.).

ABDOMINAL/GALL BLADDER SONOGRAM
Uses high frequency sound waves to exam the gall bladder which gives information about presence of tumors and patency of vessels.

1. May be required to fast.

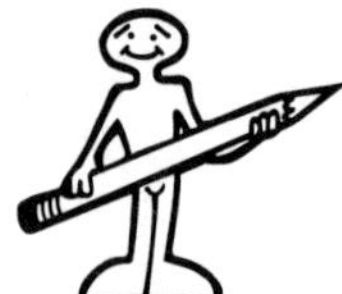

Notes

PHYSIOLOGY OF THE NERVOUS SYSTEM

A. Central nervous system (CNS).
  1. Brain.
  2. Spinal cord.
B. Peripheral nervous system (PNS).
  1. Twelve pairs of cranial nerves.
  2. Thirty-one pairs of spinal nerves.
  3. Autonomic nervous system.
    a. Sympathetic system.
    b. Parasympathetic system.

Cells of the Nervous System

A. Neuron—the functional cell of the nervous system.
B. Function/classification.
  a. Afferent neurons (sensory) transmit information to the CNS.
  b. Efferent neurons (motor) transmit information away from the CNS.
  c. Synapses or synaptic terminals are areas of chemical transmission of an impulse from the axon of one neuron to the dendrites of another neuron.
C. Supporting cells provide support, nourishment, and protection to the neuron.
D. Myelin sheath.
  a. Dense membrane or insulator around the axon.
  b. Facilitates function of the neuron.
  c. Contributes to the blood-brain barrier to protect the central nervous system against harmful molecules.
E. Nerve regeneration—entire neuron is unable to undergo complete regeneration.
  1. Neuron regeneration in the CNS is very limited, possibly due to the lack of neurilemma.
  2. Scar tissue is a major deterrent to successful cellular regeneration.
F. Impulse conduction.
  1. Reflex arc.
    a. Reflex arc is the functional unit which provides pathways over which nerve impulses travel.
    b. Passage of impulses over a reflex arc is called a reflex act or a reflex.
    c. Reflex arc—The afferent neuron carries the stimulus to the spine, integrates it into and through the spine (CNS) to the efferent neuron, and crosses the synapse with the message from the CNS to the organ or muscle which responds to the stimuli. This is the sequence of events evaluated when testing the deep tendon reflexes.
  2. Synaptic transmission.
    a. A chemical synapse maintains a one-way communication link between neurons.
    b. Chemical neurotransmitters (neuro-mediators) facilitate the transmission of the impulse across the synapse.
      (1) Acetylcholine.
      (2) Norepinephrine.
      (3) Dopamine.
      (4) Histamine.
    c. Impulses pass in only one direction.

Central Nervous System

The brain and the spinal cord within the vertebral column make up the *central nervous system*.

A. The brain and the spinal column are protected by the rigid bony structure of the skull and the vertebral column.
B. Meninges—protective membranes that cover the brain and are continuous with those of the spinal cord.
  1. Pia mater—a delicate vascular connective tissue layer that covers the surfaces of the brain and the spinal column; part of the blood-brain barrier.
  2. Arachnoid—a delicate nonvascular, waterproof membrane that encases the entire CNS; the subarachnoid space contains the cerebral spinal fluid.
  3. Dura mater—a tough membrane immediately outside the arachnoid; provides protection to the brain and spinal cord.
C. Cerebral spinal fluid (CSF).
  1. Serves to cushion and protect the brain and spinal cord; brain literally floats in CSF.
  2. CSF is clear, colorless, watery fluid; approximately 100 to 200 cc total volume, with a normal fluid pressure of 70 to 150 mm of water (average—125 cm water pressure).
  3. Formation and circulation of CSF (Figure 15-2).
    a. Fluid is secreted by the choroid plexus located in the ventricles of the brain.
    b. CSF flows through the lateral ventricles into the third ventricle, then flows through the Aqueduct

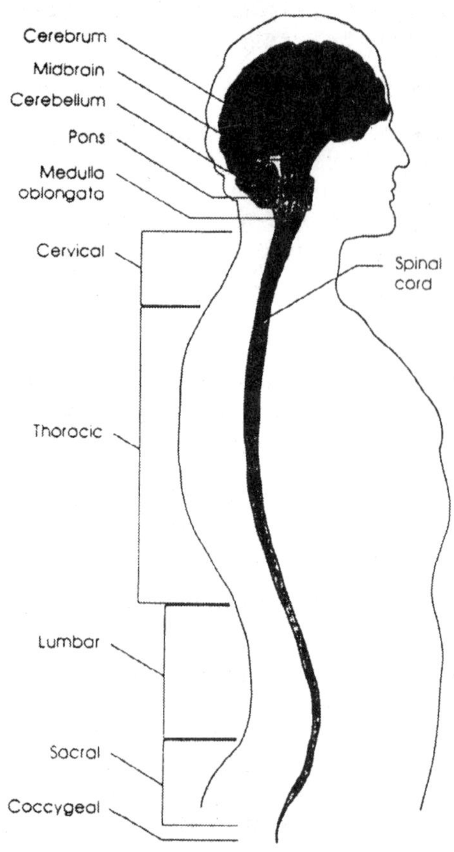

Figure 20-1:Major divisions of the central nervous system
Reprinted with permission: Phipps, WJ, Sands, JK, & Marek, JF (1999). *Medical Surgical Nursing: Concepts & Clinical Practice*, 6th ed. Philadelphia: Mosby, p 1673.

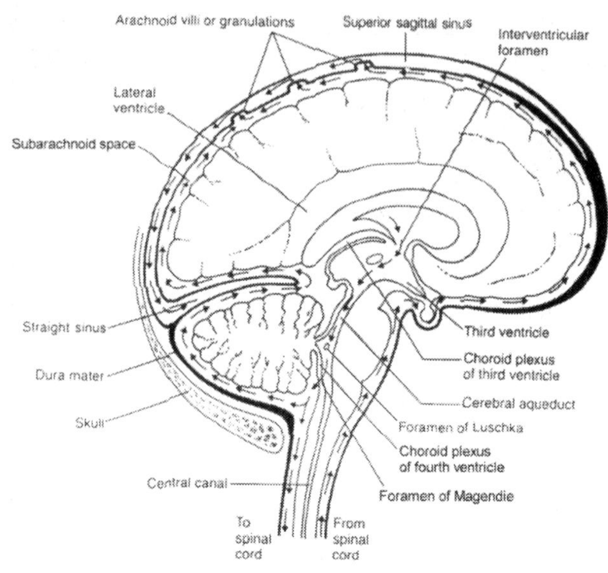

Figure 20-2: Circulation of cerebrospinal fluid.
Reprinted with permission: Ignatavicius, D., Workman,L., Mishler, M., (1995). *Medical Surgical Nursing: A Nursing Process Approach,* Phildelphia: W.B. Saunders, p. 1098.

of Sylvius into the fourth ventricle, where the central canal of the spinal column opens.

c. From the fourth ventricle, CSF flows around the spinal cord and brain.

d. Since CSF is formed continuously; it is reabsorbed at a comparable rate by the arachnoid villi.

D. Brain.

1. Cerebrum—the largest portion of the brain; separated into hemispheres; the cerebral cortex is the surface layer of each hemisphere.

2. Major lobes of the central cortex.

a. Frontal.

(1) Coordination of voluntary skeletal muscle movement.

(2) Abstract thinking, morals, judgment.

(3) Broca's area for speech, motor speech area, expressive (ability to speak and write).

b. Parietal.

(1) Interprets sensory nerve impulses (pain, temperature, touch).

(2) Maintains proprioception.

(3) Recognition of size, texture, and shape of objects.

c. Temporal.

(1) Auditory area—interprets meaning of certain sounds.

(2) Wernicke's area for speech, sensory speech area, comprehension and formulation of speech (understanding spoken and written words).

d. Occipital area—interprets vision and controls ability to understand written words.

3. Motor areas of the cerebral cortex.

a. Primary function is coordination and control of skeletal muscle activity.

b. Corticospinal tracts (pyramidal tracts).

(1) Descending tract from the motor area of the cerebral cortex to the spinal cord.

(2) Majority of motor nerves cross in the medulla to the opposite side before descending into the spinal cord.

(3) These corticospinal tracts do not cross over.

c. Brain cells and the nerve fibers in the descending tracts of the central nervous system are called upper motor neurons.

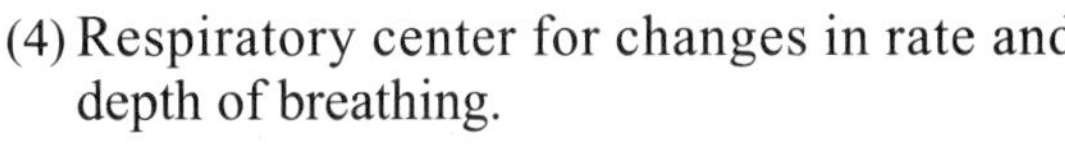

Box Text 20-1: Elderly Care Focus
Causes of Confusion in Elderly Client

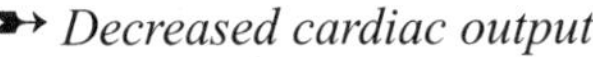

➻ *Decreased cardiac output*
- Myocardial infarction
- Dysrythmias
- CHF

➻ *Hypoxia/respiratory acidosis*
- Pneumonia
- Infection
- Hypoventilation

➻ *Neurological*
- Vascular insufficiency
- Infections
- Cerebral edema

➻ *Metabolic*
- Electrolyte imbalance
- Hypo/hyperglycemia
- Dehydration

➻ *Environmental*
- Strange surroundings
- Hypo/Hyperthermia
- Sensory overload/deprivation

4. Movement is controlled by:
   a. Cerebral cortex—voluntary initiation of motor activity.
   b. Basal ganglia—assist to maintain posture.
   c. Cerebellum—coordinates muscle movement.
5. Cerebellum—attached to the medulla and the pons.
   a. Primarily concerned with coordination of muscular activity and maintenance of equilibrium.
   b. Nerve fibers spread upward to the cerebrum and downward to the pons, medulla, and spinal cord.
      (1) Visual reflexes—pupillary constriction and movement of the eye.
      (2) Auditory reflexes—turning of the head toward sound.
6. Brain stem—consists of the pons and the medulla.
   a. Pons—contains the reticular formation, which is responsible for alertness.
   b. Medulla oblongata—a continuation of the spinal cord as it enters into the cranial vault in the brain.
      (1) Conduction center and crossing center for the upper motor neurons.
      (2) Maintains control of cardiac rate.
      (3) Vasomotor center for constriction and dilation of vessels.
      (4) Respiratory center for changes in rate and depth of breathing.
      (5) Vomiting reflex center.
      (6) Swallowing reflex center.
   c. Thalamus.
      (1) Organization and distribution of incoming sensory impulses.
      (2) Activities related to consciousness.
   d. Hypothalamus.
      (1) Regulation of visceral activities—body temperature, motility and secretions of the GI tract, arterial blood pressure.
      (2) Nerve connections with the thalamus and the cerebral cortex make it possible for our emotions to influence visceral activity.
      (3) Regulation of endocrine glands via influence on the pituitary gland.
      (4) Neurosecretion of antidiuretic hormone (ADH) which is stored in the pituitary.
7. Cerebral circulation.
   a. The internal carotid arteries enter the cranial vault at the temporal area.
   b. The circle of Willis is an arterial anastomosis at the base of the brain. The circle ensures continued circulation if one of the main vessels is disrupted.

E. Spinal cord.
1. The spinal cord is continuous with the medulla and extends down the vertebral column to the level of the first or second lumbar vertebrae.
2. Each column is divided into functional groups of nerve fibers.
   a. Ascending tracts—transmit impulses to the brain (sensory pathway).
   b. Descending tracts—transmit impulses from the brain to the various levels of the spinal cord (motor pathways).
3. Structure.
   a. Intervertebral disks lie between each vertebra to provide flexibility to the spinal column.
   b. Nucleus pulposus is a gelatin substance in the vertebral disc.
4. Upper motor neurons—originate in the brain; transmit impulses from the brain to the lower motor neuron.
5. Lower motor neurons—originate in the spinal cord; transmit impulses to the muscles and organs. These neurons form the reflex arc.
6. Reflex activity.

Table 20-1: CRANIAL NERVES

	NAME	FUNCTION
I	Olfactory	Sense of smell
II	Optic	Vision - conducts information from the retina
III	Oculomotor	Downward and outward movement of the eye Pupillary constriction and accommodation Muscle of the upper eyelid (ability to keep the eye open)
IV	Trochlear	Movement of the eye
V	Trigeminal:	
	Ophthalmic	Corneal reflex
	Maxillary	Sensory fibers of the face
	Mandibular	Motor nerves for chewing and swallowing
VI	Abducens	Inward movement of the eye
VII	Facial	Facial expression Sense of taste on anterior tongue Muscle of the eyelid (ability to close the eye)
VIII	Acoustic	Reception of hearing and maintenance of equilibrium
IX	Glossopharyngeal	Sense of taste on posterior tongue Salivation Swallowing or gag reflex
X	Vagus nerve	Assists in swallowing action Motor fibers to larynx for speech Innervation of organs in thorax and abdomen Important in respiratory, cardiac, and circulatory reflexes
XI	Accessory (Spinal)	Ability to rotate the head and raise the shoulder
XII	Hypoglossal	Muscles of the tongue

a. The reflex arc must be intact; the spinal cord serves as the connection between the afferent pathway (sensory) and the efferent pathway (motor).

b. By testing the reflex arc (deep tendon reflexes), the lower motor neuron and the sensory/motor fibers from the spinal column can be evaluated. For example, if the biceps reflex is normal, the lower motor neurons and the nerve fibers at C5 and C6 are intact.

c. Babinski reflex—normal up to one year; should not be positive in clients over one year of age.

Peripheral Nervous System (PNS)

The cranial and spinal nerves, which connect the CNS with the body parts, constitute the PNS.

A. Cranial nerves (Table 20-1).

1. Twelve pairs of cranial nerves.
2. Originate from under the surface of the brain.

B. Spinal nerves.

1. Each pair of nerves is numbered according to the level of the spinal cord from which it originates.
2. Each spinal nerve is connected to the cord by two roots.
   a. Dorsal (posterior root)—a sensory nerve carrying messages to the CNS.
   b. Ventral (anterior root)—a motor nerve carrying neuron messages to glands and to the peripheral areas.

C. Somatic nervous system—fibers which connect the CNS with the structures of the body wall.

D. Autonomic nervous system—regulates involuntary activity (cardiovascular, respiratory, metabolic, body temperature, etc.).

1. Consists of two divisions that have antagonistic activity.
2. Parasympathetic division—maintains normal body functions.
3. Sympathetic division—prepares the body to meet a challenge or an emergency (preparation for "fight/flight") (Table 20-2).
4. Most of the organs of the body receive innervation from both the parasympathetic and the sympathetic divisions. The divisions are usually antagonistic in effect on individual organs—one stimulates, the other relaxes.
5. Chemical mediators—facilitate transmission of impulses in the autonomic nervous system.
   a. Acetylcholine is released by the fibers in both divisions of the autonomic nervous system.
   b. Norepinephrine released primarily by the sympathetic division.

System Assessment

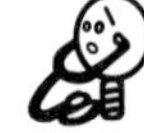

A. History.

1. Neurologic history.
   a. Avoid suggesting symptoms to the client.
   b. The manner in which the problems began and the overall course of the illness are very important.
   c. Mental status must be assessed before assuming the history data from the client is accurate.

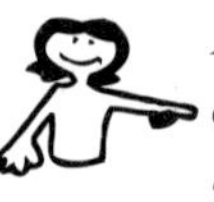

***NURSING PRIORITY:** In elderly clients assess orientation and mental status prior to continuing assessment (Box 20-2).*

2. Medical history.
   a. Chronic, concurrent medical problems.

Table 20-2: AUTONOMIC NERVOUS SYSTEM

AREA AFFECTED	SYMPATHETIC	PARASYMPATHETIC
Pupil	Dilates	Constricts
Bronchi	Dilate	Constrict
Heart	Increases rate	Decreases rate
Gastrointestinal	Inhibits peristalsis	Stimulates peristalsis
	Stimulates sphincter	Inhibits sphincters
Bladder	Relaxes bladder muscle	Contracts bladder muscle
	Constricts sphincter	Relaxes sphincter
Adrenal glands	Increases secretion of epinephrine and norepinephrine	

b. Medications (especially tranquilizers, sedatives, narcotics, etc.).

c. Pregnancy and delivery history of infants and young children.

d. Sequence of growth and development.

3. Family history—presence of hereditary or congenital problems.

4. Personal history—activities of daily living, any change in routine.

5. History and symptoms of current problem.

a. Paralysis or paresthesia.

b. Syncope, dizziness.

c. Headache.

d. Speech problems.

e. Visual problems.

f. Changes in personality.

g. Memory loss.

h. Nausea, vomiting.

B. Physical assessment.

1. General observation of client.

a. Posture, gait; coordination, check Romberg's test.

b. Position of rest for the infant or young child.

c. Personal hygiene, grooming.

d. Evaluate speech and ability to communicate.

(1) Pace of speech—rapid, slow, halting.

(2) Clarity—slurred or distinct.

(3) Tone—high pitched, rough.

(4) Vocabulary—appropriate choice of words.

Box 20-2: Elderly Focus

Assessing Neurologic Function in Elderly

Signs of Cognitive Impairment

- Significant memory loss (person, place, and time).
- Person—does he know who he is and can he give you his full name?
- Place—can he identify his home address and where he is now?
- Time—what was the most recent holiday; what month, time of day, day of the week?
- Does he show a lack of judgment?
- Is he agitated and/or suspicious?
- From his appearance, and family response, does he have probems with ADLs?
- Short-term memory—can the client recall your name, name of the President, or his doctor?
- Short term recall—ask the client to name three or four common objects and ask him to recall them within the next 5 minutes.
- Does the client have sensory deficits (hearing and vision) of which he is not aware?

e. Facial features may suggest specific syndromes in children.

2. Mental status (must take into consideration the client's culture and educational background).

NCLEX ALERT: *The level of consciousness and mental status are the most critical assessment data for the client with neurological deficits.*

a. General appearance and behavior.

b. Level of consciousness.

(1) Oriented to time, person, place.

(2) Appropriate response to verbal and tactile stimuli.

(3) Memory, problem-solving abilities.

c. Mood.

d. Thought content and intellectual capacity.

3. Assess pupillary status and eye movements.

a. Size of pupils should be equal.

b. Reaction of pupils.

(1) Accommodation—pupillary constriction to accommodate near vision.

(2) Direct light reflex—constriction of pupil when light is shone directly into eye.

(3) Consensual reflex—constriction of the opposite eye for the direct light reflex.

c. Evaluate ability to move eye.

(1) Note nystagmus—fine, jerking eye movement.

(2) Ability of eyes to move together.

(3) Resting position should be at mid- position of the eye socket.

d. PERRLA—indicates that pupils are equal, round, reactive to light and accommodation is present.

4. Evaluate motor function.

a. Assess face and upper extremities for equality of movement and sensation.

b. Evaluate appropriateness of motor movement; spontaneous and on command.

c. Movement of extremities should always be evaluated bilaterally, comparing tone, strength, and muscle movement of each side.

d. Presence of inappropriate, non-purposeful movement (i.e., posturing).

(1) Decerebrate—extension and adduction of the arms, hyperextension of the legs.

(2) Decorticate—flexion, internal rotation of the arms, extension of the legs.

(3) Presence of non-purposeful involuntary movements such as tremors, jerking, twitching.

e. Ability of an infant to suck and to swallow.

f. Asymmetrical contraction of facial muscles.

5. Evaluate reflexes.

a. Gag or cough reflex.

b. Swallow reflex.

c. Corneal reflex.

d. Babinski reflex—normal is negative in adults and children over one year; positive sign is dorsal flexion of the foot and large toe with fanning of the other toes.

e. Deep tendon reflexes (simple stretch reflex).

6. Assess vital signs and correlate with other data; changes often occur slowly and the overall trend needs to be evaluated.

a. Blood pressure and pulse—intracranial problems precipitate changes; blood pressure may increase and pulse rate may decrease.

b. Respirations—rate, depth, and rhythm are sensitive indicators of intracranial problems.

(1) Cheyne-Stokes—periodic breathing in which hyperpnea alternates with apnea.

(2) Neurogenic hyperventilation—regular, rapid, deep hyperpnea.

(3) Ataxic—completely irregular pattern with random deep and shallow respirations.

c. Temperature—evaluate changes in temperature as related to a neurological control versus infection.

DISORDERS OF THE NEUROLOGIC SYSTEM

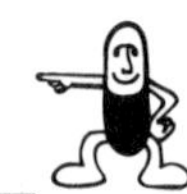

Increased Intracranial Pressure (IICP)

❑ **An increase in intracranial pressure occurs any time there is an increase in the size of the intracranial contents.**

A. The cranial vault is rigid and there is minimal area for expansion of the intracranial components.

B. An increase in any one of the components necessitates a reciprocal change in other cranial contents; this frequently results in ischemia of brain tissue. An increase in ICP results from one of the following:

1. Increased intracranial blood volume (vasodilation).
2. Increased CSF fluid.
3. Increase in the bulk of the brain tissue (edema).

C. Cerebral edema.

1. Edema occurs when there is an increase in the volume of brain tissue caused by increase in the permeability of the walls of the cerebral vessels. Protein-rich fluid leaks into the extracellular space. Most often the cause of IICP in adults; reaches maximum pressure in 48-72 hours.
2. Cytotoxic (cellular) edema occurs as a result of hypoxia. This results in abnormal accumulation of fluid within the cell (intracellular) and a decrease of extracellular fluid.

D. In compromised respiratory status (↑ $PaCO_2$) the cerebral arteries dilate with a decrease in pH and development of acidosis.

1. An acidotic state increases cerebral vascular dilatation which increases cerebral vascular blood flow and increases intracranial pressure.
2. Hyperventilation may be utilized as part of treatment to decrease the effects of acidosis on IICP.

E. Regardless of the cause, IICP will result in progressive neurological deterioration; the specific deficiencies seen are determined by the area of compression of brain tissue.

F. If the infant's cranial suture lines are open, increased ICP will cause separation of the suture lines and increase the circumference of the head.

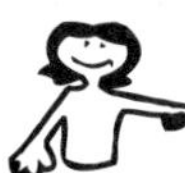

NURSING PRIORITY: There is no single set of symptoms for all clients, symptoms depend on cause, and how rapidly it develops.

Assessment

1. Risk factors/etiology.
   a. Cerebral edema secondary to the initial damage.
   b. Brain tumors.
   c. Intracranial hemorrhage due to closed head injuries.
   d. Intracranial hemorrhage due to ruptured vessels.
   e. Cerebral embolism, resulting in necrosis and edema of areas supplied by the involved vessel.
   f. Cerebral thrombosis, resulting in ischemia of the area and leading to edema and congestion of affected area.
   g. Hydrocephalus.
2. Clinical manifestations (bedside neuro checks).

NCLEX ALERT: *Determine changes in a client's neurological status. Be able to rapidly evaluate the client and recognize changes in the neuro signs that indicate an increase in the intracranial pressure.*

   a. Assess for changes in level of consciousness.

NURSING PRIORITY: The first sign of a change in the level of intracranial pressure is change in level of consciousness; this may progress to a decrease in level of consciousness.

      (1) Any alteration in level of consciousness (early sign for both adults and children)—irritability, restlessness, confusion, lethargy, difficult to arouse, etc. may be significant.
      (2) Inappropriate response, verbal and motor response to command, delayed response.
      (3) As the client loses consciousness, hearing is the last sense to be lost.

   b. Changes in vital signs.

NURSING PRIORITY: Cushing's triad—increasing systolic pressure, decreased pulse rate, and irregular respirations. IICP is well- established when this occurs.

      (1) Increase in systolic blood pressure with increase in pulse pressure.
      (2) Decrease pulse rate.
      (3) Alteration in respiratory pattern (Cheyne-Stokes, hyperventilation, ataxic).
      (4) Assess temperature with regard to overall problems, temperature usually increases.

   c. Pupillary response - pupils should be in midline, equal in size and equally reactive to direct light.
      (1) Ipsilateral—pupillary changes occurring on the same side as the lesion.
      (2) Contralateral—pupillary changes occurring on the side opposite the lesion.
      (3) Unilateral dilatation of pupils.
      (4) Pupillary response to light and accommodation, pupils equal with brisk response is normal; may change to slow, sluggish reaction then progress to fixed, dilated with no response.
   d. Decrease in motor and sensory function.
      (1) Ability to move all extremities with equal strength, no weakness or hemiplegia noted.
      (2) Failure to withdraw from painful stimuli.
      (3) Posturing - decerebrate or decorticate.
      (4) Seizure activity.
   e. Headache.
      (1) Constant with increasing intensity.
      (2) Aggravated by movement.
   f. Vomiting—projectile vomiting with no nausea.
   g. Infants.
      (1) Tense, bulging fontanel.
      (2) Separated cranial sutures.
      (3) Increasing frontal-occipital circumference.
      (4) High-pitched cry.
3. Diagnostics (Appendix 20-1).
   a. CAT scan; electroencephalogram (EEG).
   b. Magnetic Resonance Imaging (MRI) - Appendix 20-1.1
   c. Cerebral angiogram.
   d. Direct intracranial pressure monitoring.
   e. Romberg test—measures balance; stand with feet together and arms at side, first with eyes open, then with eyes closed for 20-30 seconds.
   f. Caloric testing—test is performed at bedside by introducing cold water into the external auditory canal. If the eighth cranial nerve is stimulated, nystagmus rotates toward the irrigated ear. If no nystagmus occurs, pathology is present.
   g. Doll's eyes phenomena.

(1) Doll's eye are normal when the client's head is moved side to side and the eyes move from side to side (positive test).

(2) Doll's eyes are abnormal when the client's head is moved from side to side and the eyes remain in a fixed, midline position (negative test).

h. Papilledema—edema of the optic nerve; done by examining retina area with an ophthalmoscope.

i. Lumbar puncture is generally not performed; decrease in CSF pressure could precipitate herniation of the brain stem.

Treatment

1. Treatment of the underlying cause of increasing pressure.
2. IV fluids of normal saline; D_5W tends to potentiate cerebral edema.
3. Medications.
   a. Osmotic diuretics.
   b. Corticosteroids.
   c. Anticonvulsants.
4. Maintain adequate ventilation and/or hyperventilation (mechanical ventilation) lowers $PaCo_2$ to produce vasoconstriction of cerebral vessels.
5. Placement of ventriculo-peritoneal shunt; or decompression surgery which may involve removal of brain tissue.

Complications

1. Spinal fluid leaks, especially in client with basilar skull fracture, may cause meningitis.
2. Herniation—shifting of the intracranial contents from one compartment to another; involves herniation through the tentorium; affects area for control of vital functions.
3. Permanent brain damage.

Nursing Intervention

✦ *Goal: to identify and decrease problem of IICP.*

1. Neuro checks as indicated by client status (Glasgow Coma Scale, Table 20-3).
2. Maintain semi-Fowler's position to promote venous drainage and respiratory function.

NCLEX ALERT: *Change client's position. If the client with IICP develops hypovolemic shock, do not place client in Trendelenburg position.*

Table 20-3: GLASGOW COMA SCALE

Eye opening	
Spontaneous	4
To sound	3
To pain	2
Never	1
Motor response	
Obeys commands	6
Localizes pain	5
Normal flexion (withdrawal)	4
Abnormal flexion posturing	3
Extension posturing	2
None	1
Verbal response	
Oriented	5
Confused conversation	4
Inappropriate words	3
Incomprehensible sounds	2
None	1

A score of 7 or less indicates coma.

The highest possible score is 15.

3. Change client's position slowly, avoid extreme hip flexion and extreme rotation and flexion of neck. Both these activities affect the intra-abdominal and intrathoracic pressures which can increase ICP.
4. Monitor urine osmolarity and specific gravity.
5. Evaluate intake and output.
   a. In response to diuretics.
   b. As correlated with changes in daily weight.
   c. For complications of diabetes insipidus (Chapter 13).
6. Maintain intake evenly over twenty-four-hour time period.
7. Sedatives and narcotics can depress respiration; use with caution because they mask symptoms indicating increasing IICP.
8. Client should avoid strenuous coughing, Valsalva's maneuver, and isometric muscle exercises.
9. In infants, measure frontal-occipital circumference to evaluate increase in size of the head.
10. Control hyperthermia.

✦ *Goal: to maintain respiratory function.*

***NURSING PRIORITY:** Airway is one of the most common problems in the unconscious client; position him to maintain patent airway or use airway adjuncts.*

1. Prevent respiratory problems of immobility.

Table 20-4: INCREASING INTRACRANIAL PRESSURE

Adult
Early - Restless, irritable, lethargic.
Intermediate -Unequal pupil response, projectile vomiting, changes in vital signs.
Late - Decreased level of consciousness, decreased reflexes, change in respiratory pattern, dilated pupils.

Infant, Child
Early - Poor feeding, tense fontanel, headache, nausea and vomiting, increased pitch of cry, unsteady gait.
Intermediate - less than 18mo old -increased head circumference, bulging fontanel; shrill cry, severe headache, blurred vision.
Late - same as adult.

2. Evaluate patency of airway frequently; as level of consciousness decreases, client is at increased risk for accumulating secretions and respiratory obstruction by the tongue.
3. Keep $PaCO_2$ levels within normal to low range (hyperventilation).
4. Suction as necessary, but in short duration.
5. Client may require intubation and control on a ventilator (Chapter 15-8).

✦ *Goal: to protect from injury.*

1. Maintain seizure precautions (Appendix 20-5).
2. Restrain client only if absolutely necessary; struggling against restraints will increase ICP.
3. Do not clean the ears or nasal passages of a head injury or neurosurgery client. Check for evidence of CSF leak: CSF has glucose in it; test it with a dipstix; also leaves a yellow "halo" stain.
4. Aspiration is a major problem in the unconscious client. Assess the swallow reflex and gag reflex in clients who are not fully conscious; position the client in semi-Fowler's for tube feeding.
5. Maintain quiet, nonstimulating environment.
6. Inspect eyes and prevent corneal ulceration.
   a. Protective closing of eyes if the eyes remain open.
   b. Normal saline irrigation or methylcellulose drops to restore moisture.

✦ *Goal: to maintain psychological equilibrium.*

1. Neuro checks are a continuous reminder of potential problem.
2. Encourage verbalization of fears regarding condition.
3. Give simple explanation of procedures to client and family.
4. Altered states of consciousness will cause increased anxiety and confusion; maintain reality orientation.
5. If client is unconscious, continue to talk to him/her; describe procedures and treatments; always assume that client can hear.
6. Assist parents and family to work through feelings of guilt and anger.

✦ *Goal: to prevent complications of immobility (Chapter 3).*

✦ *Goal: to maintain elimination.*

1. Urinary incontinence—may use condom catheter or indwelling bladder catheter.
2. Keep perineal area free from excoriation.
3. Monitor bowel function; evaluate for fecal impaction.

Self/Home Care

1. Teach client and family signs of IICP.
2. Call the doctor for:
   a. Changes in vision.
   b. Increased drainage from incision area or clear drainage in the ears.
   c. Abrupt changes in sleeping patterns, or irritability.
   d. Headache that does not respond to medication.
   e. Changes in coordination.
   f. Slurred speech.
3. Review care of surgical incision, wounds, or drains.

Brain Tumors

A. Brain tumors may be benign, malignant, or metastatic; malignant brain tumors rarely metastasize outside the CNS.

B. Supratentorial—tumors occurring within the anterior two-thirds of the brain, primarily the cerebrum.

C. Infratentorial—tumors occurring in the posterior third of the brain (or below the tentorium); primarily in the cerebellum or the brainstem.

D. Regardless of the origin, site, or presence of malignancy, problems of increased intracranial pressure occur because of the limited area in the brain to accommodate an increase in the intracranial contents.

Assessment

1. Risk factors/etiology.
   a. Adults—highest incidence between 55 and 70 years of age.
   b. Prognosis is generally poorer in the infant than in older children.
   c. Presence of metastatic cancer of the lung or breast.
2. Clinical manifestations—symptoms correlate with the area of the brain initially involved.

a. Headache.

(1) Recurrent.

(2) More severe in the morning.

(3) Affected by position.

(4) Headache in infant may be identified by persistent, irritated crying and head-rolling.

b. Vomiting—initially with or without nausea; progressively becomes projectile.

c. Papilledema (edema of the optic disc).

d. Seizures (focal or generalized).

e. Dizziness and vertigo.

f. Mental status changes - lethargy and drowsiness, confusion, disorientation and personality changes.

g. Localized manifestations:

(1) Focal weakness - hemiparesis.

h. Sensory disturbances.

(1) Language disturbances.

(2) Coordination disturbances.

(3) Visual disturbances.

i. Head tilt—child may tilt the head due to damage to extraocular muscles; may be first indication of a decrease in visual acuity.

j. Changes in vital signs indicative of increasing ICP.

k. Cranial enlargement in the infant under eighteen months old.

3. Diagnostics (Appendix 20-1).

a. Clinical manifestations exhibited in the neurological exam.

b. EEG.

c. CAT scan.

d. Brain scan.

Treatment

1. Medical.

a. Dexamethasone (Appendix 6-8).

b. Anticonvulsants (Appendix 20-2).

c. Radiation and chemotherapy if malignant.

2. Surgical excision—craniotomy.

Complications

Meningitis, brain stem herniation; diabetes insipidus, inappropriate ADH secretion (Chapter 13).

Nursing Intervention

✦ *Goal: to provide appropriate preoperative nursing intervention.*

1. General preoperative care with exceptions as noted (Chapter 3).
2. If there is increased ICP, do not administer an enema.
3. Prepare client, family, and parents for appearance of the client postoperatively.
4. Encourage verbalization regarding concerns of surgery.
5. Skin prep is usually done in surgery.

✦ *Goal: to monitor changes in increased intracranial pressure postoperative craniotomy.*

1. Neuro checks as necessary.
2. Maintain pulmonary function and hygiene.
3. Antiemetics to decrease vomiting and possibility of aspiration.
4. Discourage vigorous coughing.
5. Careful evaluation of the level of consciousness; regression to more lethargic or irritable state may be indicative of increasing ICP.
6. Evaluate dressing.

a. Location and amount of drainage.

b. Evaluate for CSF leak through the incision.

7. Maintain semi-Fowler's position if there is a spinal fluid leak from ears or nose.
8. Position postoperatively for infratentorial surgery.

a. Bed should be flat.

b. Position client on either side; avoid supine position.

c. Maintain head and neck in midline.

9. Position postoperatively for supratentorial surgery—semi- to low-Fowler's.
10. Trendelenburg position is contraindicated in both types of surgery.
11. Maintain fluid regulation.

a. Begin clear liquids PO after client is awake and swallow and gag reflexes have returned.

b. Closely monitor intake and output.

12. Evaluate neuro status in response to fluid balance and diuretics.
13. Evaluate changes in temperature—may be due to respiratory complications or to alteration in the function of the hypothalamus.
14. Provide appropriate postoperative pain relief.

a. Avoid narcotic analgesics.

b. Acetominophen is frequently used.

c. Maintain quiet, dim atmosphere.

d. Avoid sudden movements.

15. Prevent complications of immobility (Chapter 3).

16. Maintain seizure precautions (Appendix 20-3).

Self/Home Care

See care for client with increasing intracranial pressure.

Head Injury

A. Classification.
  1. Closed—are most often from blunt trauma.
  2. Open—injuries that penetrate the skull.

B. Children and infants are more capable of absorbing direct impact due to pliability of the skull.

C. Coup—Contre-coup injury—damage to the site of impact (coup) and damage on the side opposite of the injury (contre-coup).

D. Primary injury to the brain occurs by compression, tearing and shearing stresses on vessels and nerves.

E. Although brain volume remains unchanged, secondary injury occurs with the cerebral edema in response to the primary injury and frequently precipitates an increase in intracranial pressure.

F. Types of head injuries.
  1. Concussion—no break in skull or dura.
    a. May or may not lose consciousness for a short period of time; confusion, dizziness, amnesia, and headache are common.
    b. Glasgow Coma Scale is often normal.
    c. Usually does not cause permanent damage.
  2. Contusion (bruising).
    a. Multiple areas of petechial hemorrhages.
    b. May cause focal disturbances.
    c. Blood supply is altered in the area of injury, swelling, ischemia, and occurrence of IICP.
  3. Intracranial hemorrhage.
    a. Epidural (extradural) hematoma—a large vessel (often a meningeal artery or vein) in the dura mater is damaged; a hematoma rapidly forms between the dura and the skull, precipitating an increase in intracranial pressure.
      (1) Momentary loss of consciousness, then free of symptoms (lucid period).
      (2) Symptoms of increasing ICP may develop within minutes after the lucid interval.
      (3) Tentorial herniation may occur without immediate intervention.
    b. Subdural hematoma—bleeding between the dura and arachnoid area, usually due to the rupture of veins in the subdural space.
      (1) Develops more slowly
      (2) Subacute may not become symptomatic for several days to weeks.
      (3) Acute injury is manifested within 24 hours of the injury.
      (4) Symptoms of increasing intracranial pressure develop gradually.

Assessment

1. Risk factors/etiology.
  a. History of trauma.
  b. Epidural hematomas are uncommon in children under four years of age.
  c. Subdural hematomas are common in infants and may be the result of birth trauma.
2. Clinical manifestations—see individual types of injury.
3. Diagnostics.
  a. Neurologic history.
  b. Skull X-ray.
  c. MRI.
  d. CAT scan.
  e. EEG.

Complications

Increased intracranial pressure, meningitis, diabetes insipidus, permanent brain damage.

Treatment

***NURSING PRIORITY:** The primary objectives of treatment of the head injury client are: to maintain patent airway; to prevent hypoxia and hypercapnia resulting in acidosis; to identify occurrence of IICP.*

1. Majority of clients who experience concussion are treated at home.
2. A period of unconsciousness or presence of seizures are considered serious indications of injury.
3. Surgical intervention.
  a. Burr holes to evacuate the hematoma.
  b. Craniotomy.

Nursing Intervention

✦ *Goal: to provide instruction for care of the client in the home environment(Table 20-5).*

1. Problems frequently do not occur until 24 hours or more after the initial injury.
2. Observe the client for increased periods of sleep; if client is asleep, awaken every 2 to 3 hours to see if he can be aroused normally.

Table 20-5: DISCHARGE INSTRUCTIONS FOR HEAD INJURY CLIENTS

Arouse the person every 3-4 hours for the first 24 hours.
Anticipate complaints of dizziness, headaches.
Do not allow client to blow his nose, try to prevent sneezing.
No alcohol or sedatives for sleep.
Acetaminophen for headaches.
No exercising over next 2-3 days.

Call the doctor for:
Change in vision, blurred or diplopia.
Poor coordination -walking, grasping.
Drainage (serous or bloody) from the nose or ears.
Forceful vomiting.
Increasing sleepiness, more difficult to arouse.
Slurred speech.
Headache that does not respond to medication and continues to get worse.
Occurrence of a seizure.

3. Maintain contact with physician for re-evaluation if complications occur.
4. Doctor should be notified when there is:
   a. Any changes in LOC (increased drowsiness, confusion).
   b. Inability to arouse client.
   c. Seizures occur.
   d. Bleeding or watery drainage from the ears or nose.
   e. Loss of feeling or sensation in any extremity.
   f. Blurred vision.
   g. Slurring speech.
   h. Vomiting.

NCLEX ALERT: *Determine family's understanding of the consequences of the client's illness. Written instructions should be given to the client and to the family. Increased anxiety may affect the comprehension of verbal directions.*

✦ *Goal: to maintain homeostasis; monitor and identify early symptoms of increased intracranial pressure.*

1. Bedrest and clear liquids initially.
2. Frequent neuro checks for increased ICP.
   a. Change or decrease in level of consciousness frequently the first indication.
   b. Instruct head injury clients not to cough, sneeze or blow his nose.
3. Evaluate drainage from nose, ears and mouth.
   a. Do not clean out the ears—place loose cotton in the auditory canal and change as soiled.
   b. Check continuous clear drainage from the nose with a dextrostix; if glucose is present, it is indicative of CSF.
4. Seizure precautions (Appendix 20-5).
5. Maintain adequate fluid intake via IV or PO; do not overhydrate.
6. Assess for other undetected injuries.

✦ *Goal: to provide appropriate nursing intervention for the client experiencing an increase in intracranial pressure (see nursing goals for IICP).*

Hydrocephalus

❑ **A condition caused by an imbalance in the production and absorption of CSF in the ventricles of the brain.**

Classification

1. Noncommunicating—circulation of CSF is blocked within the ventricular system of the brain; may also be referred to as obstructive.
2. Communicating—CSF flows freely within the ventricular system but is not adequately absorbed.
3. Frequently associated with meningomyelocele in the newborn.

Assessment

1. Risk factors/etiology.
   a. Neonate—usually the result of a congenital malformation.
   b. Older child, adult.
      (1) Space occupying lesion.
      (2) Pre-existing developmental defects.
2. Clinical manifestations—infant.
   a. Head enlargement - increasing circumference in excess of normal 2 cm per month for first 3 months.
   b. Separation of cranial suture lines.
   c. Fontanel becomes tense and bulging.
   d. Dilated scalp veins.
   e. Frontal enlargement, bulging "sunset eyes."
   f. Symptoms of increasing ICP.
3. Clinical manifestations—older child, adult.
   a. Symptoms of increasing ICP.
   b. Specific manifestations related to site of the lesion.
4. Diagnostics.
   a. Same as for brain tumor.
   b. Increasing head circumference is diagnostic in infants.

Treatment

1. Noncommunicating and communicating.
   a. Ventriculoatrial shunt—CSF is shunted into the right atrium, usually done inolder children..
   b. Ventriculoperitoneal shunt—CSF is shunted into the peritoneum (preferred).
2. Obstructive—removal of the obstruction (cyst, hematoma, tumor).

Nursing Intervention

✦ *Goal: to monitor for the development of increasing ICP.*

1. Daily measurement of the frontal-occipital circumference of the head in infants.
2. Assess for symptoms of increasing ICP (Table 20-4).
3. Infant is often difficult to feed; administer small feedings at frequent intervals, as vomiting may be a problem.

✦ *Goal: to maintain patency of the shunt and monitor intracranial pressure post shunt procedure.*

1. Position supine, on the unoperative side to prevent pressure on the shunt valve and to prevent too rapid depletion of CSF.
2. Position is not a problem with children who are having a shunt revision; they have not had an increase in ventricular pressure.
3. Monitor for increasing ICP and compare with previous data.
4. Monitor for infection, especially meningitis.

Home Care

1. Teach parents symptoms of increasing ICP.
2. Have parents participate in care of the shunt prior to client's discharge.
3. Encourage parents and family to ventilate feelings regarding client's condition.
4. Refer client to appropriate community agencies.

Reye's Syndrome

❑ **This syndrome is an acute childhood illness resulting in fatty infiltration of the liver and subsequent liver degeneration.**

A. Damaged liver cells no longer adequately convert ammonia to urea for excretion from the body.

B. Circulating ammonia crosses the blood-brain barrier to produce acute neurological effects.

Assessment

1. Risk factors/etiology.
   a. Most often preceded by an acute viral infection.
   b. Primarily affects children ages six months to adolescence.
   c. Frequently, child has received salicylate (aspirin) for control of fever in the preceding viral infection.
   d. With warning labels now on aspirin, problem has significantly decreased.
2. Clinical manifestations.
   a. Initial symptom may be severe, persistent vomiting.
   b. Lethargy, listlessness.
   c. Progresses to state of increased intracranial pressure with deepening coma and posturing.
3. Diagnostics (Appendix 19-1).
   a. Elevated AST and ALT.
   b. Prolonged prothrombin time.
   c. Elevated blood ammonia levels.

Treatment

1. Primarily supportive based on stages of the disease.
2. Measures to decrease intracranial pressure.

Nursing Intervention

✦ *Goal: to monitor progress of disease state and maintain homeostasis.*

1. IV fluids.
2. Monitor serum electrolytes.
3. Maintain respiratory status; prevent hypoxia.
4. Assess for problems of impaired coagulation.
5. Decrease stress, anxiety—child may not remember events prior to the critical phase.

✦ *Goal: to monitor for and implement nursing actions appropriate for increasing intracranial pressure.*

Cerebral Vascular Accident (CVA)

❑ **Also known as a stroke or brain attack, CVA is the disruption of the blood supply to an area of the brain resulting in tissue necrosis and sudden loss of brain function.**

A. Atherosclerosis (Chapter 16)—resulting in cerebral vascular disease, frequently precedes the development of a CVA.

B. Types of stroke.
   1. Thrombosis—formation of a clot which results in the narrowing of a vessel lumen and eventual occlusion.
      a. Associated with hypertension and diabetes (i.e., conditions which accelerate atherosclerotic process).

b. Produces ischemia of the cerebral tissue and edema and congestion in surrounding areas.

2. Embolism—occlusion of a cerebral artery by an embolus.

a. Common site of origin is the endocardium.

b. May affect any age group associated with atrial fibrillation, endocarditis, and prosthetic cardiac valves.

3. Cerebral hemorrhage.

a. Rupture of a cerebral artery secondary to hypertension, trauma, or aneurysm.

b. Blood leaks into the brain tissue and the subarachnoid space.

C. The area of edema resulting from tissue damage may precipitate more damage than the vascular damage itself.

D. Transient ischemic attack (TIA).

1. Brief episode, less than 24 hours, of neurological dysfunction.

2. Should be considered a warning symptom of an impending CVA.

3. Neurologic dysfunction is present for minutes to hours, but no permanent neurological deficit remains.

E. Neuromuscular deficits resulting from a stroke are due to damage of motor neurons of the pyramidal tract.

1. Damage to the left side of the brain will result in paralysis of the right side of the body (hemiplegia—paralysis of one side of the body).

2. Both upper and lower extremities of the involved side are affected.

Assessment

1. Risk factors/etiology (See Table 20-6).

2. Clinical manifestations.

a. TIA.

(1) Visual defects - blurred vision, diplopia, blindness of one eye, tunnel vision.

(2) Transient hemiparesis, gait problems.

(3) Slurred speech.

(4) Transient numbness of an extremity.

(5) Confusion.

(6) Nosebleeds (epistaxis).

b. Completed CVA (occurs suddenly with an embolism, more gradually in hemorrhage or thrombosis).

(1) Hemiplegia—loss of voluntary movement, damage to the right side of the brain will result in left-sided weakness and paralysis.

Table 20-6: RISK FACTORS ASSOCIATED WITH CEREBRAL VASCULAR ACCIDENT

Reversible:
* Smoking
* Obesity
* Increased salt intake
* Sedentary lifestyle
* Increased stress
* Oral contraceptives

Partially Reversible:
* Hypertension
* Cardiac valve disease
* Dysrhythmias
* Diabetes mellitus
* Hypercholesterolemia

Nonreversible:
* Sex (increased incidence in men)
* Age
* Increased incidence in the black population
* Hereditary predisposition

(2) Aphasia—defect in using and interpreting the symbols of language; may include written, printed or spoken words.

(3) May be unaware of the affected side, neglect syndrome ensues.

(4) Cranial nerve impairment—chewing, gag reflex, dysphagia, impaired tongue movement.

(5) May be incontinent initially.

(6) Agnosia—a perceptual defect that causes a disturbance in interpreting sensory information; client may not be able to recognize previously familiar objects.

(7) Cognitive impairment—impairment of memory and judgment, proprioception.

(8) Hypotonia (flaccidity) for days to weeks, followed by hypertonia (spasticity).

(9) Visual defects—homonymous hemianopia: visual loss of same half of visual field of each eye, client has only half of normal vision. Horner's syndrome: ptosis of the upper eyelid, constriction of the pupil and lack of tearing in the eye.

(10) Apraxia—can move the affected limb but is unable to carry out learned movements.

(11) Increased intracranial pressure.

3. Diagnostics (Appendix 20-1).

a. Clinical manifestations elicited in the neurological exam.

b. Cerebral angiogram

c. Lumbar puncture.

d. CAT, MRI, and brain scan.

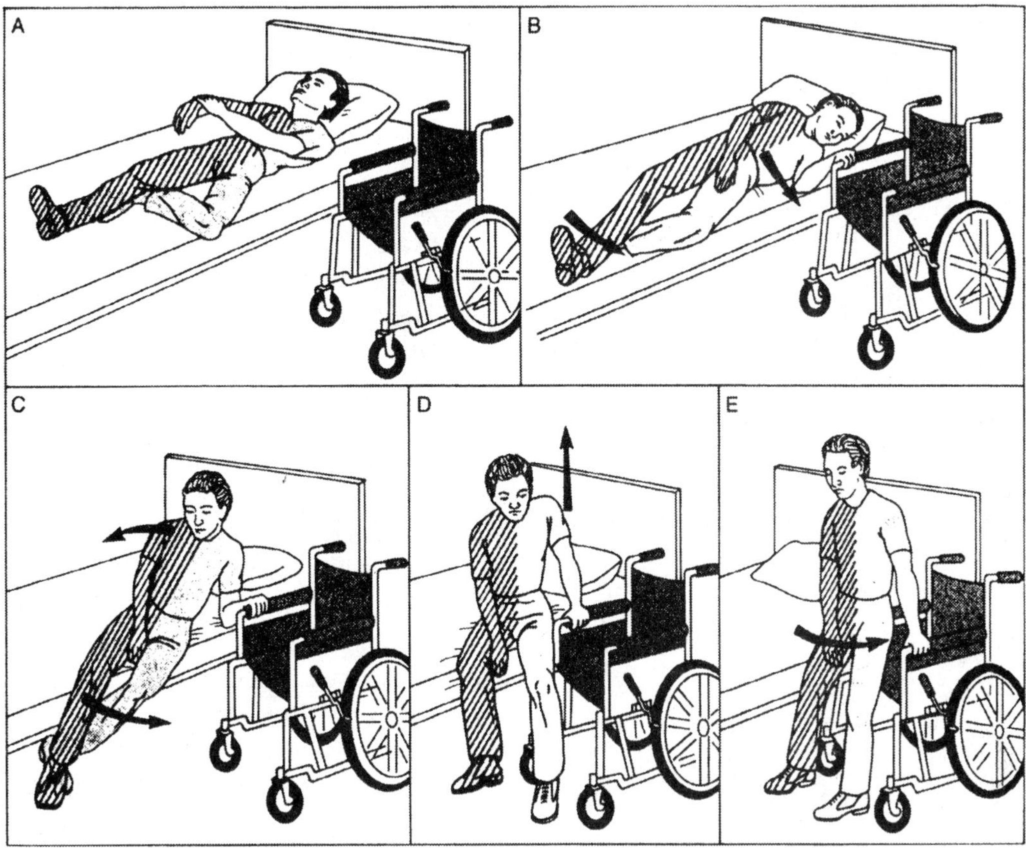

Figure 20-3: Transfer to Wheelchair
Client education guide for transfer from bed to wheelchair by a hemiplegic. (Shading indicates the affected side.) Lock the wheelchair; place it beside the bed on the nonaffected side. Use your nonaffected arm and leg (A and B) to move affected arm and leg. As your legs drop over the edge of the bed, swing your torso up to a sitting position (C). Push up to a standing position (D) by using nonaffected arm and leg. Reach across the wheelchair (E) to grasp the far arm of the chair, and turn to seat yourself.
Reprinted with permission: Black, J. And Matassarin-Jacobs, E. Luckmann and Sorensen's Medical-Surgical Nursing: A Psychophysiologic Approach, 4th ed., Philadelphia: W.B. Saunders, 1993, p. 719).

Treatment

1. Prophylactic.
   a. Aspirin.
   b. Antihypertensives.
2. Medical.
   a. Medications to decrease cerebral edema.
      (1) Osmotic diuretics.
      (2) Corticosteroids (dexamethasone).
   b. Anticonvulsants.
   c. Depending on type of stroke, anticoagulants may be used.
3. Surgical - carotid endarterectomy, especially for TIA.

Nursing Intervention

✦ *Goal: to prevent CVA through client education.*

1. Identification of individuals with reversible risk factors (Table 20-6) and measures to reduce them.
2. Appropriate medical attention for control of chronic conditions conducive to the development of CVA (Partial reversible risk factors, Table 20-6).

✦ *Goal: to maintain patent airway and adequate cerebral oxygenation.*

1. Position side-lying with head elevated.
2. Assess for symptoms of hypoxia; endotracheal intubation and mechanical ventilation may be necessary (Appendix 15-5).
3. Maintain patent airway; use oropharyngeal airway to prevent airway obstruction by the tongue.
4. Client is prone to obstructed airway and pulmonary infection; have him/her cough and deep breathe every two hours.

✦ *Goal: to assess for and implement measures to decrease intracranial pressure (see nursing goals for IICP).*

✦ *Goal: to maintain adequate nutritional intake.*

1. Administer PO feedings with caution; start after first 24 hours, check presence of gag reflex and swallowing reflex before feeding.

2. Place food on the unaffected side of the mouth, begin with non-caloric, clear foods (gelatines).
3. Select foods that are easy to control in the mouth (thick liquids) and swallow; liquids often promote coughing, as client is unable to control them.
4. Maintain high-Fowler's position for feeding.
5. Maintain privacy and unrushed atmosphere.
6. If client is unable to tolerate PO intake, tube feedings may be initiated.

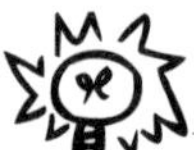

NCLEX ALERT: *Identify potenial for aspiration; assess clients ability to eat.*

✦ *Goal: to preserve function of the musculoskeletal system.*

1. Passive ROM on affected side; begin early because the exercises are more difficult if muscles begin to tighten.
2. Active ROM on unaffected side.
3. Prevent footdrop - passive exercises, rigid boots, have client out of bed as soon as possible.
4. Legs should be maintained in a neutral position; prevent external rotation of affected hip by placing a trochanter roll or sandbag at the thigh.
5. Position every two hours, but limit the period of time spent on the affected side.

NURSING PRIORITY: *Protect the client's affected side - no injections, watch for pressure areas when positioning, less time on affected side than other positions.*

6. Assess for adduction and internal rotation of the affected arm; maintain arm in a neutral (slightly flexed) position with each joint slightly higher than the preceding one.
7. Restraints should be avoided, as they often increase agitation.
8. Maintain joints in position of normal function to prevent flexion contractures.
9. Assist client out of bed on the unaffected side; this allows client to provide some stabilization and balance with the good side (Figure 20-3).

NCLEX ALERT: *Mobility - assist client to ambulate, do ROM exercises, assess for complications of immobility, encourage independence.*

✦ *Goal: to maintain homeostasis.*

1. Evaluate adequacy of cardiac output.
2. Monitor hydration status—prevent fluid overload.
   a. Carefully regulate IV intake.
   b. Evaluate response to diuretics.
   c. Assess for the development of peripheral edema.
   d. Restrict fluid intake as indicated.
   e. Assess respiratory parameters indicative of fluid overload.
3. Determine previous bowel patterns and promote normal elimination.
   a. Avoid urinary catheter if possible; if catheter is necessary, remove as soon as possible.
   b. Offer bedpan or urinal every two hours; help establish a schedule.
   c. Prevent constipation—increase bulk in the diet, stool softeners, etc.
   d. Provide privacy and decrease emotional trauma related to incontinence.

NCLEX ALERT: *Initiate a toileting schedule; the CVA client will need assistance in reestablishing a normal bowel and bladder routine.*

4. Prevent problems of skin breakdown through proper positioning and good skin hygiene.
5. Assist client to identify problems of vision.
6. Maintain psychological homeostasis.
   a. Client is very anxious due to the lack of understanding of what has happened to him/her and the inability to communicate.
   b. Speak slowly, clearly, and explain what has happened.
   c. Assess client's communication abilities and identify methods to promote communication.

Self-Care

1. Encourage independence in ADLs.
2. Provide clothing easy to get in and out of.
3. Active participation in ROM; do his/her own ROM on affected side.
4. Physical therapy for retraining of lost function.
5. Assist client to maintain sense of balance when in the sitting position; client will frequently fall to the affected side (neglect syndrome).
6. Encourage participation in carrying out daily personal hygiene.
7. Assist/teach client safe transfer from bed to wheelchair (Figure 20-2).
8. Bowel and bladder training program.

a. Go to bathroom every two hours.

b. Avoid caffeine intake.

c. High bulk in diet, avoid constipation. (Table 18-2).

9. Promote urinary continence.

10. Encourage social interaction (See Appendix 20-6)

a. Speech therapy.

b. Frequent and meaningful verbal stimuli.

c. Allow client plenty of time to respond.

d. Speak slowly and clearly; do not give too many directions at one time.

e. Do not "talk down to" or treat as a child.

f. Mental status may be normal; do not assume it is impaired.

11. Evaluate family support and need for home health services.

NCLEX ALERT: *Assist family to manage care of a client with chronic needs; determine needs of family regarding ability to provide home care after discharge.*

Cerebral Aneurysm, Subarachnoid Hemorrhage

❑ **A dilation of the wall of a cerebral artery (berry aneurysm) most often arises from an arterial junction in the circle of Willis.**

A. An aneurysm frequently ruptures and bleeds into the subarachnoid space.

B. Symptoms occur when aneurysm enlarges and exerts pressure on the brain tissue, or when it ruptures.

Assessment

1. Risk factors/etiology.

a. Congenital deformities of the vessel.

b. Atherosclerosis resulting in weakness of the vessel wall.

c. Hypertension

d. Most often occurs in middle life.

e. Head trauma may enhance the problem.

2. Clinical manifestations.

a. Rupture may be preceded by:

(1) Severe headache.

(2) Intermittent nausea.

b. Rupture frequently occurs without warning.

(1) Severe headache.

(2) Seizures.

(3) Nuchal rigidity.

(4) Hemiparesis.

(5) Loss of consciousness.

(6) Symptoms of increasing intracranial pressure.

c. Severity of symptoms depends on the site and amount of bleeding.

3. Diagnostics.

a. Lumbar puncture, revealing blood in the spinal fluid.

b. Cerebral angiogram.

c. CAT scan.

Treatment

1. Osmotic diuretics.

2. Dexamethasone (Decadron).

3. Fluids to maintain systolic blood pressure at 100-150mmHg (increase in volume and pressure increases blood flow through narrowed vessels.)

4. Surgical intervention—ligation or "clipping" of the aneurysm.

Nursing Intervention

✦ *Goal: to prevent further increase in intracranial pressure and possible rupture.*

1. Immediate, strict bedrest.

2. Prevent Valsalva's maneuver.

3. Client should avoid straining, sneezing, pulling up in bed, acute flexion of the neck.

4. Elevate head of the bed 30° to 45°.

5. Quiet, dim, nonstimulating environment.

6. Constant monitoring of condition to identify occurrence of bleeding, as evidenced by symptoms of increasing intracranial pressure.

7. Administer analgesics cautiously; the client should continue to be easily aroused in order to perform neuro checks.

8. No hot or cold beverages or food, no caffeine, no smoking.

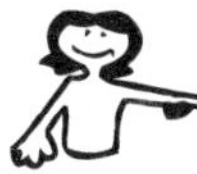

NURSING PRIORITY: *If the client survives the rupture of the aneurysm and rebleed occurs, it is most likely to occur within the next 24 to 48 hours.*

✦ *Goal: to assess for and implement nursing measures to decrease intracranial pressure (see nursing goals for increased intracranial pressure).*

✦ *Goal: to provide appropriate preoperative nursing intervention (see nursing goals for brain tumor).*

✦ *Goal: to maintain homeostasis and monitor changes in intracranial pressure postoperative craniotomy (see nursing goals for craniotomy).*

Meningitis

❑ **Meningitis is an acute inflammatory condition of the meningeal tissue covering the brain.**

A. Infectious process increases permeability of protective membrane, results in a increased protein in the CSF.

B. Inflammatory process results in the development of cerebral edema.

Assessment

1. Risk factors/etiology.
   a. Pathogenic organism most often gains entry from an infection elsewhere in the body.
   b. Meningococcal meningitis is the only form readily contagious; transmitted by direct contact via droplets from the airway of an infected person.
   c. Increased mortality in infants.
2. Clinical manifestations—older child, adult.
   a. Nuchal rigidity.
   b. Chills and fever.
   c. Headache.
   d. Increasing irritability, changes in LOC.
   e. Respiratory distress.
   f. Generalized seizures.
   g. Vomiting.
   h. Positive Kernig's sign—resistance or pain at the knee and the hamstring muscles when attempting to extend the leg after thigh flexion.
   i. Positive Brudzinski's sign—reflex flexion of the hips when the neck is flexed.
   j. Photophobia.
   k. Petechiae, purpuric rash (especially in meningococcal meningitis).
3. Clinical manifestations—neonate and infant.
   a. Fever.
   b. Apneic episodes.
   c. Bulging fontanel.
   d. Seizures.
   e. Crying with position change.
   f. Opisthotonos positioning—a dorsal arched position.
   g. Changes in sleep pattern, increasing irritability.
   h. Poor sucking, may refuse feedings.
   i. Poor muscle tone, diminished movement.
4. Diagnostics.
   a. Lumbar puncture—reveals increasing spinal fluid pressure.
   b. Examination of the spinal fluid for bacteria.

Treatment

1. Respiratory precautions until positive organism is identified.
2. IV antibiotics (Appendix 6-11).
3. Optimum hydration.
4. Anticonvulsant medications (Appendix 20-2).
5. Maintain ventilation.

Complications

1. Increasing ICP resulting in permanent brain damage.
2. Visual and hearing deficits.
3. Subdural effusion; will be absorbed when meningitis treatment is started and protein leak stops.

Nursing Intervention

✦ *Goal: to identify the organism, control spread, and initiate therapy.*

1. Maintain respiratory droplet precautions until organism is identified, place child in a private room.
2. Begin IV antibiotics after lumbar puncture and fluid sample are obtained.
3. Identify family contacts who may require prophylactic treatment.

✦ *Goal: to monitor course of infection and prevent complications.*

1. Frequent nursing assessment for increased ICP.
2. Maintain adequate hydration; may be on fluid restriction if increased ICP present.
3. Monitor infusion site for complications of IVPB antibiotics.
4. Assess for side effects of high dosage of antibiotics.
5. Decrease stimuli in environment—dim lights, quiet environment, no loud noises.
6. Avoid movement or positioning that increases discomfort; client generally assumes a side-lying position.
7. Seizure precautions.
8. Prevent complications of immobility.
9. Good respiratory hygiene.
10. Measures to decrease fever.

Encephalitis

❑ **This is an inflammatory process of the CNS.**

Assessment

1. Risk factors/etiology.
   a. May occur as a complication following a viral infection (measles, chicken pox, mumps).
   b. May be transmitted by a vector—mosquitoes and ticks.

c. Causative organism may be herpes simplex virus in middle aged adults.

2. Clinical manifestations
   a. Headache, nuchal rigidity.
   b. Fever.
   c. Seizures.
   d. Changes in LOC.
   e. Motor involvement - ataxia, dysphasia.
3. Diagnostics—examination of the spinal fluid; specific viral studies to isolate the virus.

Treatment

1. Anticonvulsants.
2. Treatment to decrease ICP.
3. Hydration.

Nursing Intervention

Same as for meningitis with the exception of antibiotic therapy. Encephalitis is caused by a viral agent and is not responsive to antibiotic therapy; antibiotic therapy may be ordered to prevent bacterial infection.

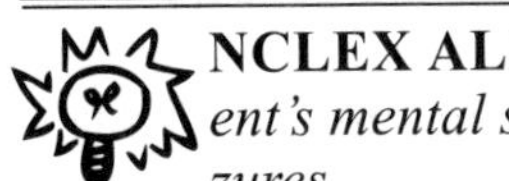

NCLEX ALERT: *Identify changes in client's mental status, manage client with seizures.*

Spinal Cord Injury

❑ **Most often occurs as a result of direct trauma to the head or neck area.**

A. Initially after the injury, the nerve fibers swell and circulation to the spinal cord is decreased; hemorrhage and edema occur, causing an increase in the ischemic process, which progresses to necrotic destruction of the spinal cord.

B. Consequences of cord injury depend on the extent of damage as well as the level of cord injury (Figure 20-1).
   1. The higher the lesion, the more severe the sequelae.
   2. Complete transection (complete cord dissolution, complete lesion)—immediate loss of all sensation and voluntary movement below the level of injury; minimal, if any, return of function.
   3. Incomplete.
      a. Central cord syndrome—center of cord is damaged; results primarily in impairment of upper extremities.
      b. Damage to one side of the cord (Brown-Séquard syndrome)—motor function and position sense may be present on one side, temperature and sensation may be lost on the opposite side.
      c. Anterior cord damage—disruption of blood flow results in a mixed loss of sensory and motor function below the level of injury.
   4. Cord edema peaks in about 2-3 days, and subsides within about 7 days after the injury.
   5. Lumbosacral injuries.
      a. Variable pattern of motor and sensory loss.
      b. Frequently results in neurogenic bowel and bladder.

C. Spinal cord shock (areflexia)—occurs predominantly in complete cord lesions. Because of the loss of communication with the higher centers of control, the muscles below the level of injury will become flaccid and all functional control will cease.
   1. Spinal cord injury interrupts the sympathetic nerve impulse transmission; the parasympathetic impulses are not counter-checked and vasodilation occurs; loss of venous return results in hypotension.
   2. There is loss of the ability of the hypothalamus to control body temperature by vasoconstriction and dilation.
   3. Condition may persist for several weeks and reverse spontaneously; resolution of spinal shock will be evident by the return of reflexes.
   4. Hyperreflexia will occur as recovery progresses. Spastic movements may be precipitated by emotion and cutaneous stimulation.

D. Autonomic dysreflexia (AD) occurs in clients with an injury at T-6 or higher.
   1. A noxious stimulus below the level of injury triggers the sympathetic nervous system, which causes a release of catecholamines, resulting in hypertension.
   2. Most common stimuli causing the response are a full bladder, fecal impaction, and skin stimulation.
   3. Severe hypertension, pounding headache, bradycardia, restlessness, skin flushed and warm are most common body responses.

E. Bladder dysfunction will occur as a result of the injury. Normal bladder control is dependent on the sensory and motor pathways and the lower motor neurons being intact.
   1. Neurogenic bladder occurs in clients with both upper and lower motor neuron disorders.
      a. Upper motor neuron disorders produce a spastic or reflex bladder.
      b. Lower motor neuron disorders produce a flaccid bladder.
   2. Management of bladder problems will depend on client's preferences and life style, as well as functional abilities.

Figure 20-4: Spinal Cord Injury.

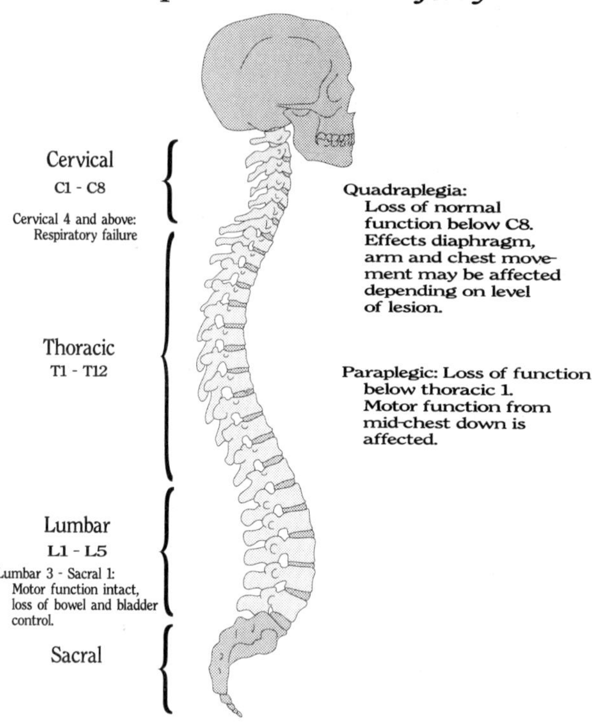

F. Long-term rehabilitation potential depends on the amount of damage done to the cord, which may not be evident for several weeks after the injury.

Assessment

1. Risk factors/etiology—accidents.
2. Clinical manifestations—depend on level of cord injury (Figure 20-1).
   a. Injury at C-3 through C-5 will cause respiratory compromise.
   b. Depending on degree of injury, varying levels of paralysis and sensory loss below the level of injury.
   c. Spinal shock.
      (1) Generally occurs within seventy-two hours and may last for several weeks.
      (2) Flaccid paralysis.
      (3) Loss of sensation and absence of reflexes.
      (4) Bowel and bladder dysfunction.
      (5) Hypotension and bradycardia.
      (6) After spinal shock, reflexes and autonomic activity return, as evidenced by development of spasticity.
   d. Autonomic dysreflexia in clients with injuries at T-6 or higher.
      (1) Severe hypertension, bradycardia.
      (2) Complaints of headache.
      (3) Flushing and diaphoresis above level of injury.
3. Diagnostics (Appendix 20-1).
   a. History of accident.
   b. Clinical manifestations.
   c. X-rays to determine level of damage.
   d. MRI.
   e. CT scan.

Treatment

1. Immobilization of the vertebral column in cervical fracture.
   a. Cervical tongs (Crutchfield, Gardner-Wells) for cervical immobility.
   b. Halo traction to promote mobility.
2. Respiratory support as necessary.
3. Immobilization of spinal column by bedrest in lumbar fracture.
4. Stabilization of spinal column by surgical procedures.
5. Corticosteroids to decrease cord edema.

Nursing Intervention

✦ *Goal: to maintain stability of the vertebral column and prevent further cord damage.*

1. Emergency care and treatment.
   a. Suspect spinal cord injury if there is any evidence of direct trauma to the head or neck area (contact sports, diving accidents, MVA).

b. Immobilize and place on spinal board with the head and neck in a neutral position; do not allow the neck to flex.

NURSING PRIORITY: *Do not hyperextend the neck in the client with a suspected cervical injury. Airway should be opened by the jaw lift method. Improper handling of the client often results in extension of the damaged area.*

c. Maintain in extended position with no twisting or turning; do not remove cervical collar or spinal board until area of injury is identified.

d. Maintain patent airway during transportation.

2. Maintain stability of the vertebral column as indicated by the level of injury.
   a. Bedrest on firm mattress with supportive devices (sandbags, skin traction, etc.); maintain alignment in the supine position; logroll without any flexion or twisting.
   b. Maintain cervical traction—tongs are inserted into the skull with traction and weights applied; do not remove weights; logroll to maintain spinal immobility.
   c. Halo vest traction—maintain cervical immobility, but allows client to be mobile.
      (1) If bolts or screws come loose—maintain the client immobilized and call the doctor.
      (2) Clean pin sites once a day, use separate sterile swab for each pin.
      (3) Roll client onto his side at the edge of the bed and allow him to push up from the mattress to a sitting position - *never* use the frame to assist the client to turn or sit up.
      (4) Correct size of wrench should be kept at bedside to remove the anterior bolts in case of emergency.
      (5) Assist client to maintain balance when standing, the traction is heavy to a person who is weak and the client is at increased risk for falling.
   d. Maintain extremities in neutral, functional position.
3. Appropriate nursing intervention when surgery is indicated for stability of the injury.

✦ *Goal: to identify level of damage and changes in neurological status.*

1. Assess respiratory function- symmetrical chest expansion, bilateral breath sounds, presence of retractions or dyspnea.
2. Motor and sensory evaluation.
   a. Ability to move extremities; strength of extremities.
   b. Sensory examination, including touch and pain.
   c. Presence of deep tendon reflexes.
3. Ongoing assessment and status of:
   a. Bladder function.
   b. Gastric function.
   c. Bowel function.
   d. Psychological adjustment to the injury.
4. Evaluate history of how injury occurred; obtain information regarding how client was transported.
5. Determine status of pain.

✦ *Goal: to maintain respiratory function.*

1. Frequent assessment of respiratory function during first forty-eight hours.
   a. Changes in breathing pattern.
   b. Client's complaints of increasing difficulty in breathing; utilization of sternocleidomastoid and intercostal muscles for respiration.
   c. Evaluate ABGs and pulse oximetry..
   d. Determine development of hypoxia.
2. Maintain adequate respiratory function as indicated.
   a. Chest physiotherapy.
   b. Incentive spirometry.
   c. Changing position within limits of injury.
   d. Assess for complications of atelectasis, pulmonary emboli, and pneumonia.
   e. Nasopharyngeal or endotracheal suctioning based on airway and level of injury.

✦ *Goal: to maintain cardiovascular stability.*

1. Spinal shock.
   a. Monitor vital signs and evaluate changes.
   b. Vagal stimulation, hypothermia, and hypoxia may precipitate spinal shock.
   c. Development of spasticity in muscles below the level of injury indicates beginning resolution of spinal shock.
2. Assess for development of autonomic dysreflexia, if it occurs:
   a. Elevate the head of the bed, and check the blood pressure.
   b. Assess for sources of stimuli—distended bladder (check foley tubing), fecal impaction, constipation, tight clothing.
   c. Relieve the stimuli and dysreflexia will subside.
   d. Maintain cardiovascular support during period of hypertension.

3. Evaluate cardiovascular responses when turning or suctioning.
4. Antiembolism stockings or elastic wraps to the legs to facilitate venous return. (Lack of muscle tone and loss of sympathetic tone in the peripheral vessels results in a decrease in venous tone and in venous return, predisposes to deep vein thrombosis).
5. Implement measures to promote venous return.

NCLEX ALERT: *Identify symptoms of DVT, apply compression stockings, and change client's position are all components of the test plan.*

✦ *Goal: to maintain adequate fluid and nutritional status.*

1. During the first forty-eight hours, evaluate GI function frequently; decrease in function may necessitate utilization of a nasogastric tube to decrease distention.
2. Prevent complications of nausea and vomiting.
3. Evaluate bowel sounds and client's ability to tolerate PO fluids.
4. Increase protein and calories in diet; may need to decrease calcium intake.
5. Evaluate for presence of paralytic ileus.
6. Increase roughage in diet to promote bowel function.

✦ *Goal: to prevent complications of immobility (Chapter 3).*

✦ *Goal: to promote bowel and bladder function.*

1. Urine is retained, due to the loss of autonomic and reflexive control of the bladder.
   a. Intermittent catheterization or indwelling catheter initially to prevent bladder distention.
   b. Nursing intervention to prevent urinary tract infection; avoid urinary catherterization if possible.
2. Determine type of bladder dysfunction based on level of injury.
3. Assess client's awareness of bladder function.
4. Initiate measures to institute bladder control.
   a. Establish a schedule for voiding; have client attempt voiding every two hours.
   b. Utilize the Credé method (in adults) for manual expression of urine.
   c. May be necessary to teach client self-catheterization.
   d. Record output and evaluate for residual urine.
5. Evaluate bowel functioning.
   a. Incontinence and paralytic ileus frequently occur with spinal shock.
   b. Incontinence and impaction are common later.
6. Initiate measures to promote bowel control (after spinal shock is resolved).
   a. Identify client's bowel habits prior to injury.
   b. Maintain sufficient fluid intake and adequate bulk in the diet.
   c. Establish specific time each day for bowel evacuation.
   d. Assess client's awareness of need to defecate.
   e. Teach client effective utilization of the Valsalva maneuver to induce defecation.
   f. Induce defecation by digital stimulation, suppository, or as a last resort, enema.

NCLEX ALERT: *Initiate a toileting schedule; the spinal injury client will need bowel and bladder retraining depending on level of the injury.*

✦ *Goal: to maintain psychological equilibrium.*

1. Simple explanation of all procedures.
2. Anticipate outbursts of anger and hostility as client begins to work through the grieving process and adjustments in body image.
3. Anticipate and accept periods of depression in client.
4. Encourage independence whenever possible; allow client to participate in decisions regarding care and to gain control over environment.

NCLEX ALERT: *Plan measures to deal with client's anxiety, promote client's adjustment to changes in body image, assist client and significant others to adjust to role changes, these items are all part of the test plan and could be tested in the client with spinal cord injury.*

5. Encourage family involvement in identifying appropriate diversional activities.
6. Avoid sympathy and emphasize client's potential.
7. Initiate frank, open discussion regarding sexual functioning.
8. Assist client and family to identify community resources.
9. Assist client to set realistic short-term goals.

Myasthenia Gravis

❑ **A neuromuscular disease characterized by a decrease in acetylcholine at the receptor sites in the**

neuromuscular junction; precipitates a disturbance in the transmission of nerve impulses.

Assessment

1. Risk factors/etiology.
   a. Autoimmune in origin.
   b. Peak incidence between ages 20 and 30.
2. Clinical manifestations.
   a. Primary problem is skeletal muscle fatigue with sustained muscle contraction; symptoms are predominantly bilateral.
      (1) Muscular fatigue increases with activity.
      (2) Ptosis (drooping of the eyelids) and diplopia (double vision) are frequently the first symptoms.
      (3) Impairment of facial mobility and expression.
      (4) Impairment of chewing and swallowing.
      (5) Speech impairment (dysarthria).
      (6) No sensory deficit, loss of reflexes, or muscular atrophy.
      (7) Poor bowel and bladder control.
   b. Course is variable.
      (1) May be progressive.
      (2) May stabilize.
      (3) May be characterized by short remissions and exacerbations.
   c. Myasthenic crisis—an acute exacerbation of symptoms of the condition, frequently preceded by some type of infection.
      (1) Decreased or absent cough or swallow reflex.
      (2) Increase in pulse and blood pressure.
      (3) Severe respiratory distress and hypoxia.
   d. Cholinergic crisis is a toxic response to the anticholinesterase medications.
      (1) Nausea, vomiting and diarrhea.
      (2) Weakness with difficulty swallowing, chewing, speaking.
      (3) Increased secretions and saliva.
3. Diagnostics.
   a. Clinical manifestations.
   b. Electromyography—shows a decreasing response of muscles to stimuli.
   c. Tensilon test—utilized for diagnosing and differentiating types of crisis (cholinergic crisis versus myasthenic crisis).

Treatment

1. Anticholinesterase (cholinergic) medications (Appendix 20-3).
2. Corticosteroids. (Appendix 6-8)
3. Plasma electrophoresis.
4. Immunosuppressive therapy.
5. Surgical removal of the thymus (thymectomy).

Nursing Intervention

(Client may be hospitalized for acute myasthenic crisis or for respiratory infection).

✦ *Goal: to maintain respiratory function.*
1. Assess for increasing problems of difficult breathing.
2. Determine client's medication schedule; when was medication last taken?
3. Assess ability to swallow; prevent problems of aspiration.

NCLEX ALERT: *Do not give the client in myasthenic crisis anything to eat or drink, as there is significant increased risk for aspirating during this time.*

4. Evaluate effectiveness of cough reflex.
5. Have emergency tracheotomy set available.

✦ *Goal: to distinguish between myasthenic crisis and cholinergic crisis.*
1. Maintain adequate ventilatory support during crisis.
2. Assist in administration of **Tensilon** to differentiate crisis.
   a. Myasthenic crisis—client's condition will improve.
   b. Cholinergic crisis—client's condition will temporarily worsen.
3. If myasthenic crisis, neostigmine may be administered.
4. If cholinergic crisis, atropine may be administered and cholinergic medications reevaluated.
5. Avoid use of sedatives and tranquilizers, which cause respiratory depression.
6. Provide psychological support during crisis.

Self-Care
1. Teach client importance of taking medication on a regular basis; peak effect of the medication should coincide with mealtimes.
2. If ptosis becomes severe, client may need to wear an eye patch to protect cornea (alternate eye patches if problem is bilateral).

3. Emotional upset, severe fatigue, infections, and exposure to extreme temperatures may precipitate myasthenic crisis.

Multiple Sclerosis

❑ **The disease is characterized by multiple areas of demyelinization of the neurons in the brain and spinal cord (CNS).**

A. The progression of the disease results in total destruction of the myelin and the nerve fibers become involved.
   1. Loss of myelin sheath causes decreased impulse conduction, destruction of the nerve axon, and a blockage of the impulse conduction.
   2. The demyelinization occurs in irregular scattered patches throughout the CNS.

B. The condition has two major courses:
   1. Exacerbating-remitting—with unpredictable remissions and exacerbations; with repeated exacerbations, there is a progressive scarring and deterioration of the neurological function.
   2. Chronic-progressive—produces a steady decline in neurologic function, may occur rapidly within a year, or may occur over several years.

Assessment

1. Risk factors/etiology - cause is unknown.
   a. More common in women.
   b. Problem of young adults.
2. Clinical manifestations.
   a. Vary from person to person, as well as within the same individual, depending on the area of involvement.
   b. Cerebellar dysfunction - nystagmus, ataxia, dysarthria, dysphagia.
   c. Motor dysfunction - weakness of eye muscles, weakness or spasticity of muscles in extremities.
   d. Sensory - vertigo, blurred vision, decreased hearing, tinnitus.
   e. Bowel and bladder dysfunction.
   f. Sexual dysfunction.
   g. Psychosocial.
      (1) Intellectual functioning remains intact.
      (2) Emotional lability—increased excitability and inappropriate euphoria.
      (3) Emotional effects of the chronic illness and changes in body image.
3. Diagnostics.
   a. No definitive diagnostic test.
   b. Diagnostics based on history and clinical manifestations.

Treatment

1. No cure; medical treatment is directed toward treatment of the disease process and symptoms.
2. Medications to decrease edema and inflammation of the nerve site.
   a. Anti-inflammatory.
   b. Immunosuppressive.
   c. Interferons.

Nursing Intervention

(Client may be hospitalized for diagnostic workup or for acute exacerbation and complications).

✦ *Goal: to maintain homeostasis and prevent complications in an acute exacerbation of disease symptoms.*

1. Maintain adequate respiratory function.
   a. Prevent respiratory infection.
   b. Good pulmonary hygiene.
   c. Prevent aspiration; sitting position for eating.
   d. Evaluate adequacy of cough reflex.
2. Maintain urinary tract function.
   a. Prevent urinary tract infection.
   b. Increase fluid intake, at least 2000cc/24 hours.
   c. Evaluate voiding—assess for retention and incontinence.
3. Maintain nutrition.
   a. Evaluate coughing and swallowing reflexes.
   b. Provide food that is easy to chew.
   c. If client is experiencing difficulty swallowing, observe closely during fluid intake.

✦ *Goal: to prevent complications of immobility (Chapter 3).*

✦ *Goal: to promote psychological well being.*

1. Focus on remaining capabilities.
2. Encourage independence and assist client to gain control over environment.
3. If impotence is a problem, initiate sexual counseling.
4. Assist client to work through the grieving process.
5. Identify community resources available.

Self-Care

1. Medical regimen and side effects of the medications.
2. Physical therapy to maintain muscle function and decrease spasticity.
3. Measures to maintain voiding, may need to perform self- catheterization.

4. Safety measures due to decreased sensation.
   a. Check bath water temperature.
   b. Wear protective clothing in the winter.
   c. Avoid heating pads and clothing that is constrictive.
5. Client should understand that relapses are frequently associated with an increase in physiological and psychological stress.

Guillain-Barré Syndrome

❑ **This condition involves segmental demyelination of nerve roots in the spinal cord and medulla. Demyelination occurs, leading to inflammation, edema and nerve root compression, which causes decreased nerve conduction and rapidly ascending paralysis. Both sensory and motor impairment; also called polyradiculitis.**

Assessment

1. Risk factors/etiology - cause is unknown, frequently a history of acute illness.
2. Clinical manifestations.
   a. Progressive weakness and paralysis begins in the lower extremities and ascends bilaterally.
   b. Paralysis ascends the body symmetrically.
      (1) Paralysis of respiratory muscles.
      (2) Cranial nerve involvement, most often facial nerve (CN VII) produces difficulty talking and swallowing.
   c. Loss of sensation and function of bowel and bladder.
   d. Manifestations may progress rapidly over hours, or occur over two to four weeks.
   e. Muscle atrophy is minimal.
   f. Paralysis decreases as the client begins recovery; most often no residual effects.

NURSING PRIORITY: Of the neuromuscular disorders, Guillain-Barré is the most rapidly developing and progressive condition. It is potentially fatal if unrecognized.

3. Diagnostics—based primarily on the clinical manifestations.

Treatment (Supportive).

1. Corticosteroids.
2. Immunosuppressives.
3. Maintain respiratory function; may require mechanical ventilation.

Nursing Intervention

✦ *Goal: to evaluate progress of paralysis and initiate actions to prevent complications.*

1. Evaluate rate of progress of paralysis; careful assessment of changes in respiratory pattern.
2. Frequent evaluation of cough and swallow reflexes.
   a. Remain with client while eating; have suction equipment available.
   b. NPO if reflexes are involved.
3. If paralysis is rapid, prepare for ET intubation and respiratory assistance.
4. Prevent complications of immobility during period of paralysis (Chapter 3).
5. Assess for involvement of the autonomic nervous system.
   a. Orthostatic hypotension.
   b. Hypertension.
   c. Cardiac dysrhythmias.
   d. Urinary retention and paralytic ileus.

✦ *Goal: to prevent complications of hypoxia if respiratory muscles become involved (Chapter 15).*

✦ *Goal: to maintain psychological homeostasis.*

1. Simple explanation of procedures.
2. Complete recovery is anticipated; residual problems are not common.
3. Provide psychological support during period of assisted ventilation.
4. Keep client and family aware of progress of disease.

Amyotrophic Lateral Sclerosis (ALS)

❑ **Involves a progressive degeneration of nerves involving the motor system; does not involve mental or sensory changes; also called Lou Gehrig's disease.**

Assessment

1. Clinical manifestations
   a. Fatigue, muscle atrophy and weakness.
   b. Progressive muscle weakness.
      (1) Begins with upper extremities and progressively involves muscles of neck and throat.
      (2) Trunk and lower extremeties are involved late in course of disease.
   c. Most often fatal in 2-5 years after onset.
2. Diagnostics - EMG and muscle biopsy.

Treatment

1. Riluzole (Rilutek) prolongs life by a few months.
2. Supportive care.

Nursing Intervention

✦ *Goal: to provide ongoing assessment in assisting client to deal with progressive symptoms.*

1. Promote independence in ADL.
   a. Conserve energy- space activities.
   b. Avoid extremes of hot and cold.
   c. Utilization of appliances to prolong independence in ambulation and ADL's.
2. Promote nutrition
   a. Small frequent feedings.
   b. Have client sit upright with head slightly flexed forward while eating.
   c. Keep suction equipment easily available during meals.
3. Encourage family and client to talk about losses and the difficult choices they face.
4. Assist family and client to identify need for advanced directives, and to complete them.

Muscular Dystrophy

❑ **The term *pseudohypertrophy* describes characteristic muscle enlargement due to fatty infiltration which occurs in muscular dystrophy.**

A. Duchenne's is the most common type and is also the most severe.

B. Condition is characterized by gradual degeneration of muscle fibers and progressive symmetrical weakness and wasting of skeletal muscle.

Assessment

1. Risk factors/etiology.
   a. Genetic—sex-linked disorder primarily affecting males.
   b. Onset generally between 3 to 5 years.
2. Clinical manifestations.
   a. History of delay in motor development, particularly in walking.
   b. Abnormal waddling gait.
      (1) Falls frequently and develops characteristic manner of rising.
      (2) Gower's sign—from sitting or squatting position, the child assumes a kneeling position and pushes his/her torso up by walking his/her hands up the thighs.
   c. Progressive muscle weakness, atrophy, and contractures..
      (1) Ambulation frequently impossible by age 9 to 11.
      (2) Ultimately destroys essential muscles of respiration; death occurs from respiratory infection or cardiac failure.
3. Diagnostics.
   a. Electromyography (EMG).
   b. Muscle biopsy.
   c. Serum enzymes - increased CPK in neonate, then gradually declines.

Treatment

No definitive therapy.

Nursing Intervention

(Child is frequently cared for at home; hospitalized only for complications).

✦ *Goal: to maintain function as long as possible.*

1. Maintain child's independence in ADLs and maintain social contact with peers as long as possible.
2. Assist parents to identify resources for assistance with physical therapy and exercise program at home.
3. Assist family to identify resources, to adapt physiological barriers within the home, and to promote mobility of the child in a wheelchair.
4. Assist family to identify methods of preventing respiratory infection;and assess for respiratory problems.

✦ *Goal: to assist parents and child to maintain psychological equilibrium and to adapt to chronic long-term illness.*

1. Assist parents to understand importance of independence and self-help skills; frequently, parents are overprotective of the child.
2. Counseling to assist parents and family members to identify family activities that can be modified to meet child's needs.
3. Mother may feel particularly guilty because of transmission of disease to her son.
4. Identify community resources available.
5. Counseling to assist family and child with chronic long-term illness and child's eventual death.

Cerebral Palsy (CP)

❑ **Damage to the motor centers of the brain; nerve impulses are not correctly sent or received. Results in impairment of muscle control.**

Assessment

1. Risk factors/etiology.
   a. Commonly results from existing prenatal brain abnormalities (kernicterus, hemolytic disease of newborn).
   b. Prematurity is single most important determinant of CP.

(1) In about 24% of cases, cause is not identifiable.

2. Clinical manifestations.
   a. Delayed achievement of developmental milestones.
   b. Increased or decreased resistance to passive movement.
   c. Abnormal posture.
   d. Presence of infantile reflexes (tonic neck reflex, exaggerated Moro).
   e. Associated disabilities:
      (1) Mental retardation; approximately ⅓ of the children affected.
      (2) Seizures.
      (3) Attention-deficit problems.
      (4) Vision and hearing sensory impairments.
3. Diagnostics.
   a. Neurological examination and contributing history.
   b. Diagnostic tests to rule out other neurological dysfunction.
   c. Frequently difficult to diagnose in early months; condition may not be evident until child attempts to walk.

Treatment

1. Maintain and promote mobility with orthopedic devices and physical therapy.
2. Skeletal muscle relaxants.
3. Anticonvulsants as indicated.

Nursing Intervention

(Child is frequently cared for at home and on an outpatient basis unless complications occur).

✦ *Goal: to assist child to become as independent and self-sufficient as possible.*

1. Physical therapy program designed to assist individual child to gain maximum function.
2. Assist child to progress according to developmental level and functional abilities; encourage crawling, sitting, and balancing appropriate to developmental level.
3. Assist child to carry out activities of daily living as age and capacities permit.
4. Speech therapy as indicated.
5. Encourage play appropriate for age.
6. Encourage appropriate educational activities.
7. Bowel and bladder training may be difficult, due to poor control.

✦ *Goal: to maintain physiological homeostasis.*

1. Maintain adequate nutrition.
   a. May experience difficulty eating, due to spasticity; may drool excessively.
   b. Encourage independence in eating; utilize self-help devices.
   c. Provide a balanced diet with increased caloric intake to meet extra energy demands.
2. Maintain safety precautions to prevent injury.
3. Increased susceptibility to infections, especially respiratory infections, due to poor control of intercostal muscles and diaphragm.
4. Increased incidence of dental problems; schedule frequent dental checkups.

✦ *Goal: to promote a positive self-image in the child and provide support to the family.*

1. Use positive reinforcement frequently.
2. Assist parents to set realistic goals.
3. Encourage recreation and educational activities, especially those involving other children with cerebral palsy.
4. Encourage child to express feelings regarding his/her disorder.
5. Do not "talk down" to child; communicate at appropriate developmental level.
6. Assist parents in problem solving in home environment.
7. Identify community resources available.

Parkinson's Disease (Paralysis Agitans)

❑ **A progressive neurological disorder causing destruction and degeneration of nerve cells in the basal ganglia; results in damage to the extra pyramidal system, causing difficulty in control and regulation of movement.**

A. Dopamine, a neurotransmitter, is responsible for normal functioning of the extra pyramidal system.

B. The condition is correlated with a depletion of, or imbalance in, dopamine and an increased activity of acetylcholine.

Assessment

1. Risk factors/etiology.
   a. General onset is after age 60.
   b. Rarely occurs in the black population.
2. Clinical manifestations.
   a. Tremor.
      (1) Affects the arms and hands bilaterally—often the first sign.

(2) Tremors usually occur at rest, voluntary movement may decreased tremor; tremors during voluntary movement not as common.

(3) Described as "pill-rolling" tremor.

(4) Aggravated by emotional stress and increased concentration.

b. Muscle rigidity.

(1) Increased resistance to passive movement.

(2) Movement may be described as "cog-wheel rigidity" due to jerky movement of extremities.

c. Bradykinesia - slow activity.

(1) Decreased blinking of the eyelids.

(2) Loss of ability to swallow saliva.

(3) Facial expression is blank or "mask-like".

(4) Loss of normal arm swing while walking.

(5) Difficulty initiating movement.

d. Stooped posture, shuffling propulsive gait.

e. May exhibit mental deterioration similar to Alzheimers.

f. Onset usually gradual.

3. Diagnostics—no specific diagnostic test.

Treatment

1. Medication to enhance dopamine secretion (Appendix 20-4).
2. Anticholinergic medications to decrease effects of acetylcholine (Appendix 20-4).

Nursing Intervention.

✦ *Goal: to maintain homeostasis.*

1. Encourage independence in ADLs utilizing self-help devices.
2. Maintain nutrition.
   a. Increase calories, protein, and easily chewed foods.
   b. Frequent small meals.
   c. Allow ample time for eating.
   d. Monitor weight loss.
   e. Provide pleasant atmosphere at mealtime; client frequently prefers to eat alone due to difficulty swallowing and inability to control saliva.
   f. Increase fluid intake with increased bulk in the diet to decrease problem with constipation.
3. Maintain muscle function.
   a. Full range of motion to extremities to prevent contracture.
   b. Decrease effects of tremors .
   c. Exercise and stretch daily.
   d. Physical therapy as indicated.

✦ *Goal: to promote a positive self-image.*

1. Encourage diversional activities.
2. Assist client to set realistic goals.
3. Explore reasons for depression; encourage client to discuss changes occurring in lifestyle.
4. Assist client in gaining control of ADLs and environment.
5. Assist client to identify and avoid activities that increase frustration levels.
6. Encourage good personal hygiene.

Headache

❑ **A symptom of an underlying disorder, rather than a disease itself.**

Assessment

1. Types of headaches.
   a. Cluster headaches—occur in numerous episodes or clustering; no aura; unilateral pain often arising in nostril spreading to forehead and eye; often begin at night.
   b. Migraine—constriction of intracranial vessels leading to an intense throbbing pain when vessels return to normal; prodromol or aura; crescendo quality; pain unilateral, often beginning in eye area; nausea, vomiting, photophobia.
   c. Tension headache (muscle contraction headache)—feeling of tightness of a band around the head; onset gradual; may have dizziness, tinnitus, or lacrimation; associated with stress and premenstrual syndrome.

Treatment

1. Migraine—sumitriptan (**Imitrex**), dihydroergotamine mesylate (**Migranal**).
2. NSAIDS.

Nursing Intervention

1. Prevention—recognize triggers, decrease stress, adjust medications during menstrual cycle.
2. Watch for signs of ominous headache: new onset unilateral headache in person over age 35; vomiting, not accompanied by nausea; pain awakens client.

Trigeminal Neuralgia

❑ **A cranial nerve disorder affecting the branches of the trigeminal nerve (cranial nerve V).**

Assessment

1. Risk factors/etiology.
   a. Onset generally between 20 and 40 years of age.
   b. Increased frequency with aging.

2. Clinical manifestations.
   a. Abrupt onset of paroxysmal intense pain in the lower and upper jaw, cheek, and lips.
      (1) Tearing of the eyes and frequent blinking.
      (2) Facial twitching and grimacing.
      (3) Pain usually brief; ends as abruptly as it begins.
   b. Recurrence of pain is unpredictable.
   c. Pain is initiated by cutaneous stimulation of the affected nerve area.
      (1) Chewing.
      (2) Washing the face.
      (3) Extremes of temperature—either on the face or in food.
      (4) Brushing teeth.
3. Diagnostics.
   a. Clinical manifestations.
   b. Test to rule out other neurologic dysfunctions.

Treatment

1. Medical management of pain.
   a. Phenytoin (**Dilantin**).
   b. Carbamazepine (**Tegretol**).
2. Surgical intervention.
   a. Local nerve block.
   b. Surgical intervention to interrupt nerve impulse transmission.

Nursing Intervention

✦ *Goal: to control pain.*

1. Assess the nature of a painful attack.
2. Identify triggering factors; adjust environment to decrease factors.
   a. Keep room at an even, comfortable temperature.
   b. Avoid touching client.
   c. Avoid jarring the bed.
   d. Allow client to carry out own ADLs as necessary.
3. Administer analgesics to decrease pain.

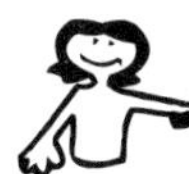

***NURSING PRIORITY**: Due to the severe pain of the condition, clients are susceptible to severe depression and suicide.*

✦ *Goal: to maintain nutrition.*

1. Frequently, client does not eat, due to reluctance to stimulate the pain.
2. Provide lukewarm food which is easily chewed.
3. Increase protein and calories.

Self-Care

1. Identify presence of corneal reflex; provide protective eye care if reflex is absent.
2. If there is loss of sensation to the side of the face, client should:
   a. Chew on the unaffected side.
   b. Avoid temperature extremes in foods.
   c. Check the mouth after eating to remove remaining particles of food.
   d. Maintain meticulous oral hygiene.
   e. Have frequent dental checkups.

Bell's Palsy

❑ **A cranial nerve disorder affecting the facial nerve (cranial nerve VII), characterized by a disruption of the motor branches on one side of the face which results in muscle flaccidity of the affected side of the face.**

Assessment

1. Clinical manifestations.
   a. Lag or inability to close eyelid on affected side.
   b. Drooping of the mouth.
   c. Decreased taste sensation.
   d. Upward movement of the eyeball when closing the eye.
2. Diagnostics—no specific diagnostic test.

Treatment

1. Corticosteroids.
2. Vasodilators.

Nursing Intervention

✦ *Goal: to assess nerve function and prevent complications.*

1. Analgesics to decrease pain.
2. Evaluate ability of client to eat.
3. Meticulous oral hygiene.
4. Prevent drying of the cornea on the affected side.
   a. Instill methylcellulose drops frequently during the day.
   b. Ophthalmic ointment and eye patches may be required at night.
5. As function returns, active facial exercises.

✦ *Goal: to assist client to maintain a positive self-image.*

1. Changes in physical appearance may be dramatic.
2. Discuss with client that the condition is usually self-limiting with minimal, if any, residual effects.
3. Client may require counseling if facial appearance is permanent.⌘

Study Questions—Neurological System

1. The nurse is assessing a client with a tentative diagnosis of a brain tumor. What would the nurse anticipate the client's primary complaint to be?

① Decreased appetite.
② Frequent insomnia.
③ Recurrent headaches.
④ Peripheral edema.

2. The nurse is caring for a client with a right sided cerebral venous accident (CVA). The nurse includes what activities in the care of this client?

① Passive ROM exercises to affected side, active on unaffected side.
② Place food on the affected side of the client's mouth.
③ Hot packs to the right leg to decrease muscle spasm.
④ Turn every 2 hours and maintain position on the right side for 2 hours.

3. A client is scheduled for an electroencephalogram. What will the nurse explain to the client regarding the purpose of this test?

① Evaluate electrical currents of skeletal muscles.
② Measure ultrasonic waves in the brain.
③ Determine size and location of brain activity.
④ Record brain electrical activity.

4. A CVA client is aphasic, it has been a week since his stroke. He is beginning to show functional improvement and demonstrates an ability to follow verbal directions. What will rehabilitation now include?

① A right-leg brace.
② Ambulation training.
③ Speech training.
④ Vocational retraining.

5. The nurse is caring for a client who is doing well after his craniotomy. What will the bowel care for this client include?

① An enema every other day to avoid Valsalva's maneuver.
② High fiber diet and stool softeners to prevent constipation.
③ Low residue diet to decrease stool formation and prevent constipation.
④ Daily checking for impaction due to loss of bowel innervation.

6. Following a grand mal seizure, what nursing action is the *highest* priority?

① Loosen or remove constricting clothing and protect client from injuring himself.
② Maintain a patent airway by turning the client's head to the side and suctioning if necessary.
③ Remain with the client and administer anticonvulsant medications as ordered by the physician.
④ Describe and record events before the onset of the seizure, during the seizure, and after the seizure.

7. A client with Parkinson's disease is experiencing anorexia and vomiting since beginning levodopa. What will be the initial nursing activity?

① Assess his food preferences.
② Monitor his blood pressure.
③ Hold his medication and notify the physician.
④ Administer his medication with food.

8. In the immediate postoperative period following a lumbar laminectomy, what is the *priority* nursing action?

① Check for bladder distention.
② Ambulate the client.
③ Change the surgical dressing.
④ Determine presence of postural hypotension.

9. When obtaining a health history, what will the nurse expect a client with a recent diagnosis of Parkinson's disease to report?

① Weight loss.
② Slowness of movement.
③ Continual motor tremors.
④ Depression.

10. In caring for a client with Parkinson's disease, what is important for the nurse to understand?

① Intellectual capabilities will decrease.
② Diversional interests may decrease.
③ Mood fluctuations may occur.
④ Communication skills may fluctuate.

11. Bronchopneumonia is a common problem in children with spastic cerebral palsy. The nurse understands this occurs because:

① There is an associated dysfunction of the respiratory center in the central nervous system.
② The immunological system is immature and does not produce adequate antibodies to fight infection.
③ Decreased mobility leads to stasis of secretions in the respiratory passages.
④ There is a weakness of the voluntary muscles that control respirations.

12. What nursing observations that would support theidentification of the early development of a chronic subdural hematoma in a 3-month-old infant?

① Posterior fontanel is closed, anterior fontanel is open.
② Retinal hemorrhages and hemiparesis.
③ Increased irritability and vomiting.
④ Papilledema and regressive behavior.

13. After a temporal craniotomy, what is an important nursing intervention?

① Take temperature orally only.
② Restrain the client as necessary.
③ Suction the client every 2 hours.
④ Do not position client with head down.

14. What will the neurological nursing assessment of an 88-year-old client with a left cranial hemisphere hemorrhage reveal?

① Spasticity, bilateral Babinski sign.
② Right side flaccidity and hemiparesis.
③ Spasticity and left foot clonus.
④ Flaccidity and bilateral foot clonus.

Answers and rationales to these questions are in the section at the end of the book entitled "Chapter Study Questions: Answers & Rationales."

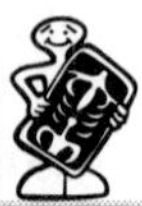

Appendix 20-1: NEUROLOGIC SYSTEM DIAGNOSTICS

NONINVASIVE DIAGNOSTICS

SKULL AND SPINE X-RAYS - simple X-rays to determine fractures, calcifications, etc.

Nursing Implications:
Explain procedure to client.

ELECTROENCEPHALOGRAPHY (EEG) - a recording of the electrical activity of the brain to physiologically assess cerebral activity; useful for diagnosing seizure disorders; used as a screening procedure for coma; also serves as an indicator for brain death.

Nursing Implications:
1. Explain to client that procedure is painless and there is no danger of electrical shock.
2. Determine from physician if any medications should be withheld prior to test, especially tranquilizers and sedatives.
3. Frequently, coffee, tea, and cola prohibited prior to examination.
4. Client's hair should be clean prior to the examination; after the exam, assist client to wash electrode paste out of hair.

MAGNETIC RESONANCE IMAGING (MRI) - Cell nuclei have magnetic properties; the MRI records the signals from the cells in a manner that provides information to evaluate soft tissue structures (tumors, blood vessels).

Nursing Implications:
1. Procedure will take approximately 1 ½ hours.
2. All metal objects should be removed from the client (hearing aids, hair clips, jewelry, buckles, etc.).
3. The client will be placed in a long magnetic tunnel for the procedure.
4. Poor candidates for MRI.
   a. Clients with pacemakers (the magnetic field interferes with the function of the pacemaker, and interferes with the test as well).
   b. Clients with implanted insulin pumps.
   c. Pregnant client, and very obese clients.
   d. Any client who requires life support equipment (the equipment will malfunction in a magnetic field).

COMPUTERIZED AXIAL TOMOGRAPHY (CAT SCAN) - computer-assisted X-ray of thin cross-sections of the brain to identify hemorrhage, tumor, edema, infarctions, and hydrocephalus.

Nursing Implications:
1. Explain appearance of scanner to client and explain importance of remaining absolutely still during the procedure.
2. Remove all objects from client's hair; fluids only for 4-6 hours prior to test.
3. Dye will be injected via venipuncture; assess for iodine allergy and advise the client he may experience a flushing or warm sensation when the dye is injected.
4. Contrast dye may discolor urine for about 24 hours.

BRAIN SCAN - A scanner traces the uptake of radioactive dye in the brain tissue. The dye is concentrated in the damaged tissue; it will take approximately 2 hours after dye is injected for the scan to be done.

Nursing Implications:
1. Determine if medications need to be withheld prior to procedure.
2. Client will be asked to change positions during the test in order to visualize the brain from different angles.
3. The client should not experience any pain.

CALORIC TESTING—Test is performed at bedside by introducing cold water into the external auditory canal. It is contraindicated in the client with a ruptured tympanic membrane and is not done on the client who is awake. If the eighth cranial nerve is stimulated, nystagmus rotates toward the irrigated ear. If no nystagmus occurs, pathology is present.

POSITRON EMISSION TOMOGRAPHY (PET) -see Appendix 17-1.

Appendix 20-1: NEUROLOGIC SYSTEM DIAGNOSTICS

INVASIVE DIAGNOSTICS

LUMBAR PUNCTURE - a needle is inserted into the lumbar area at L4 - L5 level; spinal fluid is withdrawn, and spinal fluid pressure is measured; contraindicated in presence of increased intracranial pressure; normal spinal fluid values: opening pressure - 60 to 150 mm water, specific gravity 1.007, pH 7.35, clear, protein 15 to 45 mg/dL, glucose 45 to 75 mg/dL, no microorganisms present.

Nursing Implications:
Pre-test:
1. Have client empty bladder.
2. Explain position to client (lateral recumbent with knees flexed.
3. Advise physician if there is a change in the client's neuro status prior to the test; increased intracranial pressure is a contraindication to a lumbar puncture.

Post-test:
1. Keep client flat at least 3 hours, and sometimes up to 12 hours, to decrease occurrence of headache.
2. Encourage high fluid intake.
3. Observe for spinal fluid leak from puncture site; if leakage occurs, it may precipitate a severe headache.

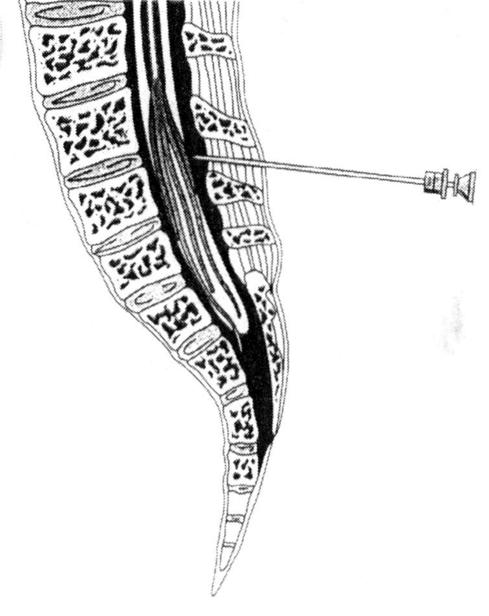

Figure 20-5: Lumbar Spinal Puncture: Position and angle of the needle.
Reprinted with permission: Phipps, WJ, Sands, JK, & Marek, JF (1999). *Medical Surgical Nursing: Concepts & Clinical Practice*, 6th ed. Philadelphia: Mosby, p 1688

MYELOGRAM — injection of dye into the subarachnoid space and utilization of X-rays of the spinal cord and vertebral column to identify spinal lesions.

Nursing Implications:
Pre-test:
1. Same as for lumbar puncture.
2. Check if client has any allergies to dye.

Post-test:
1. If amipaque, a water-soluble contrast medium is used, keep the head of the bed elevated 15 to 30 degrees to decrease dispersion of the dye to the brain; headache may occur due to irritation of the CNS; client should not receive any of the phenothiazine medications prior to or immediately after the examination.
2. If pantopaque, an oil-based contrast medium is used, most of it is removed via aspiration at the end of the test; client remains flat for 12 to 24 hours to reduce cerebral spinal fluid leakage and headache.

CEREBRAL ANGIOGRAM — injection of contrast material into the cerebral circulation; series of X-rays taken to study the cerebral blood flow; dye is usually injected via a soft catheter that is inserted and threaded through the femoral artery.
Nursing Implications:
Pre-test:
1. Client should be well-hydrated, but is NPO for 6-8 hours prior to the test; he/she should void prior to procedure.
2. Inform client he/she should remain very still during the procedure.
3. A feeling of warmth in the face and mouth and a metallic taste in the mouth common when dye is injected.

Post-test:
1. Evaluate client's neurological status; complications involve occlusion of cerebral arteries.
2. Observe injection site for hematoma formation.
3. Post-test complications can result in permanent disability.
4. Check circulation distal to area of puncture.

Appendix 20-1: NEUROLOGIC SYSTEM DIAGNOSTICS

INVASIVE DIAGNOSTICS

ELECTROMYOGRAPHY (EMG) - determines electrical potential for individual muscles. Flat electrodes or small needles are placed in the muscle. The client may be asked to move and perform simple activities; the electrical stimulus for the muscle will be recorded.

Pre-test:

1. May determine pre-test serum muscle determinations.
2. Explain to the client that small needles will be inserted into the skin.

Post-test:

1. Client may need something for pain because of muscle stimulation.
2. Assess needle sites for areas of hematomas, apply ice pack to prevent and/or relieve.

Appendix 20-2: ANTICONVULSANTS

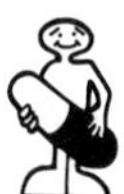

MEDICATIONS	SIDE EFFECTS	NURSING IMPLICATIONS
Phenobarbital (**Sodium Luminal**): IM, PO, rectal, IV Primidone (**Mysoline**): PO	Drowsiness, ataxia, excitation in children and in the elderly.	1. Client should avoid potential hazardous activities requiring mental alertness. 2. Sudden withdrawal may precipitate symptoms. 3. Close observation of response in children and elderly. 4. Used to treat grand mal and focal seizures. 5. See Appendix 15-5 for care of client with seizures.
Phenytoin (**Dilantin**): PO, IV	Gingival hyperplasia, skin rash, hypoglycemia Visual changes: nystagmus, diplopia, blurred vision dysrhythmias	1. Administer PO preparations with meals or milk to decrease gastric irritation. 2. Frequently used with phenobarbital for control of grand mal seizures. 3. IM injection not recommended. 4. Do not mix with any other medications when administering IV solution. 5. Promote good oral hygiene, gum hyperplasia is a problem with long term use. 6. See Appendix 15-5 for care of client with seizures.
Divalproex sodium (**Depakote**): PO	Monitor platelet counts GI, dermatologic effects, blood dyscrasias.	1. Should not be given to clients with severe liver dysfunction. 2. Potentiates action of phenobarbital, phenytoin, diazepam. 3. Use: absence seizures.

Appendix 20-3: CHOLINERGIC (ANTI-CHOLINESTERASE) MEDICATIONS

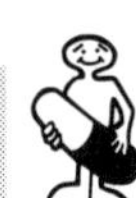

MEDICATIONS	SIDE EFFECTS	NURSING IMPLICATIONS
CHOLINERGIC MEDICATIONS: Intensify transmission of impulses throughout the CNS, where acetylcholine is necessary for transmission.		
Neostigmine bromide (**Prostigmin**): PO, SQ, IM Pyridostigmine bromide (**Mestinon**): PO, IM, IV Edrophonidum chloride (**Tensilon**): IV, IM	Excessive salivation, increased GI motility, urinary urgency, bradycardia, visual problems	1. Primary group of medications used for treatment of myasthenia gravis. 2. Atropine is the antidote for treatment of overdose. 3. In treatment of myasthenia gravis, medication is frequently administered 30 to 45 minutes prior to meals. 4. **Mestinon** is given for maintenance of the myasthenia client. 5. **Tensilon** is utilized for diagnostic purposes; not recommended for maintenance therapy. 6. Teach client symptoms of side effects and advise them to call the doctor if present.

Appendix 20-4: ANTI-PARKINSONISM AGENTS

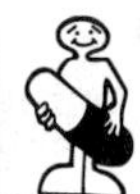

MEDICATIONS	SIDE EFFECTS	NURSING IMPLICATIONS
ANTI-CHOLINERGIC: Decreases synaptic transmissions in the CNS.		
Benztropine mesylate (**Cogentin**): PO, IM, IV Trihexyphenidyl hydrochloride (**Artane**): PO, IM, IV Procyclidine (**Kemadrin**): PO	Paralytic ileus, urinary retention, cardiac palpitations, blurred vision, nausea and vomiting, sedation, dizziness.	1. Administer PO preparations with meals to decrease gastric irritation. 2. Medications have cumulative effect. 3. Should not be used in clients with glaucoma, myasthenia gravis, GU or GI tract obstruction, or in children under 3 years old. 4. Monitor client carefully for bowel and bladder problems. 5. May be used to treat side effects of **Thorazine.**
DOPAMINERGIC: Assists to restore normal transmission of nerve impulses.		
Levodopa (**L-DOPA, Larodopa**): PO	***Early:*** anorexia, nausea and vomiting, abdominal discomfort, postural hypotension. ***Long term:*** abnormal, involuntary movements, especially involving the face, mouth and neck; behavioral disturbances involving confusion, agitation, and euphoria.	1. Administer PO preparations with meals to decrease GI distress. 2. Almost all clients will experience some side effects which are dose-related; dosage gradually increased according to client's tolerance and response. 3. Onset of action is slow; therapeutic response may require several weeks to months. 4. Vitamin B_6 (pyridoxine) is antagonistic to the effects of the medication; decrease client's intake of multiple vitamins and fortified cereals.
Carbidopa/levodopa (**Sinemet**): PO	(Same as for levodopa)	1. Same as for levodopa. 2. Utilization of carbidopa significantly decreases the amount of levodopa required for therapy. 3. Prevents the inhibitory effects of levodopa on vitamin B_6.
Amantadine hydrochloride (**Symmetrel**): PO	Orthostatic hypotension, dyspnea, dizziness, drowsiness, blurred vision, constipation, urinary retention (side effects are dose-related).	1. Less effective than levodopa; produces a more rapid clinical response.

Appendix 20-5: SEIZURE DISORDERS

❑ **DEFINITION:** Interruption of normal brain functioning by uncontrolled paroxysmal discharge of electrical stimuli from the neurons.

CLASSIFICATIONS OF SEIZURES:

Partial Seizures:

1. **Focal seizures (motor)** - confined to a specific area (hand, arm, leg).
2. **Jacksonian seizures (motor)** - activity begins slowly and progresses. May start with slow clonic movement in the hand and progress up the arm and over the side of the body. May be several minutes in duration.
3. **Complex partial** -characteristically produces automatisms (lip smacking, grimacing, repetitive hand movements). Client may become violent; period may be followed by amnesia and confusion.

Generalized Seizures:

1. **Absence (petit mal)** - characterized by a short period of time when the client is in an altered level of consciousness. Staring, blinking period (followed by resumption of normal activity) is characteristic. May occur over 100 times per day, may go unnoticed; generally, onset in children between ages of 4 and 12.
2. **Tonic-clonic seizures** - may experience an aura prior to the development of the seizure (auditory, visual, sensory, olfactory disturbances). Full recovery may take several hours; client may be confused, amnesic, and irritable during this recovery period.

Tonic phase -client may lose consciousness and fall, followed by muscle spasms. Apnea and cyanosis are common during this period; generally last for about one minute.

Clonic phase -hyperventilation, with rapid jerking movements. Tongue biting, incontinence, heavy salivation may occur during this period.

SEIZURE ETIOLOGY:

Acute Disorders:

1. Increased intracranial pressure.
2. Metabolic alterations.
3. Febrile episodes in children (generally between 6 mos and 3 yrs).
4. Infections.

Chronic (recurrent):

1. Brain injury at birth.
2. Trauma.
3. Vascular disease.
4. Brain tumors.
5. Idiopathic.

Nursing Assessment:

1. Identify any activities that occurred immediately prior to the seizure.
2. Was the client aware a seizure was going to occur? If so, how did he know?
3. Describe type of movements that occurred and the body area affected- - jaw clenched, tongue biting.
4. Presence of incontinence.
6. Period of apnea and cyanosis.
7. Presence of automatisms (lip smacking, grimacing, chewing).
8. Duration of seizure.
9. Changes in level of consciousness.
10. Condition of client post-seizure: oriented, what level of activity, any residual paralysis or muscle weakness.

NCLEX ALERT: *Report characteristics of a client's seizure, determine changes in client's neurologic status.*

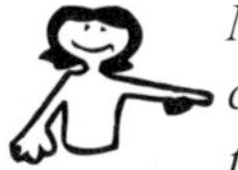

NURSING PRIORITY: *Artificial ventilation cannot be performed on a client in a tonic-clonic seizure. After the seizure is over, evaluate the airway and initiate ventilations if necessary.*

Nursing Management:

1. Remain with the client who is in seizure activity, note the time the seizure began and how long it lasted.
2. Do not attempt to force anything into the client's mouth if the jaws are clenched shut.
3. If the jaws are not clenched, place an airway in the client's mouth. This protects the tongue and also provides a method of suctioning the airway should the client vomit.
4. Protect the client from injuring himself by falling out of bed or by striking himself on bedrails, etc.
5. Loosen any constrictive clothing.
6. Do not restrain client during seizure activity; allow seizure movements to occur, but protect client from injury.
7. Evaluate respiratory status, if vomiting occurs; be prepared to suction the client to clear the airway and prevent aspiration.
8. Maintain calm atmosphere and provide for privacy after the seizure activity.
9. Re-orient client.

Client Education:

1. Identify activities/events that precipitate the seizure activity.
2. Avoid alcohol.
3. Take medications as directed.
4. Counseling for the family and for the client to assist them in maintaining positive coping mechanisms.

Appendix 20-6: APHASIA

❑ **Aphasia is a defect in the utilization and interpretation of language symbols. It may involve all aspects of language, or it may involve a specific area. The condition is precipitated by a problem of the cerebral cortex. The most common cause of aphasia is frequently a vascular problem involving the middle cerebral artery. The speech center is located in the dominant side of the cerebral hemisphere. The speech center for a right-handed person is located in the left cerebral hemisphere. Aphasic clients are often frustrated and irritable. Emotional lability is common. Accept the behavior in a manner that prevents embarrassment for the client.**

TYPES OF APHASIA

Sensory Aphasia (receptive or fluent, Wernicke's area) — Cannot understand oral or written communication. Client cannot interpret or comprehend speech or read.

Motor Aphasia (expressive, Broca's aphasia) —Inability to speak or to write; however, the client can comprehend incoming speech and can read.

Mixed —Most aphasia involves both the sensory and the motor aspect of speech. Rarely is aphasia only sensory or only motor.

NURSING IMPLICATIONS

1. Stand in front of the client, speak clearly and slowly.
2. Do not shout or speak loudly; the client can hear.
3. Be patient, give the client time to respond, do not press him for immediate answers.
4. Use nonverbal communications - touch, smile, show.
5. Assist the client with motor aphasia to practice repeating simple words - yes, no, please.
6. Listen carefully, try to understand, try to communicate; this conveys to the client that you care.
7. Provide directions as simply as possible.
8. Involve the family in practice and assist them to identify ways they can support the client.

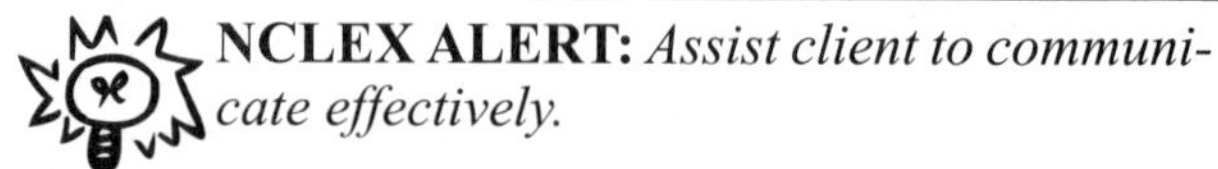

NCLEX ALERT: *Assist client to communicate effectively.*

PHYSIOLOGY OF THE MUSCULOSKELETAL AND CONNECTIVE TISSUE

Skeletal System

A. Bone structure.

1. Periosteum—dense fibrous membrane covering the bone; periosteal vessels supply bone tissue.
2. Epiphysis—a cartilage area in children which provides for longitudinal growth of the bone.
3. Articular cartilage—provides a smooth surface over the end of the bone to facilitate joint movement.
4. Red bone marrow—hemopoietic tissue located in the medullary cavity.
   a. In the fetus, almost all of the marrow is red.
   b. Red bone marrow is found in the adult in:
      (1) Ribs and sternum.
      (2) Vertebral bodies.
      (3) Portion of the hip bone.
   c. Function of red bone marrow is the formation of:
      (1) Red blood cells.
      (2) White cells.
      (3) Platelets.
      (4) Destruction of old red blood cells (phagocytosis).

B. Bone maintenance and healing.

1. Regulatory factors determining both formation and resorption.
   a. Weight-bearing stress stimulates local bone resorption and formation; in states of immobility where weight bearing is prevented, calcium is lost from the bone.
   b. Vitamin D promotes absorption of calcium from the GI tract and accelerates mobilization of calcium from the bone to increase or maintain serum calcium.
   c. The parathyroid hormone regulates the concentration of calcium in the serum partially by promoting the transfer of calcium from the bone.
   d. Calcitonin increases the production of bone cells.
2. Bone healing.
   a. When a bone is damaged or injured a hematoma precedes new tissue formation in the production of new bone substance.
   b. A callus is formed as minerals are deposited to organize a network for the new bone.
   c. The callus forms the initial clinical union of the bone and provides enough stability to prevent movement when bones are gently stressed.
   d. Continued bone healing provides for gradual return of the injured bone to its pre-injury shape and structural strength; this is frequently referred to as remodeling of the bone.

NURSING PRIORITY: *Age, displacement of the fracture, the site of the fracture, and blood supply to the area of injury are factors influencing time required for fracture healing to become complete.*

Connective Tissue—Joints and Cartilage

A. Joints.

1. The action of joints permits bones to change position and facilitate body movement.
2. The diarthrodial (synovial) joint is the most common type of joint in the body.
   a. Cartilage (hyaline) covers the end of the bone.
   b. A fibrous capsule of connective tissue joins the two bones together.
      (1) Synovium (synovial membrane) lines the capsule.
      (2) Synovial fluid is secreted by the synovium and serves to lubricate the joint and to decrease friction.

B. Cartilage is rigid, connective, avascular tissue; nourished by capillaries in adjacent connective tissue; damaged cartilage heals slowly due to lack of direct blood supply.

C. Ligaments and tendons are tough fibrous connective tissue providing stability while continuing to permit movement.

1. Tendons attach muscles to the bone.
2. Ligaments attach bones to bone joints.

Skeletal Muscle

A. Lower motor neurons control the activity of the skeletal muscle. The junction between the axon of the nerve cell and the muscle is the myoneural junction.

B. Energy is consumed when skeletal muscles contract in response to a stimulus.

Box 21-1: Elderly Care Focus
Musculoskeletal Changes

- Decreased bone density leads to more frequent fractures.
- Decrease in subcutaneous tissue results in less soft tissue over bony prominences.
- Degenerative changes in the spine alter posture and gait.
- Degenerative changes in cartilage result in decreased movement of joints.
- Decreased range of motion of extremity; may need increased assistance with ADLs.
- Slowed movement and decreased muscle strength leads to decreased response time.

1. Lactic acid, a by-product of muscle metabolism, accumulates if there is not a sufficient amount of oxygen available to the cell.
2. Muscle fatigue results from:
   a. Increased work of the muscle, with inadequate oxygen supply.
   b. Depletion of glycogen and energy stores.
   c. Accumulation of lactic acid.

C. Muscle contraction.

1. Isometric—the length of the muscle remains constant, the force generated by the muscle increases; an example is when one pushes against an immovable object.
2. Isotonic—shortening of the muscle, but with no increase in muscle tension.
3. Normal activity is a combination of both types of muscle contraction.
4. Muscles accomplish movement only by contraction.
   a. Flexion—bending at a joint.
   b. Extension—straightening of a joint.
   c. Abduction—action moving away from the body.
   d. Adduction—action moving toward the body.

NCLEX ALERT: *Do range of motion exercise for a client; know the terms used in referring to movement of joints.*

5. Hypertrophy will occur if muscle is exercised repeatedly.
6. Atrophy will occur with muscle disuse.

System Assessment

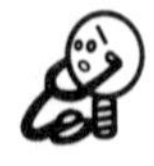

A. History.

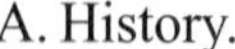

1. History of musculoskeletal injuries, neuromuscular disabilities, inflammatory, and

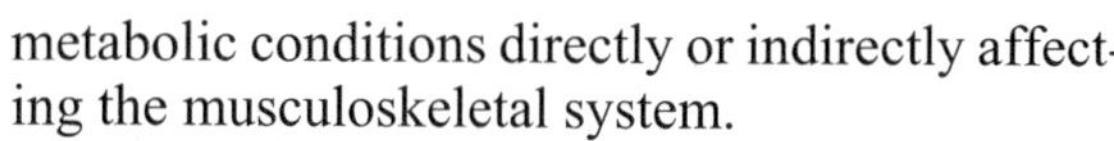

metabolic conditions directly or indirectly affecting the musculoskeletal system.
2. Familial predisposition to orthopedic problems.
3. Level of normal activity.
   a. Occupation.
   b. Exercise, recreation.
4. Existence of other chronic health problems.

B. Physical assessment.

1. Initial inspection for gross deformities, asymmetry, swelling, and edema.
2. Nutritional status—appropriateness of client's weight and body frame.
3. Joints.
   a. Movement—active and passive; examine active movement first; compare movement and range of motion to opposite side.
   b. Inflammation and tenderness—with or without movement.
   c. Presence of joint deformities and dislocations.
4. Evaluate limb length and circumference if there appears to be hypertrophy or inconsistency in bone length.
5. Evaluate client's spinal alignment, posture, and gait.
6. Evaluate skeletal muscle.
   a. Muscle strength bilaterally.
   b. Coordination of movement.
   c. Presence of atrophy or hypertrophy.
   d. Presence of involuntary muscle movement.
7. Assess peripheral pulses and peripheral circulation.
8. Assess for presence and characteristics of pain.
   a. Most musculoskeletal pain is relieved by rest.
   b. Identify precipitating activities and/or precipitating factors.
   c. Type of pain and location.

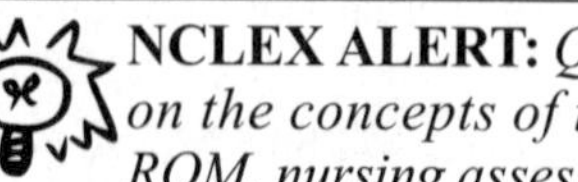

NCLEX ALERT: *Questions are often based on the concepts of immobility, performing ROM, nursing assessment of an extremity for compromised circulation, and general operative care. Pay close attention to the direction of the question.*

9. Sensory changes:
   a. Ask about back pain and injury.
   b. Assess for decrease sensation in lower extremities.

DISORDERS OF MUSCULOSKELETAL AND CONNECTIVE TISSUE

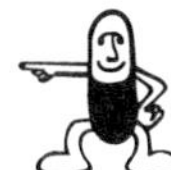

Congenital Hip Dysplasia

A. Malformations of the hip as a result of imperfect development of the femoral head, the acetabulum, or both. The structures that support the hip joint and hold the joint together are too loose or the joint cavity is too shallow.

Assessment

1. Risk factors/ etiology.
   a. Frequently associated with other congenital deformities.
   b. Prenatal factors.
      (1) Maternal hormone secretion.
      (2) Intrauterine posture, especially frank breech position.
2. Clinical manifestations.
   a. Newborn.
      (1) Ortolani's sign—infant supine, knees flexed, hips fully abducted; a click is heard or felt as the hip is reduced by abduction.
      (2) Asymmetrical gluteal and thigh folds.
      (3) Shortening of the leg on the affected side, one knee is lower than the other (Galeazzi sign).
3. Diagnostics — X-ray, CT scan.

Treatment

1. Treatment is initiated as soon as condition is identified.
2. For the newborn the dislocated hip is securely held in a full abduction position. This keeps the femur in the acetabulum and stabilizes the area.
   a. Abduction devices.
      (1) Pavlik harness—a fabric, strap harness that is secured around the infant's shoulders and waist, and is connected to straps around the lower leg. The harness maintains the legs in a flexed abducted position at the hip. The harness may be removed for bathing, but the infant will wear it full time until the hip is stable.
      (2) Hip spica cast—- most often used when adduction contracture is present. After the removal of the cast, a protective abduction brace is fitted.
   b. Closed reduction—utilized in older children 6-18 months old.
   c. Open reduction—if hip is not reducible with traction or closed reduction.
3. Successful reduction becomes increasingly difficult after age 4.

Nursing Intervention

✦ *Goal: to identify problem in the newborn prior to discharge.*

✦ *Goal: to assist parents to understand mechanism to maintain reduction.*

1. Pavlik brace—teach parents proper application of brace, undershirts should be worn under the brace; check skin under brace for irritation or pressure areas, no oils or lotions under brace.
2. Teach parents cast care if hip spica cast is applied.

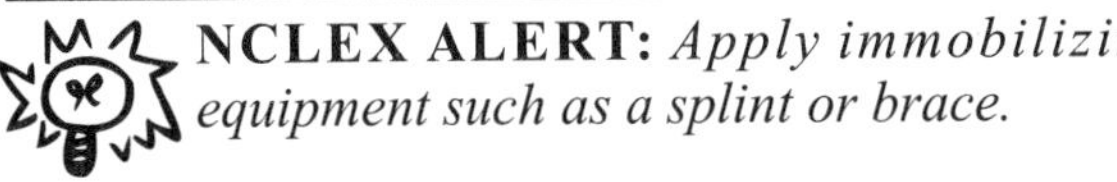

NCLEX ALERT: *Apply immobilizing equipment such as a splint or brace.*

✦ *Goal: to facilitate developmental progress.*

1. Provide appropriate stimuli and activity for developmental level.
2. Encourage parents to hold and cuddle child.
3. Maintain normal home routine.

Clubfoot (Talipes Equinovarus)

❑ **Deformity of the foot in which, adduction, plantar flexion and inversion of the foot occur in varying degrees of severity. Unilateral occurs more commonly than bilateral.**

Assessment

1. Risk factors/etiology (nonconclusive).
   a. Intrauterine compression.
   b. Decreased growth of distal tibia.
2. Assessment.
   a. Condition is apparent at birth.
   b. In true clubfoot there is severe limitation on the range of motion.
3. Diagnostics—clinical manifestations.

Treatment

Begun immediately and most often requires three stages for correction.

1. Correction of deformity—series of casts are applied for gradual stretching and straightening.
2. Maintenance of correction—clubfoot shoes.
3. Follow-up observations to prevent recurrence of deformity.

Nursing Intervention

✦ *Goal: to assist parents to understand mechanism of treatment to achieve correction.*

1. Appropriate care of cast or brace at home.
2. Follow-up care and importance of frequent cast changes.

✦ *Goal: to facilitate developmental progress and adapt nurturing activities to meet infant and parent needs (same as for congenital hip).*

Herniated Lumbar Disc

❑ **The intervertebral disc forms a cushion between the vertebral bodies of the spinal column. As stress on an injured or degenerated disc occurs, the cartilage material of the disc (nucleus pulposus) herniates inward toward the spinal column, causing compression or tension on the spinal nerve root. The problem most often occurs in the lumbosacral area.**

Assessment

1. Risk factors/etiology.
   a. Degenerative disc disease.
   b. Obesity.
   c. Injury or stress to the lower back.
   d. Muscle-strengthening exercises.
2. Clinical manifestations (lumbar disc).
   a. Low back pain radiating down the posterior thigh.
   b. Coughing, straining, sneezing, bending, and lifting aggravate the pain.
   c. Lying supine and raising the leg in an extended position will precipitate the pain.
3. Diagnostics—myelogram, MRI.

Treatment

1. Conservative.
   a. Analgesics, muscle relaxants.
   b. Weight reduction if appropriate.
   c. Ice may be used for first 48 hours after injury, then heat is better analgesic.
   d. Activity modification, good body mechanics.
2. Surgical.
   a. Laminectomy—removal of the herniated portion of the disk.
   b. Micro-laminectomy—removal of the herniated disk utilizing a microscope. There is less trauma in the disk area, improved hemostasis, minimal nerve root involvement.

Nursing Intervention

✦ *Goal: to relieve pain via conservative measures and prevent recurrence of problem.*

1. Decrease muscle spasm with analgesics and decreased activity.
2. Begin ambulation slowly and avoid having client bend, stoop, sit, or lift.
3. Instruct the client and family regarding the principles of body mechanics.
4. The client will need a firm mattress; avoid sleeping in the prone position, especially with a pillow.
5. Instruct the client and family regarding lower back exercises.
6. Encourage correct posture; avoid prolonged standing.
7. Sit in straight-backed chairs.
8. Semireclining position with forward flexion of lumbar spine (recliner) may be position of comfort.

✦ *Goal: to prepare client for laminectomy.*

1. Preoperative nursing intervention as appropriate.
2. Have client practice logrolling.
3. Have client practice voiding from supine position.
4. Discuss with client postoperative pain and anticipated methods to decrease pain.
5. Evaluate bowel and bladder function.
6. Identify specific characteristics of pain for data base postoperatively.
7. Establish a baseline neurological assessment for reference postoperatively.

✦ *Goal: to maintain spinal alignment postoperative laminectomy.*

1. Keep the bed in flat position.
2. Logroll client when turning.
3. Keep pillows between the legs when positioned on the side.
4. The client with micro-disk surgery will have less limitations on his mobility. Often he may assume a position of comfort.

✦ *Goal: to maintain homeostasis and assess for complications postoperative laminectomy.*

1. Evaluate incision area for possible leakage of spinal fluid and bleeding.
2. Analgesics may be given via PCA pump or epidural catheter.
3. Assess pain and determine if there is any pain radiation.

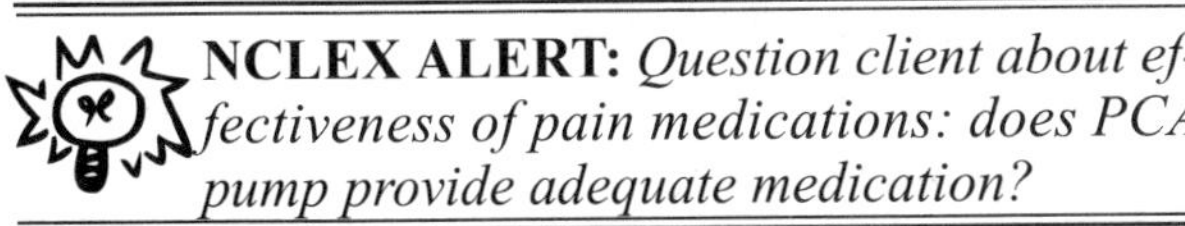

NCLEX ALERT: *Question client about effectiveness of pain medications: does PCA pump provide adequate medication?*

4. Evaluate sensation of extremities.
5. Determine ability to move feet and toes.
6. Evaluate circulatory status of legs and feet.

***NURSING PRIORITY:** The laminectomy client frequently experiences difficulty voiding; this may be due to edema in the area of surgery that interferes with normal bladder sensation.*

7. Normal bladder function returns in 24-48 hours; assess current status of voiding.
8. Ambulate as soon as indicated (frequently on first postoperative day if no fusion was done).
9. The client with the micro-laminectomy experiences less pain, is frequently out of bed the day of surgery, and has fewer complications.
10. Paralytic ileus is a common complication; assess for decreased bowel sounds and abdominal distention.

Scoliosis

❑ **A lateral curvature of the spine. If scoliosis is allowed to progress without treatment, it will severely affect the shape of the thoracic cavity and impair ventilation.**

A. Idiopathic (predominant type) occurs primarily in adolescent girls.

B. Most noticeable at beginning of growth spurt, around 10 years.

Assessment

1. Clinical manifestations.
   a. Uneven hips and shoulders.
   b. Visible curvature of the spinal column; head and hips are not in alignment.
   c. When child bends forward from the waist, there is visible asymmetry of the shoulders. The ribs and shoulder are more prominent on one side.
   d. Waist line is uneven, one hip is more prominent.
2. Diagnostics.
   a. Clinical manifestations.
   b. X-ray.

Treatment

1. Observation and monitoring for curvature less than 20°.
2. Brace if curvature shows progression.
   a. Milwaukee brace for high thoracic curvatures.
   b. Boston brace (pelvic model) for thoracic-lumbar curves.
3. Surgery—Spinal fusion and placement of a rod to prevent destruction of the fused segment. The rod may be left in place permanently unless it becomes displaced or causes discomfort.

Nursing Intervention

✦ *Goal: to identify defects early and promote effective conservative therapy.*

1. Promote health programs in school to identify condition.
2. Assist client and parents to properly utilize braces.
   a. Make sure brace is properly fitted and does not inadvertently rub bony prominences.
   b. May put light tee-shirt under brace for comfort.
   c. Initially, the brace is worn 20 to 23 hours per day.
   d. Brace is regularly adjusted to promote correction.
   e. If progress is good, child is weaned from the brace during the daytime and wears it only at night.

NCLEX ALERT: *Apply immobilizing devices such as a splint or brace.*

   f. Supplemental exercises.

✦ *Goal: to support normal growth and development and assist the child to develop a positive self-image.*

1. Continue to encourage peer socialization.
2. Encourage independence.
3. Encourage child to participate in and be independent in scheduling of activities and other aspects of care.
4. Emphasize positive long-term outcome.

✦ *Goal: to maintain spinal alignment postoperative correction (See care of client postoperative laminectomy and fusion).*

✦ *Goal: to maintain homeostasis and assess for complications postoperative correction (See postoperative laminectomy and fusion).*

Fractures

A. A disruption or break in the continuity of the bone, which occurs most often from a traumatic injury.

B. Characteristics of bones in children affecting fractures and fracture healing.

1. Presence of epiphyseal plate; if damaged in the fracture it may affect the growth of the long bone.
2. Periosteum is thicker and stronger, has an increased blood supply; therefore healing is more rapid.
3. Bones are more porous and allow for greater flexibility.

C. Pathological fractures occur secondary to a disease process.

D. Classification of fractures.

1. Type.
   a. Complete—fracture line extends through the entire bone; the periosteum is disrupted on both sides of the bone.
   b. Incomplete—fracture line extends only partially through the bone (greenstick, hairline type fractures).
   c. Comminuted—fractures with multiple bone fragments; more common in the adult.
   d. Greenstick—an incomplete fracture with bending and splintering of the bone; more common in children.
2. Classified according to location on the bone—proximal, middle, or distal.
3. Stable vs. unstable fracture.
   a. Stable—a portion of the periosteum usually remains intact; frequently transverse, spiral, or greenstick fractures.
   b. Unstable—bones are displaced at the time of injury, with poor approximation.
4. Simple, closed fracture—does not produce a break in the skin.
5. Complex, open, or compound fracture— involves an open wound through which the bone has protruded.
6. Epiphyseal injuries—if the fracture line extends through the epiphyseal plate, bone growth may be affected. Problem with children.

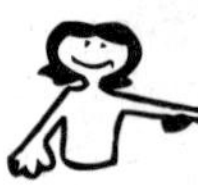

***NURSING PRIORITY:** Be familiar with the terms used to describe fractures.*

Assessment

1. Risk factors/etiology.
   a. Pathological fracture.
      (1) Osteoporosis.
      (2) Multiple myeloma.
      (3) Osteogenic sarcoma.
      (4) Metabolic diseases.
   b. Trauma.
2. Clinical manifestations.
   a. Edema, swelling of soft tissue around the injured site.
   b. Pain - immediate, severe.
   c. Abnormal positioning of extremity; deformity.
   d. Loss of function due to disruption of bone integrity.
   e. False movement: movement occurs at the fracture site; bone should not move except at joints.
   f. Crepitation—palpable or audible crunching as the ends of the bones rub together.
   g. Discoloration of the skin around the affected area.
   h. Sensation may be impaired if there is nerve damage.
   i. Loss of normal function.
3. Diagnostics.
   a. Clinical manifestations and history.
   b. X-ray of involved area.

Treatment

1. Immediate immobilization of suspected fracture area.
2. Fracture reduction.
   a. Closed reduction—manual realignment of the bones; then injured extremity is usually placed in a cast for continued immobilization until healing occurs.
   b. Open reduction—surgical correction of alignment.
3. Traction (Figure 21-2).
   a. Purposes.
      (1) Immobilization of fractures until surgical correction is done; immobilization or alignment of fracture until sufficient healing occurs to permit casting.
      (2) Decrease, prevent, or correct deformities associated with muscle diseases and bone injury.
      (3) Decrease muscle spasm by fatiguing involved muscles.
   b. Types.
      (1) Skeletal—wire or metal pin is inserted into or through the bone (Kirschner wires or Steinmann pins).
      (2) Skin—force of pull is applied directly to the skin and indirectly to the bone.
4. Cast application to maintain immobility of affected area.

a. Cast applied to immobilize joints above and below the injured area.
b. Short or long arm cast.
c. Body jacket cast for spinal injuries.
d. Hip spica cast for femoral fractures.
(1) Body jacket.
(2) Long leg cast.

5. External/internal fixation
a. Rigid external device consisting of pins placed through the bone and held in place by a metal frame.
b. Internal fixation (ORIF - open reduction, internal fixation) is done through an open incision and hardware (pins, plates, rods, screws) is placed in the bone.
c. Both methods may be used to treat a fracture.

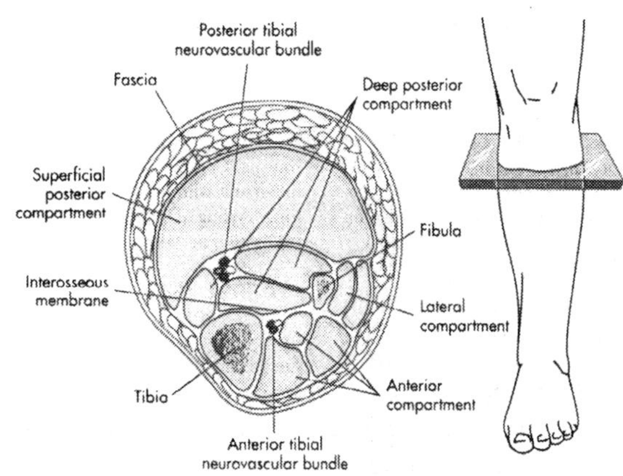

Figure 21-1: Compartments of Lower Leg
Compartments of the proximal third of the lower leg - anterior, lateral, deep posterior, superficial posterior. As the compartment swells, pressure is exerted on vessels and nerves within the compartment.
Reprinted with permission: Phipps, WJ, Sands, JK, & Marek, JF (1999). *Medical Surgical Nursing: Concepts & Clinical Practice*, 6th ed. Philadelphia: Mosby, p. 1936.

Complications

1. Direct complications.
a. Delayed union.
b. Nonunion.
c. Angulation (bone heals at a distorted angle).
2. Infection—especially in injuries resulting in an open fracture and soft tissue injury.
3. Decreased circulation resulting from pressure of cast and edema formation.
a. Decreased pulses distal to injury.
b. Pain unrelieved by analgesics and edema.
c. Decrease sensory and motor function.
d. Pallor
4. Compartment syndrome—muscle, nerves, vessel are restricted to a confined space or "compartment" within an extremity (Figure 21-1).
a. Etiology.
(1) Decreased compartment size from cast, splints, tight bandages, tight surgical closure.
(2) Increase in compartment contents caused by hemorrhage, and/or edema.
b. Clinical manifestations of compartment syndrome.
(1) Muscle ischemia occurs as a result of compression of structures in the compartment.
(2) Arterial compression may not occur, pulses may still be present.

NCLEX ALERT: *Implement measures to prevent circulatory complications; situations regarding compromised circulation in the orthopedic client are consistently included on the exam.*

(3) May cause permanent damage if not relieved immediately.
(4) Clients complain of excessive pain unrelieved by analgesics.
(5) Occurrence of complication may be decreased by elevating the extremity and applying of ice packs after initial injury.
(6) Treatment is directed toward immediate release of pressure. If the client has a cast, the cast may be "bivalved." The cast is split in half, the halves are secured around the extremity by a wrap such as an elastic bandage.
(7) Volkmann's contracture—compartment syndrome that compromises circulation; occurs most often as a result of short arm cast used to immobilize a fracture of the humerus.
(8) Can result in permanent damage in a short time (6-8 hours).
(9) Paresthesia is frequently the first sign, pulselessness is a late sign.

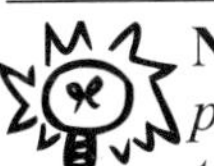

NCLEX ALERT: *Implement measures to prevent potential neurological complications.*

5. Venous stasis and thrombus formation related to immobility.
6. Fat embolism.
   a. Associated with fractures of long bones; primarily occurs in adults.
   b. Clinical manifestations generally occur within 12 to 48 hours of injury.
   c. Fat embolism producing symptoms of acute respiratory distress and hypoxia.
7. Blisters may be associated with fractures that are a twisting type of injury, or when compartmental syndrom occurs.

Nursing Intervention

✦ *Goal: to provide immobility and emergency care prior to transporting victim.*

1. Evaluate circulation distal to injury.
2. If pulses are not present or if the extremity must be realigned to apply splint for transfer, apply just enough traction to support and immobilize the fracture in a position of proper alignment. Once the traction is initiated, do not release it until the extremity has been properly splinted.
3. Splint and immobilize extremity prior to transfer.

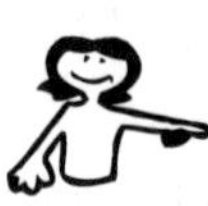

***NURSING PRIORITY:** Do not apply traction to compound fractures; traction may cause more damage to tissue and vessels.*

4. Elevate the affected extremity, if possible, to decrease edema.

✦ *Goal: to identify complications early; frequent peripheral nerve and vascular assessment distal to the area of injury.*

1. Impaired blood flow.
   a. Pulselessness.
   b. Skin pale and cool to touch.
   c. Pain, swelling, edema distal to cast.
   d. Capillary refill less greater than 3 seconds.
2. Nerve damage from excessive pressure.
   a. Paresthesia, numbness distal to cast.
   b. Motor paralysis of previously functioning muscles.
   c. Feeling of deep pain and pressure.
3. Infection.
   a. Unpleasant odor from cast.
   b. Drainage through cast (foul, purulent).
   c. Temperature elevation.
   d. Increased warmth over cast, "hot spot."

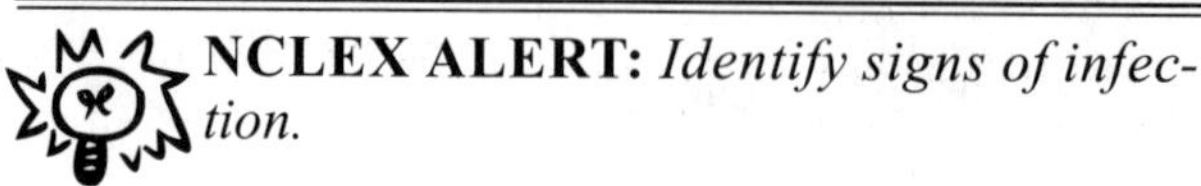

NCLEX ALERT: *Identify signs of infection.*

4. Compartment syndrome.
   a. Significant increase in pain, not responsive to analgesics.
   b. Loss of movement and sensation distal to cast.
   c. Skin is pale, cool to touch.
   d. Edema distal to cast.
   e. Pulses may be present initially.
5. Notify physician immediately if any of the above complications are present.

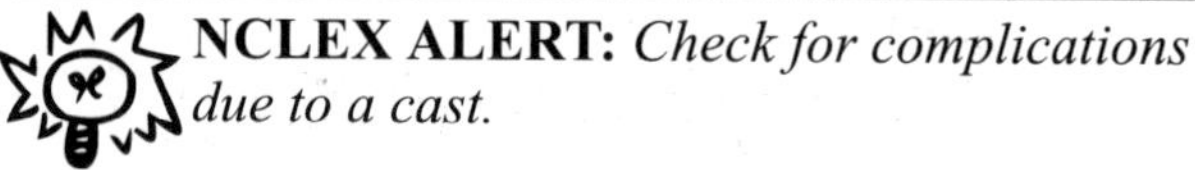

NCLEX ALERT: *Check for complications due to a cast.*

✦ *Goal: to maintain immobilization via cast.*

1. Allow plaster cast to dry adequately before handling or moving the client.
   a. Do not cover the cast with a blanket.
   b. Encourage cast to dry by utilizing fans and maintaining adequate circulation.
   c. Avoid handling wet cast to prevent indentions in the cast which may precipitate pressure areas inside the cast.
   d. Reposition client every 2 hours to increase drying on all cast surfaces.
   e. "Petaling" a cast is done to cover the rough edges and prevent crumbling of a plaster cast; edges are covered with small strips of waterproof adhesive.
   f. Do not allow cast to become excessively damp or to get wet.

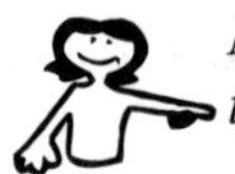

***NURSING PRIORITY:** Do not apply any type of heat to a cast to enhance drying.*

2. Synthetic cast (fiberglass, polyester cotton knit) are lighter and require minimal amount of drying time.
   a. Frequently used for upper body cast.
   b. Preferable for infants and children.
   c. Cast does not crumble around the edges and soil as easily.
   d. Cast drys rapidly if it gets damp and it does not disintegrate in water; some synthetic casts can be immersed for bathing.
3. Continue to assess for compromised circulation and compartment syndrome.

Figure 21-2: Traction
Reprinted with permission: Phipps, WJ, Sands, JK, & Marek, JF (1999). *Medical Surgical Nursing: Concepts & Clinical Practice*, 6th ed. Philadelphia: Mosby, p 1920-1921.

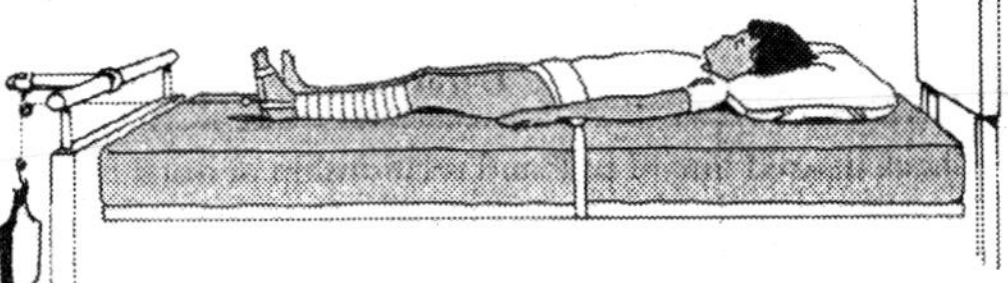

Buck extension traction.

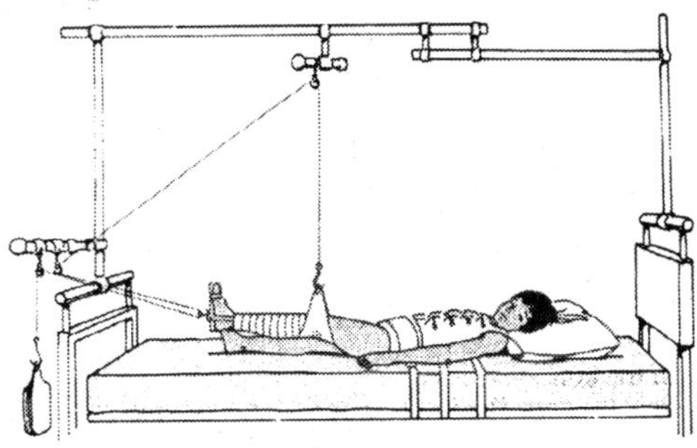

Russell traction.

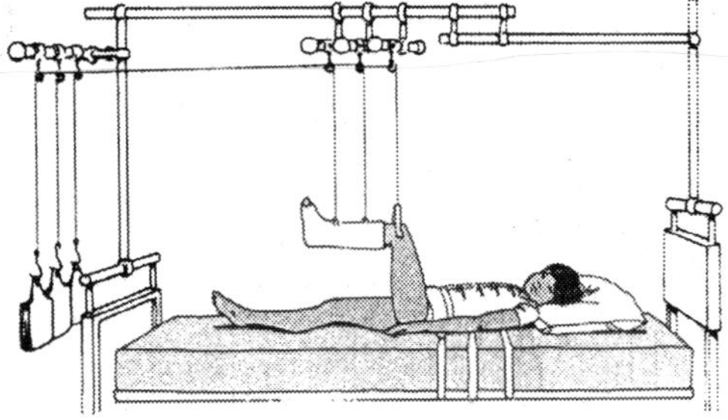

"90-90" traction.

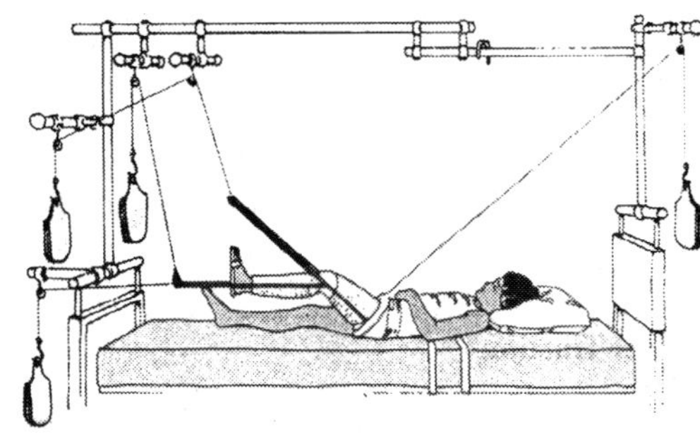

Balance suspension with Thomas ring splint and Pearson attachment.

4. Body jacket cast and hip spica cast.
   a. Evaluate for abdominal discomfort due to cast compression of mesenteric artery against duodenum.
   b. Relief of pressure via nasal gastric tube and suction, or cast removal and reapplication.
   c. Evaluate for pressure areas over iliac crest.
5. Elevate casted extremity, especially during the first 24 hours after application.
6. Apply ice packs over the area of injury during the first 24 hours.
7. Encourage movement and exercise of unaffected joints.

✦ *Goal: to maintain immobilization via traction (see Figure 21-1).*

1. Assume that traction is continuous unless the doctor orders otherwise.
2. Carefully assess for skin breakdown, especially under the client.
3. Do not change or remove traction weight on a client with continuous traction.
4. The traction ropes and weights should hang free from any obstructions.
5. Traction applied in one direction requires an equal counter traction to be effective.
   a. Do not let the client's feet touch the end of the bed; this will cause the counter traction to be lost.
   b. Do not allow the traction weights to rest on anything at the end of the bed; this negates the pull of the traction.
6. Carefully assess the pin sites in clients with skeletal traction. Osteomyelitis is a serious complication of skeletal traction.

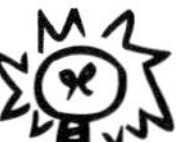

NCLEX ALERT: *Maintain traction devices.*

✦ *Goal: to prevent complications of immobility (Chapter 3).*

NCLEX ALERT: *Prevent complications of immobility - the majority of clients with fractures will experience some level of immobility.*

Box 21-2: Elderly Care Focus
Musculoskeletal Nursing Implications

- Difficulty maintaining immobility after fractures; therefore, they are frequently repaired with surgical intervention (ORIF).
- Heal more slowly, so use of extremity and weight-bearing are frequently delayed.
- Complications of immobility occur more frequently; mobilize hospitalized clients as early as possible.
- Do not rely on fever as the primary indication of infection; decreasing mental status is more common.
- Contractions are more common.
- More frequent use of assistive devices - canes and walkers.

✦ *Goal: to prevent complications from external/internal fixation.*

1. Inspect exposed skin and pin sites for infection.
2. Cleanse around pin sites.
3. Perform wound care to incisional area or area of trauma.
4. Careful observation for development of an infection.
5. Evaluate for circulatory and neurosensory impairment.

Self/Home Care

1. Client should not:
   a. Bear weight on the affected extremity until instructed to do so.
   b. Allow the cast to get wet (discuss alternatives in bathing).
   c. Insert anything under or in the cast.
2. Client should report any symptoms associated with swelling or increase in pain.
3. Assess any pin sites for evidence of infection.

Specific Fractures

A. Colles' fracture.
   1. Fracture of the distal radius.
   2. Primary complication is compartment syndrome.

B. Fractured pelvis.
   1. Frequently occurs in elderly and is associated with falls.
   2. May cause serious intra-abdominal injuries (hemorrhage) and urinary tract injury.
   3. Bedrest is utilized for stable fractures.
   4. Combination of traction, cast, and surgical intervention may be utilized in complex fractures.
   5. Turn client only on specific orders.

C. Fractured hip —may be repaired by pinning or hip joint replacement.
   1. Common in elderly women over 65 years old due to loss of postural stability and loss of bone mass.
   2. Clinical manifestations.
      a. External rotation and adduction of the affected extremity.
      b. Shortening of the length of the affected extremity.
      c. Severe pain and tenderness.
   3. Treatment.
      a. Initially, Buck's traction to immobilize fracture and decrease muscle spasms (Fig. 21-2).
      b. Surgical repair as soon as client's condition allows (permits earlier mobility and prevents complications of immobility).
   4. Nursing intervention postoperative (Box 21-2).
      a. Circulatory and neurologic checks distal to area of injury.
      b. Position to prevent flexion, adduction and internal rotation, which cause dislocation of the prosthesis.

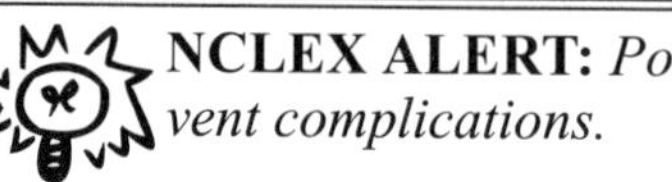
NCLEX ALERT: *Position a client to prevent complications.*

(1) Do not adduct the affected leg past the neutral position.
(2) Maintain the affected leg in an abducted position.
(3) Maintain abduction with an A-frame pillow or by keeping pillows between the knees.
(4) Avoid acute flexion of the hip.
(5) Prevent external rotation by utilizing sandbags, pillows, and trochanter rolls at the thigh.
(6) Extreme external rotation accompanied by severe pain is indicative of hip prosthesis displacement.

c. Check physician's order regarding positioning and turning.

d. Evaluate blood loss.
(1) Check under the client for hemorrhage.
(2) Measure the diameter of the thigh to evaluate the presence of internal bleeding.

NCLEX ALERT: *The client is especially prone to complications of immobility; utilize nursing interventions to minimize complications.*

D. Total hip replacement.
   1. Hip replacement may be done due to a pathological fracture or due to a disease process such as arthritis.
   2. Preoperative care.
      a. Encourage client to practice using either crutches or a walker, whichever is anticipated to be used postoperatively.
      b. Encourage client to practice moving from the bed to the chair in the same manner he will postoperatively.
      c. Assist the client to begin practicing the postoperative exercises so he will understand and be able to do them correctly.
   3. Postoperative care
      a. Maintain abduction.
      b. Quadriceps exercises,
      c. Nerve and circulation checks.
      d. Mobilized first or second postoperative day to prevent complications of immobility; may use sequential compression pumps on lower extremely to prevent venous stasis.
      e. Low molecular weight Heparin (Appendix 16-3) may be given to prevent thrombophlebitis.

NURSING PRIORITY: *Postoperatively, do not allow the repaired hip to flex greater than 90 degrees; avoid adduction and internal rotation of extremity. Flexion and adduction will dislocate the hip prosthesis.*

E. Femoral shaft fracture.
   1. Common injury in young adults and children.
   2. Treatment.
      a. Immobility via a spica cast in older children.
      b. 90°-90° traction (Fig 21-2) balanced skeletal traction for fractured femur.
      c. Older child, adult.
         (1) Internal fixation (adults).
         (2) Balanced skeletal traction for 8 to 12 weeks.
         (3) Immobilization via hip spica alone or after balanced skeletal traction.

F. Rib fractures.
   1. Usually heal in 3 to 6 weeks with no residual impairment.
   2. Painful respirations cause client's breathing to be more shallow and coughing to be restrained; this precipitates buildup of secretions and decreased ventilation.
   3. Chest taping or strapping is not usually utilized because it decreases thoracic excursion.
   4. Multiple rib fractures may precipitate the development of a pneumothorax or a tension pneumothorax (Chapter 15).

Osteoporosis

❑ **A metabolic bone disease that involves an imbalance between new bone formation and bone resorption.**

A. Primary osteoporosis is most common type. Occurs most often in women after menopause and low levels of estrogen are associated with the increase in bone resorption.

B. Bone loss occurs predominantly in the vertebral bodies of the spine, the femoral neck in the hip, and in the distal radius of the arm. The bone mass declines, leaving the bone brittle and weak (Figure 21-3).

Assessment

1. Risk factors/etiology.
   a. Incidence increases in white women after age 50 years.
   b. Accelerated post menopause bone loss (estrogen deficit).
   c. Low peak bone mass - the maximum amount of bone a person achieves.
   d. Endocrine disorders of the thyroid and parathyroid.
   e. Adolescents and young women with eating disorders.
2. Clinical manifestations.
   a. May be asymptomatic until X-rays demonstrate skeletal weakening. Bone loss of 30% to 50% must occur before osteoporosis can be identified on standard X-rays.
   b. Spinal deformity and "dowager's hump."
      (1) Results from repeated pathological, spinal vertebral fractures.
      (2) Gradual loss of height.
      (3) Increase in spinal curvature (kyphosis).
   c. Spinal fractures may occur spontaneously, or as a result of minimal trauma.
   d. Chronic low thoracic and midline back pain.
   e. Height loss may precipitate thoracic problems, decrease in abdominal capacity and exercise tolerance.
   f. Hip fractures and vertebral collapse are the most debilitating problems.
3. Diagnostics.
   a. Serum lab values of calcium, phosphorus, and alkaline phosphatase are usually normal.

b. Computed tomography or bone density scan to evaluate bone loss.

Treatment

1. Dietary—increased protein, calcium and vitamin D.
2. Medications.
   a. Calcium supplements—daily intake of calcium should be approximately 1000 mg for men, and 1500 mg for post menopausal women.
   b. Vitamin D supplements to enhance utilization of calcium. Spending 15 minutes daily in the sun will provide adequate Vitamin D.
   c. Estrogen replacement therapy as indicated.
   d. Alendronate (**Fosamax**) and Calcitonin (**Calcimar**) are medications to facilitate increased bone density.
3. Exercise—activities that put moderate stress on bones by working them against gravity (walking, racquet sports, jogging). This type of exercise is believed to decrease the development of osteoporosis and possibly increase new bone formation. Swimming and yoga may not be as beneficial, due to decreased stress on bone mass.
4. Compression fractures of the vertebrae usually heal without surgical intervention.

Complications

Bone fracture occurring in the vertebral bodies, distal radius, or the hip.

Nursing Intervention

✦ *Goal: to decrease pain and promote activities to diminish progress of disease.*

1. Pain relief.
   a. Bedrest initially.
   b. Firm mattress.
   c. Narcotic analgesics initially then followed by NSAIDs.
2. Assess bowel and bladder function; client prone to constipation and paralytic ileus if vertebrae are involved.
3. Regular daily exercise; encourage outdoor exercises (increases utilization of Vitamin D).
4. Increased calcium intake and estrogen therapy.

Self-Care

1. Decrease falls and injury by maintaining safe home environment.
2. Understand need to continue medications, even if they do not make the client feel better. Important for client to understand that the calcium supplements are to prevent further damage.
3. Do not exercise if pain occurs.
4. Avoid heavy lifting, stooping, and bending. Review and demonstrate good body mechanics with the client.

Osteomyelitis

❑ **An infection of the bone.**

A. The most common causative organism is *Staphylococcus.*

B. Inflammatory response occurs initially, with increased vascularization and edema.

C. Even though the healing process occurs, the dead bone tissue frequently forms a sequestrum which continues to retain viable bacteria; may produce recurrent abscesses for years.

D. Classified according to acute or chronic status.
   1. Acute—sudden onset; may heal in 2 to 3 weeks or progress to chronic.
   2. Chronic—a continuous, persistent problem or exacerbation of previous problem.

Assessment

1. Risk factors/etiology.
   a. Indirect entry of organism.
      (1) Hematogenic.
      (2) Injury and infection of adjacent soft tissue.
   b. Direct injury.
      (1) Trauma.
      (2) Surgical procedures.
2. Clinical manifestations.
   a. Acute.
      (1) Tenderness, swelling, and warmth of affected area.
      (2) Drainage from infected site.
      (3) Fever, chills.
      (4) Constant pain in affected area.
      (5) Circulatory impairment.
   b. Chronic.
      (1) Continuous drainage from wound or sinus tract.
      (2) Recurrent episodes of pain.
      (3) Low-grade fever.
      (4) Remission and exacerbation of problem.
3. Diagnostics.
   a. Wound culture.
   b. Blood culture.
   c. Radionuclide bone scan.
   d. Gallium scan.

e. MRI.

f. X-ray only shows soft tissue swelling; 2 to 3 weeks before irregularity of bones can be identified via X-ray.

Treatment

1. Intensive IV antibiotics.
2. Immobilization of affected area.

Nursing Intervention

✦ *Goal: to decrease pain, promote comfort, and decrease spread of infection.*

1. Administer IVPB antibiotics, frequent assessment of status of IV site.
2. Maintain correct body alignment.
   a. Move affected extremity gently and with support.
   b. Prevent contractures, especially of affected extremity.
3. If there is an open wound, maintain wound precautions. (Chapter 6).
4. Client is usually discharged with antibiotics and should maintain close follow-up care.

Osteosarcoma

A. The most common primary bone cancer; it advances very rapidly with metastasis to the lungs via the blood. (See Chapter 8).

B. Most commonly affects the long bones, most often the distal end of the femur.

Assessment

1. Risk factors/etiology.
   a. Peak incidence between 10 and 25 years old.
   b. Increased incidence in males during adolescence.
   c. Primary tumors of the prostate, breast, kidney and lung metastasize to the bone.
2. Clinical manifestations.
   a. Localized pain at site of tumor.
   b. Client may limp and be unable to function at full capacity.
3. Diagnostics.
   a. CT to determine the extent of the lesion.
   b. Radioisotope scans to evaluate for metastasis.
   c. Lung evaluation to determine if metastatic sites are present.
   d. Serum lab studies are inconclusive; client usually has an increase in serum alkaline phosphatase.
   e. X-ray will reveal the tumor location and assist in determining an appropriate biopsy site.

Box 21-3: Elderly Care Focus
Protecting Joints

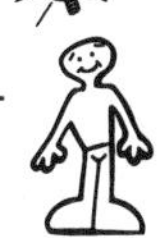

- If pain lasts longer then one hour after exercise, need to change exercises that involve that joint.
- Plan activity and work that conserves energy - do important tasks first.
- Alternate activities, do not do all heavy tasks at one time.
- Minimize stress on joints - sit rather then stand, avoid prolonged repetitive movements, move around frequently, avoid stairs or prolonged grasping.
- Use largest muscles rather then smaller ones - use shoulders or arms rather then hands to push open doors; pick up items without stooping or bending, use leg muscles; women can carry purses on their shoulders rather then in their hands.
- Painful, swollen inflamed joints should not be exercised; do basic ROM.
- Regular exercise even when joints are painful and stiff -swimming and bike riding maintain mobility without weight-bearing.

Treatment

1. Amputation of extremity and or extensive surgical resection of bone and surrounding tissue.
2. Chemotherapy.
3. Radiation therapy.

Nursing Intervention

✦ *Goal: to maintain homeostasis and prevent complications postoperatively.*

1. An extensive pressure dressing with wound drains/suction may be applied.
2. ROM is usually begun immediately; continuous passive motion (CPM) may be used immediately or on first postoperative day for both upper and lower extremity surgery.
3. Muscle toning is important prior to weight bearing.
4. Frequent neurovascular assessment due to resection of nerves and vessels in area; extremity may also be casted or splinted.

✦ *Goal: to prevent complications and promote mobility post amputation . (Appendix 21-3)*

✦ *Goal: to assist the client/child and family to cope with the diagnosis and build basis for rehabilitation.*

1. Honest, straightforward information to child/client and parents regarding the situation.
2. Allow the family and client an opportunity to express their concerns and fears; surgery is extensive and may affect body image.(See Chapter 9)
3. Anticipate sense of loss of control and anger over changes in body.

4. Encourage normal growth and developmental activities as appropriate; allow client to be as independent as possible.

✦ *Goal: to assist the child and the family to cope with the side effects of chemotherapy and radiation. (See Chapter 8).*

Rheumatoid Arthritis

❑ **A systemic disease that affects all areas of the body; inflammatory responses occur in all connective tissue. Early symptoms include inflammation of the synovial joints.**

A. Joint involvement progresses in stages; if disease is diagnosed early, permanent joint deterioration may be prevented.
   1. The synovium becomes thickened and inflamed, and fluid accumulates in the joint space; this causes a pannus to form.
   2. The pannus tissue erodes the cartilage and destroys the joint.

B. Exacerbations and remissions occur. Condition tends to be progressive with each exacerbation.

C. Condition is a problem of the connective tissue; inflammatory response may occur in organs throughout the body (heart, lungs, blood vessels, muscles).

Assessment

1. Risk factors/etiology.
   a. Significantly increased incidence in women.
   b. Occurs at any age; peak incidence occurs between 20 and 45 years of age.
2. Clinical manifestations.
   a. Symmetrical joint involvement (hands and feet).
      (1) Warm, tender, red, painful joints.
      (2) Decrease in range of motion.
      (3) Decrease in strength.
      (4) Stiffness and pain worse in the morning, decreases during the day with moderate activity.
   b. Subcutaneous nodules over bony prominence.
      (1) Painless, frequently occur on the elbow.
      (2) May be present for weeks to months.
   c. Systemic effects.
      (1) Vasculitis.
      (2) Pulmonary fibrosis.
      (3) Pericarditis.
      (4) Ocular problems
   d. Chronic deformities develop, most often in the hands.
   e. Exacerbation of symptoms may be associated with physical or emotional stress.
3. Diagnostics.
   a. Positive serum rheumatoid arthritis factor.
   b. Increased erythrocyte sedimentation rate (ESR).
   c. Increased C-reactive protein (CRP).
   d. Aspiration of synovial joint fluid.

Treatment

1. Nonsteroidal anti-inflammatory drugs (NSAIDs).
   a. Salicylate (aspirin) is primary drug.
   b. Ibuprofen, naproxen.
2. Corticosteroids.
3. Heat and/or cold applications.
4. Assistive devises to preserve joints and prevent deformity.
5. Physical and rehabilitative therapy.
6. Surgery—joint replacements.

Complications

1. Musculoskeletal.
   a. Severe joint deformity, flexion contracture.
   b. Diffuse skeletal demineralization.
   c. Stress fractures.
2. Systemic involvement

Nursing Intervention

✦ *Goal: to relieve pain and preserve joint mobility and muscle strength.*

1. Use warm, moist compresses to relieve pain and stiffness of muscle spasms.
2. If heat increases pain, cold compresses may be beneficial in an acute episode.
3. Acutely inflamed joints should be immobilized in a device that maintains a functional position.
4. Position client to maintain correct body alignment and prevent contractures, especially flexion contractures.
5. Immobility can increase the pain; range of motion exercises and weight-bearing may help decrease pain.

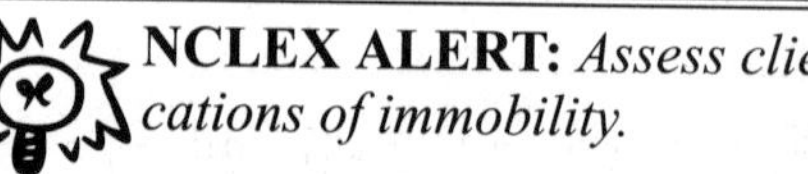

NCLEX ALERT: *Assess client for complications of immobility.*

6. Anti-inflammatory medications should be taken prior to activity and with meals or food, to decrease gastric upset.

7. If client is on steroids, he should wear an identification tag.

✦ *Goal: to assist client to prevent joint deformity, preserve joint function, reduce inflammation and pain.*

1. Regularly scheduled rest periods, (excessive fatigue is a problem); balance activities with rest.
2. Protect joints.
   a. Maintain functional joint alignment; avoid positions which precipitate joint contraction (sitting too long with knees bent).
   b. Warm moist or cold compresses to relieve pain and muscle spasm.
   c. Acutely inflamed joints may be splinted; splint should be removed periodically and joint exercised.
   d. Use large muscle groups, avoid repetitive movement of smaller joints.
   e. Do not rub or exercise joints that are acutely inflamed; rub muscle around the joint and immobilize it.
3. Demonstrate ability to carry out individual exercise program.
4. Identify medications that are effective in pain relief.
5. Discuss with client importance of identifying false advertising regarding claims of cure and relief of chronic pain.
6. Encourage client to be independent in ADLs as long as possible.

Self Care

1. Encourage client to ventilate feelings regarding chronic progression of the disease state.
2. Evaluate family support system; help family to identify measures to assist client.
3. Modify home routine to decrease stress on joints - ADLs, dressing, etc.
4. Identify measures to assist client to maintain self-esteem - what activities client can continue to participate in; focus on what client can do.
5. Assist client to set realistic goals.
6. Identify community resources available.

NCLEX ALERT: *Determine client's ability to perform self care; assist family to manage care of client with chronic needs.*

Osteoarthritis (Degenerative Joint Disease)

❑ **It is a progressive, nonsystemic, no inflammatory disease that causes a progressive degeneration of synovial joints of weight-bearing long bones.**

A. Primary is associated with aging, secondary is caused by musculoskeletal injury or conditions that cause repetitive damage to joints.

B. The cartilage at the ends of the long bones deteriorates and leaves the ends of the bones rubbing together; this produces a painful, swollen joint.

Assessment

1. Etiology/predisposing factors.
   a. Excessive use of a specific joint—knees in athletes, feet in dancers, etc.
   b. The hips are more commonly affected in men; in women it is the hands.
   c. Obesity—joints that carry excess weight are more likely to wear out earlier.
   d. Frequently associated with the older adult.
2. Clinical manifestations.
   a. Joints involved.
      (1) Primarily involves weight-bearing joints; occurs as a result of mechanical stress.
      (2) May also involve joints in the fingers and the vertebral column.
   b. Symptoms occurring in the joint.
      (1) Pain, swelling, tenderness.
      (2) Crepitus—a grating sound or feeling with movement.
      (3) Instability, stiffness and immobility.
   c. Pain occurs on motion and with weight-bearing.
   d. Pain increases in severity with activity.
   e. Heberden's nodes—bony nodules on the distal finger joints.
3. Diagnostics.
   a. No specific test to confirm.
   b. Synovial fluid analysis.
   c. Arthroscopy.
   d. X-ray.

Treatment

1. Medications (NSAIDs).
   a. Steroids are not as effective as in rheumatoid arthritis.
   b. Medication therapy directed toward relief of pain.
2. Activity balanced with adequate rest.

3. Weight reduction if appropriate.
4. Physical therapy and exercise.
5. Surgical intervention with joint replacement.

Nursing Intervention

✦ *Goal: to relieve pain, prevent further stress on the joint, and maintain function.*

1. Acutely inflamed joint should be immobilized with splint or brace.
2. Plan ADLs to prevent stress on involved joints and provide adequate rest periods.
3. Heat compresses for relief of pain; cold may be used if joint is inflamed.
4. Very important to maintain regular exercise program; decrease activity in acutely inflamed, painful joints.

✦ *Goal: to assist client to understand measures to maintain health.*

1. Identify activities requiring increased stress on involved joints.
2. Maintain regular exercise program - (walking, swimming) to promote muscle strength and joint mobility.
3. Encourage independence in ADLs.

✦ *Goal: to maintain psychological equilibrium and promote positive self-esteem.*

Juvenile Rheumatoid Arthritis

❑ **A chronic inflammatory problem of connective tissue; involves the synovial joints.**

A. Synovium becomes thick and edematous; granulation tissue turns to scar tissue and the joint is destroyed.

B. May involve other organs—spleen, liver, lungs, blood dyscrasias.

Assessment

1. Risk factors/etiology.
   a. Possibly autoimmune in origin.
   b. Peak onset between 2 and 16.
2. Clinical manifestations.
   a. Morning stiffness.
   b. May have multiple joint involvement, both large and small joints.
   c. Joint may be tender and painful to touch or may be relatively painless.
3. Diagnostics (diagnosis by exclusion of other diseases).

Treatment

1. Medications.
   a. Salicylates.
   b. Non-steroid anti-inflammatory (NSAIDs).
   c. Corticosteroids not commonly used for children.
2. Physical therapy.
3. Moist heat is used to reduce stiffness and relieve pain.
4. Exercise—especially water exercises.

Complications

1. Severe hip disease and loss of vision from iridocycitis.

Nursing Intervention (child is usually cared for at home except with severe exacerbations.)

✦ *Goal: to decrease pain and promote joint mobility.*

1. Moist heat to relieve joint stiffness and pain.
2. Therapeutic exercises incorporated into play activities.
3. Maintain good body alignment when child is at rest; prevent flexion contractures of affected joints.
4. Avoid over exercising painful joints.

✦ *Goal: to assist child to maintain normal growth and development patterns, and to promote self-esteem.*

1. Well-balanced diet without excessive weight gain.
2. Schedule regular exercise program appropriate to developmental level.
3. Encourage independence; allow child to participate in planning care.
4. Encourage school attendance and socialization with peers.

Gout

❑ **An arthritic condition resulting from a defect in the metabolism of uric acid (hyperuricemia).**

A. Uric acid is the end product of purine metabolism.

B. Condition of hyperuricemia may also occur in individuals receiving chemotherapy (secondary gout).

Assessment

1. Risk factors/etiology.
   a. Increased incidence in middle-aged men.
   b. Familial tendency.
2. Clinical manifestations.
   a. Intense pain and inflammation of one or more small joints - especially the large toe.
   b. Characterized by remissions and exacerbations of acute joint pain.
   c. Onset is generally rapid with swollen, inflamed, painful joints.
   d. Presence of tophi or uric acid crystals in the area around the large toe and the outer ear.
   e. Tophi may be present in subcutaneous tissue.
3. Diagnostics- persistent hyperuricemia >7mg/dl.

Treatment

1. Medications.

Antigout (Appendix 21-2).

a. NSAIDs for pain and also to assist in preventing attacks.

1. Decreased purine diet (Chapter 3).

Complications

1. Uric acid kidney stones.
2. Secondary osteoarthritis.

Nursing Intervention

✦ *Goal: to prevent acute attack, promote comfort, and maintain joint mobility.*

1. Medications should be given early in the attack to decrease the severity of the attack.
2. Protect affected joint.
   a. Immobilize.
   b. Elevate the joint.
   c. No weight bearing.
3. Cold packs may decrease pain.
4. Decreased purine diet.
5. Encourage high fluid intake to increase excretion of uric acid and to prevent the development of uric acid stones.
6. Assist client to identify activities and lifestyle that precipitate attacks.
   a. Dietary habits.
   b. Alcohol consumption.
   c. Increased stress.

Study Questions—Musculoskeletal System

1. Postoperatively, following a lumbar laminectomy, the client continues to complain of the same low back pain that he had prior to surgery. The nurse knows that this finding is caused by what problem?

① Failure of the surgeon to remove the client's herniated disk.
② Swelling in the operative area that compresses adjacent structures.
③ Twisting of the client's spine when he turns side to side.
④ Limitation of movement resulting from spinal fusion.

2. A seven year old boy is in the emergency room with a greenstick fracture of the ulna. How will the nurse explain the fracture to the parents?

① The bone is broken across the growth plate.
② There is a splintering of the bone on one side.
③ There is a separation of the bone at the fracture site.
④ The bone is broken into several fragments.

3. A client has a fractured hip and is currently in Buck's traction prior to surgery. How is the counterattraction in Buck's traction is achieved?

① Applying a ten-pound counterweight at the knee.
② Placing shock blocks under the head of the bed.
③ Elevating the knee gatch and elevating the head of the bed about 30°.
④ Elevating the foot of the bed frame and allowing the weights to hang freely.

4. The nursing care plan for a postoperative client who has had a right leg amputation includes what measures to decrease edema?

① Apply ice packs to the stump for 72 hours.
② Elevate the stump by raising the foot of the bed for 24 to 48 hours.
③ Wrap the stump with Ace bandages from proximal to distal ends.
④ Administer anti-inflammatory medications as ordered.

5. A client has a long leg plaster cast applied. What nursing actions are implemented while the cast is still wet?

① Use only the fingertips when moving the cast.
② Keep the client and cast covered with blankets.
③ Support the cast on plastic-covered pillows.
④ Place a heat lamp directly over the cast.

6. A client is being treated with Buck's traction. What are important nursing interventions for this client?

① Remove the traction boot every 6 hours to provide skin care.
② Check and clean the pin sites at least three times daily.
③ Check the area around the hip where the traction is applied.
④ Verify that weights are amount ordered and are hanging freely.

7. For a client with severe painful osteoarthritis, a regimen of heat, massage, and exercise will provide what response?

① Help relax muscles, pain, and stiffness.
② Restore range of motion previously lost.
③ Prevent the inflammatory process.
④ Assist the client to effectively cope with pain.

8. In taking the health history of a client with severe painful osteoarthritis, what will the nurse expect the client to report?

① A gradual onset of the disease, with the involvement of weight bearing joints.
② A sudden onset of the disease, with involvement of all joints.
③ No complaints of morning stiffness.
④ Joint pain that is not affected by exercise.

9. A 30-year-old client is on bed rest with a fracture of the left femur. He is started on subcutaneous heparin injections. What is the purpose of this medication?

① Prevent thrombophlebitis and pulmonary emboli associated with immobility.
② Promote vascular perfusion by preventing formation of microemboli in the left leg.
③ Prevent venous stasis that promotes vascular complications associated with immobility.
④ Decrease the incidence of fat emboli associated with long bone fractures.

10. What is important assessment information to obtain in a client with a fractured hip?

① Circulation and sensation distal to the fracture.
② Amount of swelling around the fracture site.
③ Degree of bone healing that has occurred.
④ Amount of pain that the fracture and healing are causing.

11. What evaluation is important in the preoperative nursing assessment of a client with a severely herniated lumbar disc?

① Movement and sensation in the lower extremities.
② Leg pain that radiates to both lower extremities.
③ Reflexes in the upper extremities.
④ Pupillary reaction to light.

12. The nursing care plan for a 2-month-old infant in a left hip spica cast includes what nursing measures?

① Palpate the left brachial artery and compare it to the right.
② Check cast for tightness by inserting fingers between skin and cast.
③ Blanch the skin of areas proximal to the casted left leg.
④ Maintain constant traction on the affected left leg.

13. Nursing care for the client in Russell's traction includes what measures?

① Keeping the client flat in bed to promote traction pull.
② Checking the distal circulation of the affected leg.
③ Turning the client every two hours to the unaffected side.
④ Allowing the client to sit in a chair at the bedside.

14. What are the priority nursing intervention(s) in the care of a 40-year-old client in a balanced suspension traction for a complete transverse fracture of the left femur?

① Increase fluid intake to prevent the development of renal stone due to the stasis of urine in the bladder.
② Frequent checks regarding level of pain and sensation distal to the affected extremity, and care of the pin site.
③ Keep an abduction device between his legs to prevent external rotation of the affected leg.
④ Encourage a diet high in calcium to promote an increase in bone strength and repair.

15. Which statement describes the callus formation stage in the phases of bone healing?

① New bone enters area, forming woven bone and beginning to knit the broken ends.
② Blood clots and forms a hematoma between broken ends of bone.
③ Granulation tissue forms and becomes firm, linking the two fragments of bone.
④ Mature cells are deposited, resulting in calcified tissue that resembles normal bone.

16. A 27-year-old client is admitted with a fractured right femur. Treatment includes: balanced traction with a Thomas splint and a Pearson attachment. What will the nursing care of a client in this traction include?

① Assessing the groin area for signs of pressure.
② Preventing pressure at the heel of the affected side.
③ Changing the compression bandages once a shift.
④ Maintaining the bed in flat position to facilitate traction.

17. The nurse is planning care for a client with a herniated disk. What intervention is considered part of conservative treatment of herniated disk?

① Left lateral Sims' position with bathroom privileges.

② Bedrest and methocarbamol (**Robaxin**) to decrease muscle spasms.

③ Small incision in the spinal column to remove the disk.

④ Daily physical therapy and ambulation with crutches.

18. A diabetic client with a right below the knee amputation tells the nurse that he feels pain in the amputated leg, even though the leg is gone. The nurse's response is based on what information?

① The condition is called phantom pain and it is experienced by most amputees.

② Phantom pain is pain the client feels is there but it is because of denial.

③ The pain is not observable or measurable therefore the nurse cannot medicate the client.

④ The nerve endings have not adjusted to the loss of the extremity, offer him pain medication.

Answers and rationales to these questions are in the section at the end of the book entitled "Chapter Study Questions: Answers & Rationales."

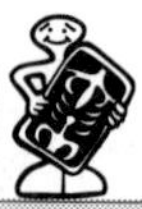

Appendix 21-1: DIAGNOSTIC STUDIES

SERUM DIAGNOSTICS

RHEUMATOID FACTOR (Latex fixation)—Used to determine presence of autoantibodies (rheumatoid factor) seen in clients with connective tissue disease; if antibody is present, it is suggestive of rheumatoid arthritis; the higher the antibody titer, the greater the degree of inflammation.

ANTINUCLEAR ANTIBODY (ANA)—Measures the presence of antibodies that destroy the nucleus of body tissue cells (i.e., those seen in connective tissue diseases); a positive test is associated with systemic lupus erythematosus.

INVASIVE DIAGNOSTICS

ARTHROSCOPY—Involves the utilization of an arthroscope inserted into a joint for visualization of the joint structure; preferably, procedure is conducted in the operating room with strict asepsis, performed under either local or general anesthesia; frequently utilized to diagnose structural abnormalities of the knee.

Nursing Implications:
1. Preoperative nursing intervention as appropriate with the level of anesthesia to be used.
2. After procedure, wound is covered with a sterile dressing.
3. A compression bandage may be applied for 24 hours post-test; teach client symptoms of vascular compromise.
4. Walking is permitted; however, excessive exercise should be avoided for a few days.
5. Teach the client signs of infection (increased temperature, local inflammation at site).

ARTHROCENTESIS—Incision of a joint capsule to obtain samples of synovial fluid; local anesthesia and aseptic preparation utilized prior to fluid aspiration. Synovial fluid is examined for infection, bleeding into the joint, and to confirm specific types of arthritis.

Nursing Implications:
1. Explain procedure to client.
2. May be done at bedside or in an examination room.
3. Compression dressing usually applied and joint rested for several hours post-test.
4. Observe dressing for leakage of blood or fluid.

ARTHROGRAM—Used to visualize soft tissue structures. Contrast medium is injected into the joint for visualization on X-ray.

LAMINOGRAM—Used to determine bone destruction, status of a bone graft, foreign bodies, etc.

MYELOGRAM—Used to determine status of vertebral disk. See Appendix 20-1.

BONE BIOPSY—May be performed in client's room or in a treatment room. After satisfactory local anesthetic, a long needle is inserted into the bone, or a small incision is made, to obtain bone tissue.

Nursing Implications:
1. Plan for analgesic to be administered prior to procedure.
2. If an incision was made, maintain a pressure dressing over the site.
3. Extremity is elevated to decrease edema and may be immobilized, for about 12 to 24 hours.
4. Assess the puncture or incision for evidence of infection.

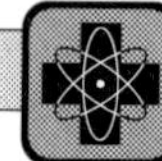

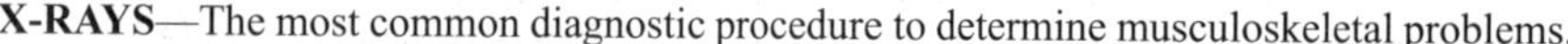

NON-INVASIVE DIAGNOSTICS

X-RAYS—The most common diagnostic procedure to determine musculoskeletal problems.
1. Identify musculoskeletal problems.
2. Determine progress of disease or condition.
3. Evaluate effectiveness of treatment.

BONE SCAN—Radioisotopes are injected intravenously and bone is scanned to determine where the isotopes are "taken up." May be used to determine malignancies, arthritis, and osteoporosis. No special precautions prior to or after test; need to encourage fluid intake to increase excretion of dye.

COMPUTERIZED AXIAL TOMOGRAPHY—(computerized tomography, CAT scan) See Appendix 20-1.

MAGNETIC RESONANCE IMAGING (MRI)—See Appendix 20-1.

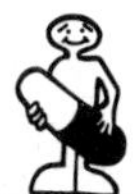

Appendix 21-2: MEDICATIONS

MEDICATIONS	SIDE EFFECTS	NURSING IMPLICATIONS
ANTIGOUT: Decreases the plasma uric acid levels by either inhibiting the synthesis of uric acid or by increasing the excretion of uric acid.		
Colchicine: PO, IV	Nausea, Vomiting, Diarrhea.	1. Take medication at earliest indication of impending gout attack. 2. Take medication with food. 3. Promote high fluid intake to promote uric acid excretion. 4. In acute attack, administer one tablet every hour until symptoms subside, or until GI problems occur, or a total of 8mg has been taken.
Allopurinol (**Zyloprim**): PO	Rash. GI distress. Fever. Headache.	1. Administer with food to decrease gastric upset. 2. Discontinue medication if rash occurs. 3. Use with caution in clients with renal insufficiency. 4. May be used to decrease serum uric acid levels in clients on chemotherapy.
Probenecid (**Benemid**): PO Probenecid Colchicine (**Colbenemid**) PO	GI disturbances, Headache, Skin rash, Fever.	1. Urate tophi deposits should decrease in size with therapy. 2. Lifelong therapy is usually required.
SKELETAL MUSCLE RELAXANTS: Relaxes skeletal muscle by depressing synaptic pathways in the spinal cord.		
Methocarbamol (**Robaxin**): PO, IM, IV Cyclobenzaprine (**Flexeril**): PO Baclofen (**Lioresal**): PO	Drowsiness, dizziness, GI upset, rash, blurred vision. Drowsiness, dizziness, headache, GI upset, orthostatic hypotension. Drowsiness, weakness, fatigue, confusion.	1. Use: muscle spasm associated with MS and spinal cord injury. 2. Caution clients to avoid activities that require mental alertness for safety (driving, power tools, etc) 3. Evaluate client for postural hypotension. 4. Advise client to avoid CNS depressants (alcohol, opioids, antihistamines).
Dantrolene (**Dantrium**): PO, IV	Hepatotoxcity, muscle weakness, drowsiness.	1. Teach clients symptoms of liver dysfunction. 2. Acts directly to relax skeletal muscle.
CALCIUM MEDICATIONS: Hormones that prevent the reabsorption of bone and decrease serum calcium.		
Calcitonin-salmon (**Calcimar**): SQ, IM	GI upset, local inflammation at injection site, flushing	1. Monitor levels of serum calcium. 2. Only given parenterally.
Aminobisphosphonate (**Fosamax**) PO (**Miacalcin**) nasal spray	GI upset, nasal ulceration due to nasal sprays, flushing, rash.	1. Have client swallow tablet whole, do not chew. 2. Take in AM with large glass of water and wait at least 30 minutes before eating or lying down. 3. Make sure client has adequate intake of Vitamin D. 4. Use: prevention of postmenopausal osteoporosis.
CORTICOSTEROIDS: (See Appendix 6-8)		

Nonsteroid anti-inflammatory: See Appendix 6-9.

Appendix 21-3: AMPUTATIONS

❑ DEFINITION: Removal of all or part of an extremity.

Indications for Amputation:

1. Peripheral vascular disease, especially vascular disease of lower extremities.
2. Severe trauma.
3. Acute chronic infection.
4. Malignant tumors.

Nursing Implications:

1. Prevent further loss of circulation to the extremity.
2. Promote psychological stability.
3. Promote comfort.
4. Promote optimum level of mobility.

POSTOPERATIVE CARE

NCLEX ALERT: *Be familiar with the nursing management of a client with an amputated extremity, especially regarding positioning to prevent contractures.*

Stump Wound Care:

1. Elevate the stump for approximately 24 to 48 hours; after that time, keep the joint immediately above the stump in an extended position. Flexion contracture hinders prosthetic utilization.

2. Discuss the phenomenon of phantom limb sensation.

3. Administer analgesics; phantom limb pain is very real to the client.

4. Evaluate stump for bleeding and healing.

5. A rigid compression dressing (plaster molded over stump dressing) may be applied to prevent injury and to decrease swelling. Controlling the edema will enhance healing and promote comfort. Changes of the rigid dressing are necessary; as the stump heals it also shrinks. The compression dressing may be changed three or four times before a permanent prosthesis is fitted. The compression dressing may be formed so that it can attach to a prosthesis.

6. If the client is not fitted with a rigid compression dressing, the stump will be shaped with a compression bandage. Ace bandage elastic wrapping is often used for compression of this type.

7. Discourage semi-Fowler's position in the client with above the knee amputation, position encourages flexion contraction at the hip.

Stump Care After Wound Has Healed:

1. Continually assess for skin breakdown; visually inspect the stump for redness, abrasions, or blistering.

2. The stump should be washed daily, carefully rinsed and dried. Soap and moisture contribute to skin breakdown.

3. Do not apply anything to the stump (alcohol increases skin dryness and skin cracking, lotions keep skin soft and hinder prosthetic use).

4. Client should put the prosthesis on when he gets up and wear it all day. The stump tends to swell if the prosthesis is not applied. The more the person wears the prosthesis, the less the swelling.

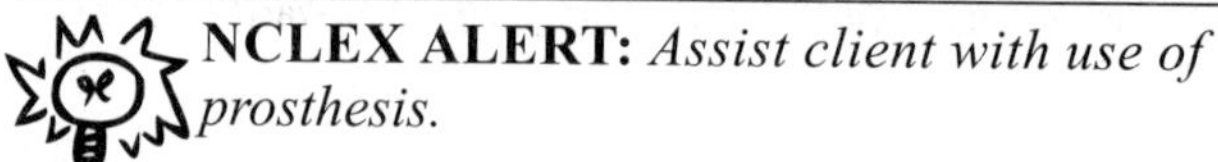

NCLEX ALERT: *Assist client with use of prosthesis.*

Appendix 21-4: ASSISTIVE DEVICES FOR IMMOBILITY

Crutches

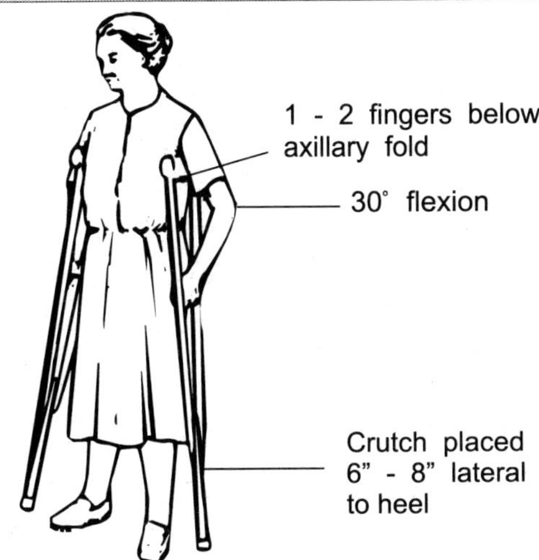

Measuring a client

- Have client lie flat in bed with arms at side.
- Measure the distance from the client's axilla (armpit) to a point 6-8 inches out from the heel.
- Adjust handbars so that client's elbows are slightly flexed.
- Have client stand, then measure distance between client's axilla and arm pieces. You should be able to put two of your fingers between client's axilla and the crutch bar.

Four-point Alternate Gait

- The four-point alternate gait is used by patients who can bear partial weight on both feet — for example, arthritic or cerebral palsy patients. It is a particularly safe gait, in that there are three points of support on the floor at all times.
- This gait provides a normal walking pattern and makes some use of the muscles of the lower extremities.

Three-point Alternate Gait

- For the three-point alternate gait the patient must be able to bear the total body weight on one foot; the affected foot or leg is either partially or totally non-weight-bearing.
- In this gait both crutches are moved forward together with the affected leg while the weight is being borne by the patient's hands on the crutches. The unaffected leg is then advanced forward.

Crutch walking

- Upstairs - unaffected leg moves up 1st, followed by the crutches and the affected leg.
- Downstairs - Crutches and affected leg move down 1st, transfer of body weight to the crutches and move the unaffected leg down.

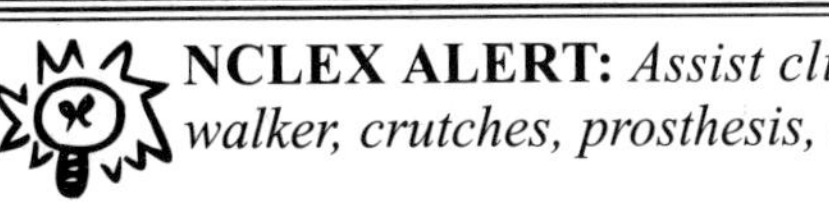
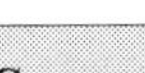

NCLEX ALERT: *Assist client with use of a walker, crutches, prosthesis, etc.*

Canes

- The cane is used on the side opposite the affected leg.
- The cane and the affected leg move together.

Walkers

- Lift the walker and place it approximately two feet in front.
- Gain balance before moving walker forward again, provides stability and equal weight bearing.

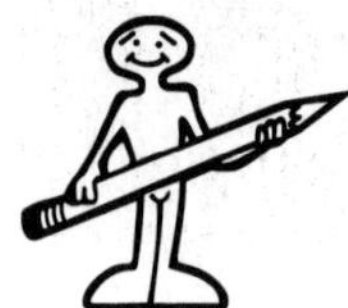

Notes

PHYSIOLOGY OF THE REPRODUCTIVE SYSTEM

Male Reproductive System

A. External genitalia.

B. Internal genitalia.

1. Testes (gonads)—spermatogenesis in a seminiferous tubule, and testosterone production by the interstitial cells.

C. Accessory glands.

1. Seminal vesicles—secrete nearly one-third of the volume of semen; also prostaglandin.
2. Prostate gland—produces a slightly alkalotic substance which contains high levels of acid phosphatase and serves as the vehicle for spermatozoa.

D. Semen.

1. Male ejaculate composed of spermatozoa and seminal plasma.
2. Alkaline pH: 7.2 to 7.4.
3. Average volume of ejaculate: 2.5 to 4 cc; may vary from 1 to 10 cc; repeated ejaculation leads to decreased volume.
4. Sterility: sperm count less than 20 million per milliliter; (normal sperm count 100 million per milliliter.)
5. Storage of sperm: varies from a period of several hours to 40 days, depending primarily on the frequency of ejaculation.

Female Reproductive System

A. External genitalia.

1. Labia majora—contains an extensive venous blood supply, which leads frequently to edema and varicosities in pregnancy.
2. Periurethral (Skene's) glands— often site of gonorrheal infection.

B. Internal genitalia.

1. Vagina—a thin-walled, muscular membranous canal that connects the external genitalia with the center of the pelvis.
   a. pH is acidic, which is maintained by a relationship between lactic acid-producing Döederlein's bacillus (lactobacillus) and the vaginal content.
   b. Bacilli break down vaginal epithelial cells; disruption of this cycle (antibiotic therapy, douching, vaginal sprays, etc.) may destroy the normal self-cleansing action of the vagina.
2. Cervix - protrudes into the vagina.
   a. Provides an alkaline environment to shelter sperm from the acidic vagina.
   b. Cervical mucus pH increases (alkaline) and becomes clear and more viscous at ovulation.
3. Uterus—a hollow, pear-shaped, muscular pelvic organ; located between the bladder and the rectum.
   a. Uterine wall—endometrium is the inner mucosal lining; undergoes cyclic changes due to hormonal level.
   b. Uterine ligaments—maintain position uterus in pelvic cavity.
4. Fallopian tubes—attached to the upper, outer section of the uterus.
   a. Distal tubules are fimbriated and bell-shaped.
   b. By their peristaltic and ciliary action, they move the egg into the uterine cavity.
5. Ovaries—located behind and below the fallopian tubes, produce ovum, estrogen, and progesterone.

C. Breasts —Divided into lobes and lobules arranged in a radial pattern, separated by fibrous tissue called Cooper's ligaments.

D. Menstrual cycle (Figure 22-3).

1. The cyclical hormonal changes occurring from menarche to menopause.
2. Phases.
   a. Menstrual phase—shedding of the superficial two-thirds of the endometrium; initiated by periodic vasoconstriction of the spiral arteries.
   b. Proliferative phase—a period of rapid growth; extends from day five to ovulation.
   c. Secretory phase—follows ovulation; large amounts of progesterone are produced; uterine lining is prepared to receive and nourish a fertilized ovum if one is available.
3. Fertilization—generally occurs in the outer third of the fallopian tube; a single ejaculation deposits 2.5 to 4.0 cc of semen, containing approximately 200 to 400 million spermatozoa.
4. Implantation—the zygote (fertilized ovum) is propelled by ciliary action of the fallopian tube into the uterine cavity; implants into the endometrium about seven to ten days after fertilization.

E. Bony pelvis structures.

System Assessment

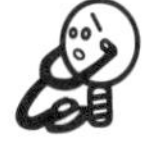

A. External assessment.

1. Assess vulvar area for discharge, erythema, or growths.
2. Assess penis for growths, masses, erosions, ulcers, or vesicles.
3. Inspect breasts for nipple inversion, retraction, secretions, nodules, lumps, or masses.
4. Determine if there is any abdominal pain or tenderness upon palpation.

B. Internal assessment.
1. Pelvic examination.
   a. Collection of a Pap smear.
   b. Bimanual examination.
2. Digital rectal examination to evaluate prostatic size.

C. History.
1. Menstrual history.
   a. Age of onset.
   b. Last menstrual period.
   c. Duration of cycle, amount of flow, and use of birth control methods.
2. Obstetric history.
3. Urinary system.
   a. Pattern of voiding—dysuria, urgency, nocturia, frequency.
   b. Difficulty starting stream, stopping stream, changing the force of stream, or a feeling of incomplete emptying of bladder.
4. Sexual function.
   a. Ability to achieve erection and ejaculation.
   b. Problems with intercourse.
   c. Bleeding after intercourse.
   d. Exposure to sexually-transmitted diseases.
   e. Change in sex drive-libido.

DISORDERS OF THE REPRODUCTIVE SYSTEM

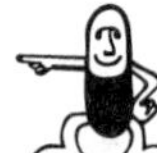

Prostate Disorders

A. Benign prostatic hypertrophy (BPH)—enlargement of prostate gland tissue.

B. Cancer of the prostate—a malignancy of the prostate gland which is a hormone, dependent adenocarcinoma; growth of the tumor is usually related to the presence of androgen hormone, but tumor develops an ability to continue to grow in the absence of hormones.

Assessment

1. Risk factors/etiology.
   a. BPH—present in at least 50% of men over age 50.
   b. Prostatic carcinoma—rarely found in men under 60 years of age; usually found in the posterior lobe of the prostate gland; increased incidence in black men and married men.
2. Clinical manifestations.

NCLEX ALERT: *Relate client's symptoms to adverse reactions of medication. Carefully assess the client with BPH in regard to anticholinergic medications (atropine) that cause urinary retention as a side effect.*

   a. Common to both disorders.
      (1) Urinary hesitancy, frequency, urgency, and dribbling.
      (2) Nocturia, hematuria, urinary retention, and a sensation of incomplete emptying of the bladder.
      (3) Post-void dribbling.
      (4) Diminished force of urinary stream.
   b. Prostatic cancer.
      (1) Tumor grows slowly and is confined to capsule, therefore prostate may appear normal thus delaying the diagnosis.
      (2) On digital rectal exam there is unilateral prostatic enlargement—"stony hard" and fixed.
      (3) Obstruction is rare unless BPH is also present.
      (4) Pain in the hip or back may be presenting symptom are a result of metastasis.
3. Diagnostics.
   a. BPH.
      (1) Digital rectal examination.
      (2) Cystoscopy and IVP.
      (3) Urinalysis with culture and sensitivity.
      (4) BUN and serum creatinine to rule out renal damage..
   b. Prostatic cancer.
      (1) Elevated serum acid phosphatase.
      (2) CT scan.
      (3) Tumor markers
      (4) Prostatic specific antigen (PSA) and prostatic acid phosphatase (PAP).
      (5) Needle biopsy of prostate.

Treatment

1. Medical
   a. BPH - finasteride (**Proscar**) to shrink prostatic tissue.
   b. Radiation, hormonal, and chemotherapy for malignancy.
2. Surgical—size of prostate and general health dictate the type of surgery.
   a. Transurethral resection of the prostate (TURP)—removal of prostatic tissue via a resectoscope, which is passed through the urethra; primary treatment for BPH.
   b. Suprapubic prostatectomy—removal of the prostate through a lower midline abdominal incision through the bladder into the anterior aspect of the prostate.
   c. Retropubic prostatectomy—a low abdominal incision is made into the prostate gland without entering the bladder.
   d. Transuretheral prostate dilation—balloon dilatation of urethra, exerting pressure on enlarged prostate to open the urethra.
   e. Perineal (radical) prostatectomy—incision is made between the scrotum and the anus; most often used with cancer of the prostate; frequently results in problems with impotence and urinary control.
   f. Orchiectomy— bilateral orchiectomy.

Complications

1. BPH.
   a. Preoperative.
      (1) Urinary tract infection.
      (2) Rupture of overstretched blood vessels in the bladder—hematuria.
      (3) Hydroureter and hydronephrosis with resultant renal failure.
   b. Postoperative.

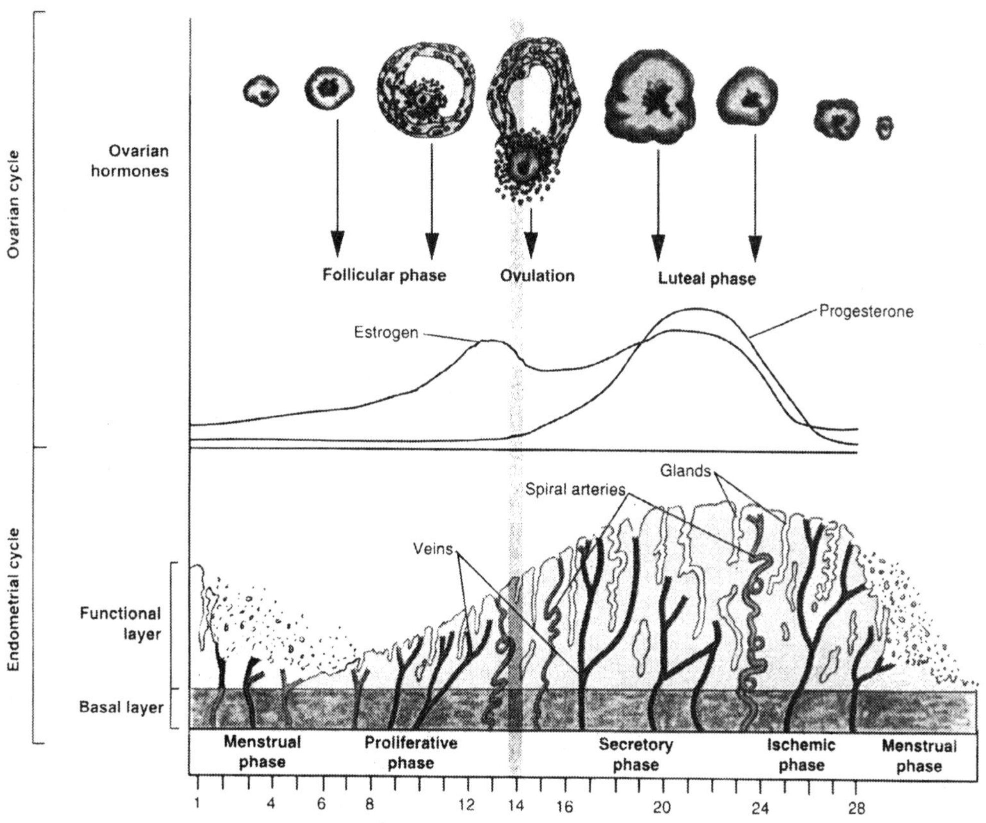

Figure 22-1: Female Reproductive Cycle
Reprinted with permission: Gorrie, TM, Mckinney, ES, & Murray, SS, (1998) *Foundations of Maternal-Newborn Nursing,* 2nd ed. Philadelphis: Saunders, p 66.

(1) Hemorrhage - especially in the first 24 hours.

(2) Urethral stricture.

(3) Bladder spasms.

(4) Retrograde ejaculation—semen passed into the bladder rather than out through the penis.

(5) Epididymitis.

(6) Absorption of irrigating fluid creating fluid overload.

2. Prostatic cancer.

a. Preoperative.

(1) Complications are similar to BPH.

(2) Cancer may spread via the perineal lymphatic system to the regional lymph nodes; from the veins of the prostate, it spreads to the pelvic bones, bladder, lungs, and liver.

b. Postoperative.

(1) Increased problems with DVT due to lithotomy position during resection.

(2) Metastases.

(3) Change in sexual functioning—impotence and failure to ejaculate.

Nursing Intervention

✦ *Goal: to promote elimination, treat urinary tract infection, and provide client education.*

1. Evaluate adequacy of voiding and presence of urinary retention. Assess need for placement of catheter.
2. Teach client to avoid bladder distention which results in loss of muscle tone.
   a. Do not postpone the urge to void; it is important to prevent overdistension of the bladder which further complicates the problem.
   b. Avoid drinking a large amount of fluid in a short period of time.
   c. Avoid alcohol because of the diuretic effect.
3. Encourage annual digital rectal examination of the prostate for all men over age 40years.
4. Examination is recommended every six months for clients who have BPH or who have had a prostectomy.

NCLEX ALERT: *Assess all male clients over 50 years old for symptoms of BPH, occurs in 80% of men over age 80.*

Box 22-1: Elderly Care Focus
Benign Prostatic Hypertrophy (BPH)

➣ ***General***

- All men over 60 years of age should be assessed for urinary retention and adequacy of bladder emptying.
- Increased problem with urinary stasis; increased straining to urinate; increased incidence of infections.

➣ ***Postoperatively***

- Closely evaluate for presence of infection, especially UTI, respiratory.
- Assess fluid balance; confusion and agitation may be symptoms of fluid overload.
- Assist the client to ambulate as soon as possible - increased risk for pooling of blood in pelvic cavity and pulmonary emboli from immobility.
- Increased risk for falls.
- Determine psychological response to physical stress (confusion, disorientation); orient to surroundings frequently.

✦ *Goal: To maintain closed irrigation postoperatively in the TURP or suprapubic prostectomy client.*

1. Continuous irrigation with sterile, antibacterial, isotonic irrigating solution (Murphy drip, CBI).
   a. Closed bladder irrigation (CBI) is done with a triple lumen catheter: one lumen for inflating the balloon (30 to 50 cc water), one for maintaining outflow of urine, one for the instillation of the continuous irrigating solution.
   b. Provides continuous irrigation to prevent infection and to flush the bladder of tissue and clots following TURP.
   c. If clots occur, the catheter may be irrigated or the rate of flow increased until the drainage outflow clears.
   d. Only use isotonic irrigating fluid in the system, symptoms of TURP syndrome -increased blood pressure, nausea, confusion.
   e. Calculate intake and output carefully, a large amount of bladder irrigation fluid must be subtracted from total output to gain client's true urinary output.
2. Blood clots are normal for first 24 to 36 hours.
3. If client has excessive bleeding, the physician may increase the size of the balloon on the indwelling catheter and put traction on the catheter to compress the area of bleeding.

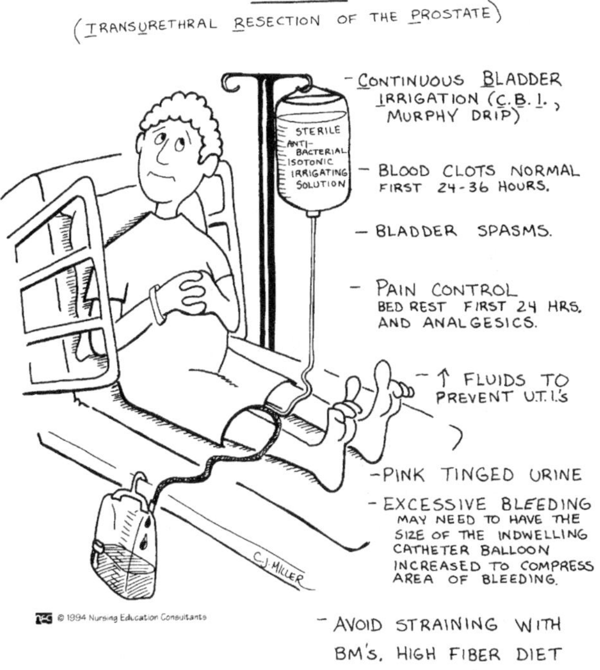

Figure 22-2: Study Graphic for Care of Client with Transurethral Resection of the Prostrate
Zerwekh, J. & Claborn, J. (1994). *Memory Notebook of Nursing*, Vol. 1, Dallas, TX: Nursing Education Consultants, Inc.

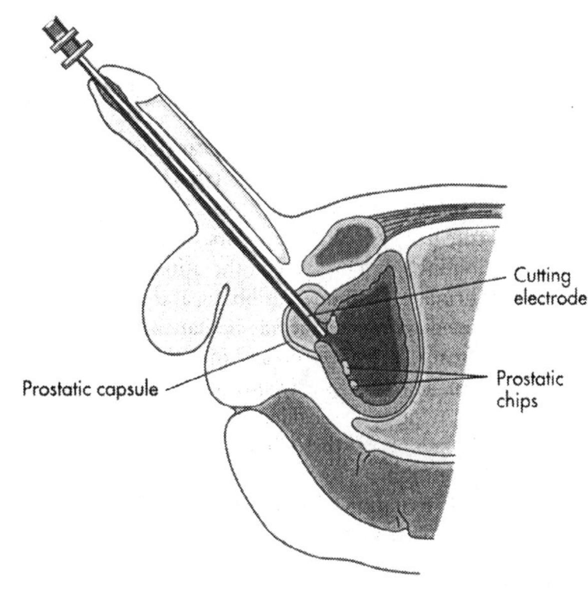

Figure 22-3: Transurethral Resection of the Prostrate
Reprinted with permission: Phipps, WJ, Sands, JK, & Marek, JF (1999). *Medical Surgical Nursing: Concepts & Clinical Practice*, 6th ed. Philadelphia: Mosby, p 1618

NCLEX ALERT: *Maintain client's continuous bladder irrigation -prevent over distention of the bladder. If client complains of pain, check the urinary drainage and make sure it is patent. Obstruction most commonly occurs in the first 24 hours, due to clots in the bladder.*

4. Bladder spasms—belladonna and opium suppositories are administered PRN (often spasms occur due to presence of clots in the catheter).
5. Bladder sensations of a full bladder are common while the irrigating catheter is in place. Explain (repeatedly) about the urinary catheter, and encourage the client to not bear down in an attempt to void.

✦ *Goal: To provide postoperative care.*

1. After client is ambulatory, encourage walking rather than sitting for prolonged periods.
2. Teach client exercises to control urinary stream and maintain continence.
   a. Contract perineal muscles by squeezing buttocks together.
   b. Practice starting and stopping the stream several times during voiding.
3. Assure client that TURP does not usually cause problems relating to sexual functioning; provide opportunity for open discussion regarding sexual concerns.
4. Dribbling post voiding is not uncommon, problem usually subsides with in a few weeks, practice perineal exercises.
5. Teach client to avoid straining during bowel movement, encourage diet high in fiber and administer stool softeners as needed.
6. Discuss with the client the importance of maintaining a high fluid intake to prevent urinary tract infections.

✦ *Goal: To provide postoperative care for a client postoperative radical prostatectomy.*

1. Maintain adequate pain control, frequently PCA device.
2. Due to surgical position and postoperative immobility, client is at high risk for DVT.
   a. Monitor sequential compression devices.
   b. Antiembolism stockings.
   c. Low-dose prophylactic Heparin.

NCLEX ALERT: *Identify symptoms of DVT.*

3. Perineal prostatectomy and total prostatectomy for cancer frequently result in impotence, due to damage to the pudendal nerves.
4. Record output from drains.
5. Emphasize importance of not straining against catheter to relieve bladder pressure.

NCLEX ALERT: *Explain procedure to client and family - it is important to clarify for the client the information the doctor gives him; however, it is the doctor's responsibility to advise the client regarding any complications he may experience with sexual functioning.*

Self-Care

1. If client is discharged with urinary catheter, teach him how to care for the catheter, and how to relieve an obstruction.
2. Avoid suppositories and enemas.
3. Return to the doctor for any signs of urinary tract infection and for follow up PSA tests.
4. After removal of urinary catheter, teach client exercised to increase urinary control (see BPH).
5. Continue high fluid intake, avoid strenuous exercise, and avoid prolonged sitting, encourage walking.

Inflammatory Disorders

A. Prostatitis—inflammation of the prostate usually caused by bacteria (*E. coli, Proteus*) or by a sudden decrease in sexual activity.

B. Epididymitis—inflammation of epididymis, often secondary to prostatitis or a urinary tract infection; often develops as a complication of gonorrhea; in men under age 35 major cause is *Chlamydia trachomatis*.

Assessment

1. Clinical manifestations.
   a. Prostatitis.
      (1) Fever and chills.
      (2) Perineal, rectal, and/or back pain.
      (3) Dysuria, urethral discharge.
      (4) Prostate is enlarged, firm, and tender when palpated.
   b. Epididymitis.
      (1) Pain and tenderness in the inguinal canal.
      (2) Swelling in the scrotum and groin.
      (3) Temperature and chills.
      (4) Pyuria and bacteriuria.
2. Diagnostics.
   a. Rectal examination.
   b. CBC.
   c. Urine and semen culture and sensitivity.

Treatment

1. Prostatitis.
   a. Antibiotics.
   b. Analgesics, stool softeners, and sitz baths.
2. Epididymitis.
   a. Bedrest with elevation of the scrotum (scrotal support or scrotal bridge).
   b. Antibiotics if indicated.
   c. Treatment of client's sexual partners (chlamydia infection).
   d. Cold compresses.

Complications

1. Chronic prostatitis can lead to recurrent urinary tract infection and epididymitis.
2. May have chronic reoccurring incapacitating infections.

Nursing Intervention

✦ *Goal: to assist client to understand measures to maintain health.*

1. Encourage early treatment to prevent complications.
2. In chronic prostatitis encourage activities that drain the prostate, such as intercourse, masturbation, and prostatic massage.
3. Antibiotics may not be effective because it is difficulty to obtain therapeutic levels in prostatic secretion.
4. Encourage treatment of sexual partners when epididymitis is of chlamydia or gonorrhea origin.

Undescended Testes (Cryptorchidism)

❑ **Undescended testes (cryptorchidism) is a condition of failure of one or both testes to descend into the scrotal sac.**

Assessment

1. Inability to palpate the testes in the scrotal sac.
2. Cremasteric reflex is the normal retraction of the testes, frequently stimulated by touch or cold. May

present a problem in attempting to determine if there is an undescended testicle or if the testicle is retractable.

Treatment

1. Surgical intervention—orchiopexy: testis is brought into the scrotal sac and secured.
   a. Prevents damage to the undescended testicle by body heat.
   b. Decreases the incidence of tumor formation.
   c. Usually done between ages of 1 and 3 years; fewer complications are encountered if repair is done prior to 5 years.
   d. Most often done on an outpatient basis.
   e. Men with a history of cryptorchidism have an increased risk of fertility problems and for development of testicular cancer as an adult.

Nursing Intervention

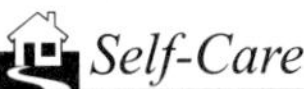

1. Long-term follow-up regarding fertility.
2. Prevent infection by careful cleansing after stool and urine, due to the close proximity of the scrotum.
3. Teach parents to teach the child how to do self-examinations when he is old enough.

Testicular tumors (Cancer)

❑ **Tumors of the testicles are often malignant and tend to metastasize quickly.**

Assessment

1. Most common cancer in men ages 15 to 35.
2. More common in clients who have had cryptorchidism and infections.
3. A mass is palpated in the scrotum; the client may or may not complain of pain; most men experience a heaviness in the scrotum.
4. For men who were born between 1940 and 1971, if possible obtain mother's medical history to determine if she was given diethylstilbestrol (DES) during pregnancy. Significant increase in testicular cancer in these clients.
5. Diagnostics.
   a. Alpha-fetoprotein and human chorionic gonadotropin are increased.
   b. Intravenous urogram.
   c. Lymphangiography.
   d. CAT scan for metastasis..

Table 22-1: TESTICULAR SELF-EXAMINATION

- ✦ Examine the testicles at same time every month, to help you remember to do it.
- ✦ Perform the examination after a bath or shower because this is when the scrotal sac is relaxed.
- ✦ Gently roll the testicle between your thumb and fingers; it should feel smooth; there should be no pain.
- ✦ If there is any lump or irregularity on the testicle, report it to the doctor as soon as possible.

Treatment

1. Surgical intervention—orchiectomy (removal of the testicle) is performed as soon as possible in order to remove the tumor and make a definite diagnosis. If there is lymph node involvement, a retroperitoneal lymph node dissection is done, which is an extensive radical abdominal surgery.
2. Medical.
   a. Postoperative irradiation to the lymphatic drainage pathways.
   b. Multiple chemotherapy medications.

Nursing Intervention

✦ *Goal: to detect any abnormality of the testes through client's self-examination (Table 22-1).*

NCLEX ALERT: *Participate in health promotion programs. Teach men how to perform self- examinations.*

1. Teach clients, especially those between ages 15 and 35, to self-examine monthly while showering or bathing to detect any abnormality of the testes.
2. Emphasize importance of follow-up of client with a history of undescended testes or a previous testicular tumor.

✦ *Goal: to assist the client to understand the implications of surgery.*

Hydrocele and Varicocele

A. Hydrocele—A collection of fluid around the testicle or along the spermatic cord. Client usually does not experience any pain. If circulation becomes impaired, then client experiences more discomfort.
B. Varicocele—A cluster of dilated veins in the scrotal sac, often just above the testis. Occurs most often in young adults; generally do not experience severe pain, but a chronic dull ache in the scrotal area. May contribute to infertility.
C. Treatment
   1. Hydrocele—needle aspiration or surgical aspiration and drainage.

2. Varicocele—surgical intervention only if there are complications with fertility; otherwise a scrotal support.

D. Nursing Intervention: provide preoperative and postoperative care (See Chapter 3).

Cystocele and Rectocele

Assessment

1. Risk factors/etiology
   a. Obesity and child bearing.
   b. Genital atrophy due to aging.
2. Clinical manifestations.
   a. Cystocele—protrusion of the bladder into the vagina.
      (1) Stress incontinence—during coughing, lifting, or sneezing.
      (2) Frequency and urgency.
      (3) Difficulty emptying bladder.
   b. Rectocele—protrusion of the rectum through the vaginal wall.
      (1) Constipation.
      (2) Incontinence of gas or liquid feces.
3. Diagnostics - bimanual pelvic examination.

Treatment

1. Medical—Kegel's exercises for mild stress incontinence (tighten and release perineal muscles several times during the day, stop urinating in midstream and hold it for a few seconds)
2. Surgical.
   a. Cystocele— anterior colporrhaphy.
   b. Rectocele— posterior colporrhaphy.
   c. Procedure is usually called "A and P repair."

Nursing Intervention

✦ *Goal: to assist client to understand the implications of and be prepared for surgery.*

1. Preoperative teaching.
2. Postoperative period.
   a. Prevent wound infection.
   b. Prevent pressure on suture line in the vagina.
   c. Perineal care BID and after each voiding or defecation.
   d. Low-residue diet after surgery to prevent pressure on incision area.

Self-Care

1. Encourage the use of mild laxatives to prevent straining at stool.
2. Prevent constipation - a low-residue diet may be ordered initially to prevent accumulation of large stool; however, after the area is healed, client needs a high-residue diet to prevent constipation.
3. Activities that are restricted include heavy lifting, prolonged standing, walking, sitting, and intercourse until area has healed.
4. Call the doctor if there is persistent pain or purulent, foul-smelling vaginal discharge.

Vaginal Inflammatory Conditions

Common predisposing factors.

1. Excessive douching.
2. Oral contraceptives, steroids.
3. Antibiotics—especially broad-spectrum, which wipe out normal vaginal flora (vagina is protected by an acidic pH and the presence of Doederlein's bacillus).
4. Improper cleaning after voiding and defecating.
5. Assess for recurrent chronic infection, there may be an underlying condition (prediabetic state, HIV) that should be further evaluated.

Bacterial Vaginosis

1. Characteristics.
   a. Causative organism—*E. coli, Haemophilus vaginalis*.
   b. Profuse yellowish discharge, "fishy smell."
   c. Itching, redness, burning, and edema, which are aggravated by voiding and defecation.
2. Treatment — antibacterial/antiprotozoal medication.

Candidiasis

1. Characteristics.
   a. Organism—*Candida albicans* (fungus).
   b. Internal itching, beefy red irritation, inflammation of vaginal epithelium.
   c. White, cheese-like odorless discharge which clings to the vaginal mucosa.
   d. Occurs frequently and is difficult to cure.
   e. Treatment — antifungal vaginal medication.

Trichomoniasis

1. Characteristics.
   a. Organism—*Trichomonas vaginalis* (protozoan).
   b. Itching, burning, dyspareunia.

c. Frothy, green-yellow, copious, malodorous vaginal discharge, strawberry spot on cervix.

d. Sexual partner needs to be treated also because of cross-infection. Men are usually asymptomatic.

2. Treatment — antibacterial/antiprotozoal medication.

Postmenopausal Vaginitis (Atrophic Vaginitis)

1. Characteristics.

a. Due to lack of estrogen.

b. Itching and burning.

c. Loss of vaginal tissue folds and epithelial covering.

2. Treatment — estrogen vaginal cream.

Nursing Intervention

✦ *Goal: to teach client regarding personal hygiene to prevent infection, decrease inflammation, and promote comfort.*

1. Appropriate cleansing from front of vulva to back of perineal area.
2. Frequently, infection is worse around the menstrual period. Teach client to change tampons at least 3 to 4 times a day.
3. Do not douche; the normal protective bacteria are washed out and other bacteria are introduced.
4. If infection is chronic, it may be necessary to have sexual partner tested; he may be reinfecting the woman.
5. Discourage use of feminine hygiene sprays, because of increased irritation.
6. Avoid constricting clothing and non-cotton underwear.

✦ *Goal: to educate the woman regarding correct utilization of medication .*

1. Vaginal suppositories, ointments, and creams are often utilized.

a. Handwashing before and after insertion of suppository or application of cream.

b. Remain recumbent for 30 minutes after application, to promote absorption and prevent loss of the medication from the vaginal area.

c. Wear a perineal pad to prevent soiling of clothing with vaginal drainage.

Dysfunctional Uterine Bleeding

❑ **Bleeding that is excessive or abnormal in the amount or frequency without regard to systemic conditions; occurs when the hormonal events responsible for the balance of the cycle are interrupted.**

Amenorrhea

1. Absence of menses - primary (no menstruation has occurred by age 16 years); secondary (woman previously had menses).
2. May be indicative of menopause.
3. May be first indication of pregnancy.
4. Occurs when woman has lost a critical fat percentage (athletes, anorexia).

Menorrhagia

1. Excessive vaginal bleeding.
2. Single episode of heavy bleeding may indicate a spontaneous abortion.
3. May be associated with IUD.
4. Hypothyroidism.

Metrorrhagia

1. Vaginal bleeding between periods.
2. May be normal menopause.
3. Ectopic pregnancy.
4. Breakthrough bleeding from oral contraceptives.
5. Cervical polyps.

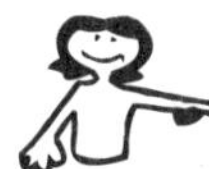

NURSING PRIORITY: *Vaginal bleeding after menopause or surgical hysterectomy is a symptom of a problem that needs to be evaluated.*

Nursing Intervention

1. Assist to determine most likely cause of problem.
2. Report excessive bleeding, abdominal pain, fever.
3. Dilation and curettage (D&C) may be done to treat abnormal bleeding

a. Often done of outpatient basis, with either general regional or local anesthesia.

b. Spotting and vaginal drainage is common for several days; if it is more then your normal period or if it lasts longer then 2 weeks, call the doctor.

c. Report any signs of infection - fever, foul, purulent discharge, increasing abdominal pain.

d. NSAIDs often used for pain control.

e. Avoid sexual intercourse and tampons for about two weeks.

Endometriosis

❑ **Endometriosis is the presence of endometrial tissue outside of the uterus. The tissue responds to hormonal stimulation by bleeding into areas within the pelvis, causing pain and adhesions.**

Assessment

1. Risk factors/etiology.
   a. Small pieces of endometrial tissue back up through the fallopian tubes into the abdomen during menstruation.
   b. Most common in premenopausal women 30 to 40 years old.
2. Clinical manifestations.
   a. Dysmenorrhea; deep-seated aching pain in the lower abdomen, vagina, posterior pelvis, and back occurring one to two days before menses.
   b. Abnormal excessive uterine bleeding and painful intercourse (dyspareunia); painful defecation.
3. Diagnostics.
   a. Laparoscopy.
   b. Ultrasonography.

Treatment

1. Medical—Danocrine (**Danazol**) a synthetic androgen, may be given over a 6-to 8-month period, or oral contraceptives. If a woman desires more children, she is encouraged to get pregnant, as the condition recedes during pregnancy.
2. Surgical intervention.
   a. Laser treatment of endometrial tissue in the extrauterine sites.
   b. Panhysterectomy (usually carried out in women close to the menopause).

Nursing Intervention

✦ *Goal: to assist client to understand measures to maintain health.*

1. Teach client about disease process; clarify any false ideas.
2. Provide emotional reassurance, potential for infertility.
3. Initiate pre- and postoperative teaching if surgery is elected.

Pelvic Inflammatory Disease (PID)

❑ **PID is an infectious condition of the pelvic cavity that involves the fallopian tubes, the ovaries, and/or the peritoneum.**

Assessment

1. Risk factors/etiology.
   a. Complication of gonorrhea, *C. trachomatis*, and staphylococcal organisms.
   b. Intrauterine devices (IUDs) are correlated with an increased incidence of PID.
2. Clinical manifestations.
   a. General malaise, fever, nausea, and vomiting.
   b. Leukocytosis.
   c. Bilateral lower abdominal pain.
   d. Vaginal discharge which is heavy and purulent.
   e. Chronic PID—persistent pelvic pain, secondary dysmenorrhea, dysfunctional uterine bleeding, and periodic episodes of acute symptoms.
3. Complications.
   a. Sterility, due to adhesions and strictures within the fallopian tubes.
   b. Ectopic pregnancy.
   c. Pelvic abscess or generalized peritonitis.
4. Diagnostics.
   a. Abdominal pain on palpation.
   b. Culture and sensitivity of drainage from the vagina, cervix, or cul-de-sac of Douglas.
   c. Ultrasonography, laparoscopy, culdocentesis..

Treatment

1. Medical: antibiotics, analgesics.
2. Surgical: incision and drainage of abscesses with or without a laparotomy.

Nursing Intervention

✦ *Goal: to prevent the spread and extension of the infection.*

1. Maintain semi-Fowler's position to promote drainage of the pelvic cavity by gravity.
2. Strict medical asepsis when in contact with discharge—wound and skin precautions.
3. Encourage oral fluids and maintain adequate nutrition.
4. Client should avoid sexual activities and douches.

✦ *Goal: to provide psychological support.*

1. Encourage expression of feelings related to guilt and possibility of sterility.
2. Explain factors relating to the long-term management of PID and the importance of maintaining medical supervision.

Sexually-Transmitted Diseases (STDs)

A. Characteristics
   1. Transmitted by sexual activity; including oral and rectal activities and between people of the same or opposite sex.
   2. One person can have more than one STD at a time.
   3. All sexual partners need to be evaluated.

B. Nursing role is to recognize and provide factual information.
   1. Mode of transmission.
   2. Prevention of transmission.
   3. Importance of contacts being identified and treated.

4. Information provided in accepting, nonjudgmental manner.
5. Oral contraceptives do not provide any protection.

C. Clients with STD's should be tested for HIV.

D. Hepatitis B is considered a sexually transmitted disease. (See chapter 19).

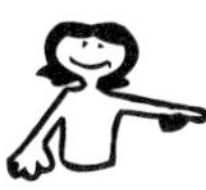

NURSING PRIORITY: *Consider all oral, genital, and rectal lesions to contain pathological organisms until documented otherwise.*

Syphilis

Characteristics

1. Causative agent: spirochete *Treponema pallidum.*
2. Incubation period: 10 to 90 days; average is 20 to 30 days.
3. Transmission: direct contact with primary chancre lesion, body secretions (saliva, blood, vaginal discharge, semen), and transplacentally to the fetus.
4. Communicability: highly infectious during the primary stage; blood contains the spirochete during the secondary stage; during the latent stage usually noninfectious after 1 year, and late (tertiary) stage is noninfectious.

Assessment

1. Primary stage.
   a. Chancre - painless lesion found on the penis, vulva, lips, vagina, or rectum.
   b. Usually heals spontaneously within 2 to 3 weeks, with or without treatment.
   c. Regional lymphadenopathy.
2. Secondary stage.
   a. Client may be asymptomatic, secondary stage usually begins anywhere from 2 weeks to 6 months after the chancre has healed.
   b. Maculopapular rash on the palms of the hands and on the soles of the feet.
   c. Lymphadenopathy; gray mucous patches in the mouth.
   d. Condylomata lata— flat lesions that may appear in moist areas; are most infectious of any syphilitic lesion (not to be confused with condylomata acuminatum in genital warts).
   e. Symptoms will disappear within two to six weeks.
3. Latent stage.
   a. Absence of clinical symptoms.
   b. Serologic tests for syphilis remain positive.
   c. Transmission through blood contact can occur.
   d. The majority of clients remain in this stage without further symptoms.
4. Congenital syphilis.
   a. Maculopapular rash over face, genital region, palms and soles.
   b. Snuffles - a mucopurulent nasal discharge.
   c. After age 2 - Hutchinson's teeth (notched central incisors with deformed molars and cusps).
5. Diagnostics.
   a. Serologic screening tests - Venereal Disease Research Laboratories (VDRL).
   b. Rapid plasma reagin (RPR).
   c. Fluorescent Treponemal Antibody Absorption (FTA-ABS) test.
   d. VDRL and FTA-ABS are based on presence of antibodies and are not positive until about four weeks after the appearance of the chancre.
6. Complications - development of late (tertiary) syphilis and the resultant systemic involvement of the cardiovascular and central nervous system.

Nursing Intervention

1. Administration of parenteral penicillin is treatment of choice. Tetracycline or doxycycline if client is allergic to penicillin.
2. If pregnant mother is treated prior to the 18th week of gestation, the fetus usually will be born unaffected.
3. Prevention education regarding sexual exposure, adequate case-finding and treatment of contacts.
4. All cases are reported to local public health authorities.

Gonorrhea

Characteristics

1. Most common venereal disease; an infection of the genitourinary tract; however, may affect the rectum, pharynx, and the eyes; caused by the bacteria *Neisseria gonorrhoeae.*
2. Incubation period: 2 to 7 days.
3. Transmission: direct contact with exudate via sexual contact or transmission to the neonate during passage through the birth canal.
4. Communicability: contagious as long as organism is present.

Assessment

1. Men.
   a. Urethritis, epididymitis, dysuria, and purulent urethral discharge.
   b. Increased evidence of asymptomatic disease in males, or a chronic carrier state.
2. Women.

a. Initial urethritis or cervicitis often go unnoticed.

b. Vulvovagnitis, vaginal discharge, dysuria.

c. If untreated, may result in pelvic inflammatory disease (PID).

3. Neonate - ophthalmia neonatorum.

4. Diagnostics.

a. Positive gram stain smear of discharge or secretion.

b. Positive culture.

5. Complications.

a. Men: prostatitis, urethral strictures, urethritis, and sterility.

b. Women: PID, Bartholin abscess, ectopic pregnancy, infertility.

Nursing Intervention

1. Prophylactic antibiotic treatment for gonorrhea eye infection in the neonate -ophthalmia neonatorum.
2. Encourage follow-up cultures 7 to 14 days after treatment, and again at 6 months.
3. Teach importance of abstinence from sexual intercourse until cultures are negative.
4. Urge client to inform sexual mate so that he or she may be treated for infection.
5. Important to take the full course of the antibiotics.

Herpes Genitalis (HVH Type II)

Characteristics

1. Infection caused by the *herpes virus hominis* (HVH) Type II, which is characterized by painful vesicles surrounded by an erythematous area; progresses to shallow ulcers, pustules, and crusts; healing occurs spontaneously in about 2 to 4 weeks during the initial infection.
2. Lesions characteristically occur below the waist, generally in the genital area. It is possible for the Type II virus to cause oral lesions.
3. Virus enters a latent phase and may be harbored by the individual for an indefinite period of time; virus may be reactivated by stress, sunburn, sexual activity, and fever.
4. Recurrent outbreaks are most often less severe than the original lesions.
5. Incubation period: unknown.
6. Transmission: by direct contact with the vesicles, increased documentation indicating asymptomatic shedding and transmission of virus.
7. Communicability: highly contagious.

Assessment

1. Initial sensation of tingling and itching prior to the rupture of the lesion.
2. Primary infection usually local inflammation, pain, lymphadenopathy, and systemic symptoms.
3. Diagnostics: confirmed by using a tissue culture technique which identifies the herpes type II virus.
4. Complications.

a. Increased incidence of cervical cancer in women.

b. Lesions in pregnant women or a positive viral tissue culture are a concern. Client will be closely monitored to determine if a problem with delivery is anticipated - possible cesarean section. .

Nursing Intervention

1. Teach importance of genital hygiene and avoidance of sexual contact while lesions are present.
2. Teach good hygiene practices, if the lesions break open, the fluid contains the virus. The virus can be spread by contact and cause a lesion in any area of the body.

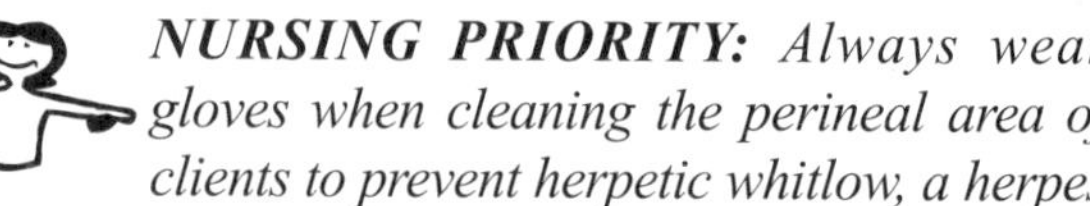

NURSING PRIORITY: *Always wear gloves when cleaning the perineal area of clients to prevent herpetic whitlow, a herpes lesion around the nail bed. Nurses are at risk for developing this because of local contact of the HVH virus on broken skin areas around the nail.*

3. If oral acyclovir (**Zovirax**) is started at the first sign of a lesion, the course of the lesion may be decreased.
4. Symptomatic treatment: sitz baths, wet compresses, and analgesics for relief of pain.

Cytomegalovirus (CMV)

Characteristics

1. A virus belonging to the herpes family which leads to very mild illnesses but can cause a wide range of serious congenital deformities in the fetus or newborn.
2. Transmission: human contact.
3. Communicability: about 4 out of 5 people over the age of 35 have been infected with CMV, usually sometime during childhood or young adulthood. Symptoms are so mild, most often the diagnosis is overlooked.

Assessment

1. Effect on the mother usually asymptomatic or with mononucleosis-type illness symptoms.
2. Effect on the neonate - serious hematologic and CNS consequences. High mortality rate in severely affected neonates.
3. Diagnostics:

a. **TORCH** screening - **T**oxoplasmosis, **O**ther (hepatitis), **R**ubella, **C**ytomegalovirus infection, **H**erpes simplex.

b. Increased lymphocytes and abnormal liver function test.

Nursing Intervention

1. Prevention is the primary goal - pregnant women, should avoid being around affected individuals and congenitally infected infants.
2. Prevention of exposure is almost impossible, as the primary infection is asymptomatic.

Chlamydia Infection

Characteristics

1. Nongonococcal urethritis (NGU) is an infectious disease caused by the *Chlamydia trachomatis*.
2. Incubation period: 2 to 35 days.
3. Transmission: direct contact sexual contact.

Assessment

1. Males.
   a. Urethritis, epididymitis, proctitis.
   b. Primary reservoir is the male urethra.
2. Females.
   a. Mucopurulent cervicitis, postpartal endometritis, salpingitis, vaginitis.
   b. Primary reservoir is the cervix.
3. Effect of maternal infection on newborn: inclusion conjunctivitis and pneumonia.
4. Both males and females are frequently asymptomatic.
5. Diagnostics: isolation of the organism in a tissue culture or serologic compliment fixation testing.

Nursing Intervention

1. Urge client to have sexual partner treated.
2. Emphasize the importance of long-term drug therapy due to the pathogen's unique life cycle that makes it difficult to cure.
   a. Antibiotics - doxycycline and azithromycin are primary antibiotics for treatment.
   b. Penicillin and its derivatives are not effective against the organism; consequently, this usually explains the persistence of infection in clients who are treated for gonorrhea and do not respond to the treatment.

Genital Warts

Characteristics.

A. Characterized by cluster of warts caused by the human papilloma virus -HPV —condylomata acuminata.

B. HPV is continually shed from the surface and reinfection is not uncommon.

Assessment

1. Warts are found in areas subject to trauma during sexual activity - penis, urethra, perianal area, anal canal; vulva, cervix, vaginal canal.
2. Diagnosed by observation and biopsy of lesions.
3. The cervix and anal canal may be involved if there are lesions on the vaginal or anal area.

Nursing Intervention

1. Education regarding transmission.
2. Close follow up with Pap smears in women - increased incidence or cervical cancer.
3. Increased incidence of squamous cell cancer of penis in men.
4. Podophylin applied topically once or twice a week, and antimitotic preparations are most common treatments.
5. Transmission is direct contact with a person who has lesions present.

Cervical Cancer

Assessment

1. Risk factors/etiology.
   a. Multiple sex partners.
   b. Early age of first intercourse.
   c. Herpes genitalis type II.
   d. History of sexually-transmitted diseases or genital warts.
2. Clinical manifestations.
   a. Clients are asymptomatic until late in disease state.
   b. Thin and watery drainage which later becomes dark and foul-smelling as the disease progresses.
3. Diagnostics.
   a. Papanicolaou smear (Pap Smear).
      (1) Women should begin having yearly Pap smears when they are 18 years old, or when they become sexually active.
      (2) Pap smears are continued after menopause and hysterectomy.
   b. Classification of Papanicolaou test - Cervical Intraepithelial Neoplasia (CIN)
      (1) Normal limits - minimal or no inflammation.
      (2) Significant inflammation - no malignant cells.
      (3) CIN grade I - suggestive of malignancy; non-conclusive.
      (4) CIN grade II - increased indications of a malignancy.
      (5) CIN grade III - strongly suggests malignancy.

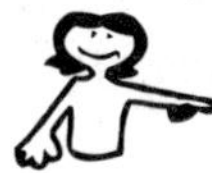

NURSING PRIORITY: If cancer of the cervix is identified prior to becoming invasive (or in situ stage), there is virtually a 100% cure rate.

c. Cervical biopsy (office procedure). Post-test, the client should:

(1) Avoid strenuous activity for 24 hours.

(2) Leave vaginal packing in for about 24 hours.

(3) Abstain from sexual intercourse for approximately 24 hours.

(4) Avoid using tampons.

(5) Avoid douching.

Treatment

1. Surgical intervention.

a. Conization (cryosurgery)—used for carcinoma in situ.

b. For cervical cancer, the following procedures may be done:

(1) Vaginal hysterectomy—removal of the uterus; fallopian tubes and ovaries remain intact.

(2) Panhysterectomy (TAH-BSO)—total hysterectomy; includes removal of fallopian tubes and ovaries.

(3) Radical hysterectomy—a panhysterectomy plus a partial vaginectomy and removal of lymph nodes.

(4) Pelvic exoneration—radical hysterectomy plus total vaginectomy, removal of bladder with urinary diversion, bowel resection, and colostomy.

c. Radiation therapy, either internal (radium implant) or external for invasive cancer.

Nursing Intervention

✦ *Goal: to provide health teaching to detect premalignant cervical dysplasia.*

1. Warning signs of cancer.
2. Importance of yearly Pap smears.
3. Encourage verbalization of feelings related to the surgery and diagnosis of cancer.

✦ *Goal: to provide pre-and postoperative teaching in preparation for a total abdominal hysterectomy.*

1. General preoperative care.
2. Postoperatively, assess for complications such as backache or decreased urine output, as this can indicate accidental ligation of the ureter.
3. Urinary retention may occur due to bladder atony and edema; explain to client the necessity for a Foley catheter.
4. Early ambulation is encouraged to prevent postoperative thrombophlebitis.
5. Determine if the doctor is going to put the client on hormonal replacement. If he does, determine type, and discuss with the client.
6. If dyspareunia occurs, she should contact her doctor.

✦ *Goal: to provide psychological support.*

1. Encourage verbalization of concerns related to body image.
2. Teach that sexual activity should be avoided until the wound is healed (about 4 to 6 weeks).
3. Avoid heavy lifting for two months.
4. Client who has had a pelvic exoneration will have many concerns regarding sexual function, as the vagina will be lost. Menopause may occur, and there will be a urinary or bowel diversion to the abdominal wall (an ileal conduit or colostomy).

Breast Carcinoma

Assessment

1. Risk factors/etiology.

a. Leading cause of death due to cancer in women ages 14-54 years.

b. Family history of breast cancer.

c. Nulliparous women or those whose first parity occurred after age 30.

d. Early menses, late menopause. Removal of the ovaries prior to age 35 years significantly decreases the risk of breast cancer.

e. The incidence of recurrence of breast cancer is significant.

f. Presence of other cancer: endometrial, ovarian, colon-rectal.

2. Clinical manifestations.

a. Asymmetry of the breasts.

b. Skin dimpling, flattening, or nipple deviation are suggestive of a lesion.

c. Skin coloring and thickening, large pores, sometimes called peau d'orange (orange peel appearance).

d. Changes in the nipple, discharge from the nipple.

e. Mass is painless, nontender, hard, irregular in shape, and nonmobile.

f. Majority of malignant lesions are found in the upper outer quadrant of the breast (tail of Spence).

3. Diagnostics.

a. Mammography.

b. Breast biopsy.

c. Serum tumor markers: CEA, hCG.

4. Complications—Metastases via the lymphatic system to the bone, lung, brain, and liver.

Treatment

(Review Chapter 8: Cancer)

1. Surgical.
   a. Modified radical mastectomy—(most common) removal of all breast tissue, axillary lymph nodes; the pectoralis major muscle remains intact. Preservation of the muscle helps to prevent the arm edema frequently associated with mastectomy.
   b. Local excision—(lumpectomy) may be done to stage the malignancy and determine appropriate chemotherapy/radiation therapy, but the breast is preserved.
   c. Radical mastectomy—(less common) removal of all of the breast tissue, the pectoral muscles, and the axillary lymph nodes of the surrounding tissue.
   d. Breast reconstruction - may be delayed until after radiation, or may be done at the time of the mastectomy.
2. Radiation—combined with surgery and chemotherapy.
3. Hormonal therapy—Breast cancers that are classified as "estrogen receptors" are less invasive tumors and respond to changes in estrogens. Hormone therapy is being used in conjunction with surgical intervention to prevent/decrease recurrence.
4. Chemotherapy—a combination of drugs will be used to treat the malignancy.

Nursing Intervention

✦ *Goal: to promote early detection of breast cancer through public education and self-breast examination.*

1. Evaluate risk factors; educate women regarding who has increased risk factors.
2. Perform self-breast examinations (SBE) on a regular basis; once a month about a week after a period, or at the same time each month if the woman has no periods.
3. Important that the SBE be done on a regular basis; this makes it easier to detect abnormalities when they occur.
4. The SBE should include:
   a. Step 1 - Inspection before a mirror to determine asymmetry or changes in size. Breast should be evaluated from three positions: with the arms relaxed at the sides; with the arms over the head pressing on the back of the head; with the hands on the hips, palms pressing inward to flex the chest muscles. Look for dimpling, differences in sizes of the breast, ulcerations, nipple retraction or increased vascularity.
   b. Step 2 - Breast should be palpated while lying down; flatten the right breast by placing a pillow under the right shoulder. With the fingers flat, use the sensitive pads of the middle three fingers of the left hand. Feel for lumps or changes using a rubbing motion. Press firmly enough to feel the different breast tissues. Examine all of the breast from the collar bone to the base of your bra and the axillary area. Pay particular attention to the upper outer quadrant of each breast. Gently squeeze the nipple to determine presence of any drainage.
   c. Step 3 - In the shower or bath examine your breasts; hands glide easier over wet skin.
5. Women over 40 should have a mammogram every 1 to 2 years; women over 50 should have a mammogram every year; those women with increased risk factors should maintain regular follow-up with a physician.
6. The American Cancer Society provides excellent teaching opportunities for nurses, as well as extensive information for women regarding early detection of breast cancer and rehabilitation after a mastectomy.

NCLEX ALERT: *Teaching women about breast cancer, risk factors, self-examinations, and preventive health care is consistently included on the exam.*

✦ *Goal: to prepare the client physiologically and psychologically for surgery (normal pre-and postoperative care, Chapter 3).*

1. Assist woman to decrease emotional stress and anxiety; encourage spiritual and social resources.
2. Provide emotional support, encourage verbalization.
3. Anticipate concerns related to sexuality and fear of rejection by husband or sex partner after the mastectomy (see Chapter 9 on Body Image).
4. Determine if any plans have been discussed for reconstructive surgery.

NCLEX ALERT: *Plan measures to assist client to cope with anxiety; assess client's response to illness; identify coping mechanisms of client and family.*

✦ *Goal: to recognize and prevent postoperative complications.*

1. Frequently, a pressure dressing is in place immediately postoperative. There may be one or more drains in the incisional area.

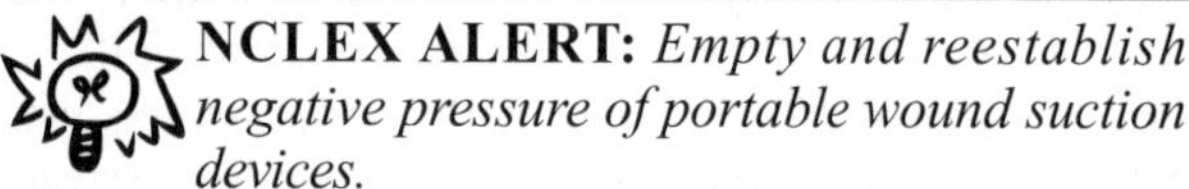

NCLEX ALERT: *Empty and reestablish negative pressure of portable wound suction devices.*

2. Position arm on affected side so that each joint is elevated and positioned higher than the more proximal joint; this promotes gravity drainage via the lymphatic and venous circulations.
3. Do not take blood pressure or perform any injections or venipuncture on the arm of the affected side.
4. Arm exercises are usually started on the first postoperative day.
   a. Assist/teach the woman to perform flexion and extension exercises with the wrist and elbow frequently throughout the day. Squeezing a ball is good exercise at this period.
   b. The affected arm should not be abducted or externally rotated in initial exercises. Encourage movement of the arm in activities of daily living (brushing her hair, eating, washing her face).
5. Active exercises are begun after wound healing is well-established. Exercises may still be done from the supine position, but more range of motion is encouraged, with some abduction and external rotation of the upper arm.
6. Approximately two to three weeks after surgery, and with good wound healing, more active exercises are begun.
   a. Pendulum arm swings.
   b. Pulley-type rope exercise to promote forward and lateral movement of the arms.
   c. "Wall climbing" with the fingers.

NCLEX ALERT: *Identify factors interfering with wound healing - the arm on the affected side will be at increased risk for developing problems of edema and infection. The arm should be protected throughout the rehabilitation and during activities of daily living for an indefinite period of time.*

✦ *Goal: to promote client's return to homeostasis and understand implications of modified life style; identify measures to maintain health.*

1. Discuss symptoms of recurrence and importance of maintaining regular visits to the physician to monitor recovery and to detect changes.
2. Promote a positive self-image and reintegration with family and loved ones.
3. Discuss with client plans for obtaining either a temporary or a permanent breast prosthesis.
4. Encourage the woman to participate in the *Reach for Recovery Program* through the American Cancer Association. Check with the physician to see if representatives may visit with the client prior to the surgery.⌘

Study Questions—Reproductive System

1. The nurse receives a report on a client's Pap smear. The result is reported in the CIN classification. The client's results are a CIN Grade III. What is the nurse's interpretation of this report?

① Highly suspicious for malignancy.

② Indicative of metastatic problems.

③ Definitive for malignancy.

④ Diagnostic of tissue dysplasia.

2. A client has been diagnosed with genital herpes type II, she asks the nurse when she is contagious. The nurse would explain to the client that she is most contagious at what stage?

① Vesicles rupture and release exudate.

② Superficial, painful ulcers appear.

③ Yellow vaginal drainage is present.

④ Pustules become inflamed and erythematous.

3. What is important to include in the discharge teaching plan for a 38-year-old client post vaginal hysterectomy?

① Do not douche with any type of solution.

② Refrain from sexual intercourse for two months.

③ Take hormone replacement therapy.

④ Anticipate heavy vaginal bleeding.

4. During a well woman physical examination a young woman is diagnosed with a primary genital herpes lesion. When completing the client's history, what will the nurse would anticipate the client to report?

① Anuria.

② Pruritus.

③ Leukorrhea.

④ Dyspareunia.

5. After a vaginal hysterectomy, what is a priority nursing action immediately postoperative?

① Assist with sitz baths tid.
② Provide a high-protein diet.
③ Teach the client exercises to strengthen the abdomen.
④ Observe the client for decreased urine output.

6. What is an important nursing action when assisting the doctor with a pelvic examination?

① Instruct the client to douche prior to the exam.
② Explain to the client that she will not feel any pain.
③ Have the client empty her bladder before the examination begins.
④ Lubricate the speculum well before handing it to the doctor.

7. A teenage boy comes to the office complaining of intense burning while urinating and gray green discharge coming from his penis. The nurse recognizes these symptoms of what problem?

① Herpes with open lesions.
② Stage 2 syphilis.
③ Urinary tract infection.
④ Gonorrhea.

8. After examining a painless sore on the penile shaft, the doctor asks the nurse to order a Fluorescent Treponemal Antibody Absorption Test (FTA-ABS). The nurse identifies the purpose of this test is to diagnose what condition?

① Herpes Genitalis Type 2.
② Trichmonasis.
③ Cytomegalovirus.
④ Syphilis Stage 1

9. The night shift nurse notes at the end of her shift that a post mastectomy client has a total of 90 cc of serosanguineous drainage after a 24 hour period. What is the best nursing action?

① Report amount of drainage to the physician.
② Start frequent BP checks and observe for hemorrhage.
③ Continue to monitor the drainage.
④ Reinforce packing at the wound site.

10. What is important nursing care for a post mastectomy client regarding the positioning of the affected arm?

① Hold the arm close against the side of her body.
② Secure the arm below the level of the heart.
③ Wrap the arm in an ace bandage and keep below the heart.
④ Elevate arm above heart level.

11. A client is admitted for benign prostatic hypertrophy, and is scheduled to have a transurethral prostate resection. What assessment data would indicate to the nurse the client is developing a complication?

① The client has difficulty emptying his bladder.
② Client states he feels like he cannot empty his bladder.
③ The client complains of frequency and nocturia.
④ Increasing complaints of flank pain and hematuria.

12. The nurse is discussing the importance of self breast examination to a client who is being discharged after a vaginal hysterectomy. What is important information for the nurse to give this client?

① Perform self-breast exam one week after her normal period.
② Examine her breast on a regular bases about the same time every month.
③ Breast should be palpated while in the sitting position.
④ Use the tips of the fingers to palpate deeply into the breast tissue.

13. The nurse is discussing testicular self-examination with a male client. What information is important for the nurse to include in the discussion?

① The best time to perform the examination is 24 hours after sexual intercourse.
② The examination should be conducted at the same time each month.
③ Every three to four months the client should perform this self-examination.
④ When the scrotum is pulled up tight against the body the testis are easier to palpate.

14. The nurse is assessing a client who had a transurethral resection of the prostate (TURP) 6 hours ago. He has a urinary catheter with a continuous bladder irrigation running. What nursing observations would indicate a complication is developing?

① Catheter drainage of 50cc the past hour and increase in suprapubic pain.
② Dark, grossly bloody catheter drainage with pieces of tissue.
③ Client complains that he feels like he needs to void.
④ Moderate amount of bloody discharge from around the catheter.

Appendix 22-1:
MEDICATIONS USED IN REPRODUCTIVE SYSTEM DISORDERS

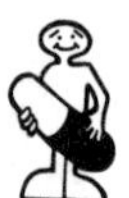

MEDICATIONS	SIDE EFFECTS	NURSING IMPLICATIONS
ALPHA -1 ADRENERGIC BLOCKER: Medications decrease the size of the prostate, therefore decreasing pressure on the urinary tract in clients with BPH.		
Doxazosin (**Cardura**): PO Terazosin (**Hytrin**): PO	Dizziness, fatigue, hypotension, dyspnea	1. Advise client of possible problems of decreased blood pressure and orthostatic hypotension. 2. Prostatic cancer should be ruled out before medications are started. 3. Medication should decrease problems of urination associated with BPH.
Finasteride (**Proscar**): PO	Impotence, decreased libido	1. Client should take contraceptive precautions or not have sexual intercourse with women who could potentially get pregnant.
ANTIFUNGAL/PROTOZOAL MEDICATIONS: Used to treat vaginal infections.		
Over-the-counter: Clotrimazole (**Gyne-Lotrimin**): intravaginally Miconazole (**Monistat 3**): intravaginally *Prescription only:* Fluconazole (**Diflucan**): PO, IV, intravaginally Terconazole (**Terazol**): intravaginally Metronidazole (**Flagyl**): PO, IV		1. Creams are not recommended to be used with tampons or diaphragms. 2. Not recommended for use in pregnancy or lactation. 3. **Flagyl** is used to treat trichomoniasis; teach client urine may turn red-brown and *to avoid alcohol*, as it can lead to serious side effects of throbbing headaches, nausea, excessive vomiting, hyperventilation, and tachycardia. 4. Suppositories or applicators are used to place medication in vagina. 5. If client does not see improvement within 3 days, she should return to her health care provider. 6. **Diflugan** can be given as a single dose for vaginal candididasis.

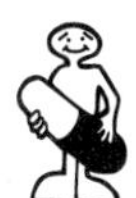

Appendix 22-2:
HORMONE REPLACEMENT

MEDICATIONS	SIDE EFFECTS	NURSING IMPLICATIONS
Conjugated estrogen (**Premarin, Ortho-est**): PO intravaginally Micronized estradiol (**Estrace**): PO, intravaginally Estradiol (**Estraderm**): transdermal patches	Nausea vomiting, break through bleeding, weight gain, swollen tender breast, increased blood pressure. Increased risk of uterine cancer.	1. Should not be given to women who have a uterus, estrogen compounds should be given with progesterin combinations. 2. Important for menopausal women to continue with increased calcium and weight bearing exercises along with estrogen replacement to prevent osteoporosis. 3. Should not be used by women who have known or suspected cancer of the breast, undiagnosed vaginal bleeding, or possible pregnancy. 4. Use: replacement hormone to treat symptoms associated with menopause - hot flashes, atopic vaginitis.
Medroxyprogesterone acetate: (**Provera**)	Menses may become more irregular	1. Use: replacement hormone for menopausal women who still have a uterus, significantly decreased risk of uterine cancer when used with estrogen therapy. 2. Medication may be given cyclical or on a daily basis with **Premarin**. 3. Women should continue with increased calcium intake to prevent osteoporosis, weight bearing exercises; yearly PAP smears and mammograms, and cholesterol series.

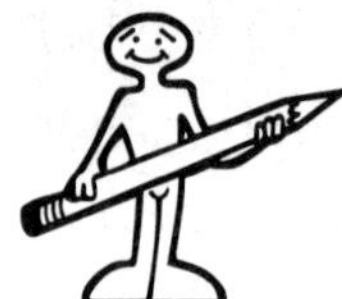

Notes

PHYSIOLOGY OF THE KIDNEY AND URINARY TRACT

A. Kidney function.

1. Excretory.

a. Rid the body of metabolic wastes.

(1) Regulate fluid volume; normally 125 cc of fluid is filtered each minute (glomerular filtration rate), however only one cc is excreted as urine; average urine output is about 1,440 cc per day.

(2) Regulate the composition of electrolytes.

(3) Assist in maintaining acid-base balance.

b. Regulation of blood pressure.

(1) Juxtaglomerular cells are located in the afferent arteriole just before it enters the glomerulus.

(2) The cells respond to a decrease in the blood flow (decrease in blood pressure) by increasing the secretion of renin.

(3) Renin acts on angiotensin I and converts it to angiotensin II, which is a powerful vasoconstrictor. Peripheral resistance is increased, therefore blood pressure is increased.

2. Endocrine.

(1) Aldosterone production is stimulated by the increase in angiotensin I, therefore sodium and water are retained to increase the circulating volume and increase the blood pressure.

(2) Regulates red blood cell production through synthesis of erythropoietin; released in response to hypoxia.

(3) Aids in calcium metabolism by activating vitamin D, which promotes normal bone activity.

B. Nephron function.

1. Filtration—occurs in the glomerulus via a semipermeable membrane. The membrane does not normally allow large protein molecules to be filtered out of the blood.

a. Glomerular filtration rate (GFR) is the amount of blood filtered by the glomeruli in a given time (approximately 120-140 mL per minute).

b. Changes in GFR occur when the pressure gradients from the glomerular capillaries across the semipermeable membrane to the glomerulus are altered.

(1) Pressure gradient changes occur when there is a variation in the systemic blood pressure (hypotension), a significant change in the pressure in Bowman's capsule in the glomerulus (edema), and when ureteral obstruction occurs.

(2) The kidney response to changes in pressures is buffered by an autoregulatory mechanism in order to maintain a stable range of blood pressure. The autoregulatory mechanism maintains renal blood flow and the GFR within wide fluctuations of blood pressure. When the pressure range is outside the autoregulatory mechanism (hypotension/hypertension), the GFR will fluctuate with the systemic blood pressure.

NCLEX ALERT: *Determine client has a decreased urinary output -urinary output should be carefully evaluated regarding blood pressure level; blood pressure must provide renal perfusion to maintain adequate urinary output. The level of blood pressure to maintain renal perfusion varies greatly from one client to another.*

(3) If the glomerular membrane is damaged, plasma proteins will escape. A decrease in serum proteins decreases the normal serum oncotic pressure; this results in water retention and edema formation.

2. Tubular reabsorption—after the glomerulus has filtered the blood, the tubules separate the water and solutes by osmosis and diffusion. Water moves across the semipermeable membrane and is reabsorbed or excreted in response to the concentration gradient of the solutes (sodium, potassium, chloride, urea, etc.). Only a small amount of the total water filtered out of the kidneys is excreted as urine. Solutes are also reabsorbed according to the concentration gradient.

3. Tubular secretion—regulates the potassium level and maintains the acid-base balance with other regulatory mechanisms.

C. Urinary tract.(Figure 23-1)

1. Ureters.

a. Muscular tubes through which urine flows from the kidney to the bladder.

b. Ureterovesical valve—located at the opening of the ureter into the bladder (ureterovesical junction); prevents back-flow of urine into the ureters when the bladder contracts.

2. Bladder.
   a. As the bladder fills, the stretch receptors are stimulated. In the adult, the first urge to void will occur when 100 cc to 150 cc have collected; approximately 400 cc of urine will initiate a feeling of bladder fullness.
   b. Bladder capacity varies from 1,000 to 1,800 cc.
3. Voiding—stimulation is sent to the sacral area of the spinal column where the micturition reflex or voiding reflex is initiated. After toilet training, the cerebral cortex (via the spinal column) allows for voluntary control of bladder contractions that initiate urination.
4. Urethra—a small, membraneous tube which conveys urine from the bladder to the exterior of the body.

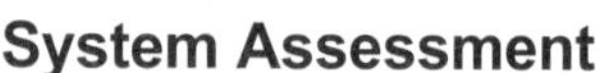

System Assessment

A. External assessment.
   1. Inspect skin for changes in color, turgor, and texture (urate crystals).
   2. Assess face, abdomen, and extremities for edema.
   3. Determine weight gain.
   4. Palpate kidneys and bladder.
      a. Landmark—for kidney palpation is the costovertebral angle (CVA), formed by the rib cage and the vertebral column.
      b. Bladder is palpated just above the suprapubic area (or symphysis pubis bone).
      c. Kidney and bladder should be non-palpable with no discomfort on palpation.

B. History.
   1. Presence of renal or urological congenital defect.
   2. Determine if client has ever been exposed to chemicals, especially carbon tetrachloride, phenol, and ethylene glycol, as these are nephrotoxic.
   3. Determine if client has received antibiotics which may be nephrotoxic—aminoglycosides, amphotericin B, and sulfonamides.
   4. Assess dietary intake—determine increased levels of calcium.
   5. Determine level of activity—immobility leads to demineralization of the bones, which can predispose to infection and calculus formation.
   6. Evaluate complaints of pain—dysuria, flank, costovertebral, or suprapubic.

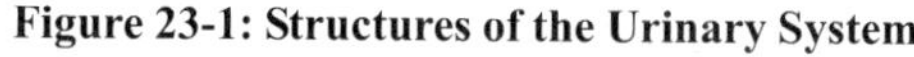

Figure 23-1: Structures of the Urinary System
Reprinted with permission: Phipps, WJ, Sands, JK, & Marek, JF (1999). *Medical Surgical Nursing: Concepts & Clinical Practice*, 6th ed. Philadelphia: Mosby, p 1396

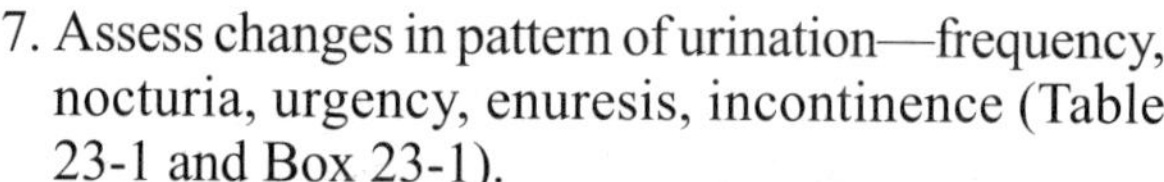

   7. Assess changes in pattern of urination—frequency, nocturia, urgency, enuresis, incontinence (Table 23-1 and Box 23-1).
   8. Assess changes in urine output—polyuria, oliguria, anuria.
   9. Assess changes in urine consistency—hematuria, pyuria, diluted, concentrated, change in color.
   10. Determine if client is on any medications that may affect urinary or renal function.
   11. Determine if client has any chronic health care problems that affect renal and urinary tract structures (diabetes mellitus, hypertension, or allergies).

DISORDERS OF THE URINARY-RENAL SYSTEM

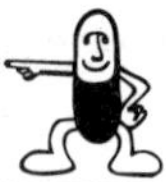

Urinary Tract Infections (UTI)

❑ **Stasis of urine in the bladder and reflux of urine back into the original reservoir are the primary factors in causing UTI.**

A. Upper urinary tract infections—***pyelonephritis***, an inflammation of the renal pelvis and the parenchyma of the kidney.

B. Lower urinary tract infection.
   1. Cystitis—inflammation/infection of the bladder.
   2. Urethritis—inflammation of the urethra.

Table 23-1: TYPES OF URINARY INCONTINENCE

TYPE OF UI	DEFINITION	PATHOPHYSIOLOGY	SYMPTOMS & SIGNS
Urge	Involuntary loss of urine associated with a strong sensation of urinary urgency.	▪ Involuntary detrusor (bladder) contractions (detrusor instability (DI). ▪ Detrusor hyperactivity with impaired bladder contractility (DHIC). ▪ Involuntary sphincter relaxation.	Loss of urine with an abrupt and strong desire to void. Involuntary loss of urine (without symptoms).
Stress	Urethral sphincter failure usually associated with increased intra-abdominal pressure.	▪ Urethral hypermobility due to anatomic changes or defects such as fascial detachments (hypermobility). ▪ Intrinsic urethral sphincter deficiency (ISD) failure of the sphincter at rest.	Small amount of urine loss during coughing sneezing, laughing or other physical activities. Continuous leak at rest or with minimal exertion (postural changes).
Mixed	Combination of urge and stress UI.	▪ Combination of urge and stress features as above. ▪ Common in women, especially older women.	Combinations of urge and stress UI symptoms as above.
Overflow	Bladder overdistention.	▪ A contractile detrusor. ▪ Hypotonic or underactive detrusor secondary to drugs, fecal impaction, diabetes, lower spinal cord injury, or disruption of the motor innervation of the detrusor muscle. ▪ In men —secondary obstruction due to prostatic hyperplasia, prostatic carcinoma, or urethral stricture. ▪ In women—obstruction due to severe genital prolapse or surgical over correction of urethral detachment.	Frequent or constant dribbling or urge or stress incontinence symptoms, as well as urgency and frequent urination.
Functional	Chronic impairments of physical and/or cognitive functioning	▪ Chronic functional and mental disabilities.	Urge incontinence or functional limitations.
Unconscious or reflex	Neurologic dysfunction.	▪ Decreased bladder compliance with risk of vesicoureteral reflux and hydronephrosis. ▪ Secondary to radiation cystitis, inflammatory bladder conditions, radical pelvic surgery, or myelomenigocele. ▪ In many non-neurogenic cases, no demonstrable DI.	Postmicturitional or continual incontinence. Severe urgency with bladder hypersensitivity (sensory urgency).

Source: Fantl, J., Newman, D., Colling, J. et al. (1996) Managing acute and chronic incontinence. *Clinical Practice Guideline: Quick Reference Guide for Clinicians*, No. 2, Rockville, MD: US Department of Health and Human Services, Public Health Servide, Agency for Health Care Policy and Research, AHCPR Pub. No. 96-0686.

C. Urinary tract infections occur in an ascending route up the urinary tract system.

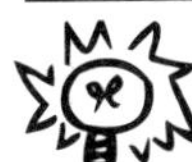

NCLEX ALERT: *Use alternative measures to promote voiding; promote bowel and bladder control.*

Assessment

1. Factors contributing to UTI.
   a. Adult female urethra is short, in close proximity to the rectum and vagina, which predisposes it to contamination from fecal material.
   b. Ureterovesical reflux—the reflux of urine from the urethra into the bladder. This causes a constant residual of urine in the bladder after voiding and precipitates UTI.
   c. Vesicoureteral reflux (ureterovesical reflux)—the reflux of urine from the bladder into one or both of the ureters and possibly into the renal pelvis.
   d. Instrumentation—catheterization or cystoscopic examination.
   e. Stasis of urine in the bladder leading to urinary retention for any reason (clients with prostate disease).

Box 23-2: Elderly Care Focus:
Urinary tract infections

- First symptom may be increasing confusion.
- A sudden onset of incontinence or increase in incontinent problem should be investigated.
- Fever, chills, tachycardia in the absence of urinary tract symptoms should be evaluated for septicemia from a urinary tract origin.
- Avoid indwelling urinary catheters.
- Encourage clients to void every 2 hours even if they do not feel a need; decreases residual and incontinence.
- Cleanse perineal area after each voiding and prevent fecal contamination of the urinary meatus.
- Women should wear cotton underwear.

f. Obstruction to urinary flow—congenital anomalies, urethral strictures, ureteral stones, or contracture of the bladder neck.

g. Bladder hypotonia; mechanical compression of the ureters, hormone changes predispose the pregnant woman to increased urinary tract infections.

h. Metabolic disorders such as diabetes.

i. Sexual intercourse promotes development of UTI.

j. Fecal contamination of the urethral meatus.

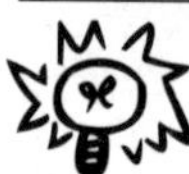

NCLEX ALERT: *Identify an infection - be able to assess and to identify pertinent data indicating a urinary tract and/or kidney infection.*

2. Clinical manifestations.

a. Cystitis.

(1) Frequency, urgency, dysuria (classic triad of symptoms).

(2) Hematuria.

(3) Nocturia, incontinence.

(4) Often asymptomatic with bacteriuria.

(5) Low back pain.

b. Pyelonephritis.

(1) Fever, chills, flank pain.

(2) Painful urination (dysuria).

(3) Pain and tenderness at the costovertebral angle.

(4) Symptoms of cystitis.

3. Diagnostics.

a. Urinalysis—pus, bacteria, and RBCs found in the urine.

Box 23-1: Elderly Care Focus
Dealing with Incontinence

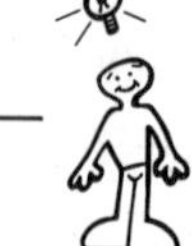

➸ *Need to determine:*

- Does client have difficulty initiating urinary flow?
- Is client aware of need to void?
- Can client empty bladder completely or is there residual?
- Is there bladder distention and overflow dribbling?
- Is stress incontinence present?
- What are usual voiding times?

➸ *Nursing Interventions*

- Assist the client to determine when he needs to urinate before an accident occurs.
- Maintain adequate fluid intake, but limit fluids before bedtime.
- Establish a voiding schedule - offer assistance and encourage voiding.
- Make sure client has easy access to the bathroom.
- Assess for presence of UTI.
- Teach client Kegel exercises.

b. Urine test for culture and sensitivity—done for recurrent or complicated infections; colony count of at least 100,000 colonies per cc of urine indicates infection.

c. Acute pyelonephritis.

(1) Elevated WBC count.

(2) Possible positive blood culture.

(3) Intravenous pyelogram, and KUB —identify stones or obstructions, or structural defects.

4. Complications.

a. A lower urinary tract infection may result in an upper urinary tract infection.

b. Chronic pyelonephritis may occur after repeated bouts of acute pyelonephritis.

Treatment

1. Medical. (See Appendix 23-2)

a. Broad spectrum antibiotics, especially the sulfonamides.

b. Urinary analgesics.

c. Antispasmodics.

2. Dietary.

a. Encourage fluid intake of 3,000 cc per day.

(1) Dilute urine causes less irritation.

(2) The increase in flow of urine through the urinary tract system decreases the movement of bacteria up the urinary tract.

(3) Discourage carbonated beverages and foods or drinks containing baking powder or baking soda.

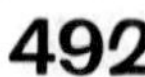

b. An acid-ash diet, to increase the acidity of the urine. (See Chapter 2).

Nursing Intervention

✦ *Goal: to obtain relief of pain, urgency, dysuria, and fever.*

1. Antibiotics need to be taken as scheduled - initially, therapy may be for 1-3 days; if problem is recurrent, 10-14 day therapy may be initiated.
2. Encourage eight to ten glasses of fluids daily.
3. Teach importance of voiding every two to three hours during the day to completely empty the bladder.
4. Sitz bath to decrease irritation of urethra.

✦ *Goal: to prevent recurrence of infection.*

1. Avoid sitting in bathtub with bubble bath additives; warm bath will decrease symptoms, but do not add anything to the water.
2. Explain importance of cleansing the perineal area from front to back after each bowel movement.
3. If intercourse seems to predispose to infection, encourage voiding immediately after intercourse.
4. Teach importance of long-term therapy if recurrent infections are problem.
5. Encourage and explain the need for follow-up care to prevent complications of chronic urinary tract infections.
6. Avoid caffeine and alcohol.

Urinary Calculi

❑ **Stones may form anywhere in the urinary tract; the most common location for stones is in the pelvis of the kidney. If the stones are small, they may be passed into the bladder.**

A. Stones in the bladder may increase in size if there is urinary stasis and alkaline pH.

B. Types of urinary calculi.

1. Calcium oxalate or phosphate stones—tend to be small; comprise 95 percent of all upper urinary tract calculi.
2. Struvite stones—contain bacteria and tend to form large stones.
3. Uric acid stones—occur most often in clients with primary or secondary problems of uric acid metabolism (gout).

Assessment

(Regardless of the type of stone formed, the clinical manifestations, diagnostics and treatment are essentially the same).

1. Risk factors/etiology.
   a. Infection.
   b. Urinary stasis.
   c. Immobility.
   d. Hypercalcemia and hypercalciuria (hyperparathyroidism, renal tubular acidosis).
   e. Excessive intake of dietary proteins, which increases uric acid production.
   f. Increased incidence in males over 40 years old.
2. Clinical manifestations.
   a. Sharp, sudden, severe pain.
      (1) May be described as "colic", either ureteral or renal.
      (2) Pain may be intermittent, depending on the movement of the stone; spasm in the ureter occurs as it attempts to move the stone toward the bladder.
      (3) Pain may radiate around the flank area, down into the genitalia, the bladder, and the thigh.
   b. Hematuria may be present from the traumatic effects of the stone on the ureter and the bladder.
   c. Nausea and vomiting are common.
3. Diagnostics.
   a. Urinalysis.
   b. CT scan
   c. KUB X-ray (kidney, ureters, bladder).
   d. Intravenous pyelogram and retrograde pyelogram.
4. Complications.
   a. Recurrent stone formation.
   b. Infection.
   c. Renal failure.

Treatment

1. Medical.
   a. Increase fluid intake to 3000cc/day to decrease urine concentration.
   b. Medications that prevent the absorption of calcium (thiazide diuretics and phosphates).
   c. Spasmolytic agents (anticholinergics).
   d. For uric acid stones, allopurinol (**Zyloprim**).
   e. Dietary.
      (1) Decrease calcium intake in client with calcium stones.
      (2) Sodium may also be restricted, since sodium increases the excretion of calcium in the urine.
      (3) Decrease in protein intake or an alkaline-ash diet for clients with uric acid stones.
2. Surgical.

a. Nephrolithotomy—incision into the kidney, with removal of the stone.

b. Ureterolithotomy—incision into the ureter to locate a stone and remove it.

3. Extracorporeal lithotripsy.

a. Client is supported on a frame and flank area is submerged in a tank of water.

(1) Sound waves travel through the water and are directed to the stone. The force of the sound wave shatters the stone and the remains are excreted in the urine.

(2) It is essential that the client remain absolutely immobile during the procedure, which lasts about 30 to 45 minutes.

(3) Depends on the doctor and the status of the client as to the type of sedation or anesthesia. Procedure is not particularly painful; however, it is difficult for client to remain immobile for the time required.

b. Percutaneous ultrasonic lithotripsy - sound waves are directed by a probe that is inserted via fluoroscopy

c. After percutaneous lithotripsy, a nephrostomy tube may be inserted.

d. Hemorrhage, infection and urinary retention are possible complications.

Nursing Intervention

✦ *Goal: to relieve pain.*

1. Administer analgesics as prescribed—morphine or meperidine (**Demerol**).
2. Hot baths or moist heat on flank area.
3. Encourage increased fluid intake (3000cc/day).
4. Strain all urine and inspect for blood clots and passage of stone.
5. If stone is passed, it should be saved and taken to the lab for analysis to determine the type of stone so appropriate therapy can be maintained.

✦ *Goal: to promote understanding of health care regimen.*

1. Dietary restrictions depending on type of stone; majority of clients will have calcium dietary restriction.
2. Discuss rationale, dose, frequency, and important information relating to medication administration.
3. Teach symptoms of recurring stone formation, such as hematuria, flank pain, or signs of infection.
4. Continue high fluid intake.
5. Promote medical follow-ups periodically to evaluate for symptoms of infection and recurring stone formation.

Hypospadias and Epispadias

A. Hypospadias—The urethral opening is located behind the glans penis, or along the penile shaft; a common anomaly.

B. Epispadias—The urethral opening is located on the dorsal or upper side of the penis; a rare problem.

Assessment

1. Clinical manifestations.

a. Visualization of defect.

b. Chordee -ventral curvature of the penis gives it a crooked appearance (hypospadias).

c. Stream of urine does not come out the end of the penis.

d. Commonly associated with cryptorchidism (hypospadias).

Treatment

Surgical correction of the defect.

1. Hypospadias—recommended repair in 6-18 months.
2. Epispadias is much more complex and frequently associated with other GU system defects, the repair may be very involved and require several stages.

Nursing Intervention

✦ *Goal: to provide emotional support and promote normal growth and development.*

1. Be sure that the infant is not circumcised, as the foreskin is used in the repair of hypospadias.
2. The infant with epipadias may be discharged home prior to repair.
3. Important not to delay repair, as child may be viewed as "different" by peers.
4. Diapers or an ileostomy bag over bladder area when infant has bladder defect. .
5. Teach parents signs of urinary tract infection.
6. Assist parents to understand realistic expectations of surgery (epispadias).

Nephrotic Syndrome

❑ **A problem with glomerular permeability to plasma proteins results in massive urinary protein loss. The most common type is a primary condition, minimal change nephrotic syndrome.**

A. Changes occur in the basement membrane of the glomeruli that allow the large protein molecules to pass through the membrane and be excreted. The loss of albumin from the serum decreases the oncotic pressure in the capillary bed and allows fluid to pass into the interstitial tissues and into the abdominal cavity (ascites).

B. The interstitial fluid shift causes hypovolemia, the renin-angiotensin response is stimulated, aldosterone secretion is increased, and the tubules begin to conserve sodium and water to increase the circulating volume.

C. In the majority of children with the syndrome, the etiology is unknown; it may be congenital, idiopathic, or secondary to another disease; frequently, there is no evidence of renal dysfunction or systemic disease.

Assessment

1. Risk factors/etiology.
   a. Often preceded by an upper respiratory disease, considered a precipitating factor, not a cause.
   b. Majority of children are male and between ages of 6 months and 7 years.
2. Clinical manifestations.
   a. Edema.
      (1) Facial edema, especially periorbital edema. May be more pronounced in the morning and subside some during the day.
      (2) Generalized edema of the lower extremities; may increase during the day.
      (3) Labia and scrotum may become very edematous.
      (4) Edema may progress to the level of severe generalized edema (anasarca).
      (5) Ascites and pleural effusion.
   b. Gradual increase in weight.
   c. Volume of urine is decreased and may be foamy and dark or tea-colored.
   d. Irritability, fatigue, lethargy.
   e. Blood pressure most often remains within normal ranges.
   f. Child is malnourished, due to decreased intake as well as loss of protein in the urine, but may not appear so due to edema.
3. Diagnostics.
   a. Decreased serum protein - hypoalbuminemia.
   b. Urinalysis—increased specific gravity, massive proteinuria.
   c. Creatinine clearance may be decreased, with normal serum creatinine.
4. Potential complications.
   a. Compromised immune system leading to increase in infections (pneumonia, bronchitis, peritonitis).
   b. With severe edema formation, child may become hypovolemic.

Treatment

1. Medical.
   a. Corticosteroids - prednisone.
   b. Diuretics—used when edema progresses despite sodium restriction.
   c. Salt-poor human albumin for vascular insufficiency and severe edema.
   d. Prophylactic broad-spectrum antimicrobial agents.
   e. Immunosuppressant therapy, usually cyclophosphamide (**Cytoxan**) used for children who are not responsive to steroid therapy.
2. Dietary.
   a. Decreased sodium intake.
   b. Protein intake should be high biological value.
   c. There is usually no fluid restriction.

Nursing Intervention

✦ *Goal: to monitor disease progress and reduce edema.*

1. Support edematous areas such as scrotum.
2. Provide and encourage a salt-restricted diet.
3. Administer salt-poor albumin; monitor closely for circulatory overload during and after administration.
4. Provide meticulous skin care; change position frequently and monitor good body alignment.
5. Cleanse and powder opposing skin surfaces frequently.
6. Daily weights, accurate intake and output, measure abdominal girth.
7. Dipstick urine for protein, check specific gravity.
8. Monitor cardiac function for complications of fluid balance (marked edema but hypovolemic).

✦ *Goal: to prevent infection.*

1. Child susceptible to infection due to decreased immune state as well as steroid therapy.
2. Protect child from upper respiratory infections; good pulmonary hygiene, check breath sounds.
3. Prevent skin excoriation and breakdown, assess carefully for indications of infection.

✦ *Goal: to promote nutrition.*

1. Encourage adequate protein intake.
2. Serve small quantities to children.
3. Encourage input from child in selecting foods from prescribed diet.

Self-Care

1. Instruct as to medical regimen - steroids, diuretics, antibiotics.

2. Reassure parents that the prognosis is good; there may be relapses that will require therapy, but few children progress to chronic disease.
3. Obtain medical assistance if relapse occurs - edema, proteinuria, fever.
4. Encourage normal growth and development activities, try to prevent social isolation.
5. Teach parents how to perform dipstick urine for protein; may need to keep a daily diary to evaluate level of proteinuria.

Glomerulonephritis

❑ **An inflammatory reaction in the glomerulus as a result of an antigen-antibody response to the beta-hemolytic *streptococcus*. An immune complex is formed as a result of the antigen-antibody formation; the complex becomes trapped in the glomerulus. As a result of the edema in the glomeruli, the GFR is significantly decreased.**

Assessment

1. Risk factors/etiology.
   a. The stimulus of the antigen-antibody reaction is most often Group A beta-hemolytic *streptococcus* infection of the throat (tonsillitis, pharyngitis), which ordinarily precedes the onset of the condition by about 10 days.
   b. Streptococcal pharyngitis, and impetigo are most common precipitating conditions..
   c. Most common in children, but all age groups can be affected.
2. Clinical manifestations.
   a. Acute glomerulonephritis.
      (1) Disease may be mild with proteinuria—asymptomatic hematuria.
      (2) Tea or cola-colored urine due to hematuria.
      (3) Facial and periorbital edema.
      (4) Decrease in urine output (oliguria).
      (5) Mild to moderate increase in blood pressure, hypertension is more severe in the adult.
      (6) Azotemia—presence of nitrogenous waste products in the blood.
   b. Chronic glomerulonephritis - symptoms reflect progressive renal failure, more common in adults.
3. Diagnostics.
   a. Urinalysis.
      (1) Proteinuria.
      (2) Increased specific gravity.
      (3) Hematuria.
      (4) Red cell casts.
   b. CBC—dilutional decrease in hemoglobin and hematocrit.
   c. Elevated BUN, creatinine.
   d. Positive complement studies and ASO titer.
4. Complications.
   a. Chronic renal failure.
   b. Circulatory overload (pulmonary edema) and CHF.
   c. Hypertensive episodes.

Treatment

1. Medical.
   a. Diuretics for severe edema and fluid overload.
   b. Antihypertensives.
   c. Antibiotics.
2. Dietary.
   a. Decrease sodium intake.
   b. Protein restriction if client is azotemic. The anorexia the child experiences frequently limits the protein sufficiently.
   c. Foods containing high potassium are often restricted during the oliguric phase.
3. Children with normal blood pressure, adequate urine output, and mild symptoms are cared for at home.
4. Fluid restriction may be implemented if urinary output is decreased.

Nursing Intervention

✦ *Goal: to protect client's kidneys by preventing secondary infections.*

1. Antibiotic therapy if cultures are positive.
2. Child usually experiences fatigue and malaise and will voluntarily restrict activity.
3. Avoid medications that are nephrotoxic.

✦ *Goal: to maintain fluid balance.*

1. Monitor intake and output; maintain diet and fluid restrictions.
2. Monitor renal function—check proteinuria, specific gravity and color of urine, weigh client daily, and if hypertensive, check blood pressure q 2 to 4 hours.
3. Monitor serum potassium levels.
4. Frequently, the first sign of improvement is an increase in the urine output, then may progress to profuse diuresis.

✦ *Goal: to prevent complications and promote comfort.*

1. Encourage verbalization of fears.

2. Decrease anxiety by explaining treatments and reassuring client and family that the majority of clients recover fully.
3. Most children recover spontaneously and uneventful.

Self-Care

1. Teach /parent/client symptoms to be reported to physician—nausea, fatigue, vomiting, decrease in urinary output, or symptoms of infection.
2. Explain the need for rest, good nutrition, and avoidance of people with respiratory infections.
3. Teach measures to prevent urinary tract infections.
4. Instruct client in regard to diet, fluid restrictions and medication therapy.
5. Teach client to dipstick urine to monitor for protein.

Wilms' Tumor (Nephroblastoma)

❑ **Nephroblastoma (Wilms' tumor) is one of the most common intra-abdominal tumors of childhood and is associated with congenital anomalies, especially those of the genitourinary tract. The treatment and survival rate are based on the stage of the tumor at the time it is diagnosed.**

1. Risk factors/etiology.
   a. Associated with congenital anomalies such as hypospadias and cryptorchidism.
   b. Peak incidence is at 3 years old.
2. Clinical manifestations.
   a. Swelling or mass within the abdomen—firm, confined to one side of the abdomen, causing vague pain.
   b. Abdominal pain as tumor enlarges.
   c. Hematuria, pallor, anorexia, weight loss and malaise are uncommon.
   d. Hypertension (63%).
3. Diagnostics.
   a. Physical exam.
   b. Abdominal and chest X-rays.
   c. CAT scan, IVP, ultrasonography, and MRI.
   d. CBC—may indicate polycythemia (elevated hematocrit).

Treatment

The survival rate greatly depends on the stage of the tumor at the time of diagnosis. If the tumor is diagnosed and treated in the early stages, there is a high survival rate.

1. Surgery.
   a. Surgery is frequently scheduled as soon as possible after the diagnosis.
   b. Nephrectomy - the adrenal gland may be spared, depending on the invasiveness of the cancer.
   c. If both kidneys are involved, the more healthy kidney is retained and the more involved one is removed.
2. Medical.
   a. Pre- and postoperative radiation therapy for large tumors.
   b. Postoperative chemotherapy.

Nursing Intervention

✦ *Goal: to provide safe preoperative care.*

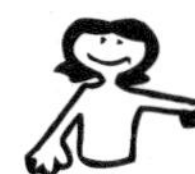

NURSING PRIORITY:** Post a sign above the bed that reads:* ***Do Not Palpate Abdomen.

1. Handle child carefully when bathing to prevent trauma to the tumor site.
2. Prepare child and family for the surgery, including anticipation of a large incision and dressing.
3. Assess vital signs, especially blood pressure, for indications of hypertension.

✦ *Goal: to assess kidney function, prevent infection.*

1. Usual postoperative care for abdominal surgery.
2. Anticipate a nasogastric tube, IV fluids, Foley catheter postoperatively.
3. Good pulmonary hygiene because child is going to be at increased risk for pulmonary infections.
4. Vincristine is frequently used in chemotherapy; closely observe the child for the development of a paralytic ileus.

Self-Care

1. Teach parents effects of chemotherapy.
2. Child has only one kidney; teach parents how to protect renal function.
   a. Signs and symptoms of urinary tract infection.
   b. Methods to prevent urinary tract infections.
   c. Advise all health care providers of compromised renal function.
   d. Prompt treatment of other infections.

Acute Renal Failure (ARF)

❑ **The abrupt loss of renal function may occur over several days or may occur over hours. The most common cause is hypotension and prerenal hypovolemia.**

Phases of Acute Renal Failure

1. Oliguric phase.

a. Urinary output decreases to *less than 400 cc per day.*

b. Increase in BUN, creatinine, uric acid, potassium, magnesium, and presence of metabolic acidosis.

c. Duration is often 8-15 days; the longer it lasts, the less favorable the recovery.

GERIATRIC PRIORITY: *The geriatric client loses his ability to concentrate urine; therefore, the urinary output may not be significantly reduced in this stage of renal failure.*

d. Non-oliguric renal failure - referred to as *high output failure;* urine is dilute and renal pathology present.

2. Diuretic phase.

a. A significant increase in urine volume; urine is very dilute.

b. BUN stops increasing.

c. Urinary creatinine clearance stabilizes.

d. May be preceded by decrease in sodium and potassium.

e. May last for two to three weeks.

3. Recovery.

a. May last from three to twelve months.

b. Usually some permanent loss of renal function, but remaining renal function is sufficient to maintain healthy life.

c. Complications—secondary infection, which is the most common cause of death.

Assessment

1. Risk factors/etiology.

a. Prerenal (renal ischemia).

(1) Circulatory volume depletion - hemorrhage.

(2) Decreased cardiac output - pump failure, CHF, especially in elderly.

(3) Decreased peripheral resistance - septic shock, anaphylaxis.

(4) Volume shifts - third spacing of fluid, gram-negative sepsis.

(5) Vascular obstruction - renal artery occlusion, dissection abdominal aneurysm.

b. Intrarenal (kidney tissue pathology).

(1) Acute tubular necrosis—hemolytic blood transfusion reaction, nephrotoxic chemicals (carbon tetrachloride, arsenic, lead, mercury), nephrotoxic medication (aminoglycosides, antibiotics, and streptomycin).

(2) Acute glomerulonephritis and pyelonephritis.

(3) Diseases that precipitate vascular changes (atherosclerosis, diabetes mellitus, hypertension).

c. Postrenal (obstructive problems).

(1) Urinary and renal calculi.

(2) Benign prostatic hypertrophy (BPH).

(3) Urethral stricture.

(4) Trauma resulting in obstruction.

NCLEX ALERT: *There are numerous disorders across the life span that can precipitate acute renal failure. It is important to know who is at increased risk for developing renal failure, and the initial symptoms. Frequently, renal failure is incorporated into a situation as a complication of the condition.*

2. Clinical manifestations (multiple body systems affected).

a. Urinary—decreased urinary output (oliguria, less than 400 cc per day, except in elderly may be 600-700 cc/day).

(1) Intrarenal and postrenal failure—fixed specific gravity is decreased, increased sodium in the urine; very little proteinuria, "muddy brown" casts.

(2) Prerenal failure—history of precipitating event; urine specific gravity may be high, high sodium concentration, and proteinuria.

(3) High output renal failure—the kidney no longer filters the urine. There is high urinary output; however, the urine is dilute and does not contain waste products from the filtering.

b. Pericarditis.

c. Respiratory.

(1) Pulmonary edema due to fluid overload.

(2) Kussmaul breathing due to metabolic acidosis.

d. Hematologic—impaired erythropoietin production leads to anemia; increased BUN precipitates bleeding tendencies.

e. Neurologic—rising BUN decreases seizure threshold.

f. Fluid and electrolyte balance.

(1) Fluid retention.

(2) Hyperkalemia.

(3) Hyponatremia (usually dilution).

(4) Metabolic acidosis from accumulation of acid waste products.

3. Diagnostics.

a. Elevated serum creatinine, BUN, and potassium.

b. Urinalysis—proteinuria, casts, RBC, WBC, specific gravity is decreased.

c. Decreased creatinine clearance (urine).

d. Increased serum phosphorous

Treatment

1. Medical.

a. Identify and treat precipitating cause of acute renal failure (management varies according to prerenal, intrarenal, or postrenal disorder).

b. Diuretic therapy may be used, with fluid challenges.

c. Decrease serum potassium -

(1) Sodium polystyrene sulfonate (**Kayexalate**) a cation exchange resin given by mouth or retention enema.

(2) IV hypertonic glucose and regular insulin to move potassium into the intracellular space; used for severe hyperkalemia.

(3) **Sorbitol**, an osmotic cathartic may be given with exchange resins to induce a diarrhea to eliminate potassium ions.

d. IV administration of sodium bicarbonate—corrects metabolic acidosis and causes electrolyte shift.

e. Decrease serum phosphate - calcium carbonate, aluminum hydroxide gel (See appendix 18-5).

f. IV dopamine to enhance renal perfusion.(**caution** - always check for correct concentration before beginning infusion - See Appendix16-6).

2. Dietary.

a. Fluid restriction; intake may be carefully calculated with output.

b. Protein, potassium, and sodium intake is regulated according to serum plasma levels.

c. Increased carbohydrate intake, protein of high biologic value.

Nursing Intervention

✦ *Goal: to maintain client in normal homeostasis and monitor renal function.*

1. Identify and monitor high-risk clients (any client with a transient or significant decrease in blood pressure, regardless of the precipitating cause).

2. Accurate intake and output.

3. Daily weight (may lose .2 to .3 kg/day during oliguric phase).

4. Assess fluid balance (hypervolemia or hypovolemia) urine specific gravity, pulmonary status, cardiac output, mental status changes.

5. Assess status of electrolytes and renal parameters - serum potassium, BUN, creatinine, phosphate levels; evaluate fluctuations of serum sodium levels.

6. Evaluate for postural hypotension.

7. Support involved body systems:

a. Cardiac dysrhythmias.

b. Pulmonary function.

✦ *Goal: to maintain nutrition.*

1. Maintain dietary restrictions on sodium, potassium and protein.

2. Encourage intake of carbohydrates.

3. Small frequent feedings, limit fluids.

4. TPN may be necessary to promote healing.

✦ *Goal: to prevent infection.*

1. Avoid indwelling urinary catheter if possible.

2. Assess for development of infectious processes. Client at increased risk due to compromised immune system.

3. Assess for and prevent UTI.

✦ *Goal: to prevent skin breakdown.*

1. Frequent turning and positioning; inspect the skin for problem areas.

2. Beds and protective devices to prevent pressure areas (See Chapter 11: decubitus ulcers).

3. Frequent range of motion and activities to increase circulation.

✦ *Goal: to provide emotional support.*

1. Always explain procedures.

2. Provide honest information regarding progress of condition.

3. Encourage client to express fears and concerns regarding condition.

Chronic Renal Failure (CRF)

❑ **CRF is a progressive, irreversible reduction in renal function such that the kidneys are no longer able to maintain the body environment. The glomerular filtration rate. (GFR)gradually decreases as the nephrons are destroyed. The nephrons left intact are subjected to an increased work load, resulting in hypertrophy and inability to concentrate urine.**

Stages of chronic renal failure.

1. Diminished renal reserve.

a. Normal BUN and serum creatinine.

b. Absence of symptoms.

c. The healthier kidney tissue compensates for the diseased tissue.

2. Renal insufficiency.

a. GFR is 25 percent of normal.

b. BUN and serum creatinine increased (azotemia).

c. Mild anemia.

d. Impaired urine concentration leading to polyuria, nocturia.

e. Headaches.

3. End-stage renal failure (uremia).

a. GFR is less than 10 percent of normal.

(1) Severe azotemia.

(2) Hyperkalemia, hypernatremia and hyperphosphatemia.

(3) Metabolic acidosis.

b. Urinary system—specific gravity of urine fixed at 1.010, proteinuria, casts, pyuria, hematuria; oliguria eventually leads to anuria.

c. Loss of normal kidney functions.

(1) Ability to regulate acid-base balance.

(2) Regulation of blood pressure.

(3) Production of erythropoietin.

d. Endocrine system—hyperparathyroidism causes hypocalcemia and hyperphosphatemia resulting in demineralization of the bones (renal osteodystrophy).

e. Hematologic system—anemia and bleeding.

f. Cardiovascular system—hypertension, CHF, uremic pericarditis, pericardial effusion.

g. Gastrointestinal system—anorexia, nausea, vomiting, ammonia (uremic fetor) odor to the breath, gastrointestinal bleeding, peptic ulcer disease.

h. Metabolic system—hyperglycemia, hyperlipidemia, gout, hypoproteinemia.

i. Neurologic system—general central nervous system depression and peripheral neuropathy.

j. Musculoskeletal system—renal osteodystrophy, tissue calcification.

k. Integumentary system— yellow/gray discoloration, pruritus, uremic frost, ecchymosis.

l. Psychological changes—emotional lability, withdrawal, depression and psychosis.

Assessment

1. Risk factors/etiology.

a. Chronic hypertension and poorly controlled diabetes account for about 60% of CRF.

b. Chronic glomerulonephritis and pyelonephritis.

c. Nephrosclerosis and renal artery disease.

d. Polycystic kidney disease.

e. Renal disease secondary to nephrotoxic drugs or chemicals.

f. Lupus erythematosus.

2. Diagnostics.

a. Increased BUN and serum creatinine level.

b. Decreased urinary creatinine clearance.

c. Elevated blood sugar and triglycerides.

d. Increased serum potassium.

e. Anemia.

Treatment

1. Medical.

a. Measures to reduce serum potassium (see discussion under acute renal failure).

b. Antihypertensives (Appendix 16-4).

c. Diuretics—thiazide diuretics may be used early.

d. Erythropoietin (**Epogen**) for treatment of anemia.

2. Dietary.

a. Problems with the client losing body weight, both adipose tissue and muscle mass.

b. Restricted protein intake; may vary from just a decrease in protein intake to a specific 20 to 40 gm per day.

c. Protein should be of a high biologic value; this enhances the utilization of the amino acids and forms less nitrogen waste products.

d. Water restriction—adjusted according to urinary output and/or dialysis.

e. Sodium and potassium restriction—based upon laboratory values.

f. Digitalis preparations to control symptoms of CHF.

3. Surgical—kidney transplant. The primary limiting factor in the number of transplants done is the availability of the kidneys.

a. Recipient criteria: candidates are evaluated on an individual basis as to how well they would benefit from the transplant.

(1) Candidates are usually under 70 years old, have a life expectancy of at least two more years, and have reasonable expectations that the transplant will improve the quality of life.

(2) Infection and active malignancy are the only absolute contraindications to transplant.

b. Donor criteria: live related donors (LRD) provide the best possible match; when they are not available, cadaver donors are considered.

Nursing Intervention

✦ *Goal: to assist the client to maintain homeostasis.*

1. Evaluate adequacy of fluid balance.
   a. Daily weight.
   b. Postural hypotension.
   c. Level of fluid intake.
   d. Discuss with the client how to monitor the fluid intake and plan for the allocated amount to be distributed over the day.
2. Encourage adequate nutritional intake within dietary guidelines.
   a. Relieve GI dysfunctions prior to serving meals.
   b. Plan diet according to client preferences if possible.
   c. Advise client that most salt substitutes contain potassium and should not be used.
3. Prevent problem of constipation.
   a. Include bran in diet.
   b. Stool softeners.
4. Avoid use of sedatives and hypnotics; increased sensitivity to these medications due to decreased ability of kidney to metabolize them.
5. Monitor electrolyte balance, especially level of potassium.
6. Assess cardiovascular status to determine how effectively the client is compensating with the increased fluid load and increased workload on the heart from the chronic anemic state.
7. Assess client for bleeding tendencies related initially to decrease in production of erythropoietin, and decreased platelet adhesiveness.
8. Evaluate client for pruritus and assist with measures to decrease skin irritation and itching.
9. Avoid products containing magnesium (antacids).
10. Assess client's activity tolerance in relation to anemia.

✦ *Goal: to provide emotional support and promote psychological equilibrium.*

1. Encourage client to express concerns.
2. Recognize that the long-term management of a chronic disease may lead to anxiety and depression.
3. Encourage ventilation of feelings regarding life-style changes.
4. Make available to client and family members support groups and community resources as well as other renal clients who are undergoing the same treatment approaches.

✦ *Goal: to provide preoperative care for kidney transplant.*

1. Maintain client's metabolic state as close to homeostasis as possible—continue with dialysis.
2. Tissue typing and antibody screening are conducted to determine histocompatibility of the donor and the recipient.
3. Immunosuppressant drugs.
4. Conduct routine preoperative procedures.

✦ *Goal: to provide postoperative care for the kidney transplant.*

1. Immunosuppressant therapy (therapy is continued indefinitely)—azathioprine, cyclosporine, and prednisone is most frequent combination of maintenance therapy.
2. Assess for renal graft failure—rejection.
   a. Acute rejection—occurs within 6 weeks, 3 months is most common time, but can be as late as 2 years.
   b. Edema – increased WBCs, fever.
      (1) Deteriorating renal function: increasing serum creatinine and BUN, increasing blood pressure, swelling and tenderness over transplant site.
      (2) Hypertension.
   c. Treatment is usually high dose steroids, and chemotherapy.
   d. Chronic rejection—occurs over months or years.
      (1) Deteriorating renal function: hypertension, increasing serum creatinine and BUN.
      (2) Graft tenderness, malaise.
      (3) Is resistant to therapy.
3. Prevent and monitor for infection (UTI, pneumonia sepsis are biggest threat in early transplant period)
   a. Important to make distinction between infection and rejection, as impaired renal function and fever occur in both.
   b. Symptoms of septicemia—infection, shaking, chills, fever, tachycardia, leukocytosis, and tachypnea.
4. Promote adaptation and psychological support in the successful transplant.
   a. Often, there is a continual fear of possible rejection.
   b. The concern of the client and the family is related to long-term usage of immunosuppressant medication, which puts a tremendous psychological stress on the family unit.
   c. Refer client to community and national agencies: National Association of Patients of Hemodialysis

and Transplantation, Inc., and The National Kidney Foundation.

Dialysis

❑ **The passage of particles (ions) from an area of high concentration to an area of low concentration across a semipermeable membrane.**

1. Water, by osmosis, will move toward the solution in which the ion concentration is the greatest.
2. When dialysis is utilized, the semi-permeable membrane used has pores large enough for waste products and water to move through, but too small for blood cells and protein molecules to pass through.

A. Indications.
1. Fluid volume overload.
2. Serum potassium greater than 6 mEq/L.
3. BUN greater than 120 mg/dl.
4. Uremia and metabolic acidosis.

B. Types of dialysis (Table 23-2).

Nursing Intervention

✦ *Goal: to remove waste products of metabolism and excess fluid; to maintain a safe level of concentration of blood components.*

1. Peritoneal dialysis.
   a. Prepare client for procedure: establish baseline criteria of lab values; weight, vital signs, bowel and bladder should be empty.
   b. Provide support and information to the client when the peritoneal catheter is inserted.
      (1) Permanent peritoneal catheters are fitted with a device to keep them in place. Example is the Tenckhoff catheter. Client should be taught how to care for the area around the catheter.
      (2) Temporary peritoneal catheters are inserted and usually a pursestring suture holds them in place.
   c. Type of peritoneal dialysis being utilized and the physical stability of the client determine how long each cycle of dialysis will take.
      (1) Cycle is initiated with the inflow of the dialysate by gravity into the abdominal cavity. The client should be carefully observed on the initial infusion to determine how well he will tolerate the additional fluid in the abdominal cavity. Initial infusion is usually 1-2 liters over 10-20 minutes (fill time).
      (2) The dialysate remains in the abdomen (dwell time), and is allowed to drain by gravity (drain time). The specific dwell time and drain time is specified in the doctor's orders.
      (3) One exchange constitutes infusion, dwell time, and drainage.
      (4) The dialysate should be warmed to body temperature before infusing (do not use a microwave oven).
   d. Insufficient outflow:
      (1) Constipation is primary cause of inflow and outflow problems.
      (2) Check the tubing for patency and keep drainage bag lower then client.
      (3) Turn client from side to side or put in semi-Fowler's position to increase abdominal pressure.
   e. Complications: possible bowel perforation from catheter insertion, peritonitis, bleeding, hypoalbuminemia, hyperglycemia in diabetic clients.
2. Hemodialysis.
   a. Vascular access site must be established. Access may be temporary or permanent.
      (1) External arteriovenous shunts—catheters are inserted into an artery and into a vein and are connected together on the outside of the arm in a "U" pattern.
      (2) Internal arteriovenous (AV) fistula, or graft—an artery and a vein in the arm are anastomosed either directly or via a graft. Access is achieved via 2 large gauge needles inserted into access site.

Table 23-2: TYPES OF DIALYSIS

Hemodialysis
Circulation of the client's blood through a compartment that contains an artificial semi-permeable membrane that is surrounded by dialysate fluid which removes excess body fluid by creating a pressure differential between the blood and the dialysate solution.

Peritoneal dialysis
Utilization of the peritoneal cavity and the peritoneum as the semi-permeable membrane that removes excess fluid.

Continuous Ambulatory Peritoneal Dialysis (CAPD)
The dialysate is infused into the abdomen and remains there for a specified time (2 to 6 hours). The dialysate is removed by gravity drainage after the prescribed time. Most clients prefer to do the dialysis at night.

Automated Peritoneal Dialysis - uses a peritoneal dialysis cycling machine. It can be done continuous, intermittent, or nightly

Intermittent Peritoneal Dialysis (IPD)—dialysis is performed on the peritoneal cycling machine for 10 to 14 hours, three to four times a week. Can be done at night.

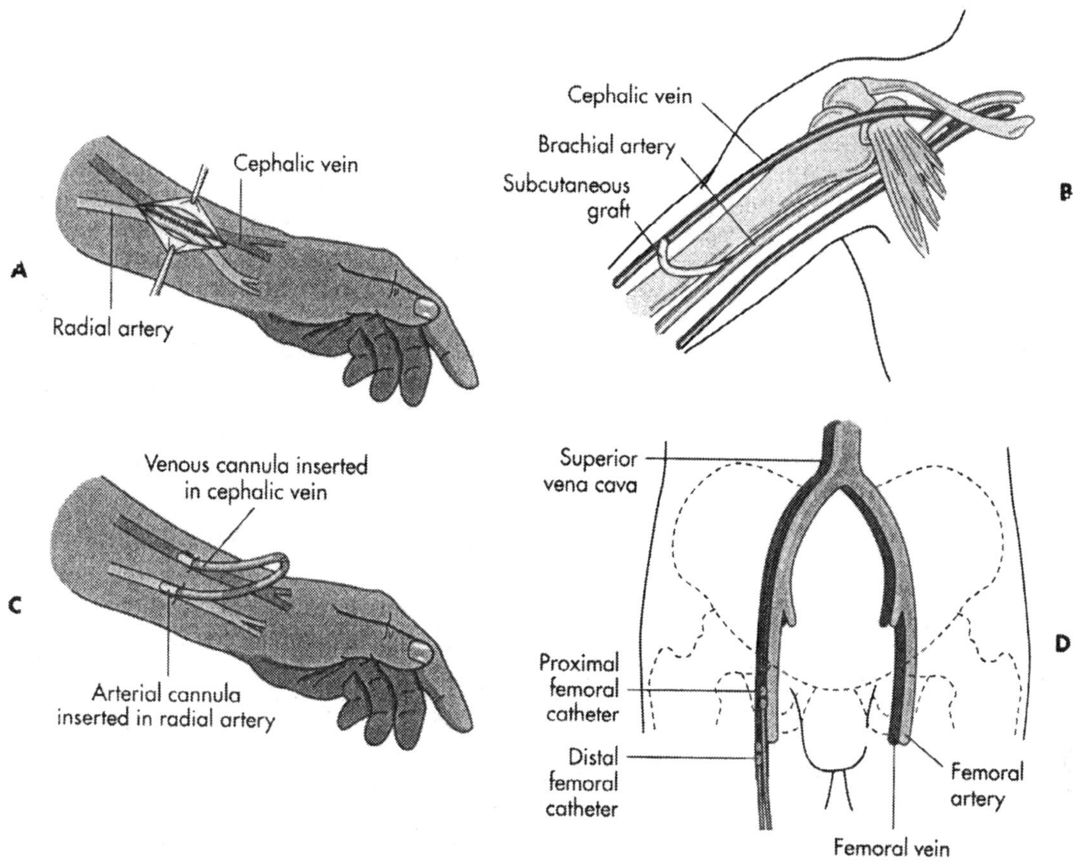

Figure 23-2: Vascular Access for Hemodialysis
A - Arteriovenous Fistula; B -Arteriovenous Graft; C - Exterior Arteriovenous Shunt; D - Femoral Vein Catheterization
Reprinted with permission: Phipps, WJ, Sands, JK, & Marek, JF (1999). *Medical Surgical Nursing: Concepts & Clinical Practice*, 6th ed. Philadelphia: Mosby, p 1483

(3) After an internal access is created, it must heal prior to being used for dialysis.

b. Evaluate access site for patency. It depends on the type of vascular access utilized as to the appropriate method to determine patency - palpate for bruit or thrill over site.

c. Do not take blood pressure, obtain blood samples, or infuse fluids and medications in the access site or the extremity that has a vascular access site.

d. Encourage range of motion and keep the extremity elevated.

e. Assess the patency of the pulses distal to the access site.

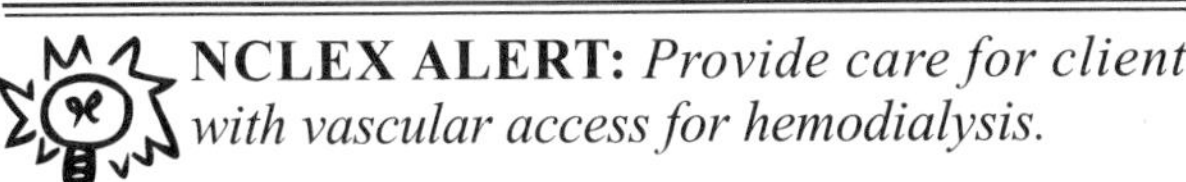

NCLEX ALERT: *Provide care for client with vascular access for hemodialysis.*

✦ *Goal: to maintain homeostasis post hemodialysis.*

1. Determine if medications need to be withheld prior to dialysis (antihypertensives).
2. Most common side effects are hypotension and headache; monitor for postural hypotension.
3. Dialysis disequilibrium syndrome - cerebral edema and neurological complications (headache, nausea vomiting, seizures); may be minimized by slower dialysis.

✦ *Goal: to maintain homeostasis during and after peritoneal dialysis.*

1. Pain is common during first few exchanges, should gradually decrease.
2. Assess for development of peritonitis - antibiotics may be added to dialysate.
3. Dialysate should return clear to slightly yellow-tinged; should not be cloudy or opaque.
4. Closely monitor blood pressure and activity after dialysis.
5. Increase protein diet to compensate for removal of protein in dialysis, low protein will impair tissue healing.

✦ *Goal: to provide emotional support and promote psychological equilibrium.*

1. Encourage client to express feelings of anger and depression. There is an increase in the rate of suicide in dialysis clients.
2. Encourage appropriate coping skills.
3. Clients on dialysis are in limbo; they do not know if they are going to get better or not. Frequently, they have ambivalent feelings about dialysis; it maintains their life, but it severely restricts their lifestyle.

Renal Tumor

❑ **The majority of renal tumors are malignant, and occur more frequently in men age 50 to 70 years of age. Most often, the tumor begins in the renal cortex, where it can actually become quite large before it begins to compress the adjacent renal tissue. The most common areas of metastasis are the liver, lungs and bone, especially the mediastinum.**

Assessment

1. Clinical manifestations.
   a. Palpable abdominal mass.
   b. Hematuria, flank pain.
   c. Weight loss, weakness anemia, hypertension.
2. Diagnostics.
   a. IVP and sonogram.
   b. CAT scan.
   c. Renal arteriography.
   d. Renal biopsy.

Treatment

1. Medical.
   a. Radiation therapy.
   b. Chemotherapy.
2. Surgical—nephrectomy.

Nursing Intervention

✦ *Goal: to provide preoperative nursing care (See Chapter 3).*

1. Instruct client that flank incision will be on affected side and that surgery will be performed in a hyperextended, side-lying position.
2. Often, client experiences muscle aches and discomfort postoperatively due to surgical positioning.
3. Radiation or chemotherapy, or both, after surgery.

✦ *Goal: to provide postoperative care.*

1. Urinary output is important to assess; catheters should be labeled and drainage recorded accurately.
2. Due to the level of the incision, respiratory complications are common. Encourage coughing and deep breathing, as well as incentive spirometry, every two hours while client is awake.
3. Assess for abdominal distention and paralytic ileus.

✦ *Goal: to provide supportive nursing care in relation to malignancy.*

(See Chapter 8 for detailed nursing management).⌘

Study Questions—Renal/Urinary System

1. The client has a nephrolithotomy for removal of a kidney stone. He returns to his room with a right nephrostomy tube after surgery. What is a priority nursing action?

① Irrigate the tube with 30 cc normal saline qid.
② Clamp the tube if drainage is excessive.
③ Advance the tube ½ inch every 8 hours.
④ Ensure that the tube is draining freely.

2. The nurse is infusing the dialysate during peritoneal dialysis. What is a nursing action to make the client more comfortable at this time ?

① Increase the rate of flow.
② Raise the head of the bed.
③ Turn the client from side to side.
④ Refrigerate the fluid prior to infusion.

3. A client has had a kidney stone removed and the nurse instructs him in measures to decrease kidney stone formation in the future. Which statement by the client indicates to the nurse he understood the teaching?

① Begin a daily 45-minute jogging program.
② Consume at least 2,500 ml fluid daily.
③ Report nocturia that occurs once a night.
④ Ingest megadoses of vitamins C and D daily.

4. During peritoneal dialysis treatment, the nurse continually evaluates the client for retention of dialysate. How will this complication be identified?

① Fractional urine ½ percent.
② Return of fecal material in the outflow.
③ An increase in sodium transfer to serum.
④ Outflows of less than 100 ml of inflow.

5. A client in renal failure is to have a serum blood urea nitrogen drawn. What will this diagnostic test measure?

① Concentration of the urine osmolarity and electrolytes.
② Serum level of the end products of protein metabolism.
③ Ability of the kidney to concentrate the urine.
④ Levels of C-reactive protein to determine inflammation.

6. A client with chronic renal failure has an internal venous access for hemodialysis on her left forearm. What action will the nurse take to protect this access?

① Irrigate with heparin and normal saline once a shift to maintain patency.
② Apply warm moist packs to the area after she returns from hemodialysis.
③ Do not use the left arm to take blood pressures.
④ Keep the arm elevated above the level of the heart.

7. What nursing measures are included in the plan of care for a client with acute renal failure?

① Observation for signs of a secondary infection.
② Provision of a high-protein, low-carbohydrate diet.
③ Urinary catheterization to determine amount of residual.
④ Force fluids to 2,000 ml in 24 hours.

8. What will the nurse identify as the goal of treatment for a client with chronic renal failure?

① Increase the urine output by increasing liver and renal perfusion.
② Prevent the loss of electrolytes across the basement membrane.
③ Increase the concentration of electrolytes in the urine.
④ Maintain present renal function and decrease the workload on the kidneys.

9. The nurse is assessing a client who had a transurethral resection of the prostate 6 months ago. What is the most common long-term complication of this procedure?

① Recurrent urinary infections.
② Continued bladder spasms.
③ Bladder neck strictures.
④ Ureteral reflux and hydronephrosis.

10. At 9 a.m. a twenty-four-hour urine specimen is started. What instructions will the nurse provide to the client?

① Place the first voided specimen in the container and continue to collect the urine until 9 a.m. the following day.
② Discard the first morning specimen, collect urine for the next 24 hours making sure to void before the sample is completed at 9 a.m.
③ Discard the first morning specimen because it may contain concentrated abnormal components.
④ Collect all urine from 9 a.m. in separate containers that are labeled for time and amount of voiding.

11. Which nursing observations indicate that a male client with a kidney stone is experiencing renal colic?

① Severe flank pain, radiating toward the testicles.
② Stress incontinence with full bladder.
③ Hematuria, severe burning on urination.
④ Enuresis with hyperalbuminuria.

12. The nurse is evaluating the client's response to hemodialysis. The laboratory values reflect the dialysis is achieving positive results. Which lab values would not reflect changes from the hemodialysis?

① Serum creatinine levels.
③ Dissolved pressure of carbon dioxide.
④ Serum potassium levels.
④ Hemoglobin levels

Answers and rationales to these questions are in the section at the end of the book entitled "Chapter Study Questions: Answers & Rationales."

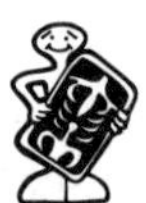

Appendix 23-1: DIAGNOSTICS OF THE URINARY-RENAL SYSTEM

SERUM LABORATORY TESTS	NORMAL	CLINICAL AND NURSING IMPLICATIONS
BUN	5 to 20 mg/dL	Common test used to diagnose renal problems; may be affected by an increase in protein intake or tissue breakdown.
CREATININE	0.6 to 1.5 mg/dL	End product of protein and muscle catabolism; more accurate determinate of renal function than the BUN; values are higher in males.
CALCIUM	10 to 20 mg/dL	Provides the matrix for bone and is important in muscle contraction, neurotransmission and clotting; in chronic renal failure, low levels of calcium lead to renal osteodystrophy.
PHOSPHORUS	2.5 to 4.8 mg/dL	Phosphorus and calcium balance are inversely related; when phosphorus level is elevated, the calcium level is decreased, which is seen in renal disease.
URINARY CREATININE CLEARANCE	Males: 21-26 mg/kg /24 hr. Females: 16-22 mg/kg /24hr	Measure of GFR; a twenty-four hour urine specimen must be collected; have client void and discard the first specimen and then begin timing the test; specimen should be kept cool or refrigerated.
URINE SPECIFIC GRAVITY	1.003 - 1.030 Children: 1.001 -1.030	May be increased when the client is dehydrated. A decrease is associated with decreased tubular absorption. In acute renal failure it may be fixed at 1.000 - 1.012. Proteinuria will increase the specific gravity.

LABORATORY DIAGNOSTICS

PROCEDURE	CLINICAL AND NURSING IMPLICATIONS
KIDNEYS, URETERS, AND BLADDER (KUB)—A flat plate x-ray of the abdomen and pelvis.	Bowel preparation may or may not be indicated.
IVP OR EXCRETORY UROGRAM—IV injection of radiopaque dye to visualize the urinary tract system.	1. Client NPO for eight hours prior to procedure. 2. Cathartic or enema given the evening prior to procedure. 3. Assess for sensitivity to iodine. 4. Instruct client that he/she will need to lie still on table while serial X-rays are taken. 5. Evaluate for iodine reaction after test and force fluids post-test to flush out the dye. 6. Be sure the elderly client is not dehydrated prior to the procedure; the contrast media is nephrotoxic and can precipitate renal failure.
RETROGRADE PYELOGRAM—An X-ray of the urinary tract which is conducted during a cystoscopic exam; ureteral catheters are inserted into the renal pelvis and dye is injected (retrograde) into the catheters.	1. Client NPO for eight hours prior to test. 2. Assess for sensitivity to iodine. 3. Explain that there may be discomfort upon insertion of the cystoscope. 4. General anesthesia may be indicated for procedure.
RENAL ARTERIOGRAM (ANGIOGRAM)—An IV injection of radiopaque dye into the renal artery (catheter is inserted into femoral artery) to visualize the renal blood vessels.	1. Client NPO after midnight. 2. Preoperative medication is administered. 3. Client should be assessed for sensitivity to iodine. 4. Evaluate venipuncture insertion site q 15 to 30 minutes after procedure to assess for bleeding. 5. Assess peripheral pulses to detect occluded blood flow. 6. Sandbag or pressure dressing may be applied to groin.

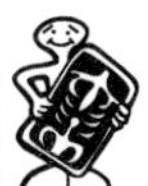

Appendix 23-1: DIAGNOSTICS OF THE URINARY-RENAL SYSTEM

Procedure	Nursing Implications
RENOGRAM—An IV injection of a radioactive nuclide (isotope) followed by a scanning device to detect radioactive emissions from the kidney; identifies renal blood flow, tubular functions, and renal excretion.	1. No specific activity or dietary restrictions. 2. Explain procedure to client.
CYSTOSCOPY—A direct method to visualize the urethra and bladder by use of a tubular lighted scope (cystoscope). Scope may be inserted via the urethra or percutaneously.	1. Force fluids or administer IV. 2. Explain lithotomy position which will be utilized. 3. Client may have general anesthesia. 4. Preoperative medication given. 5. Evaluate urine output postprocedure; check for frequency, pink-tinged color, and burning on urination (these are expected effects and will decrease with time). 6. Evaluate for orthostatic hypotension. 7. Provide warm sitz baths and mild analgesics to alleviate urethral discomfort.
CYSTOMETROGRAM—A procedure to determine the pressure exerted against the bladder wall by inserting a catheter and instilling water or saline; evaluates bladder tone.	1. Assess and evaluate for urinary tract infection postprocedure. 2. Test is often indicated for clients having difficulty with urinary control (spinal cord traumatic injuries, stroke, etc.).
RENAL BIOPSY—A percutaneous needle biopsy through the renal tissue to evaluate renal disease by obtaining a specimen of renal tissue for pathological examination.	1. Blood coagulation studies should be available on the chart prior to the biopsy procedure. 2. IVP or ultrasound studies report should be available prior to the biopsy. 3. Immediately after the procedure, pressure dressing is applied to biopsy site and checked frequently for bleeding. 4. Assess urine for gross hematuria, flank pain, or a rise or fall in blood pressure. 5. Report pain radiating from the flank area to the abdomen. 6. Encourage fluids: 3,000 cc per day unless the client has renal insufficiency. 7. Assess for complication of hemorrhage; may necessitate emergency surgical drainage or nephrectomy.
RENAL ULTRASOUND—A noninvasive procedure utilizing ultrasound waves which, with the aid of a computer, records images related to tissue density.	No specific preparation other than explanation of the procedure to the client.

Appendix 23-2:
RENAL MEDICATIONS

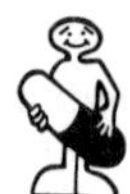

MEDICATION	SIDE EFFECTS	NURSING IMPLICATIONS

❖ **GENERAL NURSING IMPLICATIONS** ❖
—Encourage intake of 2000-3000 cc per day during treatment.
—Continue medication therapy until all medication has been taken.
—Most medications are better absorbed on an empty stomach; however, if GI distress occurs, they may be taken with food.
—Monitor intake and output, as well as symptoms of increasing renal problems.
—Check drug package insert for interactions with anticoagulants.

MEDICATION	SIDE EFFECTS	NURSING IMPLICATIONS
URINARY TRACT ANTISEPTICS: Concentrate in the urine and are active against common urinary tract pathogens. Do not affect infections in blood or tissue.		
Cinoxacin (**Cinobac**): PO Nalidixic Acid (**NegGRAM**): PO	GI upset is common, headache, rash, visual disturbances, photosensitivity.	1. Cinoxacin and nalidixic acid both cause photosensitivity.
Methenamine Mandelate (**Mandelamine, Mandameth**): PO	GI upset, bladder irritation, hepatotoxic.	1. Requires acidic urine to be effective. 2. Should not be used with sulfonamides. 3. Used for chronic UTI, rather then acute.
Nitrofurantoin (**Furadantin, Macrodantin, APO-Nitrofurantoin, Nitrofan**): PO, IM	GI upset, blood dyscrasia, pulmonary reactions.	1. Requires adequate renal function to concentrate medication in urine. 2. Should not be administered to renal transplant clients. 3. Will turn the urine a brownish-orange color.
URINARY ANALGESIC		
Phenazopyridine hydrochloride (**AZO-Standard, Pyridium, Urodine, Urogesic**): PO	Headache, GI disturbances.	1. Contraindicated in renal and liver dysfunction. 2. Advise client to report any yellow discoloration to skin or eyes. 3. Urine will turn orange. 4. Administer with caution in clients with impaired renal function.
GLYCOPROTEIN HORMONE		
Epoetin alfa. (**Epogen, Procrit**): IV, SQ	Hypertension, thromboembolic problems, headaches, seizures, iron deficiency.	1. Closely evaluate hemodialysis access ports for clotting. 2. Evaluate client's serum iron, hematocrit, and blood pressure, adequate levels are required for medication to be effective. 3. Uses: maintain hemoglobin and hematocrit in client with renal failure or who are HIV+.

Appendix 23-3: URINARY DIVERSION

❑ **A *urinary diversion* is a means of diverting urinary output from the bladder to an external device or via a new avenue.**

TEMPORARY URINARY DIVERSION:

Nephrostomy Tubes (catheters) - insertion of catheters into the renal pelvis by surgical incision or percutaneous puncture, a small catheter is inserted into the renal pelvis and attached via connecting tubing to a closed-system drainage. Tubes may be temporary or permanent.

Nursing Implications:

1. Catheter should *never be clamped* or *irrigated* (renal pelvis capacity is 3 to 5 cc).
2. Complications - infection and secondary renal calculus formation; erosion of the duct by the catheter.

Ureteral Catheters -small, narrow catheters placed through the ureters into the renal pelvis , drains each renal pelvis individually. Often client also has a Foley catheter draining the urinary bladder. The catheter splints the ureters during healing and prevents edema from occluding ureter.

Nursing Implications:

1. Check frequently for placement of ureteral catheters; tension should be avoided.
2. Ureteral catheter *should not be clamped* or *irrigated.*
3. Maintain accurate intake and output records and label all catheters.

PERMANENT URINARY DIVERSION:

Ileal Conduit (Bricker's Procedure) the transplanting of ureters into a segment of ileum, which is then brought to the abdomen and a stoma is constructed.

Nursing Implications:

1. Stoma site is marked prior to surgery, as a device must be worn continuously.
2. Mucus is present in the urine postoperatively; encourage a high-fluid intake to "flush the ileal conduit."
3. Maintain meticulous skin care and changing of appliances.
4. Provide discharge instructions in regards to symptoms of obstruction, infection, and care of the ostomy; client needs information relating to purchase of supplies, ostomy clubs, follow-up visits, enterstomal therapists, and the importance of not irrigating the ileal conduit.

Kock Pouch - a segment of the ileum is made into a reservoir; client is taught to use a catheter to drain the pouch and maintain continence.
Indiana Pouch - reservoir is created from an area of the ascending colon; makes a larger pouch to maintain continence.

Nursing Implications:

1. Client may still be incontinent and require continuous wearing of an appliance.
2. Obstruction and electrolyte problems occur with both types.
3. Continuous assessment of status of skin around stoma.
4. Client should understand how to care for the stoma prior to leaving the hospital.
   — types of appliances available.
   — increase fluid intake to decrease infections.
   — contact physician if there are changes in the color of the stoma or urine becomes dark and foul smelling.

Appendix 23-4:
NURSING PROCEDURE ■ URINE SPECIMEN COLLECTION ■

Key Points: Random sample

- May be collected at any time.
- May be specifically ordered to collect first voided specimen or to collect sample on second voiding.

Key Points: Clean catch and midstream

- Specimen is collected for culture.
- Clean urinary meatus prior to specimen collection.
- For midstream collection, tell client to start the urinary stream and collect the specimen after the voiding has begun. Regardless of how well the urinary meatus is cleaned, the specimen must be a midstream collection or the specimen is contaminated with the bacteria in the urethra.

Key Points: Catheterized specimen

- Straight in-and-out catheterization to obtain sample for culture.
- Procedure is discouraged due to introduction of bacteria and irritation producing a UTI.

Key Points: 12 to 24-Hour collection

- When the collection time is started, have the client void, discard the urine, and start the collection with the next voiding.
- Mark the collection container and collect the urine over the prescribed time frame.
- When the time frame is completed, have the client void again, add it to the specimen collection, and send to lab for evaluation.

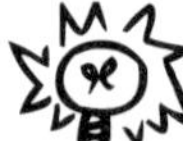

NCLEX ALERT: *Collection of urine specimens is a common nursing action; be sure to know why the sample is being obtained and what type of diagnostic test it is being collected for.*

Appendix 23-5:
NURSING PROCEDURE ■ URINARY CATHETERIZATION ■

Key Points: Insertion of a Retention Catheter

> **NCLEX ALERT:** *Insert a urinary catheter.*

- A sterile procedure.
- Lubricate catheter using sterile lubricant provided in tray.
- Cleanse the patient's meatus:

  For a female:
  a. Cleanse the patient's meatus with one downward stroke of the forceps.
  b. Repeat at least three to four times using new sterile cotton ball each time.
  c. Continue to hold the patient's labia apart until you insert the catheter.

  For a male:
  a. Hold the patient's penis upright. Hold the sides of the penis to prevent closing the urethra.
  b. Cleanse the patient's meatus with one downward stroke of the forceps.
  c. Repeat at least three to four times.
  d. Continue to hold the penis until you insert the catheter.
- Insert the catheter 2 to 3 inches beyond the point at which urine begins to flow. Inserting the catheter farther into the bladder ensures it is beyond the neck of the bladder.
- Instill sterile water into balloon after catheter is inserted.
- Anchor the catheter.
  a. ***For a female:*** Anchor or tape catheter to the side of the leg.
  b. ***For a male:*** Anchor or tape catheter to the abdomen to prevent pressure on the penoscrotal angle.
- Attach drainage bag to bed frame (not side rails), so that it hangs freely.

Key Points: Providing Catheter Care

- Maintain external clenaliness around the catheter, wash thoroughly with mild soap and water.
- Maintain closed system.
- Encourage high fluid intake to maintain constant flow of urine. Increase flow of urine inhibits the upward movement of bacteria.

Key Points: Removal of a Catheter

- Clamp catheter.
- Do not cut the catheter with a scissors. Balloon may not totally deflate if cut.
- Withdraw fluid from balloon (usually 5 to 10 cc water in balloon.)
- Pull gently on catheter to ensure balloon is deflated before attempting to remove. Damage to the urethra can occur if balloon is not totally deflated.
- Record output on I & O bedside record.
- Wash perineum with soap and water. Dry thoroughly.
- Instruct patient to drink oral fluids as tolerated and observe for signs and symptoms of urinary tract infection (burning, frequency, urgency).
- Offer bedpan or urinal at least every 2 to 4 hours after removing catheter, until voiding occurs. Keep accurate I & O record.

Appendix 23-5:
NURSING PROCEDURE ■ URINARY CATHETERIZATION ■

CLINICAL TIPS FOR PROBLEM SOLVING

1. ***If catheter is inserted in the vagina of female client:***
   - Leave the catheter in place so you do not re-introduce a new catheter into the vaginal area. Obtain a new catheter and new gloves.
   - If sterile field has been contaminated, obtain a whole new kit.
2. ***If unable to insert catheter into male patient:***
   - Obtain a new catheter kit.
     a. Hold penis vertical to patient's body.
     b. Insert catheter while applying slight traction by gently pulling upward on the shaft of the penis.
     c. If you encounter resistance, rotate the catheter, increase the traction, and change the angle of the penis slightly.
     d. When urine begins to flow, lower the patient's penis.
3. ***If pain occurs during inflation of balloon:***
   - Remove any injected water and insert the catheter farther into the bladder
4. ***If urine exceeds 1000cc with catheterization:***
   - Clamp catheter for 20 to 30 minutes and then unclamp.
5. ***If catheter comes out with balloon still inserted:***
   - Assess patient for signs of urethral trauma (i.e., bleeding, pain).
   - Obtain a new catheter and repeat the catheterization procedure, making sure that the balloon is inflated with at least 10 cc water.
   - Monitor urine output for bleeding.

FAMILY PLANNING

Infertility

❑ ***Infertility*** **is the inability to conceive a child after a year of more of regualr unprotected intercourse or the inability to carry a pregnancy to live birth (recurrent miscarriages).**

General Concepts

A. Incidence: 60 % of couples achieve pregnancy within six months; 90 % within one year.

B. Essential components for normal fertility (Table 24-1).

Assessment

A. Causes of infertility.

1. Male.

a. Coital difficulties-timing and frequency of coitus, chordee (erection curves downward), or obesity.

b. Semen factors.

(1) Sperm abnormalities-small ejaculatory volume (less than 2 ml); low sperm count (less than 20 million/ml); poor motility of sperm.

(2) Sperm autoantibodies caused by trauma, infection, or surgical occlusion (found after a re-anastomosis of the vas deferens).

c. Testicular abnormalities: undescended, atrophic, or absent testes; cryptorchidism; any trauma, irradiation, or increased temperature for prolonged periods (orchitis after mumps, gonorrhea, tuberculosis).

d. Structural abnormalities-hypospadias, urethral stricture, varicocele.

e. Chronic prostatitis; severe nutritional deficiency.

f. Social/emotional factors; the use of nicotine, alcohol, or other drugs; premature ejaculation, impotence, and coital positioning.

2. Female.

a. Hormonal dysfunction-anovulation; hyper-or hypofunction of the pituitary, thyroid, or adrenal gland.

b. Structural abnormalities-unusual size of uterus; lack of ovaries; imperforate hymen; absence or stenosis of vagina; fallopian tube blockage.

c. Coital factors-use of lubricants or douches which change the pH and may cause infection.

d. Emotional problems-severe psychoses or psychoneuroses may cause anovulatory periods.

e. Chronic infections-pelvic inflammatory disease (PID) caused by gonorrhea, previous use of intrauterine device (IUD), and other vaginal infections.

f. Immunologic reaction to sperm.

g. Social/emotional factors-use of nicotine, alcohol, or drugs.

B. Diagnostics.

1. Male.

a. Complete history and physical examination; laboratory studies such as thyroid function tests and other endocrine tests may be ordered.

b. Complete semen analysis.

NURSING PRIORITY: *Semen analysis is one of the first steps in infertility testing because it is relatively simple and does not involve any invasive procedure for the female client.*

(1) Collection of specimen-avoid ejaculation for two to three days; collect a masturbated specimen in a glass jar; transport to physician's office no later than two hours after collection (should not be warmed or chilled); sterile, unlubricated condoms can be used for collection when there are religious or cultural objections to masturbation.

NURSING PRIORITY: *Two or more abnormal samples must be obtained before a definitive diagnosis is made. Semen collections should be repeated at least 72 hours apart to allow for new germ cell maturation.*

(2) Normal values of semen: volume (1.5 to 5 ml), pH (7.2 to 8.9), density of sperm (50 million/ml, *preferably*), motility (greater than 60 percent), forward progression greater that 2+ (on a scale from 0-4), morphology of sperm (greater than 60 percent normal).

2. Female.

a. Complete history and physical examination-includes routine CBC, urinalysis, serologic studies, thyroid function studies, sedimentation rate, chest X-ray, and Pap smear.

Table 24-1: ESSENTIAL COMPONENTS FOR NORMAL FERTILITY

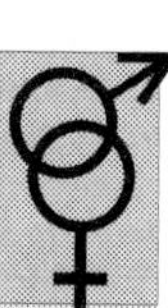

Female partner:	*Male partner:*
Vaginal and cervical mucus must be favorable for survival of spermatozoa. Clear open passage between the cervix and fallopian tubes. Patent fallopian tubes with normal peristalitic movement to allow ascent of spermatozoa and descent of ovum. Ovaries must produce and release ovum. No obstruction between the ovaries and the uterus. Endometrium must be in a normal physiologic state to allow implantation of the blastocyst and to sustain normal growth.	Testes must produce spermatozoa of normal quality and quantity. Male genital tract must not be obstructed. Secretions from genital tract must be normal. Ejaculated sperm must be deposited in the female genital tract in such a manner that they reach the cervix.

(1) Hormonal assay of LH (at mid-cycle the value is greatest) or progesterone (peaks 8 days after the LH surge).

b. Recording of basal body temperature and cervical mucus to document ovulation.

(1) Basal body temperature drops and then rises about 1° after ovulation.

NURSING PRIORITY: *Actual release of ovum occurs around 24 to 36 hours prior to the first temperature elevation;* ***BBT does not predict ovulation, only identifies that it has occurred.***

(2) A proposed time for intercourse based on serial BBT might be to recommend sexual intercourse every other day in the period of time beginning 3 to 4 days prior to and continuing for 2 to 3 days following the expected time of ovulation.

c. Cervical mucus method.

(1) Cervical mucus is thin, clear, profuse, watery, alkaline, and stringy at time of ovulation.

(2) Often estrogen secretion is inadequate for the development of a receptive cervical mucus.

(3) Supplemental estrogen therapy 6 days prior to ovulation enhances the development of *spinnbarkheit*, which means elasticity of the cervical mucus.

(4) *Ferning* is noted on a microscopic slide due to an increase in sodium chloride that crystallizes when the mucus dries on the slide.

d. Postcoital test.

(1) Conducted at time of ovulation; from one to twelve hours after coitus obtain a certical mucus specimen.

(2) Purpose is to determine sperm survival and motility along with the characteristics of cervical mucus.

e. Tubal patency tests.

(1) Hysterosalpingography or hysterogram (HSG).

(a) An instillation of a radiopaque substance into the uterine cavity.

(b) Reveals tubal patency and any distortions of the endometrial cavity.

(c) Test is scheduled during the proliferative phase, usually six days after menstrual flow.

(d) Antibiotics may be prescribed if there is a history of PID or blocked tubes.

(2) Laparoscopy.

(a) Direct visualization of the pelvic organs via an incision into the abdomen (around umbilicus).

(b) General anesthesia used.

(c) May have some discomfort from organ displacement and shoulder and chest pain caused by carbon dioxide gas in the abdomen lasting 24-48 hours after procedure.

f. Endometrial biopsy.

(1) A sample of the endometrium is obtained during days 1 to 2 before menstruation.

(2) Assesses the adequacy of the endometrium for implantation, presence of polyps, or inflammatory conditions.

C. Treatment.

1. Male.

a. Autoimmune sperm antibodies: administration of immunosuppressants, and sperm washing—dilution insemination techniques.

b. Poor quality or immotile sperm.

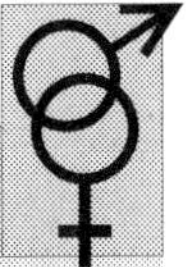

Table 24-2: FERTILITY AWARENESS

Discourage douching and artificial lubricants. They cause alteration in vaginal pH.

Encourage retention of sperm. Man using the superior position during intercourse with female remaining recumbent for at least an hour after intercourse is most effective in having sperm reach the cervix.

Prevent leakage of sperm. Woman should elevate her hips with a pillow after intercourse and avoid getting up to urinate.

Encourage intercourse at least 1 to 3 times per week. Intervals should be no more than 48 hours apart.

Promote relaxation and good nutrition to decrease stress and anxiety. Avoid emphasizing conception during sexual intercourse.

Explore other methods to increase fertility awareness. Check cervical mucus and basal body temperature.

(1) Homologous insemination (artificial insemination by husband [AIH]).

(2) Heterologous insemination (artificial insemination by donor [AID]).

2. Female.

a. Vaginal-cervical factors.

(1) Vaginal fluid is acidic; cervical mucus is alkalotic.

(2) Vaginal/cervical infections change the pH, which often destroys sperm.

(3) Treat infections with antibiotics.

b. Tubal factors.

(1) Tubal infection-treated with antibiotics.

(2) Surgery may be indicated to drain an abscess or to correct obstruction.

c. Ovarian factors—administration of fertility medications:

(1) Clomiphene citrate (**Clomid**).

(a) Indicated when ovaries are normal and pituitary gland is intact.

(b) Increases the secretion of FSH and LH, which stimulates follicle growth.

(c) Administration: take it daily for 5 days beginning on day 5 of the menstrual cycle; usually supplemental low dose estrogen is given concurrently.

(d) Side effects: vasomotor flushes, visual spots, nausea, vomiting, headache, or hair loss.

(2) Human menopausal gonadotropin (hMG) (**Pergonal**) — used when **Clomid** fails to stimulate ovulation.

(a) Potent hormone, combination of LH and FSH obtained from postmenopausal women's urine.

(b) Administration: given IM every day for varying periods of time during the first half of the cycle.

(c) Couple advised to have intercourse on the day of receiving HMG and for the next two days.

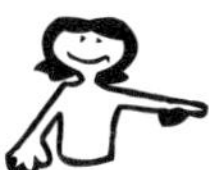

NURSING PRIORITY: *The use of fertility drugs may lead to a multiple birth rate of about 20% with 15% twins.*

d. *In vitro* fertilization ("test tube" pregnancy).

(1) First successful delivery occurred in England in 1978.

(2) Process of *in vitro* fertilization: multiple ova are stimulated by use of medication (**Clomid**, HMG therapy); mature follicles are removed by laparoscope, ova are transferred to tissue culture media, sperm are added to media under controlled laboratory conditions; if fertilization occurs, a second tissue transfer allows for division (approximately three to six days); prior to transferring the blastocysts to the uterus, the woman is maintained on progesterone therapy.

Nursing Intervention

✦ *Goal: to assist with the assessment and treatment of the couple's specific infertility problem.*

1. Provide information regarding the normal functioning of the male and female reproductive system.
2. Thoroughly explain specific examinations and diagnostic procedures to decrease anxiety and fear.

✦ *Goal: to promote fertility awareness (Table 24-2).*

✦ *Goal: to provide emotional support and encourage expression of feelings connected with infertility.*

Table 24-3: TASKS OF THE INFERTILE COUPLE

TASKS	NURSING INTERVENTION
1. Recognition of how infertility affects their lives and expression of feelings (may be negative toward self or mate).	1. Supportive: assist clients to understand and facilitate free expression of feelings.
2. Grieving the loss of potential offspring.	2. Help to recognize feelings.
3. Evaluation of reasons for wanting a child.	3. Help to understand motives.
4. Decision-making about management.	4. Identify alternative; facilitate partner communication.

1. Promote expression of feelings related to sexuality, self-esteem, and body image.
2. Assess for common reactions of surprise, denial, anger, and guilt.
3. Promote a variety of coping strategies to help deal with the uncomfortable feelings (Table 24-3: Tasks of the Infertile Couple).
4. Explore alternatives such as adoption, AID, AIH, or remaining childless.
5. Refer to supportive community agencies.

CONTRACEPTION

❑ ***Contraception* is the voluntary prevention of pregnancy. Two important factors influence the selection of the particular type of contraceptive method: acceptability and effectiveness.**

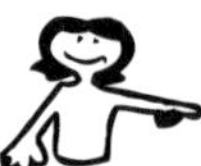

***NURSING PRIORITY:** Determine client's attitude toward and use of birth control methods.*

Assessment

A. Types of Contraception.
   1. Temporary contraception-methods used to delay or avoid pregnancy.
   2. Permanent-voluntary sterilization.

B. Contraceptive methods (Appendix 24-1).

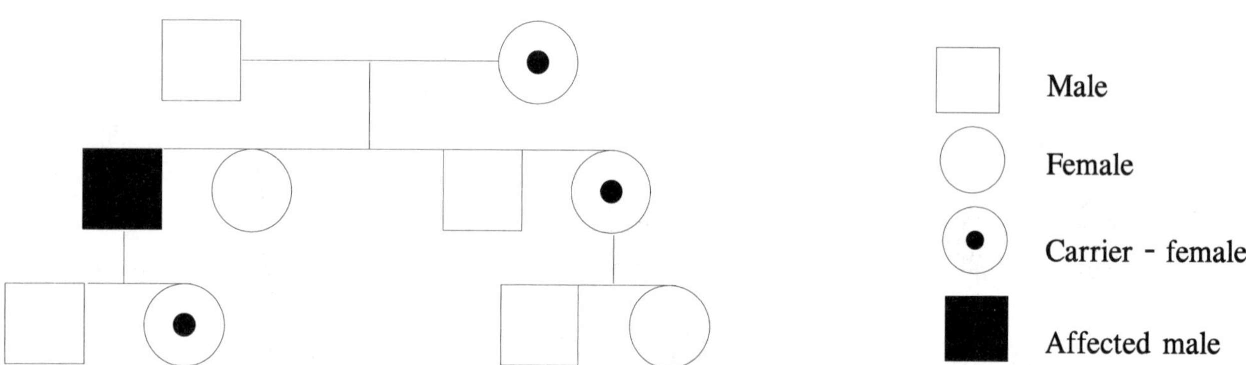

Figure 24-1: Sex-linked or X-linked Recessive Inheritance

- Affected individuals are primarily male.
- There is no male transmission.
- An affected male inherits the gene from his mother and can transmit it only to his daughters. All the daughters of an affected male are carriers.
- Unaffected male children of an affected male cannot transmit the disease.
- There is a 50 percent chance that a carrier mother will pass the abnormal gene to each of her sons, who will thus be affected.
- Common sex-linked disorders are: HEMOPHILIA, DUCHENNE MUSCULAR DYSTROPHY, and COLOR BLINDNESS.

GENETIC COUNSELING

A. Definitions:

1. Genetic (hereditary): any disorder or disease that is transmitted from generation to generation.
2. Congenital: any disorder that is present at birth that is caused by genetic or environmental factors or both.

B. Patterns of inheritance.

1. Sex-linked recessive (Figure 24-1).
2. Autosomal recessive (Figure 24-2).

Assessment

A. Families at risk.

1. Maternal factors.
   a. Increased age.
   b. Presence of disease.
      (1) Diabetes mellitus.
      (2) Epilepsy.
      (3) Mental retardation.
   c. Reproductive history of spontaneous abortions, stillborn, or previous children with birth defects.
2. Family history.
   a. Huntington's chorea.
   b. Hemophilia.
   c. Birth defects (e.g., imperforate anus, cleft lip and palate, spina bifida).
3. Ethnic backgrounds.
   a. Blacks: sickle cell trait.
   b. Eastern European Jews: Tay-Sachs.
   c. Mediterranean descendants: thalassemia.

B. Diagnostics.

1. Prenatal detection.
   a. Amniocentesis.
      (1) A simple, common, and safe outpatient procedure performed at fourteen to sixteen weeks of pregnancy.
      (2) Procedure: placenta is located by ultrasound; a needle is inserted through the abdomen (puncture site has been anesthetized); amniotic fluid is aspirated and sent to the laboratory for testing.
      (3) Indications for amniocentesis: increased maternal age, history of child with a genetic defect, mother carrying an X-linked disease, or history of either parents carrying a chromosomal abnormality (Table 24-4: Genetic Testing).
      (4) Complications: unlikely, though possible; some mild discomfort at the needle site, or rarely, abdominal wall hematoma.
   b. Ultrasound.

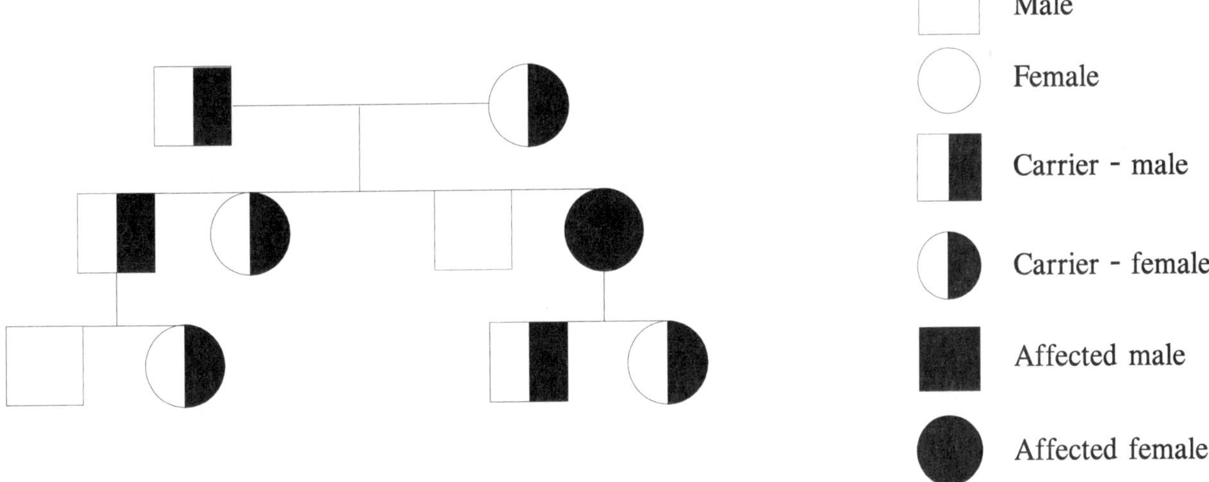

Figure 24-2: Autosomal Recessive Inheritance

- An affected individual has clinically normal parents, but they are both carriers of the abnormal gene.
- Both males and females are affected equally.
- Parents who are both carriers of the same abnormal gene have a 25 percent chance of passing the abnormal gene on to any of their offspring.
- If the offspring of the two carrier parents is clinically normal, there is a 50 percent chance that he or she is a carrier of the gene.
- Common autosomal recessive disorders are: CYSTIC FIBROSIS, PHENYLKETONURIA (PKU), SICKLE CELL ANEMIA, and TAY-SACHS disease.

(1) The use of high-frequency sound waves to assess gestational age of the fetus and position of the placenta.

(2) Often detects skeletal abnormalities, multiple births, and anencephaly.

(3) Procedure best done at 16-18 weeks when fetal structures have completed development.

2. Postdelivery detection.

a. Most institutions screen for 6 inborn errors of metabolism; these tests all use the same dried blood spot.

(1) PKU testing.

(2) Galactosemia.

(3) Hypothyroidism.

(4) Sickle cell anemia.

(5) Maple syrup urine disease.

(6) Homocystinuria.

b. Cytologic studies.

(1) Detect chromosomal abnormalities.

(2) Obtain cells from the bone marrow, skin, or blood to prepare a karyotype.

c. Dermatoglyphics.

(1) The assessment of the dermal ridges in the palm, toes, or soles of feet.

(2) Characteristic palm creases: simian line (Down syndrome).

Nursing Intervention

✦ *Goal: to allow families to make informed decisions about reproduction.*

1. Assist with detailed family history and pedigree chart.
2. Determine family's understanding and comprehension of the information.

✦ *Goal: to provide information about available diagnostic tests and treatment.*

1. Be precise and give detailed information.
2. Use familiar examples to illustrate specific risks (e.g., flipping coins).
3. Emphasize the importance of the couple making an informed decision.

✦ *Goal: to reduce incidence and impact of genetic disease by identifying families at risk and making appropriate referrals.*

1. Refer to specific agencies (e.g., Cystic Fibrosis Foundation, Muscular Dystrophy Association).
2. Provide alternatives to childbearing such as adoption and artificial insemination.

Table 24-4: GENETIC TESTING EXAMPLES

DISEASE	TEST (Amniotic fluid sample)
Cystic fibrosis	Decreased amounts of 4-methyl-umbelliferyl quanidinobenzoate (MUGB) reactive proteases
Neural tube defects: Ancephaly Spina bifida	Elevated maternal α–fetoprotein (MSAFP); decreased level may indicate Down's syndrome

NORMAL PREGNANCY CYCLE: PHYSIOLOGICAL CHANGES

Uterus

1. Increase in size due to hypertrophy of the myometrial cells (increase seventeen to forty times their prepregnant state) as a result of the stimulating influence of estrogen and the distention caused by the growing fetus.
2. Weight increases from 50 to 1,000 grams.
3. Increase in fibrous and connective tissues, which strengthens the elasticity of the uterine muscle wall.

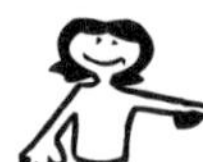

***NURSING PRIORITY:** Softening of the lower uterine segment (Hegar's sign).*

4. Irregular, painless uterine contractions (Braxton-Hicks) may begin in the early weeks of pregnancy; contraction and relaxation assist in accommodating the growing fetus.

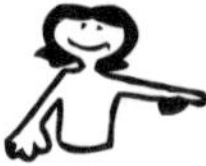

***NURSING PRIORITY:** Multigravidas tend to report a greater incidence of Braxton-Hicks contractions than primigravidas.*

5. Cervical changes.

a. Softening of the cervix due to increased vascularity, edema, and hyperplasia of cervical glands (Goodell's sign).

b. Formation of the mucous plug to prevent bacterial contamination from the vagina.

Vagina

1. Influence of estrogen leads to hypertrophy and hyperplasia of the lining along with an increase in vaginal secretions.

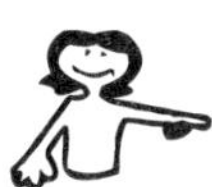

NURSING PRIORITY: A blue-purple hue of the vaginal walls is seen very early (Chadwick's sign).

2. Vaginal secretions: acidic (pH is 3.5 to 6.0) and thickish white.

Breasts

1. Increase in breast size accompanied by feelings of fullness, tingling, and heaviness.
2. Superficial veins prominent; nipples erect; darkening and increase in diameter of the areola.
3. Thin, watery secretion, precursor to colostrum, can be expressed from the nipples by the end of the tenth week.

Cardiovascular System

1. Blood volume.
    a. Increases progressively throughout pregnancy, beginning in the first trimester and peaking in the middle of the third trimester at about 45% above prepregnant levels.
    b. Normal blood pressure maintained by peripheral vasodilatation.
    c. Extra volume of blood acts as a reserve for blood loss during delivery.
2. Heart.
    a. Increase in heart rate by ten beats per minute by the end of the first trimester.

NURSING PRIORITY: Blood pressure falls during the second trimester; rises slightly (no more than 15 mm in either systolic or diastolic) during the last trimester.

    b. Increase in cardiac output.
    c. Palpitations of the heart usually due to sympathetic nervous system disturbance; later in pregnancy due to the intraabdominal pressure of the growing uterus.
    d. Cardiac enlargement and systolic murmurs.
3. Red blood cells (RBC).
    a. Stimulation of the bone marrow leads to a 20-30% increase in total RBC volume.
    b. The plasma volume increase is greater than the RBC increase which leads to hemodilution, typically referred to as physiologic anemia of pregnancy (pseudoanemia).
    c. The hematocrit, which measures the portion of whole blood to erythrocytes, decreases by 7%.
4. White blood cells (WBC): 10 to 11,000 per cu mm; may increase up to 25,000 per cu mm during labor and postpartum.

Respiratory System

1. Tidal volume increases steadily throughout pregnancy.
2. Oxygen consumption increased by 15-20% between the sixteenth and fortieth weeks.
3. Diaphragm is elevated; change from abdominal to thoracic breathing around the twenty-fourth week.
4. Vital capacity increases slightly, while pulmonary compliance and diffusion remain constant.
5. Common complaints of nasal stuffiness and epistaxis due to estrogen influence on nasal mucosa.

Urinary/Renal Systems

1. Ureter and renal pelvis dilate (especially on the right side) as a result of the growing uterus.
2. Frequency of urination (first and last trimester).
3. Decreased bladder tone (due to effect of progesterone); bladder capacity increases: 1,300 to 1,500 cc.
4. Reduced renal threshold for sugar leads to glycosuria.
5. Due to an increased glomerular filtration rate (GFR), as much as 50%, there is a decreased serum BUN, creatinine, and uric acid.

Gastrointestinal System

1. Pregnancy gingivitis—gums reddened, swollen, and bleed easily.
2. Increased saliva (ptyalism); decreased gastric acidity.
3. Nausea and vomiting due to elevated human chorionic gonadotropin (HCG).
4. Decreased tone and motility of smooth muscles; decreased emptying time of stomach; slowed peristalsis due to increased progesterone leads to complaints of bloating, heartburn, and constipation.
5. Pressure of expanding uterus leads to hemorrhoidal varicosities and contributes to continuing constipation.
6. Gall bladder—decreased emptying time, slight hypercholesterolemia, and increased progesterone level may contribute to the development of gallstones during pregnancy.

Musculoskeletal System

1. Increase in the normal lumbosacral curve leads to backward tilt of the torso.

2. Center of gravity is changed, which often leads to leg and back strain and predisposition to falling.
3. Pelvis relaxes due to the effects of the hormone relaxin; leads to the characteristic "duck waddling" gait.

Integumentary System

1. Increased skin pigmentation in various areas of the body.
   a. Facial: mask of pregnancy (chloasma).
   b. Abdomen: striae (red purple stretch marks) and linea nigra (darkened vertical line from umbilicus to symphysis pubis).
2. Appearance of vascular spider nevi, especially on the neck, arms and legs.
3. Acne vulgaris, dermatitis, and psoriasis usually improve during pregnancy.

Endocrine

1. Placenta.
   a. Functions include transport of nutrients and removal of waste products from the fetus.
   b. Produces human chorionic gonadotropin (HCG) and human placental lactogen (HPL).
   c. Produces estrogen and progesterone after two months of gestation.
2. Thyroid gland.
   a. May increase in size and activity.
   b. Increase in basal metabolic rate.
   c. Parathyroid glands-increase in activity (especially the last half of the pregnancy) due to increased requirements for calcium and vitamin D.
3. Pituitary gland.
   a. Enlargement greatest during the last month of gestation.
   b. Production of anterior pituitary hormones: FSH, LH, thyrotropin, adrenotropin, and prolactin.

NURSING PRIORITY: *Production of posterior pituitary hormones: oxytocin, which promotes uterine contractility and stimulation of milk let-down reflex.*

4. Adrenal glands.
   a. Hypertrophy of the adrenal cortex.
   b. Increase in aldosterone, which retains sodium, results in a decreased ability of the kidneys to handle salt during pregnancy; consequently, improper control of dietary sodium can lead to fluid retention and edema.

Metabolism

1. Weight gain.
   a. Normal weight gain: 20 to 30 lb (average 26 to 28 lbs.).

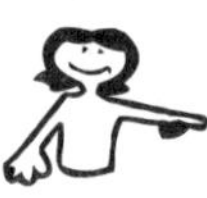

NURSING PRIORITY: *Maternal weight gain is estimated at 3 lbs., 12 lbs, and 12 lbs, for the first, second, and third trimester; approximately 1 lb per week for the second and third trimesters.*

   b. Pattern of weight gain.
      (1) First trimester-3 to 4 lb.
      (2) Second trimester-12 to 14 lb.
      (3) Third trimester-8 to 10 lb.
   c. Total weight gain is accounted for as follows:
      (1) Fetus: 7½ lb.
      (2) Placenta and membranes: 1½ lb.
      (3) Amniotic fluid: 2 lb.
      (4) Uterus: 2½ lb.
      (5) Breasts: 3 lb.
      (6) Increased blood volume: 2-4 lb.
      (7) Remaining 4-9 lb. is extravascular fluid and fat reserves.
2. Nutrient metabolism.
   a. Protein—positive nitrogen balance; fetus makes greatest demands during the last half of gestation, as it doubles weight in the last 6 to 8 weeks.
   b. Carbohydrate—increases, especially during the last two trimesters; ketosis and glycosuria occur along with lipidemia.
   c. Fat—more completely absorbed; increase in serum lipids, lipoproteins, cholesterol, and phospholipids.
   d. Increased intake of folic acid.
3. Mineral metabolism.
   a. Increased need for calcium and phosphorus especially during the last 1 to 2 months of gestation.
   b. Iron: approximately 18 mg per day is needed; a total of 1,000 mg for the pregnancy.
4. Water metabolism.
   a. Increased need for water (i.e., three liters per day) in late pregnancy.
   b. Increased water retention is frequently seen, due to the effects of hormones and the decreased plasma protein.

PSYCHOLOGICAL CHANGES OF THE EXPECTANT FAMILY

NCLEX ALERT: *Plan anticipatory guidance for developmental transitions. Pregnancy is considered a normal maturational crisis and developmental stage for the expectant couple.*

Changes in the Mother

Common Responses

A. Ambivalence.
   1. If women feels comfortable in addressing ambivalent feelings, the focus is usually on changed life-style or the career-motherhood dilemma.
   2. Indirect evidence of ambivalence:
      a. Complaints of depression or physical discomfort.
      b. Complaints of feeling ugly or unattractive.
   3. Some women may consider the possibility of abortion, if pregnancy is unwanted.

B. Acceptance.
   1. With an unplanned pregnancy, there is greater evidence of fear and conflict, along with more physical discomfort and depression.
   2. If pregnancy is well-accepted, women experiences less discomfort and more tolerance to physical discomforts during the last trimester.

C. Introversion.
   1. This "turning in on oneself" focus is normal.
   2. Helps the mother plan, adjust, adapt, build, and draw strength in preparation for childbirth.

D. Mood swings.
   1. Can cause difficulty in the relationship if couple doesn't realize what is occurring.
   2. Husband may feel exasperated with her tears and withdraw and ignore problem when she really needs him to be affectionate and supportive.

E. Changes in body image.
   1. Woman may feel negative toward body, especially during 3rd trimester.

F. Psychological tasks of the mother.
   1. Ensuring safe passage through pregnancy, labor, and birth.
   2. Seeking acceptance of this child by others.
   3. Seeking of commitment and acceptance of self as mother to the infant (binding-in).
   4. Learning to give of oneself on behalf on one's child.

Changes in the Father

A. First trimester.
   1. May feel left out of pregnancy.
   2. Confused by partner's mood swings.

B. Second trimester.
   1. Promote his involvement by his watching and feeling fetal movement.
   2. Needs to confront and resolve his own conflicts about the fathering he received as a child.
   3. Will decide on what he does and does not want to imitate from his father role figure.
   4. May react differently to partner's physical body changes.

C. Third trimester.
   1. Concerns and fears resurface.
   2. *Couvade syndrome* refers to the presence of physical discomforts in the man during their partner's pregnancy that mimic her symptoms.

PRENATAL CARE

Assessment

A. Initial visit.
   1. Complete history and physical.
   2. Obstetric history.
      a. Past pregnancies (date, course of pregnancy, labor and postpartum; information about infant and neonatal course).
      b. Present pregnancy.

B. Schedule of return prenatal visits.
   1. Frequency of return visits.
      a. Monthly for first thirty-two weeks.
      b. Every two weeks to the thirty-sixth week.
      c. After the thirty-sixth week, weekly until delivery.
   2. Subsequent assessment data follow-up.
      a. Vital signs.
      b. Urinalysis-check for protein and sugar.
      c. Monitor weight.
      d. Measurement of height of uterine fundus.
      e. Auscultation of fetal heart rate (FHR).

C. Definition of Common Terms (Table 24-5).

D. Signs and Symptoms of Pregnancy (Table 24-6).

E. Summary of the Antepartum Period (Table 24-7).

Diagnostics

A. Pregnancy tests.
   1. Immunoassay—based on antigenic property of HCG.

Table 24-5: DEFINITION OF COMMON TERMS

COMMON TERM	DEFINITION
1. Gravida*	A pregnancy regardless of the duration; includes the present pregnancy.
2. Para*	Refers to past pregnancies that continue to the period of viability (legal definition: 24 weeks gestational age).
3. Primigravida	Woman who is pregnant for the first time.
4. Multigravida	Woman who is pregnant for the second or subsequent time.
5. Nullipara (para 0)	Woman who has not had children.
6. Primipara (para 1)	Woman who has carried a pregnancy to viability; term is often used interchangeably with primigravida.
7. Multipara (para II, para III, para IV, etc.)	Woman who has given birth to two or more children.
8. Parturient	A woman in labor.

*The terms *gravida* and *para* refer to the number of pregnancies, not the number of fetuses. The woman who delivers twins on her first pregnancy remains a para 1, in spite of having two infants. She also is a para 1 if the fetus was stillborn or died soon after birth.

❑ **Another system used to describe reproductive status is the five-digit identification system characterized by the acronym GTPAL:**
G = total number of pregnancies
T = number of term infants (37 weeks of gestation)
P = number of preterm infants (before 37 weeks of gestation)
A = number of spontaneous or therapeutic abortions
L = number of living children

a. Hemagglutination-inhibition test or HAI (Neocept)—no clumping of cells when urine of a pregnant woman is added to the HCG-sensitized red blood cells of sheep 4 days after the first missed menstrual period.

b. Latex agglutination tests (Gravindex and Pregnosticon slide test)—latex particle agglutination is inhibited in the presence of urine containing HCG; accurate from 4-10 days after the first missed menstrual period.

2. Radioreceptor assay — uses radioiodine.

a. Radioreceptor Assay or RRA (Biocept-G) — uses radio-iodine labeled HCG; very sensitive test; accurate at the time of the first missed menstrual period.

b. Beta subunit radioimmunoassay or RIA (Beta Tec, Chorio Quant)—uses radioiodinated HCG that is added to urine or serum as an antigen to specific antibodies; most reliable test as it identifies the beta subunit of HCG; accurate as early as 6 days before the first missed menstrual period.

NURSING PRIORITY: *RIA is most accurate and quickest method (results in 1 hour) and it becomes positive a few days after presumed implantation, which permits earlier diagnosis.*

3. Enzyme-linked immunosorbent assay or ELISA (Pregnospia, Tandem ICON, Confidot)—uses monoclonal anti-HCG; accurate results are possible about 4 days before first missed menstrual period.

4. Home pregnancy tests (Fact, Clearblue Easy, Daisy-2)— are either HAI or ELISA type tests; best on first voided specimens; detects low levels of HCG; can be used within a few days of a missed period and give results in less than 30 minutes; false negative results should be followed up in presence of pregnancy symptoms.

B. Laboratory tests.

1. Urinalysis.
2. Complete blood count (CBC).
3. VDRL—RPR serologic screening for syphilis.
4. Rubella antibody titer—hemagglutination-inhibition test (HAI).

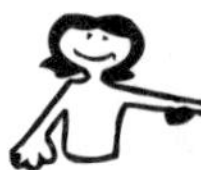

NURSING PRIORITY: *It is important to understand the rubella titer and its significance to pregnancy.*

a. Titer of 1:10 or less is considered serologically negative; titer 1:10 or greater indicates woman is immune.

b. Immunization is given within 6 weeks after delivery.

c. Teach mother who has not had rubella or a vaccination or who has a titer less than 1:10 to avoid children who have rubella or who have received a recent vaccination.

5. Blood type and Rh. If Rh is negative need to plan for administration of **Rhogam**.

C. Pelvic examination.

1. Papanicolaou smear of the cervix (Pap smear).
2. Pelvic measurements (pelvimetry).

Table 24-6: SIGNS AND SYMPTOMS OF PREGNANCY

PRESUMPTIVE/SUBJECTIVE	PROBABLE/OBJECTIVE	POSITIVE/DIAGNOSTIC
1. Amenorrhea. 2. Nausea and vomiting. 3. Excessive fatigue. 4. Urinary frequency. 5. Breast changes - tenderness, fullness, increased pigmentation of areola, pre-colostrum discharge. 6. Quickening - active movements of the fetus felt by the mother. 7. Increased pigmentation of skin and abdominal striae.	1. Positive pregnancy test (Gravindex, UCG, Pregnosticon R). 2. Enlarged abdomen. 3. Hegar's sign - softening of lower uterine segment. 4. Chadwick's sign -bluish discoloration of vagina. 5. Goodell's sign -softening of cervical lip. 6. Ballottement - pushing on fetus (4th to 5th month) and feeling it rebound back. 7. Fetal outline distinguished by palpation. 8. Braxton-Hicks contractions.	1. Fetal heart tone: 10th to 12th week -Doppler. 18th to 20th week -Fetoscope. 2. Fetal movements. 3. Fetal skeleton on X-ray (not used often). 4. Fetal sonography (after 16th week).

NCLEX ALERT: *The signs and symptoms of pregnancy are frequently tested; be sure you are able to differentiate between presumptive, probable, and positive signs.*

D. Calculation of estimated date of confinement (EDC); estimated date of delivery (EDD).

1. Naegele's rule: count back three calendar months from the first day of the last menstrual period (LMP) and add seven days.
2. Examples:
   a. LMP, April 10, 1999: EDC, January 17, 2000.
   b. LMP, September 25, 1999: EDC, July 2, 2000.

High-risk Pregnancy

1. Maternal factors.
   a. Age—under 16 or over 35.

***NURSING PRIORITY:** The pregnant adolescent is at risk both physiologically and psychologically. Physiological risks: PIH, iron deficiency anemia, sexually transmitted diseases (15-19-year-old teens have 2nd highest incidence of STD). Psychologic risks: interruption of normal growth and development for both partners, may drop out of school, adolescent fathers tend to pursue less prestigious careers and earn less income.*

   b. Parity—primigravida or greater than gravida V.
   c. Unusual stress or anxiety, single parenthood, teenage pregnancy, abusive environment.
   d. Environmental and occupational hazards—excessive exposure to radiation, handling of teratogenic chemicals.
   e. Drug use— alcohol, nicotine, cocaine, heroin, marijuana, and other addictive drugs.
   f. Delayed or absent prenatal care.
   g. Prolonged infertility or hormone treatment.
2. Preexisting medical problems.
   a. Diabetes mellitus.
   b. Hypertension and cardiovascular disease.
   c. Renal disease.
   d. Positive serology for syphilis.
   e. Viral infections: rubella, cytomegalovirus (CMV), herpesvirus type 2, HIV.
   f. Urinary tract infections.
   g. Anemia.
   h. Psychiatric disorders.
3. Obstetric factors.
   a. History of a previous high-risk pregnancy (premature labor, SGA or LGA infants, abortion, stillbirth, or maternal complications).
   b. Present pregnancy (exposure to teratogens, hyperemesis gravidarum, bleeding, toxemia, hydramnios, multiple gestation, abnormal presentation, premature labor, and isoimmune disease).
4. Nutritional factors.
   a. Underweight: (10% below for height).
   b. Overweight: (20% over normal for height).
   c. Inappropriate weight gain during pregnancy, either too little or too much.
   d. Adolescents: need additional nutrition for their own growth and development (approximately 1.5-1.7 g of protein per kg of body weight and as high as 50 calories per kg of body weight).
5. Genetic factors.

Table 24-7: SUMMARY OF NURSING MANAGEMENT DURING THE ANTEPARTUM PERIOD

WEEKS' GESTATION	PHYSICAL SIGNS AND SYMPTOMS	CHARACTERISTIC BEHAVIORS	NURSING INTERVENTIONS
0-16	Amenorrhea. Fatigue. Nausea, vomiting. Increased breast size and tenderness. Urinary frequency. Increased appetite.	Ambivalence with mood swings. Anxiety related to confirmation of pregnancy. Tells selected close persons of pregnancy.	1. Obtain complete history, including gynecologic and obstetric histories. 2. Ascertain any maternal high-risk problems such as maternal age (over 35 years) heart disease, diabetes or potential high risk neonate problems, history of congenital defects, premature births, etc.(see complete discussion in this chapter on high-risk problems). 3. Identify maternal nutritional status by assessing height, weight, and frame and compare with standardized charts of normal ranges. 4. Complete a diet history and instruction. *Important to teach about necessary changes, rather than all the concepts of good nutrition.* 5. Food cravings are usually benign and may be indulged providing a well balanced diet is maintained. *Pica is an abnormal eating pattern and requires treatment.* 6. Encourage client to express feelings about pregnancy or ambivalence. 7. Anticipatory guidance/teaching (including family) related to: Drugs, radiation, normal signs and symptoms of pregnancy as well as reportable signs of possible complications, and the normality of her mood swings.

a. History of an inheritable disorder (Down syndrome).

b. Previous infant with a congenital anomaly.

c. Parents with recessive disorders (hemophilia, cystic fibrosis).

Nursing Intervention

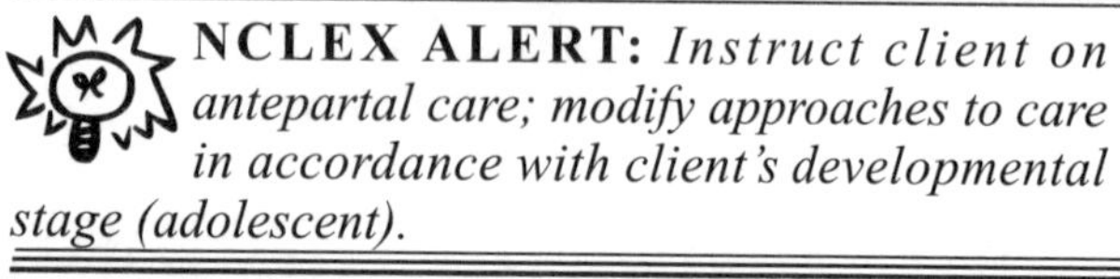

NCLEX ALERT: *Instruct client on antepartal care; modify approaches to care in accordance with client's developmental stage (adolescent).*

✦ *Goal: to educate families regarding general health practices.*

1. **Hygiene:** tub baths are permitted; during latter weeks of gestation may be awkward.
2. **Clothing:** loose, comfortable clothing with good supporting brassiere; low-heeled shoes.
3. **Breast and nipple care:** avoid rubbing nipples with towel and excessive use of soap as it dries the nipple area and removes natural secretions; creams, lotions, and ointments are not necessary on the nipple or areola and should be avoided.
4. **Employment:** no severe physical straining, heavy lifting, or prolonged periods of sitting or standing.
5. **Travel:** avoid during the last month of pregnancy; when traveling by car or airplane, frequent walking and stretching is advised; use seat belts (both lap and shoulder), positioning the lap belt under the abdomen.
6. **Rest and exercise:** adequate amounts of exercise—walking, swimming; client should stop exercising when she begins to feel tired; moderation is the key word.
7. **Sexual activity:** coital position may need to be altered to provide greater comfort; no contraindication to intercourse or any activity leading to orgasm providing that membranes are intact, no vaginal bleeding, and no history of threatened abortion or premature labor.
8. **Smoking**: not advised; associated with infants who are small for gestational age (SGA).
9. **Alcohol:** recommended not to consume any alcohol; the more consumed, the greater the risk for fetal alcohol syndrome.
10. **Dental care:** regular prophylactic care is encouraged; a soft-bristle toothbrush may be needed, due to bleeding gums; X-rays should be postponed if possible.
11. **Immunization:** live, attenuated virus immunizations (MMR) are contraindicated during pregnancy; client is cautioned against getting pregnant for at least three months following this type of immunization.
12. **Medications:** client advised to avoid medications, especially during the first trimester.

Table 24-7: SUMMARY OF NURSING MANAGEMENT DURING THE ANTEPARTUM PERIOD

WEEKS' GESTATION	PHYSICAL SIGNS AND SYMPTOMS	CHARACTERISTIC BEHAVIORS	NURSING INTERVENTIONS
16-30	Quickening. "Pregnant figure". Increased energy. Feeling of well-being. Round ligament pain.	Wears maternity clothes. Tells the world she's pregnant, begins to notice other pregnant women. Interested in learning about birth and babies - reads books, seeks out and questions friends and family, attends classes. Increased dependency as time goes on.	1. On going assessment of maternal/fetal status: FHR Vital signs Fundal height Urine test for glucose (mild glycosuria is usually benign), protein, and nitrite. Fingerstick for hemoglobin analysis (12- 14 g/dL normal) Balanced diet 2. Prevent or minimize activity intolerance and promote adequate rest by: Encouraging 8 hours sleep each day, plus one nap Scheduling rest periods at place of employment Napping at home while other small children are sleeping Using left lateral position while resting or sleeping 3. Promote adequate exercise, (e.g. Kegel, pelvic rocking, modified sit ups), sitting tailor-fashion (lotus position). 4. Anticipatory guidance/teaching (including family) related to: Libido changes, mood swings, increasing dependency, introversion, and reportable signs of possible complications.
30-40	Dependent edema. Pressure in lower abdomen. Frequent urination. Round ligament pain. Backache. Insomnia. Clumsiness. Fatigue.	Introversion. Increased dependency (craves attention and tenderness). Altered responsiveness and spontaneity as well as abdominal bulk and fatigue may decrease interest in genital sex and fatigue. Intensifies study of labor and delivery. Increasingly feeling more vulnerable. Prepares nursery - buys baby things. Decides on feeding method for baby.	1. Ongoing continued physical assessment at more frequent intervals. 2. Reassure - provide emotional support related to attractiveness and self-worth. 3. Anticipatory guidance/teaching (including family) related to: Signs and symptoms of labor, environmental modification for coming infant and providing rest for mother, teaching associated with either breast or bottle feeding, advising client concerning birthing and anesthesia options, promoting the developing parent/child attachment (encourage family to verbalize mental picture of infant and concepts of selves as parents).

✦ *Goal: to promote relief of common discomforts through client education of self-care measures (Table 24-8).*

✦ *Goal: to promote adequate nutrition.*

1. Obtain a complete diet history (See Chapter 3).
   a. Assess normal food intake.
   b. Determine prepregnant nutritional status (existence of deficiency state; severity and time at gestation in which it occurs).
2. Identify nutritional risk factors.
   a. Age: adolescents and older gravidas.
   b. Maternal weight variations.
   c. Abnormal dietary patterns: pica, fad diets, excessive use of alcohol, drugs, or tobacco.
   d. Socioeconomic status: low income, insufficient money to buy food.
   e. Preexisting medical problems: diabetes mellitus, anemia.
3. Dietary instructions and nutrient requirements.
   a. Increase calories for pregnancy (an additional 300 calories per day).
   b. Increase calories for lactation (an additional 500 calories per day).
   c. Increase protein (an additional 30 gm per day for pregnancy; an additional 20 gm per day for lactation).
   d. Increase vitamins (generally, all vitamin intake is increased, especially folic acid).
   e. Increase amount of minerals (especially iron, calcium, and phosphorous).
   f. Additional calories and protein may be recommended for the pregnant adolescent.

Table 24-8: SUMMARY OF COMMON DISCOMFORTS AND RELIEF MEASURES

DISCOMFORT	RELIEF MEASURES
1ST TRIMESTER:	
Nausea and vomiting (morning sickness)	Frequent small meals; avoid empty stomach; between meals eat crackers without fluid; take vitamin B_6 supplement.
Urinary frequency and urgency	Void frequently; decrease fluids prior to bedtime; avoid caffeinated or carbonated beverages; use perineal pads for leakage.
Breast tenderness	Well-fitting support bra; altering sleep positions; avoiding soap on the nipple and areola area.
Increased vaginal discharge	Good hygiene; use perineal or panty liner pads; cotton underwear; no douching unless prescribed.
2ND AND 3RD TRIMESTERS:	
Heartburn	Avoid fat and fried, spicy foods; eat small, frequent meals; maintain good posture; sit upright.
Ankle edema	Avoid prolonged sitting or standing; support stockings applied before rising; elevate feet while sitting.
Varicose veins	Avoid prolonged periods of standing; apply support hose before rising; elevate feet while sitting; do not cross legs at knees.
Hemorrhoids	Avoid constipation, do not strain; use ointments, bulk-producing laxatives, anesthetic suppositories as prescribed.
Constipation	Increase fluid intake (6 to 8 glasses/day); eat food and fruits high in roughage; exercise moderately; use bulk-producing laxatives as prescribed.
Backache	Correct posture; low-heeled shoes; pelvic tilt exercise.
Leg cramps	Stretch affected muscle and hold till it subsides; warm packs; maintain adequate calcium intake.
Faintness	Sit or lie down; avoid sudden changes in position; and avoid prolonged standing.
Shortness of breath	Good posture; sleep with head elevated by several pillows.

NCLEX ALERT: *Instruct client on antepartal care.*

✦ *Goal: to educate expectant family with regard to danger signs and symptoms requiring immediate attention.*

1. Vaginal discharge-blood or amniotic fluid.
2. Visual disturbances-dimness or blurring of vision, flashes of light or dots before the eyes.
3. Swelling of the face or fingers.
4. Fever and chills.
5. Severe or continuous headache.
6. Pain in the abdomen.
7. Persistent vomiting.
8. Absence of fetal movement after quickening.

✦ *Goal: to provide education and preparation for childbirth.*

1. Childbirth programs erase previous negative impressions of pregnancy, labor and delivery, promote a positive, health attitude, and teach students physical exercises and relaxation techniques.
2. Points about breathing.
   a. Slow abdominal breathing or chest breathing is practiced for the first stage of labor; concentrate on making abdominal muscles rise.
   b. Rapid chest breathing is for the active and transitional phases of labor.
   c. Panting is used to prevent pushing.

FETAL DEVELOPMENT

Developmental Stages

1. Preembryonic stage—stage of the ovum.
   a. Fertilization to the first three weeks.
   b. Fertilized ovum grows and differentiates.
   c. Formation of the three primary germ layers-endoderm, mesoderm, ectoderm.
   d. Implantation in the endometrial tissue.
2. Embryonic stage.
   a. Fourth week to the eighth week of development.

b. Period of organogenesis—differentiation of cells, organs, and organ systems.

c. Highly vulnerable time for congenital anomalies to occur.

d. At the end of this period of development, embryo has features of the human body.

3. Fetal stage.

a. Eight weeks to the time of birth.

b. Characterized by growth and development of organs and organ systems.

Summary of Growth and Development

1. 6 weeks—heart begins beating.
2. 8 weeks—brain activity begins; moves in response to touch; 1 inch long.
3. 16 weeks—begins sucking response; 31/2 inches long; sex clearly identifable.
4. 20 weeks—hearing begins to develop; can respond to external sounds in environment; 10 inches long.
5. 28 weeks—can perceive light; senses are functional; sleep-wake periods; brown fat has formed; 16 inches long; viable.
6. 30-40 weeks—increase in subcutaneous fat and weight.

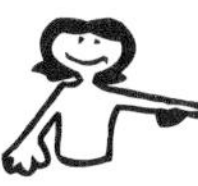

NURSING PRIORITY: At weeks thirty-four or thirty-five, surfactant production is sufficient.

Multiple Pregnancy

1. Incidence.

a. One out of ninety pregnancies is twins; one out of nine thousand pregnancies is triplets.

b. Increased incidence of twinning in the black race.

c. One out of three sets of twins is monozygotic, or identical.

2. Dizygotic or fraternal twins.

a. Fertilization of two separate ova.

b. There are two placentas; however, they may be fused.

c. Fraternal twin can be either the same sex or a different sex; also may be different gestational ages.

3. Monozygotic or identical twins.

a. One ovum and one sperm; cells of the zygote separate and form two embryos.

b. Same sex—resemble each other in appearance and structure.

c. Usually one placenta, one chorion, and two amnions; however, may have two placentas.

Placenta

A. Function.

1. Transfer of oxygen, nutrients, and metabolites.
2. Elimination of waste products from the fetus.
3. Production of hormones—human chorionic gonadotropin (HCG), human placental lactogen (HPL), estrogen and progesterone.

B. Development of the placenta.

1. Formed from the chorionic villi lying over the decidua basalis.
2. Formed by the end of the third month of gestation.
3. Separated by fifteen to thirty sections, cotyledons.
4. At term, the placenta weighs one-sixth of the fetus (6 lb fetus: 1 lb placenta).
5. Fetal surface is shiny and slightly grayish—*Schultze.*
6. Maternal side is rough and beefy red—*Duncan.*

C. Placental circulation.

1. Maternal and fetal bloodstreams are in close relationship to each other, but the circulations do not mix.
2. Approximately 500 to 700 cc of maternal blood circulates through the placenta every minute.

Fetal Circulation

A. Fetal lungs do not participate in respiratory gas exchange.

B. There are special fetal structures to bypass blood supply to the lungs.

1. Placenta.
2. Umbilical cord-length: 55 cm (22 inches); diameter: 1.0 to 2.5 cm ($\frac{1}{3}$ to 1 inch).

a. One umbilical vein carries oxygenated blood from maternal circulation to fetus.

b. Two umbilical arteries carry unoxygenated (venous) blood from fetus to placenta.

c. Wharton's jelly is a gelatinous substance which surrounds the three blood vessels providing support.

3. Foramen ovale—an opening between the right atrium and the left atrium of the heart.
4. Ductus arteriosus—connects the pulmonary artery and the aorta.
5. Ductus venosus—connects the umbilical vein and the inferior vena cava.

C. At the time of birth, the fetal circulation system begins the transition to the adult pattern of circulation; a functional closure occurs within a few days, however anatomic closure of the fetal vessels is not complete for several weeks or months.

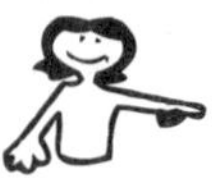

NURSING PRIORITY: This is the reason why a newborn heart murmur may not be significant (due to incomplete closure of the ductus).

FETAL WELL-BEING

Monitoring of Fetal Status

Ultrasound

❑ **A noninvasive technique utilizing high-frequency pulse sound waves which are transmitted by a transducer applied directly to the woman's abdomen.**

1. Purpose.
   a. Identifies placental location for amniocentesis or to determine placenta previa.
   b. Determines gestational age by crown-rump length (first trimester); later, biparietal diameter (BPD).
   c. Detects fetal anomalies—hydrocephalus, myelomeningocele, anencephaly.
   d. Detects multiple gestations.
   e. Monitors fetal growth to assess for intrauterine growth retardation (IUGR).
2. Procedure.
   a. Performed with a full bladder, except when ultrasound is used to localize the placenta prior to amniocentesis.
   b. Client advised to drink one quart of water two hours prior to sonogram.
   c. Requires approximately twenty to thirty minutes to perform; client must lie flat on back, which may be uncomfortable.

Chorionic Villus Sampling

❑ **A method to obtain genetic fetal tissue.**

1. Purpose—to obtain fetal tissue to establish a genetic profile as a first trimester alternative to aminocentesis.
2. Procedure.
   a. Is an invasive procedure performed under ultrasound between 9-12 weeks gestation; technique may be transvaginal or transabdominal.
   b. Allows for earlier diagnosis of genetic defects than aminocentesis.
   c. Early sampling (8-9 weeks) has been associated with an increased incidence of limb defects.

Fetal Activity Counting

1. A change in fetal activity, either a increase or a decrease, should be reported to health care provider.
2. Sandovsky method: keep a time record of fetal movements three times a day.
3. Cardiff method: keep a time record of the first ten movements felt each morning.

Nonstress Test (NST)

1. Purpose—to observe the response of fetal heart rate to the stress of activity.
2. Procedure—requires approximately twenty minutes; client in semi-Fowler's position; external monitor is applied to document fetal activity; mother activates the "mark button" on the electronic fetal monitor when she feels fetal movement.
   a. If no fetal movement-may gently rub or palpate abdomen to stimulate movement; or may be asked to eat a light meal, as increased blood sugar increases fetal activity.
3. Interpretation.
   a. Reactive: shows two or accelerations osf 15bpm or more within 20 minutes of beginning the test. Test may be rescheduled as indicated by condition; indicates a healthy fetus.
   b. Nonreactive: reactive criteria are not met. The accelerations are less than two in number, the accelerations are less than 15 bpm, or there are no accelerations. If nonreactive, then the test is extended another 20 minutes; if the tracing becomes reactive, the NST is concluded. If the NST is still nonreactive after second 20 minute trial (total 40 minutes), then additional testing, such as an amniotic fluid index (AFI) is considered. If gestation is near term, a CST may be done.

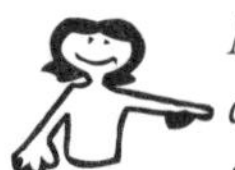

NURSING PRIORITY: Appearance of any decelerations of the FHR during NST should be immediately evaluated by the physician.

   c. Unsatisfactory: uninterpretable registration of fetal heart rate or inadequate fetal activity; reschedule NST within twenty-four hours.
4. Advantages of NST.
   a. Simple; easy to perform.
   b. Does not require hospitalization.
   c. Has no contraindications.

Biophysical Profile

1. Is the first choice for follow-up fetal evaluation.

2. Assesses ***five*** fetal variables: breathing movement, gross body movement, muscle tone, amniotic fluid volume, and FHR. First four assessed by ultrasound; the last by NST.
3. Each area has a possible score of 2—maximum score of 10. A score of 4 or below indicates need for immediate delivery.
4. Daily assessments for at risk fetus.

Contraction Stress Test (CST) or Oxytocin Challenge Test (OCT) and the Breast Self-stimulation Contraction Stress Test (BSST)

1. Purpose—to observe the response of fetal heart rate to the stress of oxytocin-induced uterine contractions; means of evaluating respiratory function (O_2 and CO_2 exchange) of the placenta.

***NURSING PRIORITY:** Many facilities now use the breast self-stimulation contraction stress test (BSST), as endogenous oxytocin is produced in response to stimulation of the breasts or nipples.*

---

2. Indications.
   a. Preexisting maternal medical conditions—diabetes mellitus, heart disease, hypertension, sickle cell disease, hyperthyroidism, renal disease.
   b. Postmaturity, IUGR, nonreactive NST, preeclampsia.
3. Contraindications.
   a. Third trimester bleeding.
   b. Previous Cesarean birth.
   c. Risk of preterm labor due to premature rupture of the membranes, incompetent cervical os, or multiple gestation
4. Procedure—BSST.
   a. Semi-Fowler's position, fetal monitor in place.
   b. Nipple stimulation begins with woman brushing her palm across one nipple through her shirt or gown for 2-3 minutes. If contractions start, nipple stimulation should stop. If contractions do not occur, bilaterial stimulation may be used for 20 minutes.
   c. Advantages: takes less time to perform, less expensive, and causes less discomfort because no IV is used.
5. Procedure—OCT.
   a. Client must be NPO, closely obseerved, either hospitalized, or on an outpatient bases.
   b. Position in semi-Fowler's to avoid supine hypotension.
   c. Intravenous administration of oxytocin—stimulates uterine contractions—uterine activity and fetal heart rate are recorded by way of external monitoring.
   d. Hypoxia is reflected in late deceleration on monitor, which indicates a diminished fetal-placental reserve.
   e. Oxytocin IV is delivered at a rate of 0.5 Mu per minute with the rate increased every fifteen minutes until contractions occur at the rate of three per ten minutes, then oxytocin is discontinued and the woman is observed until contractions stop.
6. Interpretation—OCT.
   a. Negative (reassuring): shows no late decelerations after any contraction; implies placental support is adequate.
   b. Positive(nonreassuring; abnormal): shows late decelerations with at least tow of the three contractions; may indicate the possiblity of insufficient placental respiratory reserve.

NURSING PRIORITY:** If the CST is positive and there is no acceleration of FHR with fetal movement (nonreactive NST), the positive CST is an ominous sign, often indicating a late sign of fetal hypoxia. **Most cases a negative CST with a reactive NST would be a desired result.

Amniotic Fluid Analysis

1. Purpose—analysis of the amniotic fluid obtained by the technique of amniocentesis; provides the following information:
   a. Monitoring of Rh isoimmunization process.
   b. Determination of fetal lung maturity.
   c. Genetic diagnosis (see Chapter 22).
      (1) Chromosomal abnormalities—Down syndrome.
      (2) Detection of neurotube defects through a-fetoprotein analysis (AFP).
      (3) Chorionic villus sampling involves taking a small sample of chorionic villi
2. Procedure.
   a. Amniocentesis—introduction of a needle transabdominally through the abdominal and uterine walls into the amniotic cavity to aspirate fluid for examination.
   b. Supine position with slight elevation of the head.
   c. Client should empty her bladder.

d. Location of the placenta and fetus is scanned by ultrasound to avoid trauma and injury.

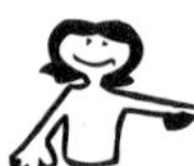

NURSING PRIORITY: FHR is monitored throughout procedure.

e. Abdomen is prepped: local anesthetic infiltrated subcutaneously; needle inserted and amniotic fluid aspirated and sent to laboratory for analysis.

3. Maturity studies.
   a. Lecithin/sphingomyelin ratio (L/S)—the components of phospholipid protein substance that composes surfactant; L/S ratio of 2:1 or greater is indicative of sufficient surfactant (occurs around ***thirty-five*** weeks).
   b. Lung profile.
      (1) Includes L/S ratio and percentages of lecithin and phosphatidyl inositol (PI) and phosphatidyl glycerol (PG).
      (2) Additional measurements allow for a more accurate picture of lung maturity.
      (3) PI increases at thirty-five to thirty-six weeks and then declines.
      (4) PG appears at thirty-five weeks and increases rapidly until term.

Fetoscopy

1. Purpose—to obtain a sample of blood or skin for diagnostic procedures.
2. Procedure— ultrasound performed prior and during; small incision made into abdomen; pierce umbilical cord and obtain blood sample.

Amnioscopy

Visualization of the amniotic fluid with an amnioscope to detect meconium staining.

COMPLICATIONS ASSOCIATED WITH PREGNANCY

High-Risk Pregnancy

A. Preexisting medical health problems complicate pregnancy.

B. Often, these problems affect the mother quite mildly; however, the effect upon the fetus is severe as evidenced by developmental anomalies and even death.

C. The medical and obstetric treatment of these conditions is described in Unit 5 under the appropriate body system.

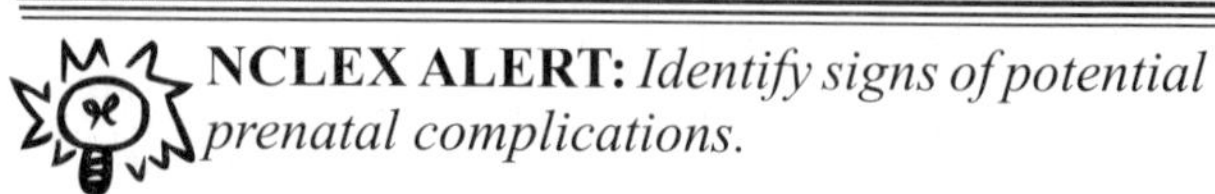

NCLEX ALERT: *Identify signs of potential prenatal complications.*

Abortion

❑ **Termination of pregnancy prior to viability (twenty to twenty-four weeks' gestation); abortions can be spontaneous (miscarriage) or induced (therapeutic or elective); approximately 75 percent to 80 percent of all spontaneous abortions occur during the second and third months of gestation.**

Assessment

1. Risk factors.
   a. Maternal: chronic infections, fibroid tumors, structural uterine anomalies.
   b. Acute infection.
   c. Endocrine disturbance: progesterone and thyroid hormone (hypothyroidism) dysfunction.
   d. Exposure to teratogens, evidence of malnutrition, and psychological factors.
2. Diagnostics.
   a. Decreased hemoglobin (less than 10.5 mg/dL if bleeding has been significant).
3. Clinical manifestations (types of spontaneous abortions.)
   a. Threatened abortion—slight bleeding, mild back and lower abdominal cramping, no cervical dilatation, no passage of the products of conception.
   b. Inevitable abortion—moderate amount of bleeding and cramping, internal cervical os dilates, and membranes may rupture.
   c. Incomplete abortion—only part of the products of conception are expelled.
   d. Complete abortion—all the products of conception are expelled.
   e. Missed abortion—fetus dies in utero, and the products of conception are retained from four to eight weeks; symptoms of pregnancy subside; if fetus is retained past six weeks, complications of disseminated intravascular coagulation (DIC) may develop due to the release of thromboplastin from the fetal autolysis process.
   f. Habitual abortion—three or more successive, spontaneous abortions.

Treatment

(Varies according to type of abortion)

1. Threatened abortion—bedrest, sedation, and sometimes progesterone therapy (may cause congenital anomalies).

2. Inevitable and incomplete abortion.
   a. Fluid replacement: IVs, type and crossmatch for possible blood transfusion.
   b. Administration of oxytocin.
   c. Dilatation and curettage or a suction evacuation to remove products of conception.
   d. Administration of **Rhogam** if mother is Rh negative (given within seventy-two hours).
3. Missed abortion.
   a. If abortion does not occur spontaneously after six weeks, suction evacuation or D&C will be done.
   b. Pregnancy past twelve weeks' gestation-induction of labor by IV Pitocin or urea or prostaglandin.
4. Habitual abortion—determination of cause, then specific therapy to correct.

Nursing Intervention

✦ *Goal: to assess or control hemorrhage.*

1. Monitoring of vital signs.
2. Accurate counting of pads to assess bleeding.
3. Assist in medical treatment—IV therapy, preparation for dilatation and curettage.

✦ *Goal: to prevent complications.*

1. Observe for shock, hypofibrinogenemia and DIC (missed abortion).
2. Prevent isoimmunization by administration of **Rhogam**.
3. Assess for infection and anemia.

✦ *Goal: to provide emotional support to the couple experiencing the loss of pregnancy.*

1. Encourage verbalization of feelings.
2. Often, verbal repetition of the experience helps one cope with the situation.
3. Be available and actively listen.

Ectopic Pregnancy

❑ **Any pregnancy that develops outside the uterus (extrauterine) is an ectopic pregnancy. Ninety percent of ectopic pregnancies are tubal; more common on the right side. Approximately one out of every three hundred pregnancies is ectopic.**

Assessment

1. Risk factors—any condition causing scarring or obstruction of the fallopian tubes (PID, gonorrheal infections, postabortion salpingitis).
2. Diagnostics.
   a. Ultrasound.
   b. Culdocentesis—assesses intraperitoneal bleeding by needle puncture of the cul-du-sac of Douglas.
   c. Laparoscope—an instrument that provides visualization of the pelvic organs via a small external incision on the abdomen; if affected tube found, a laparotomy can be performed for treatment.
3. Clinical manifestations.
   a. If tube is unruptured, usually slow, chronic bleeding with the abdomen gradually becoming rigid and very tender.
   b. If tube ruptures, sudden excruciating pain in the lower abdomen, usually over the mass; possible referred shoulder pain as the abdomen fills with blood; vaginal bleeding and shock.

Surgical treatment

1. Laparoscopy, laparotomy, salpingectomy.

Nursing Intervention

✦ *Goal: to prevent and detect early complications.*

1. Provision of nursing care for shock as indicated.
2. Prepare for surgery (IVs, oxygen, blood, etc.).
3. Administer **Rhogam** if mother is Rh negative..

✦ *Goal: to provide emotional support (loss of pregnancy and reproductive organ).*

Incompetent Cervical Os

❑ **An incompetent cervical os is a defect, usually related to trauma of the cervix, which leads to habitual abortion and premature labor.**

Assessment

1. Risk factors—cervical trauma related to D&C, conization, or cervical lacerations from previous deliveries.
2. Clinical manifestations.
   a. Cervical dilatation without painful uterine contractions.
   b. Membranes rupture, labor begins, and premature fetus is delivered.

Treatment

1. Surgical.
   a. Reinforcement of the weakened cervix by a purse-string suture which encircles the internal os.
   b. Shirodkar-Barter cerclage (permanent suture that allows the cervix to remain closed for all pregnancies, but must have a cesarean delivery).
   c. McDonald cerclage (left in place until term then removed prior to labor).

Nursing Intervention

✦ *Goal: to provide client education as to presence of purse-string suture.*

1. Advise that some vaginal spotting may occur for several days after placement of suture.
2. Should abstain from intercourse and douching, along with reduced activity level for two weeks postoperatively.
3. During labor, the suture will be removed for a vaginal delivery, or it may be left in place for a Caesarean delivery.

Gestational Trophoblastic Disease

❑ **Is a spectrum of diseases resulting from abnormal proliferation of the placenta — hydatidiform moles, gestational trophoblastic neoplasia, choriocarcinoma.**

Assessment

1. Risk factors.
   a. Found more commonly in Southeast Asia and the Far East.
   b. Once have a molar pregnancy, have a 20-40 times higher risk to having it again.
   c. Increased incidence with advanced maternal age.
2. Diagnostics.
   a. Ultrasound reveals no fetal skeleton.
   b. Elevated HCG level.
3. Clinical manifestations.
   a. Exaggerated symptoms of pregnancy—uterus too enlarged for pregnancy, excessive nausea and vomiting, early symptoms of PIH.
   b. Discharge of brownish-red fluid (like prune juice) from vagina around the twelfth week; fluid may contain vesicles.
   c. Anemia due to loss of blood.
   d. Absence of fetal heart sounds.
4. Complications.
   a. Infection.
   b. DIC.
   c. Trophoblastic embolization occurring after evacuation of molar pregnancy.
   d. Possible choriocarcinoma.

Treatment

1. Surgical—D&C to empty uterus.
2. Medical—follow-up supervision for one year.
   a. Weekly serum HCG level until they are negative; then every other week for 3-4 months; then monthly for a year; pelvic exams may be required every 2 weeks during the early period after the D&C.
   b. Rising titers of HCG indicate pathology-choriocarcinoma.

NURSING PRIORITY: *For the treatment of increasing or rising HCG levels which often indicate choriocarcinoma, the chemotherapeutic agent given is methotrexate.*

   c. Pregnancy should be avoided for at least one year.
   d. Oral contraceptive use to prevent pregnancy is controversial, as it may delay the fall in the HCG level.

Nursing Intervention

✦ *Goal: to assess for complications associated with hemorrhage and the possibility of uterine rupture.*

✦ *Goal: to provide emotional support and assist in selection of a contraceptive method.*

1. Provide simple explanations and determine understanding of course of treatment.
2. Encourage ventilation of fears associated with molar pregnancy and increased incidence of choriocarcinoma.

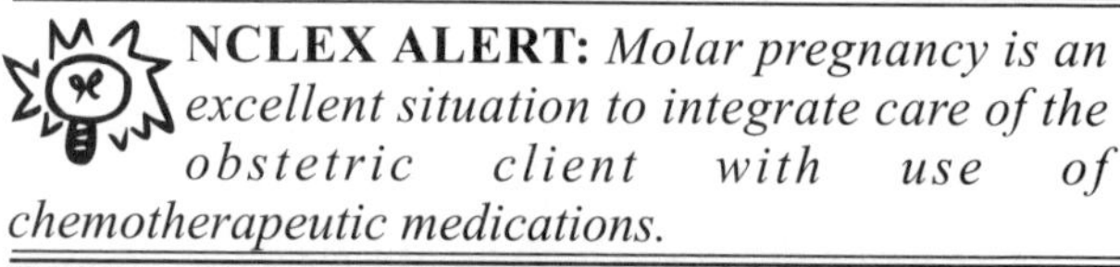

NCLEX ALERT: *Molar pregnancy is an excellent situation to integrate care of the obstetric client with use of chemotherapeutic medications.*

Hyperemesis Gravidarum

❑ **This disorder is intractable vomiting during pregnancy that results in dehydration and electrolyte imbalance. It occurs in one out of every one thousand pregnancies; the cause is uncertain.**

Assessment

1. Risk factors—none known.
2. Diagnostics—by symptoms.
3. Clinical manifestations
   a. Severe, persistent vomiting which leads to dehydration or nutritional deficiency; progresses to fluid electrolyte imbalance and alkalosis from loss of HCl.
   b. If untreated, ketoacidosis (from loss of intestinal juices), hypovolemia, hypokalemia, jaundice, and hemorrhage.
   c. Hypothrombinemia and decreased urine output.

Treatment

1. Medical—replacement of parental fluids, electrolytes, and vitamins, along with a tranquilizer or an antiemetic.
2. Dietary—NPO for first 48 hours; after condition improves, six small feedings alternated with liquid nourishment in small amounts every one to two hours; if vomiting reoccurs, NPO and IV fluids restarted.
3. May require placement of central line for extended nutritional us of TPN or lipids.

Nursing Intervention

✦ *Goal: to assist with the medical and dietary management.*

1. Accurate recording of vomitus.
2. Daily weight checks and maintenance of intake and output.
3. Desired urine output is 1000 cc in 24 hours; usually, administration of IVs at 3000 cc in first 24 hours after admission to correct hypovolemia.
4. Oral hygiene measures.
5. Clear liquids with gradual progression of small meals.

✦ *Goal: to detect and treat complications.*

1. Initial acid-base imbalance is alkalosis from the loss of hydrochloric acid; however, with prolonged vomiting and loss of alkaline intestinal juices, a ketoacidotic state occurs.
2. Protracted hyperemesis gravidarum may necessitate termination of the pregnancy.

Hypertensive Disorders

❑ **Pregnancy-induced hypertension (PIH) is the term used for hypertensive disorders that are specifically associated with pregnancy, preeclampsia and eclampsia. Previously, the term toxemia of pregnancy was used, as it was believed that toxemia was caused by toxins derived from the products of conception circulating in the blood; as a result of newer theories, this term is no longer appropriate.**

Incidence

A. Occurs in 5 percent to 7 percent of all pregnant women.

B. Seen more often in primigravidas, teenagers of lower socioeconomic class, African-Americans, women over 35 years, especially if they are primigravidas.

Etiology

A. Cause is unknown.

B. Various theories and contributing factors have been identified, but none conclusively.

Pathophysiology

A. Synthesis of prostaglandin PGE2 and prostacyclin (PGI2) is decreased, both PGE2 and PGI2 are potent vasodilators. Possible decreases in these factors may lead to increased sensitivity to angiotensin II and maybe responsible for most of the pathophysiology associated with PIH.

B. Arteriolar **vasospasm** and hypovolemia: renoglomerular lesions lead to loss of serum pro-

Table 24-9: CLINICAL MANIFESTATIONS OF PREGNANCY-INDUCED HYPERTENSION

MILD PREECLAMPSIA	SEVERE PREECLAMPSIA	ECLAMPSIA
Elevated BP - systolic increase of 30 mm Hg and 15 mm Hg increase in diastolic over baseline.	Increased hypertension - systolic at 160 mm Hg; diastolic at 110 mm Hg or more.	Elevated temperature (101°F); may precede convulsion (104°F is a grave sign).
Proteinuria - 1 gm/24 hour (1+ proteinuria).	Proteinuria - 5 gm/24 hours (3+ to 4+ proteinuria).	Tonic (15 to 20 sec) and clonic (60 sec) convulsions.
Edema -generalized especially digital and periorbital.	Edema - excessive.	Coma (lasts from few minutes to several hours).
Weight gain - 1 lb/week in 3rd trimester.	Elevated BUN, serum creatinine, uric acid.	Hypertensive crisis or shock.
	Oliguria - less than 400 cc in 24 hours.	Renal shutdown.
	Cerebral or visual disturbances.	
	Severe headache.	
	Vomiting.	
	Epigastric pain (due to edema of liver capsule, usually indicative of impending convulsion).	

Table 24-10: NURSING MANAGEMENT OF CLIENTS WITH PREGNANCY-INDUCED HYPERTENSION

✦ *Goal: Recognize the early signs of PIH and increased BP.*

1. Check BP and perform roll-over or pressor response test at weeks 28-32 in the high-risk client. Take BP in left lateral recumbent position; repeat BP after turning to supine position.
2. Monitor urine for proteinuria. Usually the last of the triad of symptoms to appear.
3. Monitor for nondependent pathologic edema, (e.g., periorbital and hands).

✦ *Goal: Recognize progression of PIH symptoms and minimize or control their sequelae.*

1. Institute weight controls. Check for sudden increases of 2 lb/week or 6 lb/month.
2. Increase protein intake in the diet. Maintain normal sodium intake; avoid use of diuretics.
3. Institute bedrest.
4. Monitor for ominous signs of deteriorating condition: headache, visual disturbances, hyperreflexia, markedly decreased urine output, epigastric or right upper quadrant pain, dyspnea, vaginal bleeding (abruptio placentae) or any change in fetal activity.
5. Administer **Apresoline**, a vasodilator, check maternal BP, pulse, and FHR.

✦ *Goal: Prevent or control seizures.*

1. Administer IV $MgSO_4$.
2. Have emergency items readily available, (e.g., O_2, suction, airway, sedatives, antidote-calcium gluconate).
3. Modify environment to ensure rest and quiet.
   a. Eliminate noise, bright lights, other harsh stimuli.
   b. Minimize number of personnel giving care.
   c. Initiate painful and/or intrusive procedures after sedation.
   d. Promote comfort at bedrest.

NURSING PRIORITY: *Diastolic increases of 20 mm Hg or more may be predictive of PIH.*

✦ *Goal: Recognize alterations in fetal well-being and promote safe delivery of the infant.*

1. Auscultate and record FHR pattern, noting presence of variability or accelerations, and report decelerations.
2. Instruct and support during amniocentesis.
3. Collect specimen for estriol determination.
4. Assist with NST and/or OCT.
5. Give instructions about induction of labor and electronic fetal heart rate monitoring.

tein, (e.g., albumin and globulin); sodium reabsorption is elevated and water is retained.

C. Oliguria results from decreased glomerular filtration rate and renal blood flow.

D. **Coagulation disorder**: decreased platelet count, increased intravascular coagulation, and fibrinogen deposits.

E. Central nervous system effects (hyperactivity): headaches, cerebral edema, hyperreflexia, and convulsions.

Assessment

A. Risk factors.
   1. Diabetes mellitus.
   2. Hypertension.
   3. Renal disease.
   4. Hydatidiform mole.
   5. Multiple pregnancy.
   6. Polyhydramnios.
   7. Age (less than seventeen or over thirty-five).
   8. Primarily a disease of the primigravida.
   9. Low socioeconomic status (malnutrition, low-protein diet).

B. Clinical manifestations of PIH (Table 24-9).

NCLEX ALERT: *The triad of symptoms for PIH is hypertension, edema, and proteinuria.*

C. Complications: *maternal.*
   1. Increased intraocular pressure leading to retinal detachment.
   2. Syndrome called **HELLP** has been associated with severe preeclampsia (**H**emolysis, **E**levated **L**iver function tests, **L**ow **P**latelet count) — findings are associated with mild DIC.
   3. Thrombocytopenia.

D. Complications: *fetal.*
   1. Usually small for gestational age.
   2. May be born prematurely.
   3. Newborn may be born oversedated due to maternal medications.
   4. May have hypermagnesemia due to maternal treatment with $MgSO_4$.

Treatment

A. Medical.
   1. Mild preeclampsia: bed rest.
   2. Severe preeclampsia: absolute bedrest, sedatives (**Valium**), antihypertensives (**Apresoline**), anticonvulsants (magnesium sulfate), prepare for

preterm delivery via cesearean section if HELLP syndrome begins (See Appendix 25-4).

3. Eclampsia: seizure precautions (vital signs, oxygen, suction, positioning).

B. Dietary: high-protein diet, moderate salt, and fluid intake of six to eight glasses of water per day.

Nursing Intervention

✦ *Goal (mild preeclampsia): to initiate preventative measures.*

1. Instruction as to home care—encourage bedrest, provide dietary instruction, and regular prenatal checkups.
2. Tests to evaluate fetal status, (e.g. fetal movement record, ultrasound, NST, estriol & creatinine levels).

A. Goals and nursing intervention for the severely preeclamptic and eclamptic client are outlined in Table 24-10.

Hydramnios

❑ ***Hydramnios* is an excessive amount of amniotic fluid. A normal amount of fluid is 500 to 1,000 cc. Any amount over 2,000 cc is considered excessive.**

Assessment

1. Risk factors (increased incidence occurs).
   a. Diabetes.
   b. Erythroblastosis fetalis.
   c. Presence of congenital anomalies.
   d. Twins.
   e. Pregnancy induced hypertension.
2. Diagnostics.
   a. Observation of abdomen (enlarges excessively).
   b. Ultrasound.
3. Clinical manifestations.
   a. Shortness of breath.
   b. Pedal edema.
   c. Generalized abdominal discomfort.

Treatment

1. Amniocentesis.

Nursing Intervention

✦ *Goal: to anticipate, detect, and prevent complications associated with polyhydramnios.*

1. Assess for history of risk factors.
2. Anticipate premature labor.
3. Provide comfort measures.⌘

Study Questions—Prenatal

1. How can a primigravida client most readily meet her increased daily iron requirements?

① Consuming at least four glasses of milk daily.
② Adding an extra source of red meat to her daily diet.
③ Taking an iron supplement with a vitamin C source.
④ Including an extra source of fruits or vegetables.

2. A primigravida client is experiencing Braxton-Hicks contractions. Which statement is true concerning this type of contraction?

① Are intensified by walking about.
② Are confined to the low back.
③ Do not increase in intensity or frequency.
④ Result in cervical effacement and dilation.

3. Which statement would the nurse explain to the client about striae gravidarum?

① Occur in 100 percent of pregnancies.
② Are silvery streaks which appear especially during the last trimester.
③ Can be decreased by a local application of cocoa butter or other types of emollient creams.
④ Will fade from their present reddish appearance.

4. Which statement about the results of a stress test (oxytocin challenge test) are considered accurate?

① Negative if no fetal heart rate accelerations occur with accompanying fetal movements.
② Nonreactive if there are no late decelerations in more than half of the contractions.
③ Positive if late decelerations occur in more than half of the contractions.
④ Reactive if the fetal heart rate accelerates with accompanying fetal movement.

5. At the beginning of her third trimester, a client reports she is having some discomfort in her lower back. What would the nurse check?

① Her posture and type of shoes she usually wears.
② Her bowel habits.
③ With the doctor for his advice.
④ The amount of milk that she drinks.

6. A client is 37 weeks pregnant and is admitted to the hospital with bright red vaginal bleeding, complaining of abdominal discomfort, but

nocontractions. After assessing the client's vital signs and determining the fetal heart rate, what is the most important information to obtain?

① The amount of cervical dilatation that is present.
② The exact location of her abdominal discomfort.
③ The station of the presenting part.
④ At what time the client last ate.

7. A young woman calls the clinic and reports missing her period. She states that she has used a home pregnancy test last night and the results were negative. She tells the nurse that her breasts are tender and that she feels nauseated most of the day. What does the nurse understand about home pregnancy tests?

① They are RIA type tests which are quick and most accurate.
② Home pregnancy tests are more reliable if collected on a random specimen.
③ The test is accurate and she is not pregnant.
④ False negative results should be followed up in the presence of pregnancy symptoms.

8. An 18-year-old primigravida attends the prenatal clinic for the first time when she is 12 weeks pregnant. Her examination and assessment proceed normally. The nurse begins to give her some instructions concerning her diet. The client says, "Please don't tell me to drink milk. I can't stand to drink it." What should the nurse do?

① Find ways to make milk more palatable.
② Give her some substitutes for milk.
③ Assess further her dislike for milk.
④ Emphasize how important milk is for the benefit of her baby.

9. A positive pregnancy test is related to the presence of which hormone?

① Chorionic gonadotropin.
② Progesterone.
③ Lactogen.
④ Estrogen.

10. A client reports that her last menstrual period was November 10. She asks the nurse, "When will my baby be due?" What is the best answer?

① "July 3."
② "August 30."
③ "Around the middle of September."
④ "The first or second week of August."

11. An L/S ratio (lecithin-sphingomyelin) is ordered for a primigravida at 35 week's gestation. What is the goal of this test?

① To determine fetal lung maturity and is done by amniocentesis.
② To evaluate the level of maternal-fetal estriol production.
③ To check the position of the fetal head.
④ To test the intrauterine fetal-placental circulation.

Answers and rationales to these questions are in the section at the end of the book entitled "Chapter Study Questions: Answers & Rationales."

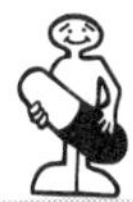

Appendix 24-1: CONTRACEPTIVE METHODS

METHODS/DESCRIPTION	NURSING IMPLICATIONS / CLIENT TEACHING
NATURAL METHODS:	
Calendar (rhythm) Basal body temperature (BBT) Ovulation (Billings) Symptothermal Cervical mucus Fertility awareness	***Client Teaching:*** *Calendar (rhythm) method*: calculate the days of fertility; considered to be days 10 to 17 of a 28-day menstrual cycle. *BBT method*: a slight decrease then an increase of about 0.4 to 0.8 degrees in temperature when ovulation occurs; fertile period ends three days after temperature elevation. *Cervical mucus method*: prior to ovulation, mucus becomes clear and stringy; nonfertile period occurs when mucus becomes thick, cloudy, and sticky, or no mucus apparent.
INTRAUTERINE DEVICE: (IUD)	
Progestasert, Copper T 380 A	***Client Teaching*** 1. Discuss the technique and the experience of IUD insertion and removal. 2. Emphasize the need for yearly Pap smears. 3. Encourage client to check IUD string, especially after each period. 4. Make sure the woman understands which type of IUD she has and when to return to have it checked or replaced.
ORAL CONTRACEPTIVES:	
Pill: (combination of estrogen and progesterone) **Minipill:** (progesterone only -0.35 mg norethindrone)	***Client Teaching:*** 1. Instruct as to the correct use of medication, the need for periodic checkups every six months, and the importance of taking the pill the same time each day. 2. Explain if a pill is forgotten one day, she should take it when she remembers, then take the next pill as scheduled the following day. 3. If two pills are missed, she should take them as above and use some other form of contraception for the remainder of the month. 4. Review common side effects, serious complications, and the reporting of any of the following symptoms: abdominal pain, chest pain, shortness of breath, headaches, eye problems, and severe leg pain.
CHEMICAL BARRIERS:	
Spermicides: jellies, creams, foams, suppositories, sponge.	***Client Teaching:*** 1. Instruct as a proper insertions of spermicide. 2. Explain how to wash applicator in warm water with a mild soap, making sure plunger is separated from barrel; do not boil applicator. 3. Advise not to douche for 6 to 8 hours after intercourse. 4. Educate about alternative methods of contraception.
MECHANICAL BARRIERS:	
Diaphragm: a dome-shaped rubber device that fits over the cervix. **Condom:** "rubbers" are thin sheaths of rubber which fit over an erect penis.	***Client Teaching:*** Diaphragm: 1. Should be refitted after every pregnancy or when there is a weight gain or loss of 20 lbs. 2. Instruct client to use spermicidal jelly or cream around diaphragm rim and in the dome. 3. Instruct that diaphragm is left in place 6 to 8 hrs. after intercourse. 4. Explain the proper method for cleansing (use Ivory soap only), storing (dry thoroughly and dust with constarch , not baby powder), and checking for defects or holes in the diaphragm. 5. Allow for sufficient practice of insertion/removal techniques. Condom: 1. Advise client to apply condom to erect penis by rolling the sheath along the entire shaft, and leaving enough slack at the end of the penis to receive the semen. 2. Explain importance of holding the condom in place while withdrawing the penis to prevent emptying of sperm into the vagina. 3. Condom should be applied prior to any penetration as the pre-ejaculatory seminal fluid may contain sperm.

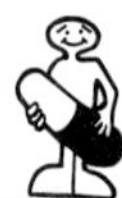

Appendix 24-1: CONTRACEPTIVE METHODS

METHODS/DESCRIPTION	NURSING IMPLICATIONS / CLIENT TEACHING
UNRELIABLE PRACTICES:	
Withdrawal (coitus interruptus) **Douching** *Description:* Coitus interruptus: withdrawal of penis prior to ejaculation. Douching: the act of cleansing/washing the semen out of the vagina.	*Nursing Implications:* Requires absolute cooperation and control of partner. Associated with high level of sexual frustration. *Client Teaching:* Encourage use of a more reliable contraceptive practice.
PERMANENT STERILIZATION:	
Tubal ligation	*Client Teaching:* 1. Discuss the permanence of the sterilization procedure with the couple. 2. Explain that often after surgery, referred shoulder pain is common due to CO_2 insufflation during laproscopy.
Vasectomy *Action:* Surgical ligation and resection bilaterally of the vas deferens.	*Client Teaching:* 1. Discuss with couple the permanence of vasectomy; even if the vas deferens is reconnected, the fertility varies between 5 percent to 60 percent. 2. Activity level should be moderate for 2 days; skin sutures are usually removed within a week. 3. Encourage the use of a scrotal support and apply ice for pain or swelling. 4. Follow-up visit for sperm sample is usually done in 4 to 6 weeks. 5. Advise couple to use another form of birth control until ejaculate contains no sperm.

LABOR AND DELIVERY

Intrapartal Factors

A. The passenger.

1. Fetal head.
 a. Bones of the skull—two frontal, two parietal, two temporal, and one occipital.
 b. Suture—membranous tissues between the bones.
  (1) Mitotic (frontal)—lies between the two frontal bones.
  (2) Sagittal—lies anteriorly between the parietal bones.
  (3) Coronal—lies between frontal bones and parietal.
  (4) Lambdoidal—located between the two parietal bones and the occipital.
 c. Fontanel.
  (1) Anterior, large fontanel (bregma) is located at the juncture of the coronal suture, sagittal suture, and frontal suture; diamond-shaped, closes at 12 to 18 months.
  (2) Posterior, or small fontanel—triangular space located at the junction of the sagittal and lambdoidal sutures; closes at approximately 2 to 3 months.
 d. Areas of the skull.
  (1) Occiput—lies behind small fontanel.
  (2) Vertex—lies between the anterior and posterior fontanels.
  (3) Bregma—area of the large fontanel.
  (4) Sinciput—the brow area.
2. Fetal attitude—relationship of the various parts of the fetal body to one another in utero; characteristic uterine posture is one of moderate flexion of the head, extremities on the abdomen and chest.
3. Fetal lie—relationship of the fetal axis to the maternal axis.
 a. Longitudinal lie—long axis of the fetal body is parallel to the long axis of the maternal body; vertex or breech presents; 99 percent of all lies.
 b. Transverse lie—long axis of the fetus is at right angles to the long axis of the mother; shoulder presentation is a serious obstetric complication.
4. Presentation and presenting parts—that part of the fetus that lies close to or has entered the true pelvis.
 a. Cephalic.
  (1) Most common (96 percent).
  (2) Usually vertex, head sharply flexed with chin near chest.
  (3) Face.
  (4) Brow.
 b. Breech (buttocks).
  (1) Complete breech or full breech presentation—legs flexed on thighs and thighs flexed on abdomen with buttocks and feet presenting.
  (2) Frank breech presentation—flexion of the hips and extension of the legs with buttocks presenting.
  (3) Footling—presentation of either single foot, both feet, or knee.
 c. Shoulder—most commonly seen with transverse lie.
5. Position—relationship of the landmark on the presenting part to a specific part of the maternal pelvis.
 a. Maternal pelvis divided into six segments—anterior, transverse, posterior segments on the right side; anterior, transverse, and posterior segments on the left side.
 b. Fetal landmarks—occiput (O) vertex presentation, mentum (M) in a face presentation, sacrum (S) in breech presentation, acromion process of the scapula (Sc) in a shoulder presentation.

Example: *LOA—left occiput anterior (very common); LSP—left sacrum posterior (frank breech); LSCA—left scapula anterior (shoulder presentation, transverse lie).*

6. Station of the presenting part-the relationship between the presenting part and the maternal ischial spines.
 a. Determined by rectal or vaginal examination.
 b. Engagement-presenting part has descended into the maternal pelvis to the level where its widest, largest diameter has passed through the pelvic inlet.
 c. Terms used to describe descent of the presenting part into the pelvis.
  (1) *Engagement* of the presenting part is when it has reached the level of the ischial spines (O station).
  (2) *Station* refers to the relationship of the presenting part to an imaginary line drawn be-

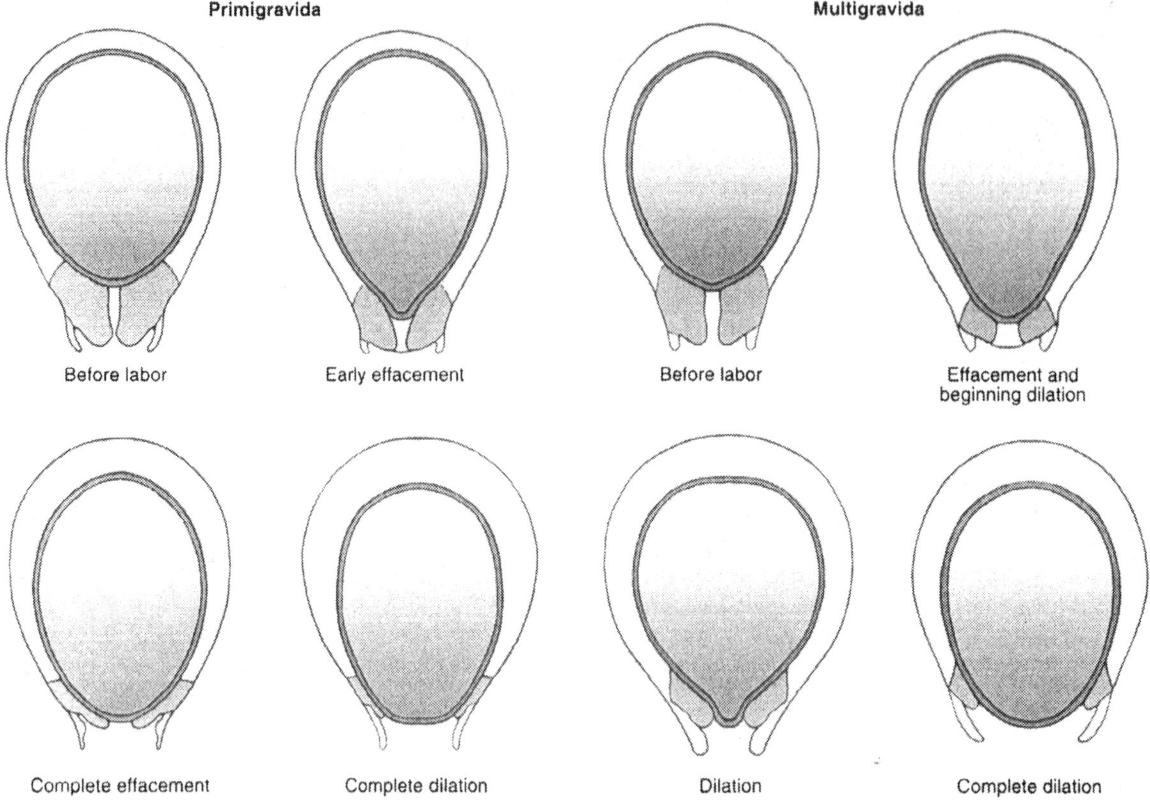

Figure 25-1: Cervical Dilatation and Effacement.
Reprinted with permission: Gorrie, TM, Mckinney, ES, & Murray, SS, (1998) *Foundations of Maternal-Newborn Nursing,* 2nd ed. Philadelphia: Saunders, p 272

tween the ischial spines of the maternal pelvis.

(3) *Floating* is when the presenting part is freely moveable about the pelvic inlet (-4,-3,-2,-1 stations).

***NURSING PRIORITY:** If presenting part is higher than the ischial spines, a negative number is assigned, noting centimeters above 0 station. As labor progresses, the presenting part moves from the negative stations to the midpelvis at 0 station into the positive stations (Sequence as follows: -5, -4, -3, -2, -1, 0, +1, +2, +3, +4,+5).*

B. The passage.

1. Types of pelvis.

a. Gynecoid-normal female pelvis; inlet is rounded.

b. Android-normal male pelvis; inlet is heart-shaped.

c. Anthropoid-inlet is oval.

d. Platypelloid-flat female pelvis; inlet is transverse oval.

2. Soft tissues.

a. Ability of the lower uterine segment to dilate and efface.

b. Ability of the vaginal canal to distend for delivery.

C. The powers—involuntary, intermittent contractions of the uterine muscle.

1. **Duration** of the contraction—the time between the first tightening sensation of the muscle and its subsequent complete relaxation.

2. **Frequency** of the contraction—time interval from the beginning of one contraction to the beginning of the next.

3. **Intensity** of the contraction—the firmness of the uterine muscle during the contraction.

4. Abdominal muscle contractions are the second power and during the second stage of labor push the fetus to the outside.

Assessment of the Labor Process

Maternal Assessment

1. Signs and symptoms *prior* to true labor.

a. Lightening—descent of the fetal head into the pelvis, experienced as "dropping" of the baby.

b. Increased vaginal mucous discharge.

c. Softening of the cervix.

d. Braxton-Hicks contractions may become uncomfortable, especially at night; discomfort is usually located in the abdomen.

e. Sudden burst of energy approximately 24 to 48 hours prior to labor.

f. Weight loss of 1 to 3 pounds; sometimes diarrhea, indigestion, nausea and vomiting.

g. Rupture of membranes.

(1) If rupture occurs before onset of labor, it is called premature rupture of the membranes.

(2) Delivery should occur within 24 hours, to decrease incidence of infection.

(3) Test with phenaphthazine (nitrazine) paper; amniotic fluid is alkaline—nitrazine paper turns blue; normal vaginal and urinary secretions are acidic.

2. Signs and symptoms of *true* labor.

a. Cervical dilatation and effacement (Figure 25-1).

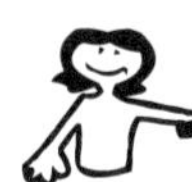

NURSING PRIORITY: *The two most important signs indicative of **true labor** are cervical dilatation and effacement.*

b. Contractions occur at regular intervals and increase in duration and intensity; intensity usually increases with walking (Figure 25-2).

c. Pain in the back which radiates around to the abdomen.

d. Bloody show—expulsion of the mucous plug; labor begins 24 to 48 hours after bloody show or bloody show may be observed at the onset of labor.

3. Mechanism of labor—sequence of passive movements of the presenting part as it moves through the birth canal.

a. Engagement.

b. Descent.

c. Flexion.

d. Internal rotation.

e. Extension.

f. External rotation—sometimes called restitution.

g. Expulsion.

4. Stages of labor.

a. First stage (stage of cervical dilatation)—begins with onset of regular contractions and ends with complete cervical dilatation and effacement, divided into phases—latent, active, transitional.

b. Second stage (stage of expulsion)—begins with complete cervical dilation and ends with delivery of the fetus.

c. Third stage (placental stage)—begins immediately after the fetus is born and ends when the placenta is delivered.

(1) Signs of placental separation—discoid to globular shape of uterus, gush of blood, lengthening of umbilical cord, and rise of uterine fundus.

d. Fourth stage (maternal homeostatic stabilization stage)—begins after the delivery of the placenta and continues for one to four hours after delivery.

Fetal Assessment

1. Determining fetal position by performing Leopold's maneuvers.

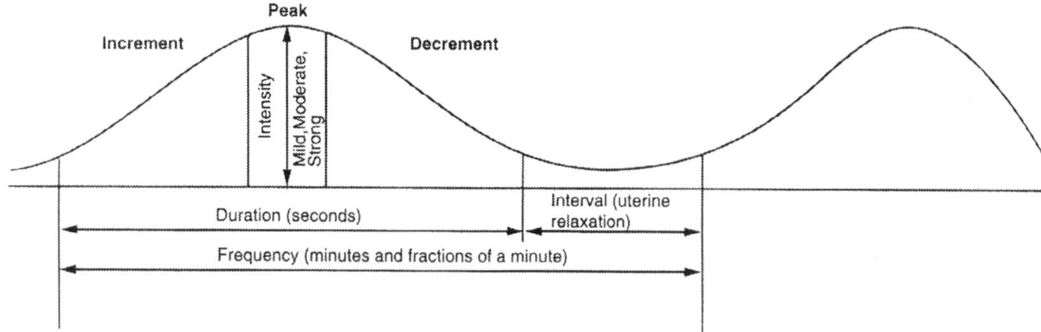

Figure 25-2: Labor Contraction Cycle
Reprinted with permission: Gorrie, TM, Mckinney, ES, & Murray, SS, (1998) *Foundations of Maternal-Newborn Nursing,* 2nd ed. Philadelphia: Saunders, p 270

Table 25-1: SUMMARY OF OBSERVATIONS AND NURSING CARE DURING LABOR

PHYSICAL FINDINGS	NURSING INTERVENTION
STAGE 1: **Latent Phase:**	
Cervical dilatation: 0 to 3 cm Cervical effacement in primipara is usually complete before dilatation; in multipara, it occurs with dilatation Duration of latent phase: 8 to 10 hours Uterine contractions are mild, 5 to 30 minutes apart, and last 10 to 30 seconds Membranes ruptured or intact Scant brown or pink vaginal discharge or mucous plug Station: primipara - usually 0; multipara -0 to -2 Fetal heart rates (FHR): clearest at level of or below umbilicus, dependent on fetal position	1. Orient to hospital environment and personnel. 2. Assess history and physical status. 3. Assess attitudes, past experiences, expectations. 4. Teach about labor. 5. Practice breathing and relaxation techniques. 6. Monitor physical status: Vital signs including FHR. 7. Voiding. 8. Amount and character of vaginal discharge. 9. Oral hygiene.
Active Phase:	
Cervical dilatation: 4 to 7 cm Duration of active phase: approximately 6 hours Uterine contractions are moderate, 3 to 5 minutes apart, and last 30 to 45 seconds Scant to moderate bloody mucus Station: 0 to +1 FHR: heard slightly below umbilicus or lower abdomen	1. Anticipate needs: Sponge face. Keep bed clean and dry. Care for dry, cracked mouth. Check bladder for fullness. 2. Stay at bedside working through each contraction with client; praise woman's efforts, point out progress. 3. Reinforce supportive efforts of the father. 4. Use touch to soothe, relax, comfort. 5. Check FHR q 15 min, B/P q 30 min. 6. Observe for hyperventilation. 7. May need analgesia to enhance coping.
Transition Phase:	
Cervical dilatation: 8 to 10 cm Duration of transition phase: 1 to 2 hours Uterine contractions of transition phase: strong, 2 to 3 minutes apart, and last 45 to 60 seconds Copious bloody mucus Station: +2 -+3 FHR: clearest directly about symphysis pubis	1. Continue physical and supportive care. 2. Use palpation or uterine contraction monitor to help patient define contractions and rest periods. 3. Observe perineum for bulging.

a. First maneuver—upper abdominal palpation to discover contents of uterine fundus.

b. Second maneuver—location of fetal back in relationship to right and left sides of mother, accomplished by sliding the hands down to a slightly lower position on sides of the abdomen.

c. Third maneuver—location of presenting part at pelvic inlet and determination as to whether the presenting part is floating or has engaged; spread hand is applied to the abdomen above the symphysis pubis; gentle palpation of the part of the fetus that lies between thumb and fingers.

d. Fourth maneuver—palpation in a downward and slightly inward direction, toward the pelvic inlet; done to determine how far the presenting part has descended into the pelvis.

2. Fetal heart rate monitoring.

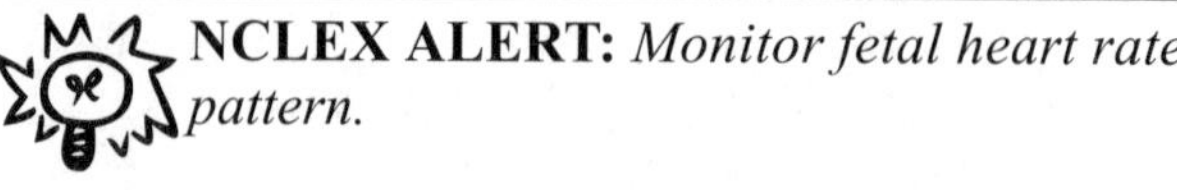

NCLEX ALERT: *Monitor fetal heart rate pattern.*

a. ***Fetoscope***—very common, inexpensive, easy-to-use method; does not give any information regarding contractions or periodic changes in FHR.

b. ***Doppler***—uses ultrasound; FHR can be heard as early as 10 to 12 weeks; no information is gathered regarding contractions or periodic changes in FHR.

c. ***External monitoring*** —a noninvasive procedure which utilizes high-frequency sound

Table 25-1: SUMMARY OF OBSERVATIONS AND NURSING CARE DURING LABOR

PHYSICAL FINDINGS	NURSING INTERVENTION
STAGE 2: **Expulsion of Fetus:**	
Cervical dilatation complete at 10 cm Cervical effacement 100% Duration of Stage 2: 20 to 50 minutes Uterine contractions are strong, 2 to 3 minutes apart, and last 60 to 90 seconds; fetal bradycardia during contraction may occur Membranes may rupture; copious bloody mucus Station: fetal descent continues at a rate of 1 cm/hr in primiparas and 2 cm or more in multiparas until perineal floor is reached Urge to push begins Perineum flattens, bulges Crowning occurs Infant is born	1. Direct pushing efforts with father for each contraction. 2. Provide comfort measures and facilitate rest between contractions: Cool cloth to face. Keep perineum clean and dry. 3. Encourage efforts; point out progress. 4. Explain preparations being made for delivery. 5. Check FHR with each contraction. 6. Help with panting for delivery of head and shoulders.  **NCLEX ALERT:** *Monitor client in labor.*
STAGE 3: **Expulsion of Placenta:**	
Usually within 5 to 10 minutes of delivery Uterine shape globular, usually firmer; fundus rises Dark vaginal bleeding - gush or trickle Umbilical cord protrudes further from introitus Placenta intact: shiny presentation of fetal side of placental separation occurs from inner to outer margins (Schultze mechanism); rough presentation of maternal side of placental separation occurs from outer margins inward (Duncan mechanism.)	1. Congratulate. 2. Initiate contact with infant. 3. Coach in relaxation for delivery of placenta and perineal repair. 4. May adminiser oxytocics after placenta has delivered. (Appendix 27-2)
STAGE 4:	
Fundus firm or becomes firm when massaged, in midline at level of umbilicus Moderate lochia rubra Episiotomy or laceration repair clean without ecchymosis or discharge, minimal edema; tenderness commensurate with analgesia, usually mild; edges well-approximated Possible extrusion of hemorrhoids	1. Facilitation of attachment - assure parents time with newborn, mother may initiate breast-feeding. 2. Ongoing assessment (q 15 min x 1 hr, then q 30 min x 2 hr) of vital signs, fundus, lochia, episiotomy and bladder function. 3. Encourage rest for both parents.

waves to detect FHR; transducer belt is held in place around maternal abdomen; monitor processes signal and prints heart rate on graphic record; advantage is its noninvasiveness; disadvantage is its being subject to half- and double-counting.

d. ***Internal monitoring*** —also called direct fetal monitoring; invasive, but provides accurate, continuous information using a stainless steel spiral electrode inserted into the fetal scalp, where it picks up electrical impulses from the fetal QRS complex; major disadvantage is membranes must be ruptured, which increases possibility of infection to mother and fetus.

3. Fetal scalp sampling - blood sample drawn from fetal scalp to assess acid-based status; pH 7.25 or above is considered normal.

Nursing Intervention During Labor and Delivery

Maternal

✦ *Goal: to monitor changes during each stage of labor (Table 25-1).*

✦ *Goal: to provide relief from pain and discomfort.*

1. Administer analgesic medication.

   a. Meperidine (**Demerol**).

      (1) Widely used.

Table 25-2: SUMMARY OF FHR PATTERNS

FHR PATTERN	CHARACTERISTICS/ PATHOPHYSIOLOGY	THERAPEUTIC INTERVENTION
BASELINE CHANGES:		
Tachycardia	*Baseline over 160 bpm or a rise of 10% of previous baseline. ***Pathophysiology***: Mild fetal hypoxia. Maternal fever. Maternal tachycardia. Fetal neurologic immaturity.	1. Monitor maternal vital signs. 2. Change maternal position. 2. Continue to watch closely.
Bradycardia	*Baseline under 120 bpm or a drop of 10% of previous baseline. ***Pathophysiology***:Congenital heart abnormalities. Fetal distress (when accompanied by periodic changes).	1. Inform neonatal personnel. 2. Change maternal position. 3. Administer oxygen to mother. 4. Prepare for immediate delivery.
Loss of variability	*Smooth baseline as recorded by *internal* fetal monitor. ***Pathophysiology***: Maternal medication. Fetal acidosis (especially if accompanied by late decelerations). Fetal neurologic immaturity.	1. Note time and dose of medication on record. 2. See "late decelerations" below.
PERIODIC CHANGES:		
Early deceleration	*Uniform shaped dip. Onset, maximal fall, and recovery coincides with onset, peak, and end of contraction. ***Pathophysiology***: Head compression.	1. Distinguish from late deceleration. 2. Observe mother for progress in labor, as these are usually indicative of cervical dilatation of 4 - 6 cm or more.
Late deceleration	*Uniform shaped dip. Onset coincides with peak of contraction with recovery occurring at the end or after the end of the contraction. ***Pathophysiology***: Uteroplacental insufficiency.	1. Correct underlying cause such as: Supine hypotension - change maternal position. Conduction anesthesia -elevate legs, increase hydration with IV fluids, apply elastic stockings or leg wraps. Uterine hyperactivity - reduce or discontinue dosage of oxytocin. 2. Left lateral position during labor. 3. Administer oxygen to mother. 4. Fetal scalp sampling. 5. Be prepared for operative delivery if fetal condition warrants.
Variable deceleration	*Variably shaped dip. Usually shaped like a V or a squared U. May occur any time during contraction cycle. May be nonrepetitive. ***Pathophysiology***: Cord compression.	1. Change maternal position. 2. If severe, lasting more than one minute - attempt upward displacement of presenting part; help mother into knee-chest or Trendelenburg position; prepare for immediate delivery if pattern does not improve. 3. Administer oxygen to mother.

(2) May cause nausea and vomiting in the mother and central nervous system depression in the fetus.

(3) Is not given when delivery is imminent.

NURSING PRIORITY: *Analgesics are generally administered to nulliparas when the cervix has dilated 5-6 cm and to multiparas when the cervix has dilated 3-4 cm.* ***Narcan*** *should be available in the delivery room to reverse the possible respiratory depression caused by narcotics.*

Table 25-3: APGAR SCORING SYSTEM

SIGN	0	1	2
Rate	Not detectable	Slow (below 100)	Over 100
Respiratory Effort	Absent	Slow, irregular	Good, crying
Muscle Tone	Flaccid, limp	Some flexions of extremities	Active motion
Reflex Irritability	No response	Grimace, extremities	Cough, sneeze, or cry
Color	Blue, pale	Body pink, extremities pale	Completely pink

b. Tranquilizers—diazepam (**Valium**), hydroxyzine (**Vistaril**), and promethazine (**Phenergan**).

(1) Are often given as adjuncts to analgesia to relieve tension and anxiety.

(2) May decrease maternal blood pressure and cause fetal central nervous system depression.

2. Assist with regional or general anesthesia (See Table 3-7 for nursing care).

a. Pudendal.

(1) Perineal anesthesia of short duration (30 minutes).

(2) Does not depress the fetus.

(3) May eliminate bearing-down reflex.

b. Paracervical.

(1) May be given in 1st stage of labor with good contractions and 3-8 cm dilation.

(2) May be repeated, or may be followed by other regional anesthesia.

(3) May cause temporary fetal bradycardia.

c. Epidural.

(1) Given in first and second stage of labor (can be administered at 4-6 cm in active phase.

(2) May cause maternal hypotension, labor dysfunction, and inability to push effectively.

(3) Onset of analgesia may be delayed from 20-30 minutes.

(4) Variability of FHR may decrease, which makes interpretation of FHR difficult.

Fetal

✦ *Goal: to monitor fetal status and detect early complications (Table 25-2).*

✦ *Goal: to provide immediate care to the normal newborn.*

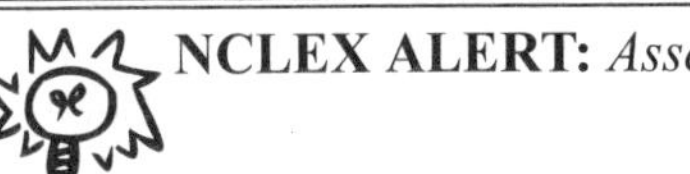

NCLEX ALERT: *Assess a newborn.*

1. Airway: clear air passages to establish respirations.
2. Body temperature: maintain warmth.
3. Apgar scoring: immediate appraisal of newborn's condition taken at 1 minute and again at 5 minutes (Table 25-3).

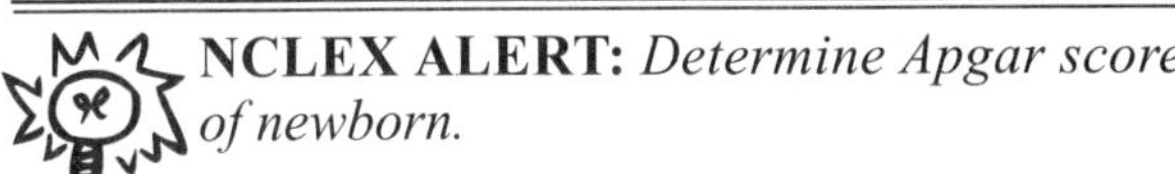

NCLEX ALERT: *Determine Apgar score of newborn.*

4. Care of the umbilical cord: clamped after pulsation ceases; examine for number of vessels and record (one umbilical artery indicates increased incidence of congenital anomalies, especially renal and genitourinary); no dressing is applied to cord.
5. Care of the eyes: prophylaxis against ophthalmia neonatorum; ophthalmic penicillin ointment, tetracycline, erythromycin, or instillation of 1 percent silver nitrate solution.
6. Identification: wristbands fastened to both infant and mother, and appropriate footprints and fingerprints are taken.
7. Administration of vitamin K (**Aqua-mephyton**): 0.5 mg to 1.0 mg IM injected into the upper outer aspect of the thigh for prevention of neonatal hemorrhagic disease due to lack of *E. coli*, necessary for the synthesis of vitamin K in the intestines.
8. Inspection for gross abnormalities: clubfoot, imperforate anus, birthmarks, etc.

9. Attachment: provide contact of newborn with mother as soon as possible after birth.

OPERATIVE OBSTETRICS

Episiotomy

❑ **An episiotomy is an incision through the perineal body to facilitate delivery by enlarging the vaginal orifice.**

Types

A. Median—midline.
  1. Easy to repair; heals well.
  2. Increased chance of extension through the rectal sphincter muscle (3rd, 4th degree laceration).

B. Mediolateral—made at a 45° angle on either right or left side.
  1. More painful healing; increased blood loss.
  2. Less risk of extension into sphincter ani muscle.

Assessment

A. Observe perineal site for bleeding, swelling, redness, or any discharge.

B. Evaluate for pain and discomfort; should be minimal discomfort for episiotomy; pain may indicate hematoma or abscess formation.

Nursing Intervention

✦ *Goal: to alleviate pain and swelling and promote comfort.*
  1. Ice pack (first eight hours; leave in place at 20 minute intervals); later followed by hot sitz baths, peri light (heat lamp treatment for 20 minutes, 3 to 4 times per day).
  2. Analgesic sprays, ointments, or foam as ordered.
  3. Teach importance of perineal cleansing (i.e., use of the spray bottle; direct flow from front to back; and change perineal pad after each elimination).

Forceps Delivery

❑ **Forceps delivery is the use of an instrument to extract the fetal head during delivery.**

Types

A. Low or outlet forceps—fetal head has reached the perineal floor.

B. Mid-forceps—head is at or below the level of the ischial spine.

C. Piper forceps—used in breech deliveries.

Indications

A. Fetal conditions—distress, prolapsed cord, premature separation of placenta.

B. Maternal conditions—heart disease, acute pulmonary edema, exhaustion, or infection.

Assessment

A. Determine criteria for forceps delivery.
  1. Head fully engaged.
  2. Complete dilatation of the cervix.
  3. Membranes have ruptured.
  4. Empty bowel and bladder.

B. Monitor fetal heart rate, as forceps may compress umbilical cord.

Nursing Interventions

✦ *Goal: to assist with forceps delivery.*
  1. Provide physician with type of forceps required.
  2. Assess for conditions necessitating forceps application.

✦ *Goal: to briefly explain procedure to couple.*
  1. Monitor fetal heart rate.
  2. Provide emotional support.

✦ *Goal: to detect complications for forceps application.*
  1. Maternal: lacerations to birth canal and rectum.
  2. Fetal: cephalhematoma, lacerations and bruising to face, facial paralysis, skull fracture, umbilical cord compression, and brain damage.

Cesarean Birth

❑ **An incision into the abdominal and uterine walls to deliver the fetus.**

Types

A. Low-segment transverse incision.
  1. Preferred and most common method.
  2. Decreased blood loss; less chance of uterine rupture with subsequent pregnancy as incision is made into lower uterine segment.
  3. Fewer complications—peritonitis and postoperative adhesions.

B. Classic cesarean incision.
  1. Used in cases of placenta previa when there are adhesions in the lower uterine segment or transverse fetal lie.
  2. Vertical incision is made between the umbilicus and symphysis pubis.

Indications

A. Maternal.
  1. Uterine dystocia.
  2. Preexisting maternal disease—heart disease, diabetes, genital herpes, gonorrhea.
  3. Severe preeclampsia and eclampsia.

4. Previous cesarean birth or surgery on the uterus.
5. Tumors of the uterus.
6. Postterm pregnancy.
7. Placenta previa and abruptio placentae.

B. Fetal.
1. Fetal distress.
2. Prolapsed cord.
3. Fetal abnormalities (e.g. hydrocephalus).

Assessment

A. Assess for possible indication for cesarean birth.

B. "Once a section always a section"—trend is to examine the condition surrounding the previous or original section; often if original section was in lower uterine segment, a trial labor may be recommended.

C. Cesarean may be planned for a specific date or may occur as an emergency procedure; common elective reasons are previous repeat cesarean section, breech presentation, or cephalopelvic disproportion.

Nursing Intervention

✦ *Goal: to provide preoperative preparation.*
1. Preparation is similar to any abdominal surgery operation.

✦ *Goal: to provide postoperative care.*
1. Cesarean birth includes both normal abdominal postoperative care and postpartum care.

Induction of labor

Indications

A. Presence of preexisting maternal disease: diabetes mellitus, hypertension, and renal disease.

B. Premature rupture of membranes, postterm pregnancy.

C. Hemolytic disease, fetal death, congenital anomaly, (i.e., anencephaly).

D. Elective.

Procedure

A. Aminotomy—artificial rupture of membranes (bag of water [AROM]); often labor begins spontaneously.

B. Oxytocin (**Pitocin**) is administered intravenously with physician in attendance.
1. Oxytocin is always piggybacked to a primary line in case it needs to be discontinued and hooked up to an infusion pump.
2. Oxytocin is administered by slow IV drip with the use of a continuous infusion pump, as it gives an accurate, constant rate.
3. Nursing management and information regarding **Pitocin** is covered in Appendix 25-2.

C. Prostaglandin (PGE_2) gel (inserted vaginally to soften cervix).

Assessment

A. Careful assessment of uterine contractions is priority; tetanic contractions could result in uterine rupture, premature separation of placenta and fetal hypoxia.

B. Fetal heart rate (FHR) check q 15 minutes along with mother's vital signs.

Nursing Intervention

✦ *Goal: to monitor and evaluate uterine response and fetal response to induction.*
1. Frequent vital sign checks and FHR (q 15 minutes); indirect or direct fetal monitoring may be used.
2. Discontinue **Pitocin** infusion if:
   a. Contractions are more frequent than every 2 minutes.
   b. Contraction duration exceeds 75 to 90 seconds.
   c. Uterus does not relax; remains contracted and tetanic.
   d. Fetal distress occurs.

✦ *Goal: to provide basic intrapartal nursing care as previously outlined in Table 25-1.*

EMERGENCY DELIVERY BY THE NURSE

A. The most important aspect of nursing care is for the nurse to remain calm and support the mother; the delivery process *cannot* be stopped.

B. *Never* force or hold back the oncoming fetal head.

C. As the head appears in the vaginal introitus, the nurse should apply gentle, even pressure with the hand on the emerging head to slow down the baby's process through the birth canal and to protect the mother's perineum from lacerations.

D. If the membranes have not ruptured when the head is delivered, they should be broken immediately to minimize aspiration of amniotic fluid.

E. Support the head after it is delivered, it will drop towards the mother's rectum and external rotation (restitution) will take place.

F. Check around the neck of the infant for the umbilical cord. If found around the infant's neck, gently slip it over the head.

G. Hold infant's head between the palms of both hands, and with a gentle downward motion, the anterior shoulder can be brought under the symphysis pubis.

Table 25-4: NURSING MANAGEMENT OF HEMORRHAGE IN THE PREGNANT CLIENT

CAUSES AND SOURCES	SYMPTOMS	NURSING INTERVENTIONS
ANTEPARTAL PERIOD:		
Abortion	Vaginal bleeding Intermittent uterine contractions Rupture of the membranes	1. Obtain history of onset, duration, amount of bleeding, and associated symptoms. 2. Observe perineal pads for amount of bleeding (blood loss can be measured by weighing perineal pads, approximately 1gm = 1ml blood). 3. Monitor vital signs of mother and fetus(frequency is determined by severity of clinical symptoms).
Placenta previa	Painless vaginal bleeding after the 7th month	
Abruptio placentae	Vaginal bleeding Extreme tenderness in abdomen Rigid, board-like abdomen Increase in size of the abdomen	**NCLEX ALERT:** *Recognize the occurrence of hemorrhage and assess new mother for complications.*
INTRAPARTAL PERIOD:		
Placenta previa	Bright vaginal bleeding	1. Insert IV and provide volume replacement. 2. Request type and crossmatch for blood. 3. Administer fluids and blood as prescribed. 4. Monitor intake and output. 5. Minimize chances for further bleeding 6. *NO* vaginal or rectal exams. 7. Bedrest in position of comfort. 8. Anticipate delivery by cesarean section.
Abruptio placentae	Symptoms same as above	
Uterine atony in stage III	Bright red vaginal bleeding Ineffectual contractility	
POSTPARTAL PERIOD:		
Uterine atony	Boggy uterus	1. Massage fundus of uterus and anticipate oxytocin medication for uterine atony client. 2. Reduce anxiety. 3. Keep woman and family advised of treatment plan. 4. Record amount of bleeding in a specific amount of time. 5. Monitor VS—overt hypotension and shock will not be seen until the woman has lost almost one third of her blood volume (1500-2000mL); watch for tachycardia and orthostatic BP changes first.
Retained placental fragments	Dark vaginal bleeding Presence of clots	
Lacerations of cervix or vagina	Firm uterus Bright red blood	
		NURSING PRIORITY: *Frequent, accurate assessment and documentation of blood loss is a priority in postpartum care; two-thirds of postpartum hemorrhage occurs without any predisposing risk factors.*

Then with a gentle upward motion the posterior shoulder can be delivered.

H. The rest of the body follows easily.

I. Immediately position with head dependent to facilitate clearing of the airway passages; if no spontaneous cry or respirations.

J. Keep infant warm by placing on mother's abdomen, skin to skin, then cover both with a warm dry blanket.

K. Palpate the uterus and assist in the delivery of the placenta.

L. Transfer both as soon as possible to a hospital facility; it is *not* necessary to hasten to cut and tie the umbilical cord unless there is sterile equipment available.

COMPLICATIONS ASSOCIATED WITH LABOR AND DELIVERY

Premature Labor

❑ ***Premature labor* is defined as labor occurring prior to thirty-seven weeks' gestation.**

Assessment

A. Risk factors.
  1. Maternal infection.
  2. Multiple gestations.
  3. Polyhydramnios.
  4. Hypertension.
  5. Third-trimester bleeding.
  6. Premature rupture of the membranes (PROM)—bag of water ruptures prior to the onset of labor.
  7. Incompetent cervical os.

B. Clinical manifestations.
  1. Contractions occurring in increasing frequency and intensity.
  2. Premature rupture of the membranes.

Treatment

A. Medications (Appendix 25-3).
  1. Tocolytics.
  2. Prostaglandin synthetase inhibitors.

Nursing Intervention

✦ *Goal: to assist in delivery if maternal complications are present.*
  1. Maternal complications—diabetes, pre-eclampsia, hemorrhage.
  2. Prepare for delivery of premature infant—if indicated, administer betamethasone (**Celestone**) to prevent respiratory distress syndrome in the newborn.
    a. Most effective if delivery is delayed forty-eight hours after administration.
    b. Do not administer if there is an adequate L/S ratio or in the presence of maternal diabetes, infection, hypertension, or if gestational age is greater than thirty-four weeks.
    c. Administered IM.

✦ *Goal: to provide emotional support.*
  1. Encourage expression of feelings related to anxiety and guilt.
  2. Identify and support coping mechanisms for couple.

✦ *Goal: to minimize fetal complications.*
  1. Promote fetal oxygenation.
    a. Avoid supine position during labor—risk of venocaval syndrome.
    b. Avoid maternal hyperventilation—leads to maternal alkalosis, which may decrease oxygen to fetus.
  2. Avoid respiratory distress in the newborn.
    a. Conduct labor with minimal analgesia or anesthesia.
    b. Assist with breathing techniques and provide support to the laboring woman.

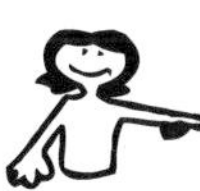

***NURSING PRIORITY:** Encourage left lateral Sims' position—promotes placental perfusion.*

Dystocia

Assessment

A. Types of uterine dysfunction.
  1. Prolonged or arrested labor—labor lasting for more than twenty-four hours after onset of regular contractions.
    a. Maternal complications: intrauterine infection, postpartum hemorrhage, fatigue, exhaustion, and dehydration.
    b. Fetal complications: fetal distress and infection.
  2. Precipitous delivery—a very rapid, intense labor of two to four hours duration.
    a. Maternal complications: trauma to the soft tissues of the cervix, vagina, and perineum, and loss of self-control.
    b. Fetal complications: fetal hypoxia.
  3. Hypotonic contractions—slow, infrequent, weak contractions occurring more than three minutes apart and lasting less than forty seconds.
    a. Causes—uterine overdistention due to large fetus or twins, polyhydramnios, and grandmultiparity.
    b. Complications—relate to prolonged or arrested labor.
  4. Hypertonic contractions—frequent, strong, painful contractions occurring two to three minutes apart, lasting sixty seconds or more.
    a. Occur more frequently in latent phase of labor.
    b. Cause: cephalopelvic disproportion (CPD) or abnormal fetal position.
    c. Tetanic contractions—uterus stays contracted for more than ninety seconds; often due to misuse of oxytocin, or mechanical obstruction.
    d. Maternal complications—exhaustion, excessive pain, and uterine rupture.
    e. Fetal complications—fetal distress.

B. Cephalopelvic disproportion (CPD)—disproportion between the size of the fetus and that of the birth canal.
  1. Usually due to a contracted pelvis—structure of the bony birth canal may delay the process of labor.
  2. Types of pelvic contractions.

a. Inlet contraction—most often is due to rickets (vitamin D deficiency).

b. Midpelvic contraction—usually prolongs labor; may need to use forceps for delivery.

c. Outlet contraction—usually a forceps delivery and often a mediolateral episiotomy to facilitate delivery.

3. Excessive size of fetus—maternal pelvis may not accommodate fetal head.

a. Fetus weighing over 4,500 gm (10 lb)—fetal macrosomatia occurring in diabetic women and postmaturity.

b. Hydrocephalus.

c. Fetal malformations—abdominal distention, incomplete twinning.

C. Faulty presentation.

1. Persistent occiput position.

2. Face, brow, or breech presentation.

3. Transverse lie—shoulder presentation.

Treatment

A. Mechanical dystocia relating to CPD, or faulty presentation, is treated by a cesarean delivery.

B. Hypotonic uterine contractions or prolonged labor is treated by administration of **Pitocin** IV.

C. Hypertonic uterine contractions are treated by sedation and rest.

Nursing Intervention

✦ *Goal: to monitor level of fatigue and ability to cope with pain.*

1. Provide basic comfort measures, back rubs, change of position, clean dry linen.

2. Provide emotional support to mother and significant other.

3. Give reassurance and stay with client continually.

✦ *Goal: to assist in the medical management of dystocia.*

1. Explain procedures to rule out cause of dystocia—sonogram, X-ray studies, etc.

2. Monitor **Pitocin** if indicated for hypotonic dysfunction or prolonged labor.

3. Prepare client for cesarean delivery (indicated in CPD and faulty presentation).

4. Administer broad-spectrum antibiotics to decrease incidence of infection.

5. Maintain hydration, monitor intake and output, and administer oxygen if indicated.

✦ *Goal: to detect early complications associated with dystocia.*

1. Monitor maternal vital signs.

2. Assess mother for signs of exhaustion, dehydration, increasing temperature, and acidosis.

3. Assess fetal heart tones frequently through fetal electronic monitoring.

Supine Hypotensive Syndrome

❑ **Supine hypotensive syndrome or venocaval syndrome occurs when the weight of the uterus causes partial occlusion of the vena cava, leading to decreased venous return to the heart.**

Assessment

A. Shock-like symptoms seen when pregnant woman assumes a supine position.

B. Risk factors: nullipara with strong abdominal muscles, gravidas with polyhydramnios or multiple pregnancies and obese women.

Nursing Intervention

✦ *Goal: to decrease supine hypotensive syndrome episode.*

1. Educate mother to turn to left side; preferred position because pressure is removed from vena cava.

2. Administer oxygen if needed.

3. Assess fetal heart rates.

NCLEX ALERT: *Recognize occurrence of a hemorrhage. It is important to be able to plan nursing management for the pregnant client who has bleeding or hemorrhage (See Table 25-4). General nursing diagnoses for the hemorrhaging client are included.*

Placenta Previa

❑ ***Placenta previa* is the abnormal implantation of placenta in the lower uterine segment; it occurs in less than 1 percent of all pregnancies.**

Assessment

A. Types of placenta previa.

1. Complete—placental totally covers internal cervical os.

2. Partial—placenta only partially covers internal cervical os.

3. Marginal, or low-lying—placenta approaches rim of internal os but does not cover it.

B. Diagnostic.

1. Ultrasonography—ascertains position of placenta.

2. Ultrasound is repeated usually during the third trimester because of the so-called migrating placenta phenomenon—the placenta gives the illusion of moving up in the uterus.

C. Clinical manifestations.

1. *Painless, bright red vaginal bleeding* beginning in the seventh month.
2. Bleeding may stop spontaneously and reoccur without warning during labor and delivery.

Treatment

A. Medical—if gestation is less than thirty-seven weeks, a conservative management of rest, and monitoring status of hemoglobin and hematocrit.

B. Surgical—if fetus is mature, delivery via cesarean section (possible vaginal delivery for marginal placenta previa if bleeding is not excessive).

Nursing Intervention

✦ *Goal: to provide nursing care associated with hemorrhage (Table 25-4).*

✦ *Goal: to detect complications associated with placenta previa.*

1. Increased risk for postpartum hemorrhage due to friable, fragile lower uterine segment.
2. Uterine rupture.

Abruptio Placentae

❑ ***Abruptio placentae* is the premature separation of a normally implanted placenta, leading to hemorrhage.**

Assessment

A. Types of abruptio placentae.

1. External—blood escapes from the vagina with separation of the placenta.
2. Concealed or internal—hemorrhage occurs within the uterine cavity.
3. Partial separation—may occur with external bleeding or be associated with concealed bleeding.
4. Complete separation—most severe, with profound symptoms of shock.

B. Risk factors.

1. Pregnancy-induced hypertension.
2. Trauma.
3. Polyhydramnios.
4. Multiple pregnancies and increased parity of mother.

C. Clinical manifestations.

1. Hemorrhage.
2. Board-like abdomen.
3. Cramp-like abdominal pain.
4. Hypovolemic shock.
5. Coagulation problems-hypofibrinogenemia.

Treatment

A. Medical—treatment of blood loss and shock; prior to surgery, type and crossmatch for blood transfusion.

B. Surgical—emergency cesarean delivery.

Nursing Intervention

✦ *Goal: to provide nursing management associated with hemorrhage (See Table 25-4).*

✦ *Goal: to detect early complications.*

1. Disseminated intravascular coagulation (DIC)—occurs as a result of concealed uterine hemorrhage and damage to the uterine wall leading to large amounts of thromboplastin released into the maternal bloodstream which leads to hypofibrinogememia.
   a. Assess for indications of DIC—bleeding from injection sites, epistaxis, bleeding gums, purpura, and petechiae.
   b. For ↓ platelet and fibrinogen levels—administer packed red cells, frozen plasma, and cryoprecipitate.
   c. Administration of heparin (to decrease thrombin generation and activity) is controversial for obstetric client.
2. Hypovolemic shock—fluid volume loss due to hemorrhage, concealed or apparent; monitor vital signs and perineal area.
3. Couvelaire uterus—bleeding into the myometrium, which causes the uterine muscle to lose its power to contract; hysterectomy is usually indicated.

Ruptured Uterus

❑ **A *ruptured uterus* is characterized by a tearing or splitting of the uterine wall during labor; it is usually a result of a thinned or weakened area that cannot withstand the strain and force of uterine contractions.**

Assessment

A. Risk factors.

1. Multiparity.
2. Obstructive labor.
3. Improper use of **Pitocin**.
4. Large fetus.
5. Weakened, old cesarean section scar.
6. External forces such as trauma.

B. Clinical manifestations.

NURSING PRIORITY: *Monitor the following warning signs of impending uterine rupture: restlessness and anxiety, no indication of labor progress, ballooning out of the lower uterine segment (which simulates a full bladder), appearance of a pathologic retraction ring (an indentation across the lower abdominal wall with acute tenderness above the symphysis pubis).*

1. Pain above the symphysis pubis.
2. Sudden, acute abdominal pain during a contraction.
3. Vaginal bleeding, shock; fetal distress.

Treatment

A. Surgical—laparotomy to remove fetus followed by a hysterectomy.

B. Medical.

1. Blood transfusions.
2. Prophylactic antibiotics.

Nursing Intervention

✦ *Goal: to provide nursing management associated with hemorrhage (Table 25-4).*

✦ *Goal: to assess for early diagnosis.*

1. Maternal mortality is high.
2. Prognosis for fetus is poor; usually dies due to anoxia caused by placental separation.

Amniotic Fluid Embolism

❑ **This problem occurs when amniotic fluid enters the maternal circulation through open venous sinuses in the placenta, at an area of placental separation, or through cervical tears under pressure from the contracting uterus. The fluid travels to the maternal pulmonary arterioles; prognosis is poor, and mortality is extremely high for the mother.**

Assessment

A. Risk factors.

1. Increased incidence in multiparas.
2. Increased incidence in a difficult, rapid labor.

B. Clinical manifestations.

1. Sudden respiratory distress (dyspnea, cyanosis, pulmonary edema).
2. Profound shock and vascular collapse.
3. Decreased fibrinogen (hypofibrinogenemia) and DIC.

Treatment

A. Medical-management is similar to pulmonary embolism.

1. Medications: fibrinogen replacement and intravenous heparin.
2. Insertion of CVP line, blood transfusions, and cardiopulmonary resuscitation as indicated.

Nursing Management

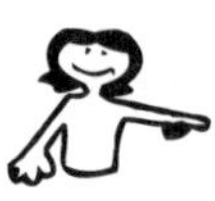

NURSING PRIORITY: *The nurse needs to be particularly observant for symptoms of amniotic fluid embolus in any client who has had a short or difficult labor.*

✦ *Goal: to assist in emergency resuscitation and provide critical care.*

1. Assist with ventilation.
2. Prepare for CVP insertion.
3. Administer medications and blood to treat DIC and shock.

✦ *Goal: to provide emotional support to father and significant others.*

Abnormal Fetal Position

Assessment

A. Occiput-posterior position (most common).

1. Dysfunctional labor pattern.
2. Prolonged active phase of labor.
3. Intense back pain.

B. Breech presentation.

1. Increased incidence with premature birth, placenta previa, polyhydramnios, multiple pregnancies, and grand multiparity.
2. FHRs usually auscultated above the umbilicus.
3. Often, passage of meconium is seen.
4. Increased danger of prolapsed umbilical cord, especially in incomplete breech presentation.

C. Transverse lie (shoulder presentation).

1. Increased incidence with placenta previa, neoplasms, fetal anomalies, and preterm labor.
2. Dysfunctional labor patterns are seen.

Treatment

A. Occiput-posterior position.

1. Vaginal delivery is possible; forceps may be needed.
2. If CPD is present, cesarean delivery is necessary.

B. Breech presentation.

1. Cesarean delivery is most often performed.
2. Vaginal delivery; for a frank breech, use of Piper forceps to assist in the extraction of the aftercoming head.

C. Transverse lie (shoulder presentation).

1. Cesarean delivery is the treatment of choice.
2. External version and extraction may be attempted.
   a. No presence of CPD.
   b. BOW intact.
   c. Fetus moveable and contractions mild.

Nursing Intervention

✦ *Goal: to provide reassurance and explanations of procedures as indicated.*
1. Explanation of possible cesarean delivery.
2. In occiput-posterior position-encourage positioning on the side or in a modified knee-chest to decrease pressure on the sacral nerves.
3. Assess for complications relating to prolonged labor and possible infection.

Multiple Pregnancy

Assessment

A. Risk factors.
   1. Increased incidence of dizygotic twinning (fraternal twins) dependent on race, heredity, advanced maternal age, and parity.
   2. Maternal risks.
      a. Spontaneous abortions are more common.
      b. Anemia occurs.
      c. Increased incidence of PIH, abruptio placentae, placenta previa, and polyhydraminos.

B. Diagnostics.
   1. Auscultation of two fetal heart tones.
   2. Measurement of fundal height exceeds gestational age.
   3. Sonography.

C. Clinical manifestations.
   1. Increased experience of more physical discomfort-shortness of breath, dyspnea on exertion, backaches, and leg edema due to excessive size of uterus.
   2. Complications occurring during labor include:
      a. Uterine dysfunction due to overstretched uterus.
      b. Abnormal fetal presentations.
      c. Preterm labor.

Treatment

A. Medical.
   1. Bedrest in lateral position to treat hypertension.
   2. Antiemetic for nausea and vomiting past the first trimester.

B. Dietary-increase of three hundred calories along with increased protein, iron, folic acid, and vitamin supplements.

C. Serial ultrasound to evaluate for IUGR.

D. NST starting at 30-34 weeks, usually done every 3-7 days till delivery.

Nursing Intervention

✦ *Goal: to provide anticipatory guidance during the antepartal period.*
1. Second trimester-prenatal visits every two weeks.
2. Third trimester-weekly visits if there are no complications.
3. Discourage travel, as labor may begin without warning.

✦ *Goal: to provide psychological support.*
1. Often, twin births are undiagnosed at the time of labor.
2. Provide assistance and advice regarding care of twins at home.
3. Since the twins are apt to be small, anticipate nursing care for a premature neonate.
4. Assess for maternal complications (e.g., postpartum hemorrhage).
5. Ensure correct identification, Baby A and Baby B.

Prolapsed Cord

❑ **A *prolapsed cord* is the washing down of the cord in front of the presenting part.**

Assessment

A. Risk factors.
   1. Shoulder presentations.
   2. Footling breech presentations.
   3. Increased incidence with prematurity (due to small size of fetus).

B. Clinical manifestations.
   1. Commonly occurs following rupture of the membranes.
   2. Cord is washed through the birth canal with a gush of amniotic fluid.
   3. Visualization of the cord—FHR is decreased, with variable decelerations noted.

Treatment

A. Medical.
   1. Insert a gloved finger into the vagina and lift the fetal head off the cord to relieve the pressure.
   2. Administer oxygen to the mother; initiate bladder filling; start an IV.
   3. Place in knee-chest position or in Trendelenburg position (head of bed or table is lowered).
   4. Any prolapsed cord outside the vagina should be kept moistened with a saline soaked gauze.

B. Surgical.

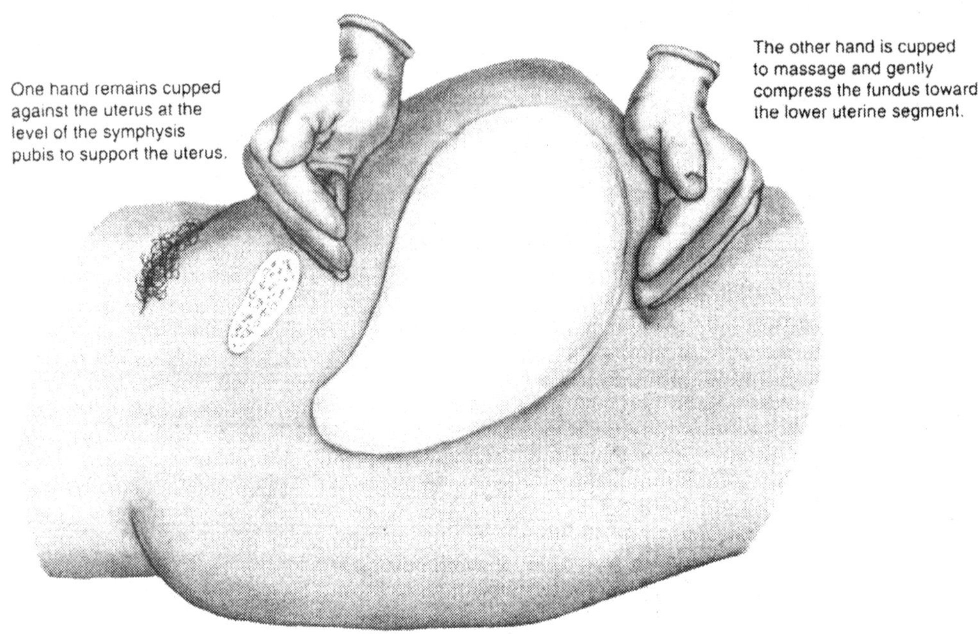

Figure 25-3: Technique for Fundal Massage
Reprinted with permission: Gorrie, TM, Mckinney, ES, & Murray, SS, (1998) *Foundations of Maternal-Newborn Nursing,* 2nd ed. Philadelphis: Saunders, p 579

1. If incomplete dilatation, cesarean delivery necessary.
2. Occasionally, if dilatation is complete, vaginal delivery possible.

Nursing Intervention

✦ *Goal: to maintain fetal oxygenation and assist with immediate delivery.*

1. Continuing assessment of FHR.
2. Maintain woman in one of the positions described previously to alleviate compression of the cord.
3. Offer emotional support to the couple.

Severely Depressed Neonate

❑ **A neonate with hypoxia and significant acidosis is a *severely depressed neonate* (Apgar score is 0 to 6).**

Assessment

A. Risk factors.

1. Preexisting maternal disease—diabetes, hypertension, preeclampsia.
2. Placental insufficiency due to:
   a. Maternal hypotension, hypertension, or hemorrhage.
   b. Umbilical cord compression.
   c. Polyhydramnios.
   d. Postmaturity.
3. Rh isoimmunization disease.
4. Uterine dystocia.

B. Clinical manifestations.

NCLEX ALERT: *Initiate actions in response to signs and symptoms of fetal distress. During fetal monitoring indications of fetal distress are often late or severe variable decelerations, lack of variability, and progressive acceleration in the FHR baseline.*

1. Severe hypoxia and acidosis.
2. Pale, flaccid, apneic neonate.
3. Heart rate less than one hundred beats per minute.
4. Slightly reactive or unresponsive to stimulation.

Treatment

A. Medical.

1. Administration of oxygen, possibly **Narcan** to reverse narcotic respiratory depression.
2. Laryngoscopy and airway suctioning; administration of oxygen.

3. Cardiopulmonary resuscitation as indicated.
4. Insertion of an umbilical artery catheter (UAC); administration of glucose to alleviate hypoglycemia and calcium gluconate to alleviate hypocalcemia.

Nursing Intervention

✦ *Goal: to identify and initiate treatment quickly in the severely depressed neonate.*

1. Assess for fetus at risk.
2. Initiate resuscitation procedures.

Intrauterine Fetal Death

❑ **Also called fetal demise.**

Assessment

A. Absent FHRs and movement.
B. Decrease in the size and tenderness of the woman's breast.
C. Negative pregnancy test and decreased maternal estriol level.
D. Diagnosis: ultrasound determines absence of FHR and occurence of fetal skull collapse.
E. Monitor for complications: hypofibrinogenemia from fetal breakdown products.

Nursing Intervention

✦ *Goal: to support the couple through the grieving process.*

1. Objectively listen; encourage expression of feelings; do not minimize the situation or event.
2. Anticipate the steps of the grieving process (denial, anger, bargaining, depression, and acceptance).
3. Provide the opportunity for the couple to spend time with the stillborn infant, if they so desire.
4. Prepare the parents to return home by providing ways to inform the siblings, other family members, and friends about the death.
5. Offer information regarding resource or support groups for parents who have lost an infant.
6. Monitor for complications.

POSTPARTAL ASSESSMENT

NCLEX ALERT: *Assess client for post partal complications. The puerperium is the period of time spanning the first six weeks following delivery. It is often referred to as the "fourth trimester." It is the period of time in which the body adjusts both physically and psychologically to the process of childbearing.*

Physiological Changes

A. Uterus.
1. Uterine involution-process by which the uterus returns to its normal prepregnant condition.
2. Immediately after delivery, top of fundus is several finger breadths above the umbilicus.
3. Twelve hours after delivery fundus of uterus is one finger breadth above umbilicus.
4. Fundus recedes/descends into the pelvis approximately one finger breadth per day.
5. By day ten, fundus is below the symphysis pubis and not palpable.
6. Afterpains-alternate contraction and relaxation of the uterine muscle.
   a. Occur primarily in multiparas.
   b. May be severe, requiring analgesics.
   c. Usually subside in forty-eight hours.
7. Lochia.

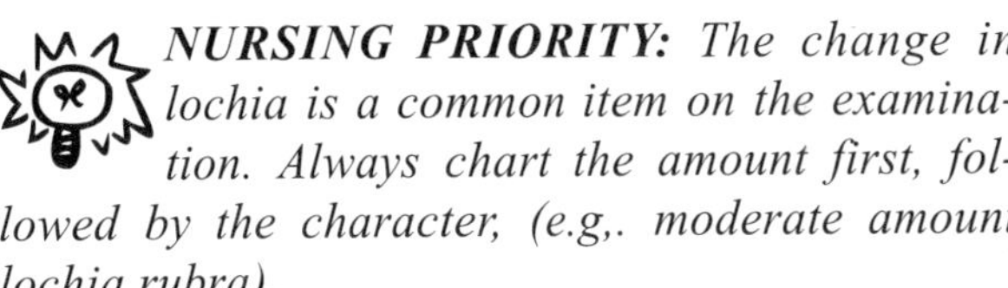

NURSING PRIORITY: *The change in lochia is a common item on the examination. Always chart the amount first, followed by the character, (e.g,. moderate amount lochia rubra).*

   a. Lochia rubra—dark red discharge; occurs the first three days.
   b. Lochia serosa—pinkish, serosanguinous discharge; lasts approximately three to ten days.
   c. Lochia alba—creamy or yellowish discharge; occurs after the tenth day and may last a week or two.
   d. When lochia subsides, uterus is considered closed; postpartal infection less likely.

B. Cervix.
1. May be stretched and swollen.
2. Small lacerations may be apparent.
3. External os closes slowly; end of first week, the opening is fingertip size.

C. Vagina.
1. Does not return to its original prepregnant state.
2. Rugae reappear in three weeks.
3. Labia majora and minora are more flabby.

D. Perineum.
1. May be bruised and tender.
2. Pelvic floor and ligaments are stretched.
3. Muscle tone is restored by Kegel exercises.

E. Ovulation and menstruation.
1. Non-breast-feeding women.
   a. Menstruation resumes in six weeks.

b. Ovulation—50 percent may ovulate during the first cycle.

2. Lactating women.

a. Varies.

b. 45 percent resume menstruation within twelve weeks after delivery.

F. Abdomen.

1. Soft and flabby.

2. Possible separation of the abdominal wall—diastasis recti.

3. Muscle tone can be restored within two to three months with exercise.

G. Breasts.

1. Anterior pituitary releases prolactin, which stimulates secretion of milk.

2. Engorgement may occur approximately thirty-six to forty-eight hours after delivery.

3. Colostrum released—thin, yellowish fluid.

a. Contains antibodies (IgA is 90% of the immunoglobulin present) along with more protein, fat-soluble vitamins (E, A, K), and more minerals such as sodium and zinc.

b. Colostrum has a laxative effect on the newborn, promotes expulsion of bilirubin-laden meconium.

c. Also encourages the colonization of the intestine with *Lactobacillus bifidus* which are bacteria that inhibit the growth of pathogenic bacteria, fungi, and parasites. The *bifudus* factor can be interfered with by food supplements given to the newborn in the first few days of life.

H. Gastrointestinal system.

1. Immediately after delivery, hunger is common.

2. GI tract is sluggish and hypoactive, due to decreased muscle tone and peristalsis.

3. Constipation may be a problem.

I. Urinary tract.

1. Urinary tract infection risk, if client has been catheterized during labor and delivery.

2. May have bruising and swelling due to trauma around the urinary meatus.

3. Increased bladder capacity, along with decreased sensitivity to pressure, leads to urinary retention.

4. Diuresis occurs during the first two days postpartum.

5. Bladder distention may displace the uterus, leading to a "boggy" uterus and increased bleeding.

J. Vital signs.

Table 25-5: POSTPARTUM HIGH RISK FACTORS

- ✦ Preeclampsia
- ✦ Diabetes
- ✦ Cardiac disease
- ✦ Cesarean birth
- ✦ Overdistention of uterus (multiple gestation)
- ✦ Abruptio placentae and placenta previa
- ✦ Precipitous or prolonged labor
- ✦ Difficult delivery
- ✦ Extended period of time in lithotomy position (legs in stirrups)
- ✦ Retained placenta

1. Temperature may be slightly elevated (100.4°F) after a long labor; should return to normal within twenty-four hours.

2. Blood pressure may be slightly decreased after delivery; however, should remain stable.

3. Pulse rate slow after delivery; puerperal bradycardia rate is fifty to seventy beats; usually returns to normal within ten days.

K. Blood values.

1. Leukocytosis is present—WBC of 20 to 30,000/mm.

2. Hemoglobin, hematocrit, RBC return to normal within two to six weeks.

3. Rule of thumb: four-point drop in hematocrit equals one pint of blood loss.

4. Pregnancy-induced increase in coagulation factors during the first week following delivery—leads to increased risk of development of thrombophlebitis and thromboembolism.

L. Weight loss.

1. Initial ten to twelve pound loss occurs due to the weight of the infant, placenta, and amniotic fluid.

2. Diuresis leads to an additional five pounds weight loss.

3. Six to eight weeks postpartum-return to prepregnant weight if an average of twenty-five to thirty pounds was gained.

Attachment—Psychosocial Response

A. Phases.

1. Taking-in phase.

a. First few days postpartum.

b. Characterized by passiveness and dependency.

c. Preoccupied with own self needs, food, attention, and physical comforts and care.

d. Talkative.

2. Taking-hold phase.

a. Occurs about two to three days postpartum; characterized by increase in physical well-being.

b. Emphasis on the present; woman takes hold of the task of mothering; requires reassurance.

c. Very receptive to teaching.

B. Attachment behaviors.

1. Exploration and identification pattern.

a. Touch—begins by stroking the extremities and the outline of the head with the fingertips; gradually moves toward using the entire surface of the hand; touches and observes first at arm's length, then on lap, or slightly away from the body; finally enfolds infant close to body with both arms.

b. Eye-to-eye contact—*en face position* (gazing into the eyes of the infant).

2. Factors influencing maternal-infant attachment.

a. Relationship with own parents.

b. Previous experience with infants.

c. Social, economic, and developmental level of mother.

d. Acceptance of pregnancy as a positive event.

e. Anesthetic/analgesic used in labor; type of delivery.

f. Support of significant others.

g. Amount of time of initial contact between mother and infant.

h. Health and responsiveness of infant.

C. Postpartum blues.

1. Transient period of depression (occurring during the puerperium).

2. Complaints of anorexia, insomnia, tearfulness, and a general let-down, sad feeling.

3. Thought to be caused by fatigue, discomfort, sensory overload or deprivation, and hormonal changes.

4. Woman needs support and reassurance that it is a transient and self-limiting experience.

5. A very small percentage of new mothers are at risk for developing postpartum psychosis.

POSTPARTUM NURSING CARE

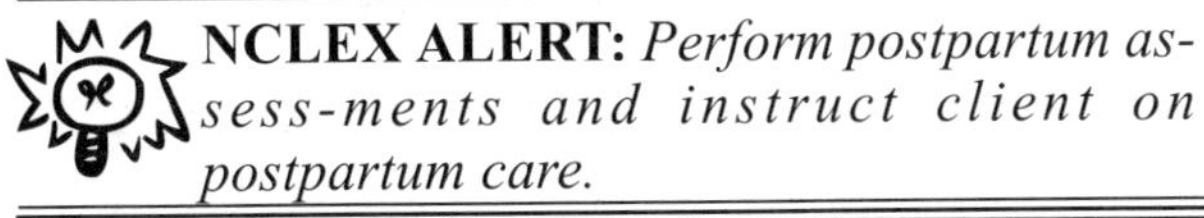

NCLEX ALERT: *Perform postpartum assess-ments and instruct client on postpartum care.*

✦ *Goal: to initiate routine postpartum assessment.*

Table 25-6: BREASTFEEDING

Types of feeding positions:

- Cradle position, side-lying, football or clutch position, and modified clutch position.

Teach mother to:

- Bring infant to level of the breast — don't lean over.
- Turn infant completely on side with arms embracing the breast on either side.
- Bring infant in as close as possible with legs wrapped around the mother's waist and the tip of the nose touching the breast.
- Bring infant's lips to nipple, when infant opens mouth to its widest point, draw the infant the rest of the way on to the nipple for him to latch-on.
- Break the suction by placing a clean finger in the side of the infant's mouth before removing the infant from the breast.

Should be put to breast 8-12 times per 24 hours.

Nipple shields or bottle nipples should be avoided.

1. General observations of mood, activity level, and feelings of wellness; routine vital sign assessment.

2. Inspection of breasts—check for beginning engorgement and presence of cracks in nipples, any pain or tenderness, and progress of breast-feeding.

3. Check uterine fundus—determine height of fundus in relation to umbilicus; should feel firm and globular (Figure 25-3).

4. Assess for bladder distention, especially during the first twenty-four to forty-eight hours.

5. Perineal area.

a. Observe episiotomy site.

(1) Evaluate healing status of episiotomy.

(2) Apply anesthetic sprays or ointments to decrease pain.

b. Determine presence of hemorrhoids and provide relief measures.

6. Lochia—record color, odor, and amount of discharge.

7. Lower extremities—assess for thrombophlebitis; checking for Homan's sign is controversial and can lead to release of a thrombus in a suspicious extremity.

8. Abdomen and perineum.

a. Initiate strengthening exercises for both abdominal wall and perineum (e.g., isometric Kegel exercises for strengthening pelvic floor, and leg raises).

✦ *Goal: to provide comfort and relief of pain.*

Table 25-7: Evaluating Breastfeeding

How do you know that an infant is getting enough breastmilk?

- Hear infant swallow and make soft "ka" or "ah" sounds.
- See smooth nutritive suckling, smooth series of sucking and swallowing with occassional rest periods, not the short, choppy sucks that occur when baby is falling to sleep.
- Breast gets softer during the feeding.
- Nursing 8-12 times per day—produce more milk with frequent nursing.
- Infant has at least 2-6 diapers/day for first 2 days after birth; 6-8 diapers/day by the 5th day.
- Infant has at least 3 bowel movements daily during the first month and often more.
- Infant is gaining weight and is satisfied after feedings.

1. Episiotomy—ice packs, first few hours; followed by peri light, sitz baths.
2. Perineal care—use of "peri bottles" to squirt over perineum (front to back) to prevent contamination and avoid use of toilet tissue.
3. Afterpain—use of analgesics (preferably one hour before feeding, especially for breast-feeding mothers).
4. Hemorrhoidal pain.
   a. Sitz baths, anesthetic ointments, rectal suppositories, Tucks.
   b. Encourage lying on side, and avoiding prolonged sitting.
   c. Stool softeners or laxatives may be indicated; usually normal bowel movement by 2nd or 3rd day after delivery.
5. Breast engorgement—well-fitting bra to provide support.

✦ *Goal: to promote maternal-infant attachment and facilitate integration of the newborn into the family unit.*

NCLEX ALERT: *Facilitate parental attachment with newborn.*

1. Use infant's name when talking about him or her.
2. Serve as a role model; be cautious not to appear so expert in handling infant because it may lead to feelings of discouragement in the mother.
3. Assist parents in problem solving and meeting their infant's needs. Explain ways to distinguish different types of cries related to hunger, illness, or discomfort.
4. Encourage parents to provide as much of the care to the infant while still hospitalized.
5. Accept parents' emotions and encourage expression of feelings.
6. Help parents understand sibling behavior and to plan for the arrival of the new family member.

✦ *Goal: to establish successful infant feeding patterns.*

1. Nonlactating mother.
   a. Provide supportive bra.
   b. Explain proper position for feeding.
   c. Formulas—ready-to-feed in disposable bottles, often with disposable nipples.
2. Lactating mothers.
   a. Avoid the use of nipple creams, ointments, or any topical preparations.
   b. Teach mother to refrain from using sunlamps or hair dryers to dry nipples.
   c. Application of expressed breast milk to nipples after each feeding has a bacteriostatic effect and may provide protection to damaged skin.
   d. Assess breasts for engorgement, nipple inversion, cracking, inflammation, or pain.
   e. Explain process of lactation and refer to community resources such as La Leche League.

✦ *Goal: to prevent infection and detect potential complications.*

1. Recognition of postpartum high risk factors in the new mother (Table 25-5).
2. Encourage 4-6 weeksafter delivery a postpartum checkup visit.
3. If symptoms of excessive bleeding, temperature elevation, pain in the calves, foul-smelling vaginal discharge, swollen breasts, or general feelings of malaise and illness occur, woman should contact care provider immediately.

✦ *Goal: to prepare and plan for discharge.*

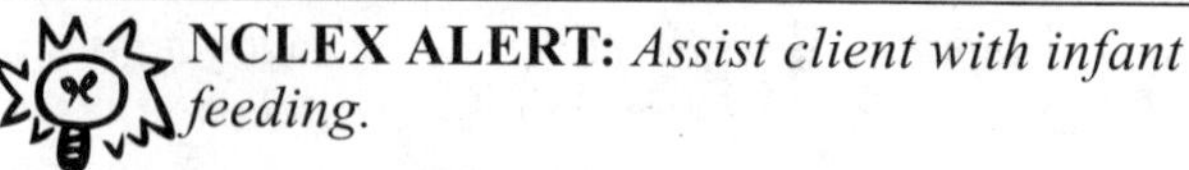

NCLEX ALERT: *Assist client with infant feeding.*

1. Determine if mother will need household help (especially important in birth of twins or after cesarean delivery).
2. Explain and teach the following infant care skills.
   a. Infant feeding (Table 25-6).
      (1) Hold bottle so that air does not get into nipple.
      (2) Method of making or preparing formula.

(3) How to break the infant's suction on the nipple.

(4) Positioning for burping and bubbling.

(5) Teach how to determine if infant is getting enough milk (Table 25-7).

b. Diapering.

(1) Frequent changing to prevent diaper rash.

(2) **Vaseline** or **Desitin** ointment to prevent irritation.

(3) Use of disposable diapers.

c. Bathing.

(1) Use of a mild soap.

(2) Kitchen sink is often a good place to bathe infant.

(3) Lotions can be applied; best advice is to avoid use of powders.

d. Umbilical cord.

(1) Apply alcohol daily and after every diaper change.

(2) Stump usually falls off in a week to ten days.

e. Pacifiers.

(1) May be used to meet infant's sucking need.

(2) Usually discontinued around four to six months, due to infant's lack of interest.

f. Sleeping.

(1) Usually sleeps through the night at around two to three months of age.

(2) Encourage mother to sleep while infant is sleeping to avoid sleep deprivation.

g. Illness.

(1) Common behavior changes are irritability, crying, loss of appetite, and fever.

(2) Explain how to take an infant's temperature.

h. Taking the infant outside.

(1) Dress infant as you would dress yourself; don't bundle infant up.

(2) Traveling—use a car seat.

i. Explain important of follow-up well-baby checkup visits with pediatrician.

COMPLICATIONS OF THE PUERPERIUM

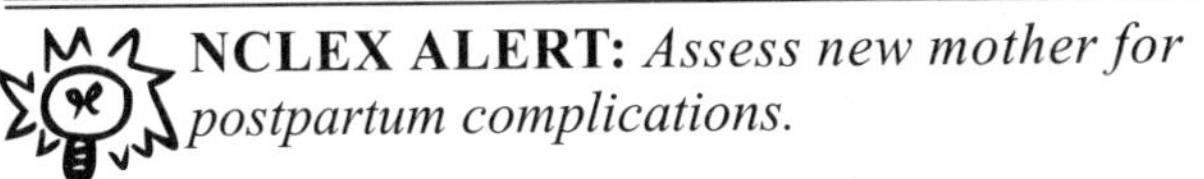

NCLEX ALERT: *Assess new mother for postpartum complications.*

HEMORRHAGE

Assessment

A. Risk factors.

1. Precipitous labor.
2. Dystocia.
3. Premature separation of placenta.
   a. Abruptio placentae.
   b. Placenta previa.
4. Forceps delivery.
5. Multiple pregnancy.
6. Large fetus.
7. Polyhydramnios.

B. Causes.

1. Uterine atony.
2. Lacerations.
3. Retained placental tissue.

C. Clinical manifestations.

1. Early postpartal hemorrhage—blood loss greater than 500 cc within the first 24 hours after delivery.
2. Late postpartal hemorrhage—blood loss greater than 500 cc after the first 24 hours.
3. Symptoms of shock—weak, rapid pulse, low blood pressure, pallor, restlessness, etc.

Treatment

A. Medical.

1. Uterine atony.
   a. Oxytocic medications.
   b. Bimanual compression of the uterus.
   c. Fluid and blood replacement.

B. Surgical.

1. Lacerations—suturing the bleeding edges.
2. Retained placenta—D&C to remove retained fragment.

Nursing Intervention

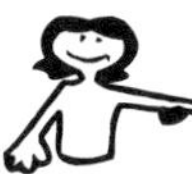

NURSING PRIORITY: *The key to successful management of hemorrhage is prevention, which includes adequate nutrition, good prenatal care, early diagnosis and management of any complications as they arise, and avoidance of traumatic procedures.*

✦ *Goal: to control and correct the cause of the hemorrhage.*

1. Uterine atony.
   a. Massage uterus to stimulate contractions.
   b. Administer oxytocic medications.
2. Lacerations.

a. Inspect perineal area.

b. Hematoma formation.

(1) Vulvar hematoma may appear as a discoloration of the perineal area.

(2) Any complaint of pain in the perineal area should be inspected carefully.

3. Retained placenta.

a. Inspect placenta at the time of delivery for intactness.

b. Never force the expulsion of the placenta.

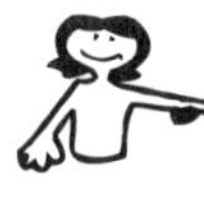

NURSING PRIORITY: *Careful observation of vaginal bleeding, doing pad count or weighing the perineal pad, is very important.*

Nursing Intervention

✦ *Goal: to maintain adequate circulating blood volume to prevent shock and anemia.*

1. Type and crossmatch blood for women at high risk to develop postpartum hemorrhage.
2. Anticipate replacement of IV fluids and blood.
3. Check hemoglobin and hematocrit values.
4. Treat for shock.
5. Monitor vital signs and amount of lochia.

✦ *Goal: to prevent postpartal infection.*

1. Maintain aseptic technique.
2. Administer prophylactic antibiotics.
3. Monitor vital signs.

✦ *Goal: to prevent postpartal hemorrhage.*

1. Identify women at increased risk.
2. Monitor hematocrit levels throughout pregnancy.
3. Encourage supplemental iron to prevent anemia.
4. Promote good nutrition.
5. Instruct client to palpate uterus for firmness and teach how to massage fundus.

Puerperal Infection

❑ **(Also called "Childbirth Fever")**

Assessment

A. Predisposing factors.

1. Antepartal infection.
2. Premature rupture of the membranes.
3. Prolonged labor.
4. Laceration.
5. Anemia; postpartum hemorrhage.
6. Poor aseptic technique.

B. Clinical manifestations.

1. Temperature elevation 38°C (100.4°F), if taken at least four times daily on any two of the first ten postpartum days, with the exception of the first 24 hours.
2. Symptoms vary according to system involved.
3. Area of involvement characterized by five cardinal symptoms of inflammation.
4. Tachycardia, chills, abdominal tenderness common.
5. Headache, malaise, deep pelvic pain.
6. Profuse, foul-smelling lochia.

C. Area involved.

1. Uterus is most often affected—endometritis.
2. May have localized infection of the perineum, vulva, and vagina.
3. Local infection may extend via the lymphatics into the pelvic organs resulting in:

a. Thrombophlebitis.

b. Salpingitis.

c. Oophoritis.

d. Peritonitis.

e. Septicemia.

4. Urinary system.

a. Pyelitis.

b. Cystitis.

Treatment

A. Medications.

1. Antibiotics.
2. Antipyretics.
3. Oxytocics.

B. Dietary.

1. High-protein, high-calorie, high-vitamin diet.
2. Encourage 3,000 to 4,000 cc of fluid per 24 hours.

Nursing Intervention

✦ *Goal: to prevent puerperal infection.*

1. Maintain meticulous aseptic technique during labor and delivery.
2. Assess and treat antepartal infection.
3. Detect anemia—check hematocrit during prenatal visits.
4. Avoid prolonged labors.

✦ *Goal: to promote mother's resistance to infection.*

1. Administer antibiotic, antipyretic, and oxytocic medications.
2. Encourage good nutrition.
3. Isolate client from other maternity clients.

4. Use semi-Fowler's position to promote free drainage of lochia and prevent upward extension of infection into pelvis.

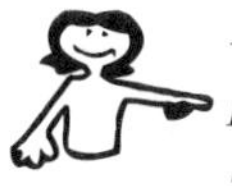

NURSING PRIORITY: The pathophysiology related to maintaining semi-Fowler's position to localize infection is important to remember, not only for obstetric clients, but others with contaminated drainage.

Mastitis

❑ ***Mastitis* is the invasion of the breast tissue by pathogenic organisms.**

Assessment

A. Predisposing factors.
   1. Fissured nipples.
   2. Erosion of the areola.
   3. Causative agent most frequently *Staphylococcus*, which is transmitted from the nasopharynx of the nursing infant.

B. Clinical manifestations.
   1. Occurs most often between the first and fourth weeks of the postpartal period.
   2. Chills and tachycardia.
   3. Red, swollen, painful breast/breasts.
   4. Fever of 39.4° C (103° F) or 40° C (104° F).

Treatment

A. Medication.
   1. Antibiotics for 10-14 days.
   2. Antipyretics.
   3. Analgesics.

Nursing Intervention

✦ *Goal: to prevent the complication of mastitis.*
   1. Teach mother how to care for breasts and nipples.
   2. Explain importance of wearing a support bra.

✦ *Goal: to promote comfort and maintain lactation.*
   1. Frequent nursing starting on the affected side.
   2. Breast massage before and during each feeding to thoroughly drain any blockages (or use a breast pump if the infant is unable to do this).
   3. Encourage good nutrition and adequate rest.
   4. Moist heat, increased fluids and vitamin C.
   5. Administer antibiotics as ordered.

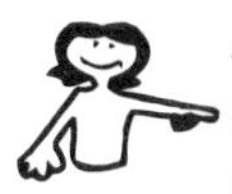

NURSING PRIORITY: Mother should continue to nurse on the affected side, because failure to do so increases the risk for abscess formation and relapse.

Postpartum Psychosis

A. Assessment.
   1. Psychotic complication is uncommon.
   2. Most mothers who suffer from postpartum psychosis have a previous history of psychiatric disturbance.
   3. Pregnancy is usually the precipitating event that leads to the crisis.
   4. Depression is the most common type of psychiatric disorder seen after childbirth.

B. Treatment and nursing intervention are outlined in Chapter 11.

Thrombophlebitis

❑ **There is an increased risk (5 times) for *thrombophlebitis* and *pulmonary* embolism during the puerperium. The reason for the increased incidence is due to a change in blood coagulation during pregnancy and a decrease in partial thromboplastin time, along with engorgement of the veins of the lower extremities and pelvis leading to pooling of blood and venous stasis. Assessment and nursing intervention are discussed in Chapter 16.**

Cystitis and Pyelitis

❑ ***Cystitis* and *pyelitis* occur as a result of trauma to the bladder mucosa, the temporary loss of bladder tone, and an increased bladder capacity. All three lead to distention and incomplete emptying of urine, predisposing the postpartum client to cystitis and pyelitis (See Chapter 23).**

Parent Reaction to Preterm, Ill Newborn, or Infant with Congenital Anomaly

Assessment

A. Period of disorganization.
   1. Grief reaction characterized by guilt, anger, and sorrow.
   2. Feelings of exhaustion, emptiness, and frequent crying.

B. Period of information seeking and resource utilization.
   1. Anxiety decreases; problem-solving begins.
   2. Begins to resolve the crisis.
   3. Often information seeking leads to further anger and sorrow followed then by a period of denial or disbelief.

C. Resolution of the crisis situation.
   1. Development of new coping strategies.
   2. Acceptance and coming to terms with the situation.

Nursing Intervention

✦ *Goal: to provide emotional support to the parents.*

1. Encourage verbalization of feelings and expression of grief.
2. Promote parent-infant contact; point out normal characteristics.
3. Encourage parents to visit, touch, and care for their infant as much as possible.
4. Refer parents to social and community agencies.⌘

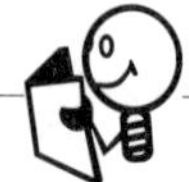

Study Questions—Intrapartum and Postpartum

1. A 20-year-old primigravida has been in the first stage of labor for 20 hours and now has hypotonic uterine dysfunction. What is the cause of this problem?

① Minor degrees of pelvic contraction.
② A vertex presentation.
③ Small amounts of analgesics.
④ Rupture of the membranes.

2. The labor monitor tracing shows repeated, mild, variable decelerations. What would the nurse expect is occuring?

① Cord compression.
② Fetal hypoxia.
③ Placental insufficiency.
④ Head compression.

3. The nurse is assessing a client 12 hours after a prolonged labor and delivery. What assessment data would cause the nurse the most concern?

① Oral temperature of 100.6°F.
② Moderate amount dark red lochia.
③ Episiotomy area bruised with small amout of serosanganeous drainage.
④ Uterine fundus palpated to the right of the umbilicus.

4. The nurse is caring for a client in labor. How are contractions timed?

① End of one to the beginning of the next.
② Beginning of one to the end of the next.
③ End of one to the end of the next.
④ Beginning of one to the beginning of the next.

5. Since bonding begins at the time of birth, the nurse would be concerned if she observed in the mother:

① Disinterest in breast-feeding following birth.
② Discomfort with postdelivery vaginal examination.
③ She did not want to see the infant at birth.
④ Worry about newborn acrocyanosis and molding.

6. The nurse is monitoring a client during labor and observes erratic fetal heart pattern on the monitor at the height of the contraction. What is the first action of the nurse?

① Position the mother on her right side.
② Check the monitor leads for placement.
③ Begin oxygen at 4L/min and observe mother's respirations and FHR.
④ Determine if contractions are increasing in duration, intensity, and frequency.

7. A client is 37 weeks pregnant and is admitted with bright red vaginal bleeding. She complains of abdominal discomfort, but she is not having contractions. After assessing the client's vital signs and FHR, what is the most important information to obtain?

① The amount of cervical dilatation that is present.
② The exact location of her abdominal discomfort.
③ The station of the presenting part.
④ At what time the client last ate.

8. The pelvic examination reveals the fetus to be at 1-station. What information does this indicate to the nurse about the presenting part of the fetus?

① Is visible on the perineum.
② Has not yet entered the true pelvis.
③ Is above the ischial spines.
④ Is too large to fit through the opening into the true pelvis.

9. A client complains to the nurse of "after-pains" following breast-feeding. What does the nurse explains to the client about these type pains?

① All women experience afterpains during the postpartum period.
② Breast-feeding causes the release of oxytocin, which causes utrine contractions.
③ Afterpains are a possible symptom of endometriosis.
④ Afterpains are a sign of subinvolution and may occur for 3 to 4 weeks.

10. What is the length of time of the second stage of labor in a woman who is a primipara?

① 20 to 30 minutes.
② 50 to 60 minutes.
③ 2 hours.
④ 3 hours.

11. What is an important nursing action when administering an enema to a postpartum client?

① Uses a small catheter.

② Administers no more than 100 cc of solution.

③ Is careful not to irritate the perineum when inserting the catheter.

④ Encourages the client to administer her own so she will know how to do it at home.

12. What is the name of the process by which the cervix becomes thin and indistinct from the body of the uterus?

① Dilation.

② Attitude.

③ Effacement.

④ Transition.

13. The client complains of severe perineal pain the first hour after delivery. What should the nurse assess for?

① Uterine atony.

② A hematoma.

③ A cervical laceration.

④ Retained placental fragments.

14. The nurse is checking a laboring client. Her assessment reveals the head at +3 station. What will the nurse do?

① Prepare for the delivery of the infant.

② Begin oxygen at 6L/minute.

③ Determine if contractions are increasing.

④ Determine the FHR.

15. A mother who is 3 weeks postpartm calls the nurse to ask what she should do for her sore, cracked nipples. What with the nurse tell her to do?

① Take the infant off of breastfeeding till the nipples heal.

② Make sure all of the areola is in the infant's mouth.

③ Cleanse the nipples with half strength perioxide and air dry.

④ Place a cool compress on the nipples after nursing.

Answers and rationales to these questions are in the section at the end of the book entitled "Chapter Study Questions: Answers & Rationales."

Appendix 25-1: MAGNESIUM SULFATE

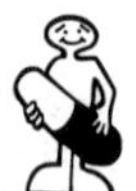

MEDICATIONS	SIDE EFFECTS	NURSING IMPLICATIONS
ANTICONVULSANT: **Magnesium Sulfate** ($MgSO_4$)		
IV: Given via an IV pump; preferred route. **IM:** 4 to 5 gm into each buttock (deep IM); 1 percent procaine may be added to decrease pain of injection.	**Maternal**: sweating, flushing, muscle weakness, depressed or absent reflexes, oliguria, respiratory paralysis. **Fetal:** crosses placenta, lethargy, hypotonia, and weakness. **Contraindications:** maternal-impaired renal function.	1. Criteria for administrations: a. Respirations - greater than 12/min. b. Presence of patellar knee-jerk movement. c. Urinary output - greater than 30 cc/hour. 2. Check blood pressure frequently for symptoms of hypotension. 3. Antidote of magnesium sulfate is *calcium gluconate*; should be available at bedside in case of respiratory paralysis. 4. Monitor fetal heart rate. 5. $MgSO_4$ is continued at least 24 hours after delivery to reduce risk of seizure activity postpartum. 6. May be used as a tocolytic agent. 7. IM administration: a. Use deep IM or Z track into ventrogluteal muscle. b. Massage site after injection. c. Apply warm, dry pack to promote absorption and increase comfort. 8. **Uses:** prevention or control of eclampsia.

Appendix 25-2: OXYTOCIC MEDICATIONS

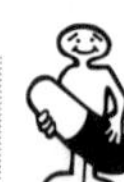

MEDICATION	SIDE EFFECTS	NURSING IMPLICATIONS
OXYTOCIC MEDICATIONS: Stimulate contraction of uterine muscle fibers; have a mild antidiuretic effect; stimulate postpartum milk flow, but not amount.		
Oxytocin (Pitocin): IM, IV, intranasal Ergonovine **(Ergotrate)**: PO, IM, IV Methylergonovine (**Methergine**): PO, IM, IV	***Maternal*** - tetanic uterine contractions, hypertension, tachycardia. ***Fetal*** - hypoxia, irregularity and decrease in fetal heart rate, possible hyperbilirubinemia. ***Contraindications:*** Severe preeclampsia or eclampsia. Predisposition to uterine rupture or CPD. Preterm infant, or the presence of fetal distress.	1. Apply fetal monitor - assess fetal heart rate pattern throughout oxytocin administration. 2. Assess maternal vital signs prior to increasing oxytocin infusion rate. 3. Discontine IV oxytocin and turn on primary IV solution, if any of the following occurs: a. Fetal distress (decreasing FHR). b. Sustained uterine contractions over 2 minutes. c. Insufficient relaxation of the uterus between contractions. 4. **Pitocin** is the only oxytocic used to induce labor; others are used after delivery to control bleeding (**Ergotrate** and **Methergine**). 5. Uses—uterine dystocia; induction of labor for diabetes mellitus, preeclampsia, eclampsia clients; control of hemorrhage and uterine atony; uterine involution.

Appendix 25-3: TOCOLYTIC AGENTS TO SUPPRESS LABOR

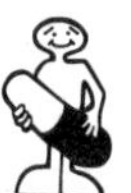

MEDICATIONS	SIDE EFFECTS	NURSING IMPLICATIONS
TOCOLYTIC AGENTS: Relaxes myometrial cells of the uterus leading to inhibition of labor. Also results in bronchial dilation and cardiac output		
Terbutaline (**Brethine**): IV, SQ, PO	***Maternal:*** tachycardia (very little effect on blood pressure), nervousness and tremors, headache, and possible pulmonary edema. ***Fetal:*** tachycardia, hypoglycemia.	1. Assess maternal (especially pulse) and fetal vital signs frequently; fetal monitoring is necessary; notify physician if maternal pulse is greater than 120 beats/min or FHR is *greater than 180 beats/min.* 2. Encourage left lateral position (Sims') to decrease hypotension and increase placental perfusion. 3. IV: use a pump for continuous infusion; infusion is continued for 12 hours after labor has stopped. 4. Watch for signs of pulmonary edema, assess blood glucose with Ritrodrine IV administration and do not give in presence of an infection. 5. ***Use:*** premature labor.
Ritodrine (**Yutopar**): IV, PO	***Maternal:*** altered pulse and blood pressure (dose related), widening pulse pressure, tachycardia, hypotension, nausea and vomiting, hyperglycemia, nervousness and tremors, and skin rash. ***Fetal:*** Altered FHR (dose-related), increased serum glucose, acidosis, hypoxia, and hypotension at birth. ***Contraindications:*** severe preeclampsia, hypovolemia, cardiac disease, used with caution in diabetic mothers.	***NURSING PRIORITY:*** *Terbutaline usually preferred over Ritodrine because of minimal effects on blood pressure and on maternal/fetal heart rate.*
Calcium Channel Blockers: Nifedipine (**Procardia**): PO or sublingual	Facial flushing, mild hypotension, reflex tachycardia, headache, nausea	1. No reported fetal side effects. 2. Not in common usage as a tocolytic agent.
Prostaglandin Synthesis Inhibitors: Indomethacin (**Indocin**): PO or rectally NSAIDS	***Maternal***: Nausea, vomiting, dyspepsia ***Fetal:*** oligohydramnios, premature closure of the ductus arteriosus in utero	

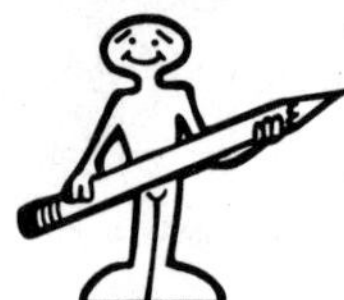

Notes

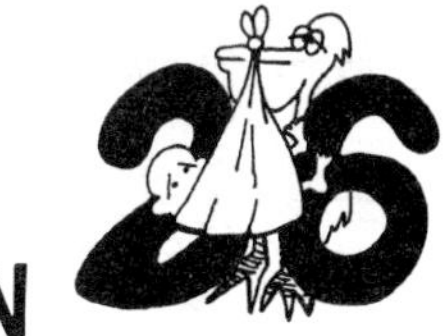

NORMAL NEWBORN

Biologic Adaptations in the Neonatal Period

Assessment

A. Respiratory system.
1. Lung maturation process.
a. Development of a functioning lung does not occur until at least 26 weeks' gestation.
b. Pulmonary surfactant usually of sufficient quantity at 35 weeks' gestation; acts to stabilize respirations and prevent atelectasis.
2. Respiratory effort.
a. Respirations are usually established within one minute after birth; often within the first few seconds.
b. Lusty cry usually accompanies good respiratory effort.
c. Newborn respiration should be quiet; no dyspnea or cyanosis.
d. Cyanosis may be apparent in the hands and the feet (acrocyanosis); circumoral cyanosis (around the mouth) may persist for an hour or two after birth, but should subside.
e. Average respiratory rate: 30-60 respirations per minute.
f. Respiratory movements: diaphragmatic and abdominal muscles are used; very little thoracic movement.
g. Neonate breathes through the nose (obligate nose-breather); consequently, nasal obstruction or mucus will lead to respiratory distress.

***NURSING PRIORITY:** Oxygen transport in the newborn is significantly affected by the presence of greater amounts of HbF (fetal hemoglobin) than HbA (adult hemoglobin), which holds O_2 easier but releases it to the body tissues only at low PO_2 levels.*

B. Circulatory system.
1. Cessation of blood flow through the umbilical vessels and placenta.
2. Closure of the ductus arteriosus, the foramen ovale, and the ductus venosus.
3. Increase in and shift to pulmonary circulation.
4. Circulatory changes are not always immediate and complete-usually complete in a few days; often this period is called *transitional circulation.*
5. Anatomic closing of the fetal blood vessels may not be complete for weeks or months; functional closure is usually adequate to produce normal circulation.
6. Heart.
a. May hear transitory heart murmurs.
b. Assess for dextrocardia—auscultated heart sounds are heard louder on right side of chest.
c. Pulse rate: 120 to 140 beats per minute.
7. Blood pressure.
a. Measured by auscultation or palpation or with the use of the doppler.
b. Blood pressure varies with size and age.
c. Recognition of hypotension.
(1) Full-term infants: systolic less than 55 mm Hg. Large preterm infants: systolic less than 50 mm Hg.
(2) Any infant: systolic less than 40 mm Hg.

C. Body temperature and heat production.
1. Loss of body heat.
a. Evaporation: heat loss as water evaporates from skin and from lungs; occurs when infant's body is wet with amniotic fluid at birth.
b. Convection: movement of body heat to flow of cool air; infant loses heat to the cool air in the delivery room.
c. Conduction: direct transfer of heat to a surface on which the infant is lying; infant loses heat to a cool sheet or blanket.
d. Radiation: heat loss from the infant's warm body as it travels through the air to cooler objects in the room; often occurs during the days following birth, especially an unclothed infant in an incubator.

***NURSING PRIORITY:** Excessive heat loss occurs from radiation and convection because of the newborn's larger surface area when compared to body weight. It is important to remember that conduction loss occurs due to the marked difference between core body temperature and skin temperature.*

e. Body temperature changes.

(1) Body temperature at birth is 0.5° C higher than mother's.

(2) Body temperature may drop to 94° F (34.4° C) or even as low as 92° F (33.3° C) after birth unless the infant is adequately protected.

2. Production of body heat.

a. Heat generated immediately by *shivering*; infant shivering is characterized by increased muscular activity, restlessness and crying.

b. Infant shivering activity is not as apparent as adult shivering activity.

c. Metabolism of brown fat.

(1) Functions to produce heat under the stress of cooling.

(2) Brown fat is located in the intrascapular region, in the posterior triangle of the neck, and in the axillae.

(3) Brown fat is metabolized and utilized within several weeks after birth.

d. Increase in metabolic rate.

(1) Stimulation of the thyroid gland leads to increased general metabolism; usually takes 12 to 24 hours.

(2) Metabolic rate remains elevated for 7 to 10 days, even after warming.

(3) Effect of chilling on the neonate.

(a) Increased heat production leads to increased oxygen consumption.

(b) Increased oxygen consumption utilized glucose and brown fat.

(c) When heat production is high, caloric need is high.

(d) Tendency to develop metabolic acidosis occurs.

(e) Production of surfactant is inhibited by cooling and respiratory distress syndrome may occur.

(f) Increased risk with smaller infants, since they have low reserve of glycogen and low reserve for increasing ventilation; leads to the tendency to become more acidotic.

General Characteristics

NCLEX ALERT: *Assess a newborn; monitor a newborn for complications.*

A. Length.

1. Average length of full-term neonate: 45.2 cm to 55 cm (17.8 inches to 21.7 inches).

2. Infant is measured by being placed flat on the back and determining the distance from head to heel by using a pencil to mark the distance and then measuring the distance when the infant is removed.

B. Weight.

1. Average birth weight for a full-term neonate: 3,400 grams (7 lb 8 oz).

2. Low birth weight: less than 2,500 grams (5 lb 8 oz).

3. Excessive weight: greater than 4,080 grams (9 lb).

4. Weight loss: between 5 percent and 10 percent of birth weight within the first few days of life; usually regain weight within 10 to 14 days.

C. Head.

1. Molding.

a. Head may appear elongated at birth; usually, molding disappears within 24 to 48 hours.

b. Occurs due to abnormal fetal posture in utero and pressure during passage through the birth canal.

2. Caput succedaneum.

a. Edema of the scalp due to the pressure occurring at the time of delivery.

b. Disappears within 1 to 2 days.

3. Cephalhematoma.

a. A collection of blood between the periosteum and the skull.

b. Usually results from trauma during labor and delivery.

c. Absorbed in a few weeks.

4. Head measurement.

a. Average circumference of the full-term neonate: 34.2 cm; usual variation ranges between 32 to 36 cm.

b. Head circumference is approximately 2-3 cm. greater than the chest circumference.

NCLEX ALERT: *Compare physical development of client to norms.*
Extremes in size may indicate microcephaly, hydrocephaly or increased intracranial pressure.

5. Fontanel.

a. Palpated for size and tension.

b. Increase in tension may indicate increasing intracranial pressure or hydrocephaly.

c. Decrease in tension (sunken fontanel) may indicate dehydration or shock.

D. Umbilical cord.

1. Determination of number of blood vessels; two arteries and one vein surrounded by Wharton's jelly.
2. Cord atrophies and sloughs off by day 6 to 10.

Behavioral Characteristics

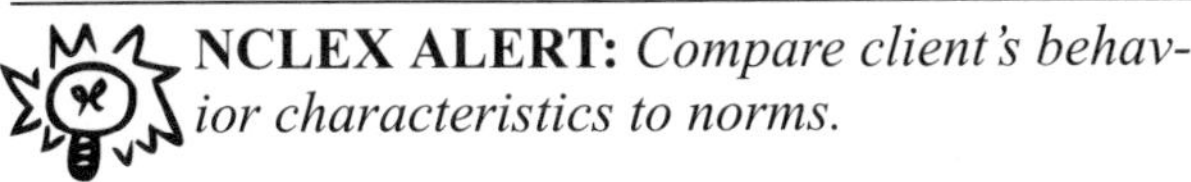

NCLEX ALERT: *Compare client's behavior characteristics to norms.*

A. Sleep and awake states.
  1. Newborn sleeps an average of 16 to 20 hours a day during the first two weeks of life, with an average of 4 hours at a time.
  2. May vary from a drowsy or semi-dozing to an alert state to a crying state.

B. Infants vary a great deal in how they respond to stimuli.
  1. Infants move easily from one state of sleep to another state of consciousness.
  2. As the infant develops he/she will reduce the total amount of sleeping time; wakeful periods will lengthen; sleeping will shift from daytime to nighttime.

Specific Body System Clinical Findings

A. Nervous system.
  1. Nervous system is relatively immature and characterized by the following:
    a. Poor nervous control; easily startled.
    b. Quivering chin.
    c. Tremors of short duration of the lower extremities.
  2. Reflex activity—the presence or absence of certain reflexes are indicative of ongoing normal development.
  3. Presence of positive Babinski sign.
    a. Normal findings until age one year.
    b. Dorsiflexion of big toe and fanning of the other toes.
  4. Neonatal reflexes. (Table 26-1).

NURSING PRIORITY: *Intactness of the neonate's nervous system is indicated by the state of alertness, resting posture, cry, and quality of muscle tone and motor activity.*

B. Hematologic system.
  1. At birth.
    a. Increased number of RBC—5,000,000 per cubic mm of blood.
    b. Hemoglobin 14 to 19 grams per 100 ml of blood.
    c. Hematocrit 48 percent to 60 percent.
  2. Leukocytosis is present at birth (9,000 to 30,000 WBC).
    a. Considerable decrease in WBC occurs within a few days after birth.
    b. Shift in the type of cells occurs—neutrophils decrease and lymphocytes increase until they predominate by the end of the first week.
  3. Anemia.
    a. Erythropoiesis slows down during the first six to eight weeks of life; RBC break down and their life span ends with resultant anemia.
    b. This drop in hemoglobin and RBC is termed *physiologic* anemia of the newborn.
    c. After the third month, a slow rise begins.
  4. Physiologic jaundice—jaundice occurring on the second or third day of life due to increase in serum bilirubin level.
    a. Pathophysiology.
      (1) Inability of the liver to clear bilirubin from the plasma.
      (2) Increased level of RBC from the maternal circulation at birth leads to increased breakdown and bilirubin production.
    b. Criteria for physiologic jaundice.
      (1) Does not appear until *after* 24 hours following birth.
      (2) Total serum bilirubin is less than 12 mg per 100 ml.
      (3) Direct serum bilirubin is less than 1 to 2 mg per 100 ml.
      (4) Infant does not show any sign of illness or cardiac decompensation.
      (5) Total serum bilirubin does not increase more than 5 mg per 100 ml per 24 hours.
      (6) Clinical evidence of jaundice disappears within one week in the full-term infant and by the end of the second week in the premature infant.
    c. Treatment - phototherapy.
      (1) Place infant nude under bili-lights exposing all areas to the light except for eyes and genitalia—cover infant's eyes with an opaque mask or eye patch.
      (2) If a *fiberoptic blanket* is used, infant's eyes *do not* need to be covered. This method is starting to replace the traditional phototherapy both for hospital and home care.

Table 26-1: MAJOR NEONATAL REFLEXES

REFLEX	DISAPPEARS	HOW TO ELICIT	RESPONSE
Rooting	3 to 4 months; May persist during sleep until 7 to 8 months	Stroke cheek.	Head turns toward side that is touched.
Babinski	1 year	Lightly stroke lateral side of foot from heel to toe across the foot.	Infant's toes fan, with dorsiflexion of great toe.
Sucking	10 to 12 months	Touch or stroke lips.	Baby sucks.
Moro (Startle)	3 to 4 months	Make a loud noise or suddenly disturb infant's equilibrium.	Infant stiffens, briskly abducts and extends arms with hands open and fingers extended to C-shape. Infant's legs flex and abduct, and arms return to an embracing posture. Crying is usual.
Grasp:			
Palmar	3 to 4 months	Press a finger against infant's palm	Infant's fingers momentarily close around object.
Plantar	8 to 10 months	Press an object against ball of infant's foot.	Infant's toes curl down and around object.
Tonic neck (Fencer's position)	6 months	Turn supine infant's head over the shoulder to one side.	Infant's arm and leg partially or completely extend on side to which head is turned; opposite arm and leg flex.

(3) Monitor skin temperature to prevent hyperthermia or hypothermia.

(4) Chart pertinent information relating to time phototherapy was started and stopped, maintenance of shielding of the eyes for bili-light, type and intensity of lamp used, distance of light to infant, whether used in combination with an isolette or an open bassinet, and any side effects.

5. Transitory coagulation defects.

a. Occurs between the second and fifth postnatal day.

b. Due to the lack of intestinal synthesis of vitamin K as a result of insufficient bacterial flora in the GI tract.

c. Administration of vitamin K (0.5 to 1.0 mg IM) is ordered to prevent complications.

C. Gastrointestinal tract.

1. Able to absorb proteins and carbohydrates quite well.

2. Stomach produces hydrochloric acid immediately after birth.

3. Digestive enzymes are present except for pancreatic amylase and lipase; this results in the inability to absorb fat adequately.

4. Stools.

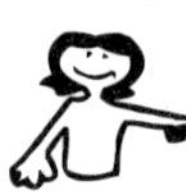

***NURSING PRIORITY:** Monitor the passage of the first meconium stool.*

a. Meconium—sticky, black, odorless, sterile stool which occurs within the first 24 hours after birth; if no stool is passed, possibility of imperforate anus may exist.

b. Stools change according to infant feeding.

(1) Transitional stools—period between second and fourth day; consist of part meconium and part milk; greenish brown or greenish yellow in color; loose and often contain mucus.

(2) Stools of the breast-fed infant are golden yellow in color, a pasty consistency, and occur more frequently than stools of formula fed infants.

(3) Formula-fed infant stools are dryer, more formed, and a paler color.

D. Genital-urinary system.

1. Urinary.

a. Urinary output is low during the first few days of life or until fluid intake increases.

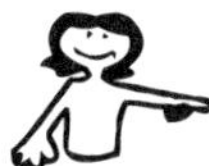

NURSING PRIORITY: Most newborns void within the first 24-48 hours after birth.

b. 30 to 60 cc voided per day during the first two days of life; followed by 200 cc per day by the end of the first week.

c. Frequency of voiding—average of 2 to 6 times per day, increasing up to 10 to 15 times per day.

2. Genitalia.

a. Female—labia majora are underdeveloped; may see bloody discharge from the vagina due to maternal hormone.

b. Male—scrotum may be edematous; testes should have descended; smegma, a cheese-like substance, collects under the foreskin and requires cleansing to reduce irritation.

E. Integumentary system.

1. Vernix caseosa—a white cheesy-like material covers the skin at birth; particularly noted in the folds and creases.

2. Petechiae—pinpoint bluish discolorations primarily on the skin and face as a result of pressure from delivery; may see bruising of tissues.

3. Lanugo—downy, fine covering of hair that may be present on the shoulders, back, earlobes, and forehead; disappears during the first week.

4. Milia—pinpoint white bumps seen over the bridge of the nose and on the cheeks during the first two weeks of life.

5. Erythema toxicum—splotchy pink papular rash appearing anywhere on the body; disappears within the first few days of life; no treatment necessary.

6. Mongolian spots—bluish darkened pigmented areas seen on the back or buttocks of dark-skinned infants (of black, oriental, and Mediterranean descent); usually disappears by school age.

7. Hemangiomatous area (stork bites)—area on the upper eyelids, between the eyebrows, upper lip, or at the nape of the neck which are light red in appearance; fade and disappear between one and two years of age.

F. Endocrine system.

1. Due to maternal hormones, breast enlargement, menses, and vulvar or prostatic enlargement; may occur in the neonate.

2. Thymus gland is normally large; grows rapidly till age 5, remains the same until about age 10, and then finally diminishes in size.

G. Sensory system.

1. Vision—visual acuity 20/150 to 20/290; retinal development is advanced.

a. Eyes appear large and pupils small.

b. All infants' eyes are blue or slate blue at birth; become their permanent color at age 3 months.

c. Tears do not develop until three to four months.

d. Eyes close to bright light; red reflex is present.

2. Hearing.

a. Sudden loud noises may elicit startle response.

b. Usually able to locate the general direction of sounds.

3. Smell developed at birth.

4. Taste.

a. Differentiates between pleasant and unpleasant tastes.

b. Rejects especially salty, sour, or bitter tastes by grimacing, and stops sucking.

5. Tactile senses.

a. Most sensitive area is around the mouth.

b. Searches for food when cheek is touched, or begins sucking movement when lips are touched.

H. Musculoskeletal system.

1. Assumes the position of comfort, which is usually the position he/she assumed in utero.

2. Normal palmar crease is present (simian crease indicative of Down's syndrome).

3. Spine is straight and flat when in prone position.

4. Creases and fat pads present on ⅔ of the soles of the feet.

5. Digits present on hands and feet; fingernails present.

Nursing Intervention

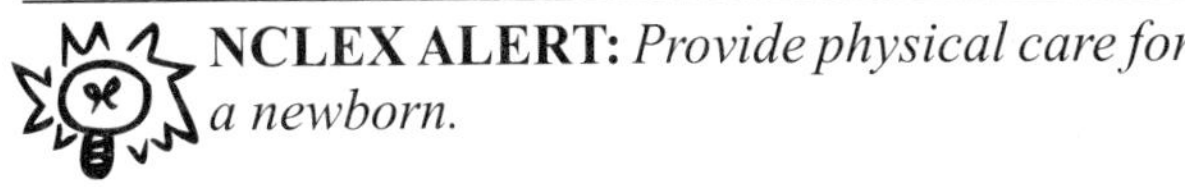

NCLEX ALERT: *Provide physical care for a newborn.*

✦ *Goal: to establish and maintain a patent airway and good oxygenation.*

1. Position infant with head slightly lower than chest; may use postural drainage or side-lying position.

2. Suction nostrils and oropharynx with bulb syringe or a De Lee Mucus trap.

3. Observe for apnea, cyanosis and mucus collection and be ready to use oropharyngeal suctioning, stimulation, oxygen administration, or resuscitative procedures if necessary.

NURSING PRIORITY: *During the admission period (first 4 hours after birth) the priority nursing goals are to: maintain a clear airway, maintain a neutral thermal environment, prevent hemorrhage and infection, and initiate bathing and oral feedings.*

✦ *Goal: to protect against heat loss from the body.*

1. Immediately after birth, dry off amniotic fluid from body using a warm blanket.
2. Replace wet blanket with warm dry blanket.
3. Cover wet hair and head with a blanket or cap.
4. Place baby on a warm padded surface, preferably under a radiant heater or in an incubator, or with skin-to-skin contact with the mother's body.
5. In the nursery, place in a heated bassinet until body temperature is stable.
6. Avoid any unnecessary procedures until body temperature is stable.

✦ *Goal: to collect data and assess physical condition and behavior.*

1. Apgar at 1 minute and then 5 minutes (See Table 25-3 for Apgar scoring).

NCLEX ALERT: *Assess a newborn, determine APGAR score of newborn. The 1 minute APGAR is a rapid evaluation of the status of the neonate's intrauterine oxygenation; the 5 minute APGAR evaluates the neonate's response to any resuscitation efforts, as well as cardiorespiratory adaptation after birth.*

2. Monitor vital signs q 15 minutes for one hour, q 30 minutes for one hour, q 1 to 2 hours x 4 until stable; also record incubator temperature.
3. Weigh and measure infant.
4. Assess for gestational age and intrauterine growth.
5. Determine special needs and high-risk category.
6. Perform Accucheck or dextrostix to detect hypoglycemia—if blood sugar is below 47-50 mg/dl feed newborn 10% dextrose in water.

✦ *Goal: to assess for periods of reactivity.*

1. First period of reactivity.
   a. Lasts approximately 30 minutes.
   b. Newborn is alert, awake, and usually hungry.

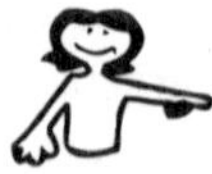

NURSING PRIORITY: *Periods of reactivity are excellent opportunities to promote attachment response.*

2. Sleep phase.
   a. First sleep usually occurs an average of 3-4 hours after birth, and may last from a few minutes to several hours.
   b. Newborn is very difficult to awaken during this phase.
3. Second period of reactivity.
   a. Infant alert and awake.
   b. Lasts approximately 4-6 hours.

NURSING PRIORITY: *Important to monitor infant closely as apnea, decreased heart rate, gagging, choking, and regurgitation may to occur and require nursing intervention.*

✦ *Goal: to protect against infection.*

1. Proper handwashing before handling infant.
2. Administer prophylactic treatment to eyes soon after birth.
   a. 1 to 2 percent silver nitrate solution, penicillin, or erythromycin antibiotic eye ointment in the conjunctival sac.
   b. Prevents ophthalmia neonatorum.
3. Avoid contact by various personnel in nursery area; avoid exposure to people with upper respiratory, skin or gastrointestinal illness.

✦ *Goal: to prevent hypofibrinogenemia.*

1. Administration of .5 to 1.0 mg of vitamin K (**Aqua Mephyton**) IM into the upper third of the lateral aspect of the thigh.

✦ *Goal: to properly identify infant.*

1. Secure identification bands to wrist, or ankles of both infant and mother in the delivery room.
2. Prints of infant's foot, palms or fingers may be obtained according to hospital policy; also mother's palm or fingerprints may be obtained.

NCLEX ALERT: *Identify a client*

✦ *Goal: to promote maternal-infant attachment to parents immediately after birth..*

1. Wrap infant snugly in warm blanket and allow parents to hold him. Do not allow chilling to occur.
2. Encourage touching and holding..

✦ *Goal: to initiate and evaluate feeding ability and provide nutrition.*

✦ *Encourage breast feeding, if desired immediately after delivery or in recovery room.*

Figure 26-1: Clinical Estimation Of Gestational Age

Ballard scale for newborn maturity rating. From: Ballard, J.L. And others; New Ballard Score, J. Pediatrics, 119:413, 1991.

NEUROMUSCULAR MATURITY

	-1	0	1	2	3	4	5
Posture							
Square Window (wrist)	> 90°	90°	60°	45°	30°	0°	
Arm Recoil		180°	140° - 180°	110° 140°	90° - 110°	< 90°	
Popliteal Angle	180°	160°	140°	120°	100°	90°	< 90°
Scarf Sign							
Heel to Ear							

A

PHYSICAL MATURITY

Skin	sticky friable transparent	gelatinous red, translucent	smooth pink, visible veins	superficial peeling &/or rash, few veins	cracking pale areas rare veins	parchment deep cracking no vessels	leathery cracked wrinkled
Lanugo	none	sparse	abundant	thinning	bald areas	mostly bald	
Plantar Surface	heel-toe 40-50 mm: -1 <40 mm: -2	>50 mm no crease	faint red marks	anterior transverse crease only	creases ant. 2/3	creases over entire sole	
Breast	imperceptible	barely perceptible	flat areola no bud	stippled areola 1-2 mm bud	raised areola 3-4 mm bud	full areola 5-10 mm bud	
Eye/Ear	lids fused loosely: -1 tightly: -2	lids open pinna flat stays folded	sl. curved pinna; soft; slow recoil	well-curved pinna; soft but ready recoil	formed & firm instant recoil	thick cartilage ear stiff	
Genitals (male)	scrotum flat, smooth	scrotum empty faint rugae	testes in upper canal rare rugae	testes descending few rugae	testes down good rugae	testes pendulous deep rugae	
Genitals (female)	clitoris prominent labia flat	prominent clitoris small labia minora	prominent clitoris enlarging minora	majora & minora equally prominent	majora large minora small	majora cover clitoris & minora	

MATURITY RATING

score	weeks
-10	20
-5	22
0	24
5	26
10	28
15	30
20	32
25	34
30	36
35	38
40	40
45	42
50	44

1. Assess ability to feed; assess for active bowel sounds, absence of abdominal distention, rooting, sucking, swallowing reflexes and alertness.

2. First feeding or test feeding—administer 10 to 15 cc of sterile water, followed by a 5 percent or 10 percent glucose solution.

✦ *Goal: to provide daily general care.*

1. Ongoing assessment and observation of vital signs, activity, appearance, color, bowel and bladder function.

2. Care of the umbilical cord.

   a. A drying solution of alcohol, triple dye or **Merthiolate** is applied to the cord.

   b. Clean the umbilical cord several times a day, especially after voiding (for a male infant).

   c. To encourage drying of the cord, expose to air frequently and position diaper below umbilicus.

   d. Observe for bleeding, oozing, or foul odor.

3. Circumcision care.

   a. Keep area clean.

   b. Observe for bleeding.

   c. A sterile gauze dressing with petroleum jelly may be applied to the area during the first 2-3 days.

NURSING PRIORITY: Teach the parents that a whitish-yellow exudate around the glans is granulation tissue and is normal and not indicative of infection. It may be observed for 2-3 days and should not be removed.

4. Neonate's bath.
   a. Bath is delayed until vital signs and temperature are stabilized.
   b. Mild baby soap and warm water is used, do not immerse infant in water until cord has released.
   c. Apply principles of clean-to-dirty area—eyes, face, ears, head, body, genitals, buttocks.
   d. Head is an area for significant heat loss.
5. Assess and observe daily weight and record gain or loss.
6. Assess stools.
   a. Meconium stools.
   b. Transitional stools.

✦ *Goal: to detect complications and provide early treatment.*

1. Order newborn screen after 1st 24 hours for a formula-fed infant or neonate; if mother is breast-feeding, explain importance of returning when infant is one week old to obtain blood sample; newborn screening includes: galactosemia, homocystinuria, maple syrup urine disease, hypothyroidism, and sickle cell anemia.
2. Administration of 1st hepatitis B vaccine prior to discharge; also, hepatitis B immune globulin (IM) is given, if mother is hepatitis B carrier.
   a. Encourage follow-up visits for 2nd and 3rd dose of hepatitis B vaccine and other immunizations.
   b. Infants are tested at 9 months for HBsAg and anti-HBsAg.

NURSING PRIORITY: It is important to explain to parents to have a second newborn blood screening performed at 7-14 days to ensure against a possible false negative result on the first screening.

✦ *Goal: to promote infant feeding.*

1. Considerations in infant feeding.
   a. Infants should always be placed on their side after feeding to decease problem with aspiration.
   b. Infant will require more frequent feeding initially, generally will establish a routine of feeding every 3-4 hours.
2. Breastfeeding.
   a. First feeding should occur immediately or within a few hours after birth.
   b. Stimulates release of prolactin to initiate milk production.
   c. Assess the mothers knowledge of breast feeding on the first feeding.
   d. Assist the mother to hold the infant at the breast with the infants ear, shoulder and hips in a straight line.
   e. Have the mother touch the infants lower lip with the nipple to stimulate the latch-on reflex.
   f. Most of the aerola should be in the infant's mouth.
   g. Frequent feedings are important initially to establish milk production, often every 1.5-2 hours.
   h. One of the primary reasons mothers stop breast feeding is the perception that their milk supply is not sufficient.
   i. Encourage mother to not offer the infant a bottle until lactation is well established, generally about 4 weeks.
   j. Engorgement and nipple soreness are the most common problems the mother experiences.
3. Bottle feeding.
   a. It is not necessary to sterilize the water used to reconstitute infant's formula.
   b. The infant should be positioned in a semi-upright position for feeding.
   c. Never prop the bottle, always hold the infant.
   d. Mother should not coax infant to finish all of the bottle every time, any unused formula should be discarded.
   e. Do not warm bottles in the microwave, it results in uneven heating of the formula.

HIGH-RISK NEWBORN

Gestational Age Variation

Assessment

A. The etiology, physical characteristics at birth, goals of nursing care, and possible complications and problems related to the premature, small-for-gestational-age, postterm, and large-for-gestational-age newborn are outlined in Table 26-2.

B. Clinical estimation of gestational age (Fig. 26-1).

C. Respiratory parameters.
   1. Observe respiratory rate, rhythm, and depth.
      a. Initially, rate increases without a change in rhythm.
      b. Flaring of nares and expiratory grunting are early signs of respiratory distress.

2. Increase in apical pulse rate.
3. Subcostal and xiphoid retractions progressing to intercostal, substernal, and clavicular.
4. Color.
   a. Progresses from pink to circumoral pallor to circumoral cyanosis to generalized cyanosis.
   b. Increased intensity of acrocyanosis.
5. Progressive respiratory distress.
   a. Chin tug (chin pulled down and in with mouth opening wider— auxiliary muscles of respiration are used).
   b. Abdominal seesaw breathing patterns.
   c. Distinguish between apneic episodes (15 seconds or longer), and irregular breathing (cessation of breathing for 5-10 seconds.).
6. Falling body temperature.
7. Progressing anoxia leading to cardiac decompensation and failure.
8. Increase muscle flaccidity—frog-like position.

D. Nutrition.
1. Assess readiness and ability to feed—swallowing, gag reflexes.
2. Screen for hypoglycemia.
3. Observe for congenital dysfunction and anomalies related to tracheoesophageal fistula, anal atresia, and metabolic disorders.
4. Check amount and frequency of elimination pattern.
5. Assess for vomiting or regurgitation; a preterm infant's stomach capacity is small, and overfeeding can occur.
6. Check mucous membranes, urine output and skin turgor to recognize fluid and electrolyte imbalance.
   a. Skin turgor over abdomen and inner thighs.
   b. Sunken fontanel.
   c. Urinary output less than 30 cc per day.

E. Temperature regulation.
1. Assess infant's temperature—frequently done with a skin probe for continuos monitoring of temperature in infants at high risk.
2. Check coolness or warmth of body and extremities.
3. Detect early signs of cold stress.
   a. Increased physical activity and crying.
   b. Respiratory rate increases.
   c. Increased acrocyanosis or generalized cyanosis along with mottling of the skin (cutis marmorata).
   d. Male with descended testes—presence of cremasteric reflex (testes are pulled back up into the inguinal canal upon exposure to cold).
4. Monitor infant's temperature.
   a. Axillary temperature: 36.5° C (97.7° F).
   b. Place a temperature skin probe on infant while he is in the radiant warmer or isolette.

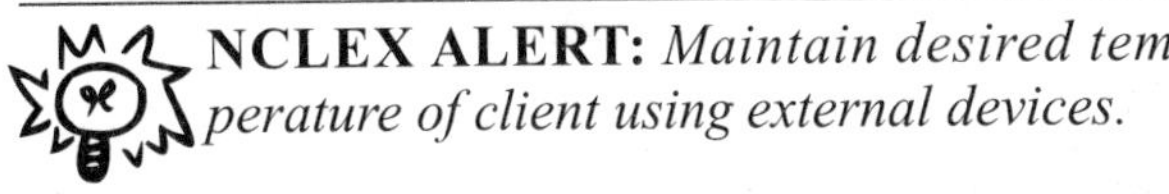

NCLEX ALERT: *Maintain desired temperature of client using external devices.*

Nursing Intervention for the High-Risk Newborn

✦ *Goal: to maintain respiratory functioning.*
1. Provide gentle physical stimulation to remind infant to breathe.
   a. Gently rub the infant's back.
   b. Lightly tap the infant's feet.

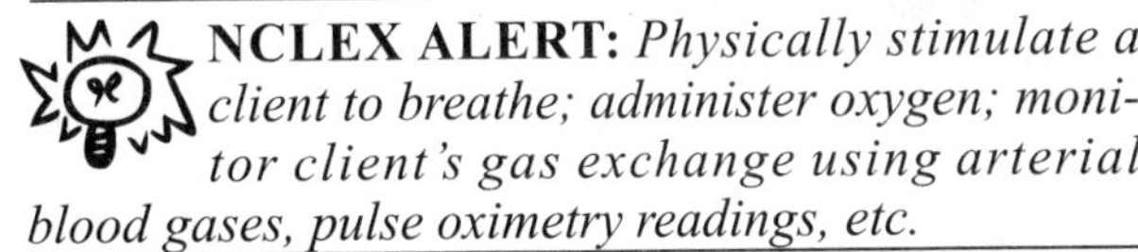

NCLEX ALERT: *Physically stimulate a client to breathe; administer oxygen; monitor client's gas exchange using arterial blood gases, pulse oximetry readings, etc.*

2. Ensure patency of respiratory tract.
   a. Maintain open airway by nasal, oral, or pharyngeal suctioning.
   b. Position to promote oxygenation.
      (1) Elevate head 10° with neck slightly extended by a small folded towel under the shoulders.
      (2) Flex and abduct infant's arms and place at side.
      (3) Avoid diapers or pin them loosely.
      (4) Turn side to side q 1 to 2 hours.
      (5) Do not place in prone position.
3. Assist infant's respiratory efforts.
   a. Monitor oxygen pressure.
      (1) Anywhere from 21 percent to 100 percent oxygen is administered to maintain the PO_2 around 50 to 80 mm Hg.
      (2) Avoid high concentrations of oxygen for prolonged periods—leads to complications of retrolental fibroplasia and bronchopulmonary dysplasia.
   b. Positive end expiratory pressure (PEEP) helps keep alveoli open at the end of expiration by providing positive pressure.

Table 26-2: GESTATION AGE VARIATIONS

PREMATURE (PRETERM - 37 WK OR EARLIER)	SMALL FOR GESTATIONAL AGE (SGA)	POSTTERM (OVER 42 week)	LARGE FOR GESTATIONAL AGE (LGA)
ETIOLOGY:			
Multiple pregnancy Premature rupture of the membranes Placenta previa Polyhydramnios PIH **Maternal diseases:** Diabetes Cardiovascular-renal problems Acute infectious problems UTI (Urinary tract infection) Genital tract abnormalities	**Chromosomal problems:** Down's syndrome Congenital anomalies **Infections:** Rubella Toxoplasmosis **Maternal factors:** Malnutrition PIH Advanced diabetes Preeclampsia Smoking Grand multiparity Alcoholism	**Postterm:** uncertain **Postmaturity syndrome:** can occur any time after 38 weeks' gestation and continue to 44 to 46 weeks' gestation; usually placental insufficiency is involved.	Maternal diabetes Multiparity Excessive maternal weight gain Genetic predisposition
PHYSICAL CHARACTERISTICS AT BIRTH:			
Inadequate amount of surfactant Poorly developed sucking and gag reflexes Unstable heart regulation Low resistance to infection Immature CNS, renal and liver systems Increased capillary fragility Excessive lanugo	Birth weight below 10th percentile on intrauterine growth curve Reduced sub q fat Loose dry skin Decreased muscle mass, especially over buttocks Sunken abdomen Sparse hair growth Wide skull sutures	**Postterm:** can be large, small, or appropriate size; usually in good condition - alert, active **Post maturity:** long and thin appearance Dry, cracked, desquamating skin Nails extending beyond fingertips Absent vernix and lanugo Malnourished and dehydrated Depleted sub q fat - "old man" wrinkled appearance Often meconium-stained skin, nails, and cord Alert	Overweight for gestational age - birth weight at or above 90th percentile on the intrauterine growth curve (over 4,000 gm or 9 lb.)
POSSIBLE COMPLICATIONS AND PROBLEMS:			
Respiratory Distress Syndrome (RDS) Patent ductus arteriosus Hypothermia and cold stress Retrolental fibroplasia due to O_2 toxicity Neonatal necrotizing enterocolitis Feeding difficulties Marked insensible water loss and loss of buffering agents through the kidneys Infection - low WBC Apnea and intraventricular hemorrhage Hypoglycemia Jaundice	Perinatal asphyxia Hypothermia Hypoglycemia Hypocalcemia Polycythemia Congenital anomalies Intrauterine infections and increased susceptibility to infections Aspiration syndrome	CPD (shoulder dystocia) Birth traumas Exposed to hazards of OCT (hypoxia) and amniocentesis (infection, bleeding, and direct trauma) Tolerate stress of labor poorly Meconium aspiration Cold stress Hypoglycemia Seizures	Hypoglycemia Polycythemia Hypervisicosity CPD - dystocia; prolonged stressful labor Fractures - shoulder CNS trauma - nerve damage to cervical or brachial plexus
LONG TERM PROBLEMS:			
Broncho-pulmonary dysplasia (BPD) Speech deficits Sensorineural hearing loss Neurologic deficits	Growth and learning difficulties	Poor weight gain Low IQ scores	Permanent nerve damage to cervical or brachial plexus

c. Continuous positive airway pressure (CPAP) counteracts the tendency of the alveoli to collapse by providing a continuous distending airway pressure.

(1) CPAP is administered either by endotracheal tube or nasal prongs.

(2) CPAP must be regulated in regards to humidification, temperature, and pressure; 6 to 10 cm of water pressure is equal to the therapeutic range for keeping the alveoli open.

4. Monitor oxygen therapy.

a. Transcutaneous oxygen tension monitoring ($TcPO_2$)—measures O_2 diffusion across the skin.

b. Pulse oximeter—monitors beat-to-beat arterial saturation; less dependent on perfusion than $TcPO_2$ or $TcPCO_2$; gives a more rapid "real time" reading.

✦ *Goal: to provide adequate nutrition.*

1. Detect hypoglycemia and treat immediately.

a. Dextrostix done frequently.

b. IV of D_5W if infant unable to tolerate oral feeding.

2. Oral feeding—initial feeding.

a. Use sterile water—1 to 2 cc for a small infant.

b. Use premie nipple to conserve infant's energy.

c. Due to small size of stomach, feedings are small in amount and increased in frequency.

3. Orogastric tube feedings.

a. Usually administered by continuous flow of formula with an infusion pump (kangaroo pump) when the infant is:

(1) Having severe respiratory distress.

(2) Too immature and weak to suck.

(3) Tired and fatigues easily using a premie nipple.

b. Placement and insertion of orogastric feeding tube.

(1) Position infant on the back or toward the right side with the head and chest slightly elevated.

(2) Measure correct length of insertion by marking on the catheter the distance from the tip of the nose to the ear lobe to the tip of the sternum.

(3) Lubricate tube with sterile water and slowly insert catheter into mouth and down the esophagus into the stomach.

(4) Test for placement of the tube by aspirating stomach contents or injecting 0.5 to 1.0 cc of air for the premature, up to 5 cc for larger infants, and auscultating the abdomen for the sound.

(5) Prior to infusing feeding by gravity into stomach, may need to check for residual; this is done by aspirating and measuring amount left in stomach from previous feeding; often the residual amount is subtracted from the current feeding so that overfeeding does not occur.

(6) If feeding is not continuous, remove tubing by pinching or clamping it and withdrawing it rapidly.

(7) Burp infant after feeding by turning head or positioning him or her on the right side.

(8) Always check to see if mother wants to pump her breast to provide the milk supply to the infant for gavage.

4. Hyperalimentation (TPN) may be ordered to provide complete nutrition through an indwelling catheter threaded into the vena cava.

5. Detect complications that arise with feeding the preterm infant as a result of the following:

a. Weak or absent sucking and swallowing reflexes.

b. A very small stomach capacity creates necessity for high caloric content of food.

c. Poor gag reflex, leading to aspiration.

d. Incompetent esophageal cardiac sphincter.

e. Increased incidence of vomiting, regurgitation, and development of abdominal distention.

f. Inability to absorb essential nutrients.

g. Excessive loss of water through evaporation from the skin and respiratory tract.

✦ *Goal: to maintain warmth and temperature control.*

1. Prevent and minimize cold stress.

a. Dry infant quickly, wrap, and place in warm incubator; may be unwrapped under a radiant heat shield.

b. All surfaces that touch the infant should be warm.

c. Oxygen and air should be warmed and humidified.

2. Maintain abdominal skin temperature at 36.1 to 36.7° C (97° to 98° F); axillary temperature 36.5° C (97.8° F).

3. Monitor infant's temperature continuously; make sure that temperature probe is set on control panel,

probe is in contact with infant's skin, and all safety precautions are maintained.

4. Prevent rapid warming or cooling, as this may cause apnea and acidosis; warming process is increased gradually over a period of 2 to 4 hours.
5. Infant may need extra clothing or need to be wrapped in an extra blanket for additional warmth; studies have shown that a clothed infant does not dissipate heat as easily as a nude one.
6. Because of the relatively large surface area of the infant's head, a cap or cover will reduce loss of body heat from the head.

Respiratory Distress

A. Types of respiratory distress.

1. Respiratory distress syndrome (RDS): Occurs as a result of the deficiency of surfactant which lines the alveoli; alveoli collapse at the end of each expiration, retaining little or no residual air, thus leading to a generalized atelectasis.
2. Meconium aspiration syndrome.
   a. Often, a fetus in utero passes meconium.
   b. Associated with fetal growth retardation (SGA) and with postmaturity.
   c. Meconium plugs small air passages and leads to inflammation of the lung tissues; areas of atelectasis there are, because of obstruction and consolidation of the meconium; secondary infection frequently occurs in the lungs.
3. Pneumonia—often associated with premature rupture of the membranes or a prolonged labor.
4. Central nervous system depression—often associated with excessive maternal analgesia or anesthesia.

Diagnostics

1. Chest x-ray.
2. Blood gases.
3. Electrocardiogram.
4. Possible lumbar puncture (to rule out central nervous system problems).
5. Determine the L/S Ratio.

Clinical Manifestations

1. Tachypnea—more than 60 respirations per minute.
2. Apneic spells.
3. Abnormal breath sounds—rales and rhonchi.
4. Chest retraction.
   a. Indicative of increased respiratory work.
   b. Begins as a mild sinking of the intercostal spaces or xiphoid retraction on each inspiration.
   c. Severe distress characterized by seesaw breathing—abdomen rises and chest sinks on inspiration; abdomen falls and chest expands on expiration.
5. Chin tug—noticed on inspiration; mouth open, lips apart.
6. Flaring of the nares.
7. Expiratory grunt.

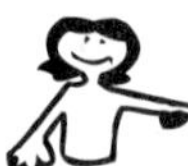

***NURSING PRIORITY:** Grunting is an ominous sign and indicates impending need for respiratory resuscitative efforts.*

   a. Protective reflex mechanism that prolongs end expiration, which increases oxygenation.
   b. Grunting sound occurs due to air pushing past a partially closed glottis.
   c. Often, it is accompanied by whining or moaning sound.
8. Prolonged expiration—air flows in easier than it flows out.
9. Cough due to excessive secretions in the respiratory tract.
10. Generalized cyanosis—usually is not observed until PO_2 is less than 42 mm Hg.

Complications

1. Hypoxia continues to increase, leading to decreased lung compliance.
2. Respiratory acidosis due to alveolar hypoventilation.
3. Metabolic acidosis occurs as a result of hypoxia → anaerobic metabolism → ↑ lactate levels and resultant base deficit.
4. Retrolental fibroplasia due to high levels of oxygen.
5. Bronchopulmonary dysplasia—chronic stiff, noncompliant lungs.

Treatment

1. Respiratory distress syndrome.
   a. Lack of surfactant and poor lung functioning lead to decreased PO_2, increased PCO_2, and a decreased pH.
   b. As condition worsens, metabolic acidosis may be superimposed upon a respiratory acidosis and lead to a severe decrease in the pH.
   c. CPAP is the primary treatment.
   d. Administration of surfactant through the airway into the infant's lungs.
2. Meconium aspiration.
   a. Oxygen with humidification.

b. Postural drainage and percussion.

c. Antibiotic therapy.

d. Acid-base imbalance correction if needed.

Nursing Intervention

✦ *Goal: to promote oxygenation and respiratory functioning.*

1. Administer a glucocorticoid (**Celestone**) to stimulate surfactant production at least 48 hours prior to delivery.
2. Refer to nursing intervention for the high-risk newborn.

✦ *Goal: to prevent respiratory distress.*

1. Assess for infants at high risk related to gestational age and predisposing factors.
2. Monitor L/S ratio of infants at risk.

Cleft Lip

Pathophysiology

1. A fissure of the upper lip to the side of the midline, which may vary from a slight notch to a complete separation extending into the nostril; may be unilateral or bilateral.
2. Caused by failure of the maxillary process to close in early fetal life; usually occurs during the sixth week of gestation.
3. Increased incidence in males; occurs in about 1:800 live births.

Assessment—visible at birth on an incompletely formed lip.

Treatment

1. Surgical—closure of lip defect usually done within a few weeks of birth.

Nursing Intervention

✦ *Goal: to provide preoperative care.*

1. Maintain nutrition.
   a. Use a large-holed nipple, a soft regular cross-cut nipple, lamb's nipple (which is longer and softer).
   b. Feed slowly.
   c. Bubble and burp frequently (after every 15 to 30 cc).
   d. Rinse cleft with water after each feeding to help prevent infection.
   e. Do not place infant on pillow, elevate HOB, or put the pillow under the mattress.
2. Prepare parents for newborn's surgery.
   a. Encourage parent to position infant on back frequently to accustom him or her to the postoperative positioning.
   b. Encourage parents to place infant in arm restraints periodically prior to admission, so that he/she becomes familiar with restriction of arm motion after surgery.
   c. Encourage parents to feed infant with the same method that will be used postoperatively.

✦ *Goal: to provide postoperative care.*

1. Prevent trauma to suture line.
   a. Position on back or side.
   b. Restrain arms with soft elbow restraints.
2. Maintain a patent airway and facilitate breathing.
   a. Use side-lying position or in an infant seat.
   b. Assess for respiratory distress, swelling of the nose, tongue, and lips.
3. Provide adequate nutrition.
   a. Feed in an upright, sitting position.
   b. Feed slowly and burp/bubble at frequent intervals.
   c. Cleanse suture line after each feeding; use cotton-tipped applicator and roll along suture line using half strength H_2O_2 and rinse with normal saline, may apply antibiotic ointment.
   d. Prevent any crust or scab formation on lip and suture line.
4. Provide discharge teaching to parents.
   a. Encourage parents to cuddle and play with child as this will decrease crying and prevent trauma to suture line.
   b. Teach feeding, cleansing, and restraining procedures.
   c. Refer to local community agencies for continued support.

Cleft Palate

Pathophysiology

1. Failure of fusion of the secondary palate; may involve the soft and hard palate along with the alveolar (dental) ridge.
2. Generally associated with a low-birth-weight infant; increased incidence of other malformations, especially GI tract defects.
3. Increased incidence in females.

Assessment

1. Opening in roof of mouth; usually associated with a cleft lip.
2. Sucking difficulties.
3. Breathing problems.

4. Later problems include increased incidence of upper respiratory infection and otitis media.
5. Later problems related to speech and hearing difficulties, and self esteem issues.

Treatment

1. Surgical.
   a. Surgery is done in 3 stages, may begin at birth or within a few weeks.
   b. As child grows, surgical correction to maxillary area is done, usually last surgery is 12-18 years old when the permanent teeth are present and correction can be done for alignment and spacing.
2. Long-term care management.
   a. Extensive orthodontics to correct problems of malpositioned teeth and maxillary arches.
   b. Speech therapy.
   c. Hearing problems related to chronic, recurrent otitis media; varying degrees of hearing loss may occur.

Nursing Intervention

✦ *Goal: to provide preoperative care.*

1. Maintain nutrition.
   a. Use a lamb's nipple or Duckie nipple.
   b. Encourage toddler to drink from a cup.
   c. Feed child in semi-upright position.
   d. Cleanse mouth with water after feeding.
2. Prevent infection.
   a. Teach parents symptoms of otitis media.
3. Provide support and teaching to parents.
   a. Teach use of arm restraints prior to hospitalization.
   b. Teach about various methods to meet infant's sucking needs.

✦ *Goal: to provide postoperative care.*

1. Maintain patent airway.
   a. Observe for respiratory distress and have emergency equipment available at bedside (endotracheal tube, suction, and laryngoscope).
   b. Position on side or back to provide for drainage of mucus and prevent trauma to the suture line.
2. Prevent injury and trauma to the suture line.
   a. Maintain age appropriate restraints.
   b. Avoid use of any objects in the mouth (e.g., straws, suction catheters, tongue depressors, pacifiers, or spoons).
   c. Avoid crying, if possible, by providing attention and affection or diversional activities if child is older.
3. Maintain nutrition.
   a. Fluids initially, then advance to soft diet based on age.
   b. Older child is not allowed to eat hard items such as cookies, potato chips, toast, etc.
   c. Cleanse suture line after each feeding by rinsing mouth with water.
4. Provide guidance to parents in relationship to long-term rehabilitation.
   a. Provide for emotional support.
   b. Encourage verbalization regarding infant with defect.
   c. Refer to appropriate community resources.

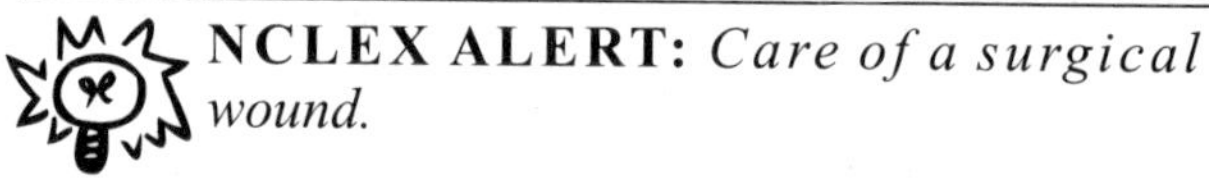

NCLEX ALERT: *Care of a surgical wound.*

Esophageal Atresia with Tracheoesophageal Fistula

Assessment

1. Risk factors.
   a. Prematurity.
   b. History of maternal hydramnios.
   c. Associated with other anomalies, especially congenital heart defects, anorectal problems (imperforate anus), and genital anomalies (exstrophy of the bladder).
   d. Incidence 1:3,000 births; occurs equally in both sexes.
2. Types.
   a. Esophageal atresia and tracheoesophageal fistula.
      (1) Most common form—80 to 95 percent of cases.
      (2) Proximal end of esophagus ends in a blind pouch and the lower segment connects to the trachea.
      (3) Characterized by the classic 3 Cs: *choking, coughing*, and *cyanosis*.
      (4) Excessive mucus secretion and constant drooling.
      (5) Aspiration is a complication, especially during feeding.
3. Diagnostics.
   a. Inability to pass a catheter into the stomach.
   b. Chest x-rays with use of radiopaque catheter.

Treatment

1. Surgical correction (for esophageal atresia with tracheoesophageal fistula).
   a. Thoracotomy with ligation of the tracheoesophageal fistula and an end-to-end anastomosis of the esophagus.
   b. If infant is in poor condition or premature, a temporary gastrostomy may be performed to allow for adequate nutrition, and the defect will be repaired at a later date.
   c. Often, a colon transplant is done if a segment of the esophagus is too short to anastomose.
   d. Surgical repair is done in stages.

Nursing Intervention

NURSING PRIORITY: *When there is any suspicion of possible esophageal problems, infant should be placed NPO until further evaluation.*

✦ *Goal: to provide preoperative care.*

1. Maintain patent airway.
   a. Supine position with head elevated on an inclined plane of at least 30°.
   b. Suction nasopharynx.
   c. Observe for symptoms of respiratory distress.
2. Early recognition of defect is important.
   a. Assess for the classic 3 Cs.
   b. Excessive salivation and drooling may occur along with gastric distention.
3. Prepare parents for infant's surgery.

✦ *Goal: to provide postoperative care.*

1. Maintain respirations and prevent respiratory complications.
   a. Pneumonia, atelectasis, pneumothorax, laryngeal edema are common complications.
   b. Administer oxygen as needed.
   c. Suction secretions and position for optimum ventilation.
   d. Maintain care of chest tubes.
   e. Administer antibiotics as ordered.
   f. Place in warm, high humidity isolette.
2. Provide adequate nutrition.
   a. Gastrostomy feedings are withheld until the second or third postoperative day.
   b. Oral feedings are delayed until two weeks or until the esophageal anastomosis is healed.
   c. Meet oral sucking needs by offering a pacifier.
3. Prepare parents for discharge.
   a. Teach techniques such as suctioning, gastrostomy tube feeding, and progression of diet.
   b. Explain signs of respiratory difficulty and indicators of esophageal constriction (e.g., difficulty in swallowing, coughing).

Imperforate Anus

Assessment

1. More common in males; often associated with neurological defects.
2. Types.
   a. A membrane over the anal opening, with a normal anus just above the membrane.
   b. Complete absence of anus (anal agenesis), with the rectal pouch ending some distance above.
   c. Rectum may end blindly or have a fistula connection to the perineum, urethra, bladder, or vagina.

Diagnostics

1. Visual examination of absent anal opening.
2. Abdominal ultrasound
3. Voiding cystourethrogram—identifies any urinary fistula malformation.

Clinical Manifestations

1. Absence of meconium.
2. No anal opening.
3. Gradual increase in abdominal distention.

Treatment

1. Surgery.
   a. Anoplasty—reconstruction of the anus.
   b. Abdominal-perineal pull-through.
   c. Colostomy.
2. Medications—antibiotics prophylactically.

Nursing Intervention

✦ *Goal: to identify and detect anal malformation.*

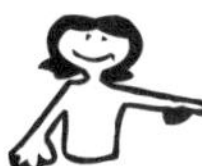

NURSING PRIORITY: *Record the first passage of meconium stool—if infant does not pass stool within twenty-four hours, further assessment is required.*

1. Detect increasing abdominal distention.
2. Inspect anal area for opening.

✦ *Goal: to provide postoperative care.*

1. Prevent infection by maintaining good perineal care and keeping operative site clean and dry, especially after passage of stool and urine.

Table 26-3: DISORDERS ACQUIRED DURING AND AFTER BIRTH

	TRAUMA	PERIPHERAL NERVE INJURIES	NEONATAL SEPSIS
ASSESSMENT	Soft tissue injury. Caput succedaneum. Cephalhematoma. Injury to bone.—fractured clavicle is the most common; often occurs with a large-sized infant.	Temporary paralysis of the facial nerve is the most common. Affected side of the face is smooth. Eye may stay open. Mouth droops at the corner. Forehead cannot be wrinkled. Possible difficulty sucking. Brachial palsy - a partial or complete paralysis of the nerve fibers of the brachial plexus. Cannot elevate or abduct the arm. Abnormal arm position or diminished arm movements.	Apathy, lethargy, low-grade temperature. Poor feeding, abdominal distention, diarrhea. Cyanosis, irregular respirations, apnea. Hyperbilirubinemia. Infant often described as "not acting right" Complete blood count, chest X-ray, and viral studies (**TORCH**) —an acronym for **T**oxoplasmosis, **R**ubella, **C**ytomegalovirus, and **H**erpes virus blood screening.
NURSING INTERVENTION	1. Place affected arm against chest wall with hand lying across chest. 2. Position is held by a figure 8 stockinette around the arm and chest. 3. Pick infant up carefully; shoulder should not be pressed toward the middle of the body. 4. Affected side should not be placed in a gown or undershirt.	1. Facial nerve palsy Eye patch and possible use of artificial tears to prevent corneal irritation. Provide support during feeding; may not nipple well. 2. Brachial nerve palsy Arm is kept abducted and externally rotated with elbow flexed Arm is raised to shoulder height, and elbow is flexed 90 degrees.	1. Prenatal prevention, maternal screening for sexually transmitted diseases, and assessing rubella titers. 2. Maintenance of sterile technique. 3. Prophylactic antibiotic treatment. 4. Cesarean birth for mother with genital herpes.

2. No rectal temperatures.
3. Side-lying prone position with hips elevated to prevent stress on perineal sutures.
4. Instruct parents as to care of colostomy (e.g., frequent dressing changes, meticulous skin care, placement of collection device, avoidance of tight diapers and clothes around stoma).

Spina Bifida

Assessment

1. A neural tube defect which results in midline defects and closure of the spinal cord (may be noncystic or cystic); most common site is lumbosacral area.
2. Types.
   a. Spina bifida occulta.
      (1) Noncystic spina bifida which results in failure of the spinous processes to join posteriorly in the lumbosacral area, usually around L5 and S1.
      (2) Neuromuscular disturbances may be apparent with foot weakness, bowel and bladder sphincter disturbance, and numbness and tingling of the extremities.
      (3) May be no apparent clinical manifestations.
   b. Spina bifida cystica.
      (1) Meningocele—a sac-like cyst of meninges filled with spinal fluid that protrudes through a defect in the bony part of the spine.
      (2) Myelomeningocele—a sac-like cyst containing meninges, spinal fluid, and a portion of the spinal cord with its nerves that protrudes through a defect in the vertebral column; most frequently associated with this is hydrocephalus (approximately 90 percent).
3. Diagnostics.
   a. Spinal X-ray films, tomograms, and skull X-rays.
   b. CT scan.
   c. Myelogram.
   d. Prenatal diagnosis - elevated αalpha-fetoprotein (obtained from amniotic fluid).

Treatment

1. Surgical—closure of defect with twenty-four to forty-eight hours to decrease infection, relieve pressure, repair sac, and possibly insert a shunt.
2. Medications—antibiotics.
3. Decreased in neuro tube defects with an increase in folic acid intake during pregnancy.

Nursing Intervention

> **NURSING PRIORITY:** *Correct positioning the infant is of paramount importance in preventing damage to the sac, as well as in providing nursing care after surgery.*

✦ *Goal: to provide preoperative care.*

1. Prevent and protect sac from drying, rupturing, and infection.
   a. Position prone on abdomen.
   b. Avoid touching sac.
   c. Meticulous care following voiding and bowel movements.
   d. Often, sterile, normal saline soaks with antibacterial solution may be used to prevent drying.
2. Detect early development of hydrocephalus.
   a. Measure head and check circumference frequently.
   b. Check fontanel for bulging and separation of suture line.
3. Monitor elimination function.
   a. Note whether urine is dripping or is retained.
   b. Indwelling catheter or intermittent catheterization is done.
   c. Assess for bowel function—glycerin suppository may be ordered to stimulate meconium passage.

✦ *Goal: to provide postoperative care.*

1. Prevent trauma and infection to the surgical site.
   a. Position as stated preoperatively.
   b. Continue to provide scrupulous skin care as listed under preoperative goals.
2. Assess neurological status frequently for indications of increasing intracranial pressure, the development of hydrocephalus or early signs of infection.
   a. Continue to measure head circumference daily.
   b. Neuro checks frequently.
3. Provide parent education in regard to positioning, feeding, skin care, elimination procedures, and range of motion exercises.
   a. Encourage and facilitate parent bonding to prevent emotional trauma to the newborn.
   b. Refer to community and social agencies for financial and social support.
   c. Encourage long-range planning and support of parents for long-term rehabilitation of infant.

Necrotizing Enterocolitis (NEC)

Pathophysiology

1. Occurs usually in the first week of life; increased incidence in preterm infants, especially those who have had fetal distress, hypoxia, intestinal mucosal injury, or shock.
2. Characterized by ischemic necrosis of the GI tract which leads to perforation.
   a. Right colon, cecum, and terminal ileum are most involved.
   b. Bowel is often dilated and surface is hemorrhagic.
   c. Ileus often develops and bowel may perforate.
   d. Peritonitis and neonatal sepsis ensue.

Assessment

1. Problems associated with feeding and elimination.
2. Abdominal distention and rigidity may be seen.
3. Bowel sounds may be absent.
4. Bile-stained emesis and blood-streaked diarrhea stool or guaiac positive.
5. Other symptoms: apnea episodes, temperature instability, jaundice, and shock-like symptoms.
6. Diagnostics-abdominal X-ray.

Treatment

1. Medical.
   a. All enteric feedings are discontinued.
   b. Nasogastric suctioning is initiated.
   c. Intravenous therapy and TPN.
2. Medications—antibiotics.
3. Abdominal X-rays to check for peritonitis, obstruction, or pneumoperitoneum (free air in peritoneum).
4. If condition is severe, surgery indicated for intestinal perforation, obstruction, and peritonitis: temporary or permanent colostomy.

Nursing Intervention

✦ *Goal: to assist with the medical and surgical management.*

1. Check nasogastric suctioning; keep infant NPO.
2. Administer antibiotics, IV, and TPN.

✦ *Goal: to detect early complications.*

1. Assess vital signs for indicators of shock.
2. Check for bowel sounds, as absence may indicate obstruction.
3. Measure abdominal girth q 4 to 6 hr to detect abdominal distention.
4. Avoid pressure on abdomen by not diapering the infant and placing them in supine or side position.

5. Consequences of NEC include: short bowel syndrome, stenosis of GI tract, recurring intolerance to feedings, with vomiting, abdominal distention, water-loss diarrhea, and failure to gain weight.

✦ *Goal: to provide support and teaching to the family.*

1. Explanation of treatment and, if surgery is done, postoperative management.
2. Assist in teaching how to care for infant's ileostomy or colostomy as necessary.

Neonatal Sepsis

Cause

1. Predisposing factor is prematurity.
2. Immature immunologic system.
3. Maternal antepartal infection: rubella, toxoplasmosis, cytomegalic inclusion disease (CMV), herpes virus type II (HVH II).
4. Intrapartal maternal infections: amnionitis, premature rupture of membranes, precipitous delivery, bacterial (*beta-hemolytic Streptococcus, Gonococcus, Staphylococcus*), fungal (*Candida albicans*), or viral (*Herpes*) vaginal infection.

Assessment

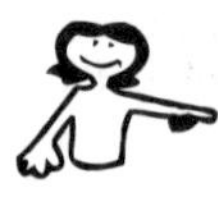

***NURSING PRIORITY:** Neonate often has very subtle behavioral changes which make it more difficult to assess a gradual onset of sepsis.*

1. Clinical manifestations.
   a. Apathy, lethargy, fever may be absent in neonates, low-grade temperature.
   b. Poor feeding, abdominal distention, diarrhea.
   c. Cyanosis, irregular respirations, apnea.
   d. Hyperbilirubinemia.
   e. Infant often described as "not acting right".
2. Diagnostics.
   a. Two blood cultures obtained from different peripheral sites.
   b. Lumbar puncture and spinal fluid for culture and sensitivity.
   c. Cultures from every orifice: urine, fecal, ear, nose, etc.
   d. Complete blood count, chest X-ray, and viral studies (TORCH, See table 26-3.).

Treatment

1. Medications.
   a. Antibiotics.
   b. Antiviral.
   c. Antifungal.

Nursing Intervention

✦ *Goal: to prevent neonatal sepsis by prenatal prevention, maternal screening for sexually transmitted diseases and assessing rubella titers.*

1. TORCH syndrome is discussed as it relates to the infant and adult in Chapter 8 and on Table 26-3.

✦ *Goal: to prevent infection during the intrapartal period.*

1. Maintenance of sterile technique.
2. Prophylactic antibiotic treatment.

Disorders of Maternal Origin

Isoimmune Hemolytic Disease of the Newborn

Pathophysiology

1. An antigen-antibody response causing destruction of fetal RBCs due to maternal sensitization of fetal red cell antigens and subsequent transfer of the resulting antibodies to the fetus.
2. Types.
   a. ABO incompatibility—results when the mother's blood group is type O (contains anti-A and anti-B antibodies) and the fetus' blood group is either type A, B, or AB.
      (1) Most often, the affected group with an ABO incompatibility is mother blood group type O and infant blood group type A.
      (2) Milder form of isoimmunization.
      (3) Can occur in the first pregnancy.
      (4) Does not necessarily increase in severity with each subsequent gestation.
      (5) Does not require intrauterine therapy (intrauterine blood transfusion).
   b. Rh incompatibility—Rh antigens enter the blood of an Rh negative mother and she produces Rh antibodies; these cross the placenta into the fetal circulation; if the fetus is Rh positive, the antibodies destroy the fetal RBCs (Figure 26-2).
      (1) Occurs with an Rh negative mother and an Rh positive father with an Rh positive fetus.
      (2) Affects the second or subsequent pregnancies, rarely the first pregnancy.
      (3) Severity of disorder progresses with each pregnancy if prophylactic treatment with Rhogam is not administered.
      (4) The hemolysis of fetal RBCs can vary in severity from anemia to icterus neonatorum or kernicterus to hydrops fetalis.

Figure 26-2: Maternal Sensitization to Rh Factor
Reprinted with permission: Gorrie, T.M., McKinny, E.S., and Murray, S.S. (1998) *Foundations of Maternal-Newborn Nursing, 2nd ed.* Philadelphia, Saunders, p. 704.

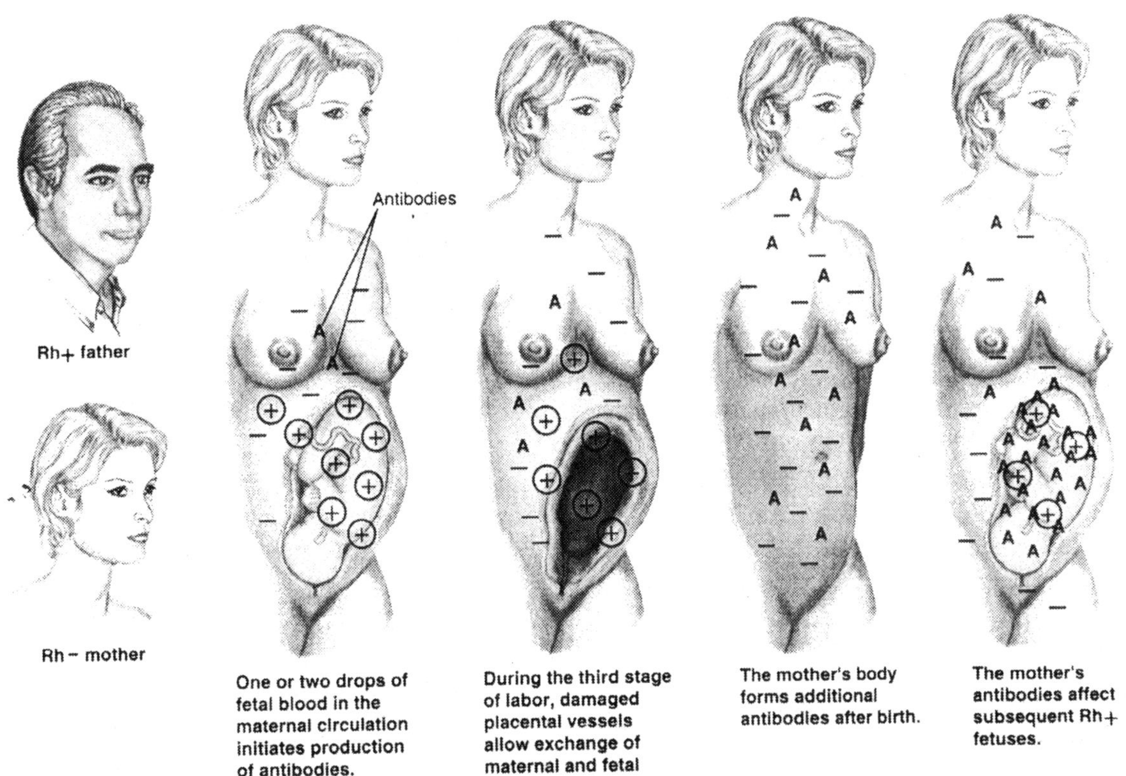

(5) If transfusion is necessary, O negative blood is used.

Assessment

1. Clinical manifestations.

a. Jaundice within twenty-four hours.

(1) Begins at the face and advances downward on the body to trunk and extremities, and finally to the palms and the soles of the feet.

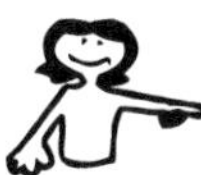

NURSING PRIORITY: *Press skin against a bony prominence (i.e., chin, nose) to detect early color change.*

(2) Bilirubin levels rises above 12 mg/100 ml of blood; may reach 30 to 40 mg/100 ml within a few days if treatment is not initiated immediately.

b. Anemia—usually evident within twelve hours; increased amount of immature RBCs (reticulocyte).

c. Placental enlargement.

d. Enlarged liver and spleen.

e. Hydrops fetalis (severest form of erythroblastosis fetalis)—characterized by hypoxia, cardiac failure, and generalized edema (anasarca).

2. Diagnostics.

a. Prenatal screening.

(1) Indirect Coombs' test—performed on the mother's serum to measure the number of Rh+ antibodies; critical level is usually defined as greater than a titer of 1:8.

(2) Antibody re-screening is usually done at 24, 28, and 34 weeks' gestation to detect any developing sensitization during the pregnancy.

b. Obtain prenatal history.

(1) Check to see if mother has had previous abortions, pregnancies terminated beyond eight weeks, or has received a blood transfusion.

c. Post delivery detection.

(1) Direct Coombs' test—reveals presence of maternal antibodies attached to the RBCs of an Rh+ infant.

(2) Umbilical cord blood is obtained.

(3) If titer is 1:64, indicates an extreme degree of hemolytic disease.

d. Other tests.

(1) Hemoglobin and hematocrit may be decreased.

(2) Increased reticulocyte count.

(3) Elevated bilirubin.

Treatment

1. Preventative.

a. Administration of RhIgG (**RhoGAM**) to prevent Rh sensitization in the pregnant woman.

(1) MICRhoGAM (50mg) is the first dose given at 28 weeks' gestation to prevent possible sensitization from a transplacental bleeding episode.

(2) Second dose: given within the first seventy-two hours postpartum.

(a) Has no effect against antibodies already present in maternal bloodstream.

(b) Provides passive immunity.

(c) Not a treatment for women who are already sensitized—recommended only for non-sensitized Rh negative women at risk of developing Rh isoimmunization.

(d) Administered after abortion, ectopic pregnancy, amniocentesis (second trimester), or blood transfusion.

(3) MICRhoGAM (50 mg of RhIgG) administered as a mini-dose following pregnancies terminated prior to twelve weeks' gestation, as a prophylaxis after amniocentesis (first trimester), and may be recommended at 28 weeks' gestation to prevent sensitization as the fetus grows.

b. Intrauterine blood transfusion.

(1) Procedure: amniocentesis with the use of ultrasound to identify peritoneal cavity of the fetus.

(2) Treatment: injection of Rh negative type O packed RBCs to improve fetal oxygenation and decrease anemia; may be done repeatedly at approximately two-week intervals until fetus lung maturity is achieved and delivery can occur.

2. Phototherapy.

a. Involves the use of high-intensity (fluorescent or blue light range) on the infant's exposed skin.

b. Causes unconjugated bilirubin to be converted into conjugated (water-soluble) form which can be excreted.

c. Indication for bili-lights varies according to the maturity of the fetus. May be started at a bilirubin level of 5 mg/100 ml of blood for a very small premie.

d. Effects.

(1) Vasodilatation of the skin.

(2) Increased insensible water loss.

(3) Decreased GI transit time—frequent loose, green stools.

(4) Skin rash—flea-bite dermatosis.

(5) Bronze-baby syndrome—serum, urine, and skin becomes a blackish brown color; cause is unknown, usually newborn recovers without complications.

e. Phototherapy may be used as an adjunct to exchange transfusion; it is not recommended for treatment of Rh incompatibility due to the excessive rate of hemolysis of RBCs.

f. Effectiveness determined by:

(1) A decrease of 3 to 4 mg/100 ml of blood in the serum bilirubin after 8 to 12 hr of therapy.

(2) A gradual diminishing of jaundice.

3. Exchange transfusion.

a. Purpose.

(1) Decrease serum bilirubin levels.

(2) Correct anemia.

(3) Remove the antibodies, the sensitized erythrocytes that are responsible for hemolysis.

(4) Prevent cardiac failure and severe erythroblastosis fetalis (hydrops fetalis).

Nursing Intervention

✦ *Goal: to identify and recognize jaundice of the physiologic type (which occurs within 48 to 72 hrs) ver-*

sus the pathologic type (occurs within twenty-four hours).

NURSING PRIORITY: *It is important for the nurse to differentiate between pathologic and physiologic jaundice in order to detect early problems.*

1. Prenatal monitoring of maternal-fetal status.
2. Monitor bilirubin levels in the newborn.
3. Identify high-risk mother.

✦ *Goal: to assist in the medical treatment.*

1. Phototherapy.
2. Exchange transfusion.
   a. Physician is in attendance during the procedure.
   b. Nurse maintains records of volumes of blood exchanged.
   c. Vital signs are monitored frequently.
   d. Observe and assess for indication of transfusion reaction.
   e. Assess umbilical site or other insertion site for signs of infection or bleeding.

Infant of the Diabetic Mother

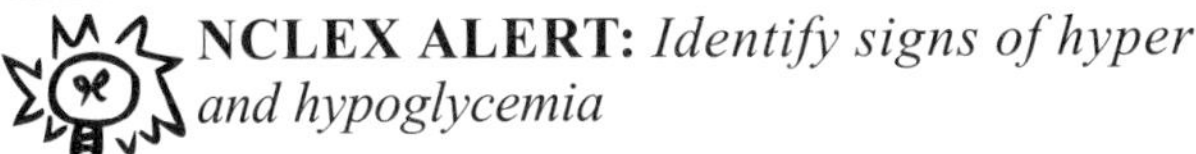

NCLEX ALERT: *Identify signs of hyper and hypoglycemia*

Assessment

1. Perinatal hazards.
   a. Large for gestational age due to receiving a great deal of glucose because of maternal hyperglycemia or infant may be small for gestational age due to insufficient placental perfusion.
   b. Size is inconsistent with gestational age; usually less mature.
   c. Maternal hyperglycemia stimulates increased fetal insulin production. Because insulin does not transfer across the placental barrier freely, and glucose does, the fetus is left with excessive insulin during the neonatal period after maternal blood glucose has been withdrawn.
2. Clinical manifestations.
   a. Puffy, cushingoid appearance, with round cheeks and stocky neck.
   b. Enlarged heart, liver, and spleen.
   c. Rapid, irregular respirations.
   d. Increased Moro reflex and irritability upon slight stimulation, or lethargy at times.
3. Common complications.
   a. Hypoglycemia—blood glucose (40mg/dL in the first 72 hours).
      (1) Lethargy, irritability, hypocalcemia.
      (2) High-pitched cry.
      (3) Twitching, jitteriness.
      (4) Seizures.
      (5) Apneic spells and abdominal distention.
   b. Respiratory distress syndrome.
   c. Polycythemia.
   d. Birth trauma due to excessive size.
   e. Congenital defects, specifically, cardiac (patent ductus arteriosus most common) and central nervous system defects (anencephaly, myelomeningocele, and hydrocephalus).

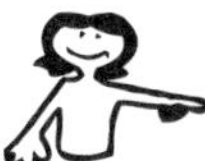

NURSING PRIORITY: *Prolonged hypoglycemia can cause irreversible brain damage.*

Treatment

1. Administration of glucose either IV or 10 percent dextrose solution orally, depending on severity of hypoglycemia.

NURSING PRIORITY: *A rapid infusion of 25-50% glucose is contraindicated because it may lead to profound rebound hypoglycemia following an initial brief increase in blood sugar.*

2. Hydration.
3. Blood glucose determinations on cord blood and done subsequently at thirty minutes, one hour, two hours, and four hours after birth.

Nursing Intervention

✦ *Goal: to identify infant at risk.*

1. Careful antepartal assessment of maternal diabetic status.
2. Treat infant at high risk and monitor continuously.

✦ *Goal: to monitor glucose levels.*

1. Blood glucose levels using glucose strips or glucometer are done frequently.
2. Minimize trauma to heel site by performing heel stick correctly.
   a. Use lancet or Accujet.
   b. Warm heel for 5-10 minutes prior to stick.
   c. Cleanse site with alcohol and dry before sticking.
   d. The lateral heel is the site of choice; however, the toes can be used if needed.⌘

Study Questions—Newborn

1. The nursing assessment of an infant reveals expiratory grunting, substernal retractions, and temperature of 99°. What is the first nursing action?

① Position the infant in Trendelenburg.
② Begin 40% humidified oxygen via hood.
③ Increase the temperature of the environment.
④ Perform a complete assessment for congenital anomalies.

2. Postoperatively, what is effective equipment to use for feeding an infant postop cleft lip/cleft palate repair?

① Premature-type nipple.
② Rubber-tipped Asepto syringe.
③ Newborn nipple.
④ Nasogastric tube.

3. Which statement best describes the problem of regulation of body temperature in a 3 ½ lb. premature infant?

① The surface area of the premature infant is relatively smaller than that of a normal, full-term infant in proportion to body size.
② There is a lack of subcutaneous fat which furnishes insulation.
③ There are frequent episodes of diaphoresis causing loss of body heat.
④ There is a limited ability to produce body proteins.

4. The nurse is caring for an infant with an unrepaired tracheoesophageal fistula. In planning care, the nurse will identify what priority nursing goal?

① Promote oxygen exchange.
② Prevent lung infection.
③ Promote bonding.
④ Replace fluid and electrolytes.

5. The nurse would identify which situation as an indication for the administration of RhoGAM?

① A woman who has been Rh-sensitized in the past two pregnancies.
② An infant with increased hemolysis of red cells due to ABO incompatibility.
③ An infant with increase in the serum bilirubin levels secondary to Rh factor antibodies.
④ A primigravida who is Rh negative is pregnant with an infant who is Rh positive.

6. While in the recovery room, the *best* immediate postoperative position for a postop cleft lip/cleft palate repair client is:

① Prone with the head turned to one side.
② Left Sims' position.
③ Supine with the head turned to the side.
④ Flat.

7. An infant is born at 28 weeks, gestation; he weighs 4 pounds 3 oz. What does the initial nursing care of this infant include?

① Place the infant in protective isolation due to the underdeveloped immune system.
② Administration of Lofenalac formula to increase digestion and utilization of calories.
③ Gavage feedings every 2 hours due to an inadequate sucking and swallow reflex.
④ Place the infant in an regulatory heater to maintain regulation of body temperature.

8. Retrolental fibroplasia is a potential hazard of preterm newborns. What causes this problem?

① Only oxygen levels of 40 percent or more.
② Short exposures to 40 percent oxygen.
③ Immaturity of the retinal vessels.
④ PaO_2 levels of 50 to 70 mm Hg in the preterm.

9. During the third day of life, the nursery nurse notices that a baby girl is jaundiced. A bilirubin level is drawn and it is 11.4mg/percent. What causes this bilirubin level?

① Physiologic jaundice.
② Hemolytic disease.
③ Erythroblastosis fetalis.
④ Sepsis.

10. A neonate is being discharged home with a fiberoptic blanket for treatment of physiologic jaundice. What is important for the nurse to include in the discharge instructions?

① Cover the infant's eyes during the treatment.
② Reduce the daily number of formula feedings.
③ Encourage fluids and increase daily feedings.
④ Expect a constipated stool until jaundice clears.

Answers and rationales to these questions are in the section at the end of the book entitled "Chapter Study Questions: Answers & Rationales."

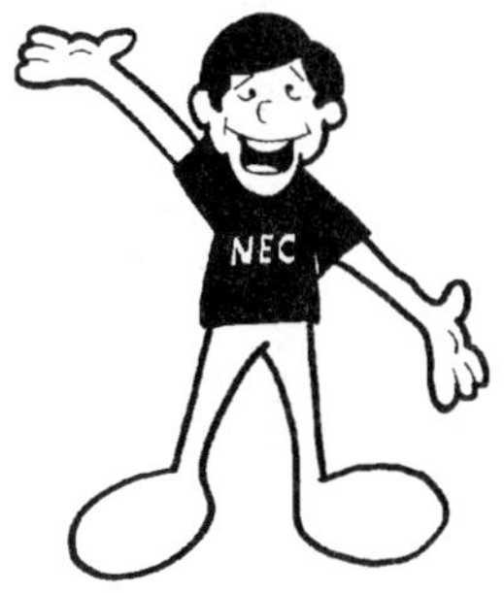

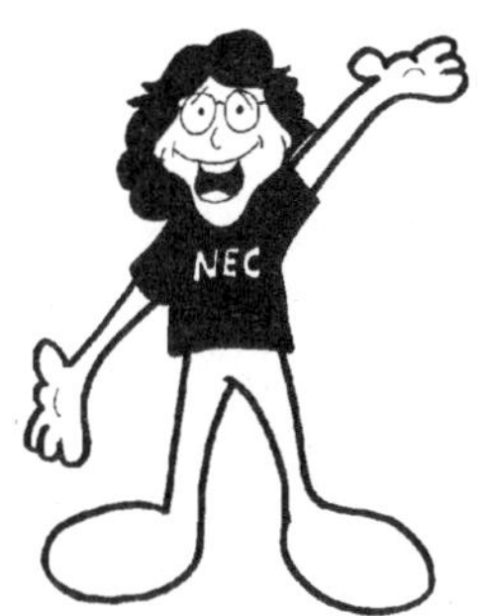

Chapter Study Questions Answers & Rationales

Chapter 2: Health Implications Across The Lifespan

1. ② Usually the toddler clings to the mother. As separation anxiety becomes intolerable, the child ignores the parent—at this stage the child relates better to the staff and doesn't mind the absence of the parent.
2. ① By the age of 9 or 10, the child has developed the mental and emotional security to express an understanding of death as a final and inevitable outcome of life.
3. ② When interviewing an older client, auditory acuity is the most common age-related aspect to take into consideration.
4. ② Children at this age are prone to anemia, especially when milk is offered frequently. Therefore, holding liquids till after solid food is offered prevents the child from "filling up" on the liquid.
5. ② Stacking rings are a good manipulative toy for a toddler and will not be adversely affected by the humid environment.
6. ② Foods high in calcium include milk products, leafy green vegetables, fish, dried beans and peas, and citrus fruit. Yellow vegetables are not high in calcium. Pasta and breads are high in sodium.
7. ② The increased potassium found in dried peaches and apricots are contraindicated in client with increased potassium and increased BUN. Dried fruit is high in potassium.
8. ③ The older adult finds meaning in life and adjusts to the death of a spouse or loved one. They are aware of death as an inevitable part of living and often react to dying as a time of reflection, rest, and peace.
9. ④ Immunizations are started as early as 1 month (recommended to be given first dose prior to discharge from the hospital) with Hepatitis B. The DPT and OPV series are started at 2 months.
10. ④ The varicella zoster vaccine can be administered any time after 12 months of age.
11. ① Varicella is an acute viral disease characterized by a maculopapular rash with vescular scabs in multiple stages of healing. Most erythematous rashes start on face and progress to rest of body.
12. ① Deep, penetrating wounds that are contaminated by soil, dust, excreta that contains *Clostridium tetani* are the cause of tetanus or lockjaw. First the wound should be thoroughly cleansed, then determination of when client received last tetanus immunization. As a rule, clients will receive a booster (Td) just as a safeguard.

Chapter 3: Concepts of Nursing Practice

1. ③ To obtain an accurate reading in an adult, the blood pressure cuff should cover the upper two-thirds of the client's arm; it should be positioned approximately 2" above the antecubital space. The systolic reading is obtained with the first of the Korotkoff sounds.
2. ④ The nurse knows that secondary prevention efforts are directed toward promoting early case finding so that prompt intervention can be instituted.

   ③ The client should be taught to pick something up from the floor by squatting down rather than bending over.
4. ② Tepid sponge baths reduce temperature by promoting evaporation. Ice or alcohol baths may reduce temperature too rapidly, leading to vascular collapse or vasoconstriction, which defeats the purpose of the cool applications. Do not allow the child to become chilled, as this will increase heat production and raise the temperature.
5. ④ The eleventh and twelfth thoracic nerve roots carry sensory fibers from the uterus. Motor fibers going to the uterus leave the spinal cord at the seventh and eighth thoracic vertebrae. The separation of motor and sensory levels permits

the use of epidural and spinal anesthesia in labor.

6. ② Weight bearing increases the vascular tone and decreases venous stasis, thereby preventing thrombi from developing; the increase in activity increases respiratory expansion and quality of breathing.
7. ④ The nurse knows that primary prevention activities are directed toward decreasing the probability of encountering illness or stressors.
8. ③ The first priority is to clear the airway and free it from any mechanical obstruction.
9. ② The apical heart rate is best counted at the point of maximum impulse (PMI). This is at the level of the apex of the left ventricle, which is located at the fifth intercostal space, midclavicular line on the left side.
10. ④ When a child with cerebral palsy or any chronic illness is hospitalized, routines utilized at home should be followed to provide continuity of care.
11. ② Children may withdraw and sleep to be able to deal with pain. The mother is the best judge of the young child's pain.
12. ④ Importance is placed on creating a comprehensive picture of the client's medical history by placing events in their proper chronological order.
13. ② The best approach to a good interview is to start with the easy less personal questions while building a rapport.
14. ④ Consent forms must be signed by the client, family, or guardian with medical power of attorney before any procedure can done on the client.

Chapter 4: Control Functions and Management

1. ③ Errors in charting should never be obliterated, recopied, or covered with "white out." When the erroneous information is not legible, it raises questions as to what the person was trying to "cover up."
2. ④ Legal reporting laws are exceptions under the invasion of privacy. Communicable diseases, gunshot, knife wounds, and child abuse are reportable.
3. ② Conversation is confidential. It is covered under invasion of privacy which states that the client has the constitutional right to be free from undesired publicity and exposure to public view.
4. ③ The client needs to show an understanding of the informed consent by giving an explanation in the clients own words.
5. ② Any suspected child abuse should be reported to the appropriate agencies.
6. ③ The nurse needs to keep skills and nurse knowledge current to deliver competent safe care.
7. ① The chart is considered a legal document. Any illegal alterations can be considered fraud.
8. ③ By knowing the history of the client, the nurse would notify the physician of the client's history and ask for a change in medications.
9. ④ Offering the physician to meet with the nursing supervisor would be the most appropriate approach giving the physician enough time to rethink his position. Giving the med would place the nurse in a position of liability, while not signing for it would increase the legal liability. Arguing with the physician would only escalate the issue.
10. ② In a quality assurance program, there must be standards from which to measure progress. Criteria are established in order to obtain objective measurement.

Chapter 5: Pharmacology

1. ③ Until the child walks or is one year of age, the vastus lateralis is the preferred muscle group site.
2. ② Only one antibiotic should be administered at a time. Both drugs should be administered at the time ordered by the doctor for greatest effectiveness.
3. ① The calculation would be 100/30 x 10 = 33.3 or 33 gtt/min.
4. ① A elderly client on multiple medications with simultaneous doses is at risk for negative drug interactions. At times more than one physician may be ordering medications without consideration to medications the client is already taking.
5. ③ The first step of drug delivery to a client is to check the order with the medication administration sheet for possible discontinuance, dose, route, or time change.
6. ③ The dose should be recorded as "not taken" and waste the poured dose. If the dose is a controlled substance the wasted dose must be witnessed. Checking the medication order for changes before accessing the medication helps to eliminate waste.
7. ② Liquid oral medications are already in solution and are thus absorbed more rapidly.
8. ④ Ingestion of oral medications mixes the substance with body fluids which in turn allows the liquefied substance to be absorbed by the mucosa of the GI tract.
9. ④ Check the physician's orders in the chart to verify giving the drug.

10. ③ By drawing up 0.3cc of air you will be able to clear the total amount of drug from the needle and seal the site from leakage.

Chapter 6: Homeostasis

1. ④ The nurse would expect to see a decreased pH and increased PCO_2 in a client with respiratory acidosis. Normal pH is 7.35-7.45 and normal PCO_2 is 35-45mm/Hg.
2. ③ The priority assessment for a client fluid problems is to the daily weight. Weight gain and loss is the most accurate measurement of fluid gain and loss.
3. ① The cost-effective and safest decision is to finish the current liter of fluid. The second and fourth answers are not relevant to the ordered fluid. The third answer does not recognize whether the client has voided and is least cost-effective. The liter of Ringer's lactate has already been considered in the daily intake.
4. ① Symptoms of lead toxicity appear insidiously, progressing from hyperirritability, anorexia, lethargy, intermittent gastrointestinal distress, constipation, and weakness to increased nervousness, ataxia, continual vomiting, impaired consciousness, and encephalopathy with seizures and coma.
5. ③ Any client on steroid therapy should understand that abrupt discontinuance can be dangerous and that a tapering off process is used to safely discontinue steroid use.
6. ② Long-term steroid use depresses the immune system making the client susceptible to infection.
7. ① The renal system controls the excretion of sodium and potassium through the countercurrent mechanism.
8. ③ With dehydration or fluid deficit, the skin becomes flush with increased blood flow to the surface capillaries; the skin then becomes dry and warm.
9. ① The body's response to fever is to bring fluid to the surface areas which have increased temperature creating a diaphoretic state and thus a loss of body fluids.
10. ④ With a continuos flow at 125cc/hr, a small guage intercath is appropriate. IVs should be started on the large vessels of the hand and progress upward. The anticubital area is not a preferred area.
11. ② The client needs a balanced solution for maintenance of electrolytes, which is the Ringer's lactate. The normal saline may be used, but most often potassium is added to the infusion.

Chapter 7: The Immune System

1. ② The presence of ANA antibodies, decreased serum complement fixation, bone marrow suppression, and increased level of LE cell formation correlates with the progress of SLE.
2. ③ Live viruses are contraindicated. Other vaccines are safe and encouraged to be given.
3. ② Cell-mediated immunity occurs when T cells are sensitized to an antigen from a previous exposure, such as the TB skin test. The itching and erythema are characteristic of the delayed hypersensitivity.
4. ④ Cytotoxic medications, like methotrexate or cyclophosphamide, are given in serious, refractory cases of SLE.
5. ① Anaphylaxis is a massive antigen-antibody response causing a physiological system shutdown and possible death.
6. ④ When the body develops a defensive response to itself, it is considered an autoimmune response.
7. ① When the immune system is depressed, weak, or compromised and is unable to defend the body from invading microorganisms. The system is consider immunodeficient.
8. ④ Actively acquired immunity occurs when the client receives an immunization. Natural active immunity occurs when the client contracts and has the disease and develops antibodies. Passive acquired immunity is when antibodies or antitoxin is administered to the client to give him a temporary immunity.
9. ④ The immune system develops antibodies in response to exposure to foreign antigens.
10. ③ The stomach defends the body from ingested bacteria and germs through secretion of gastric acids which creates a barrier to invading organisms.
11. ④ Clients usually develop symptoms within 6-12 weeks, however they may not develop until 6 months.
12. ① Category A is when the primary condition is identified or the client has recently been infected. He may be asymptomatic at this time or he may have symptoms of early non-specific change is characterized by fatigue, weight loss, persistent fever, diarrhea, night sweats, and generalized lymphadenopathy.

Chapter 8: Abnormal Cell Growth

1. ② The main goal is to get the client into remission. Medications are usually discontinued after 3 years of remission.
2. ② Due to the skin receiving radiation, erythema, desquamation, and abnormal pigmentation may develop after the radiation treatment.

3. ④ Once the implant is in place, keeping it in the exact measured position without disruption is a primary goal of care. In order to accomplish this, the head of the bed should only be slightly raised.
4. ④ Skin markings are utilized by the radiotherapist to delineate the exact area of the body to be irradiated. Treatments are completed daily in a series and do not require fasting or any form of isolation.
5. ③ A common side effect of chemotherapy medications is stomatitis. It may be manifested as inflammation of the gums and ulcerations in the mouth.
6. ③ A colposcopic exam is a microscopic exam of the cervix and is a common diagnostic test associated with cervical cancer.
7. ③ Irritation at the insertion site is a problem in a client who is immunocompromissed. Checking the IV site and surrounding area for signs of infection is a priority nursing action.
8. ③ The most common area for cancer to develop in the female body is the uterine cervix.
9. ④ Congestive heart failure (dyspnea, tachycardia, peripheral edema) is an adverse effect of doxorubicin **(Adriamycin)**.
10. ① Pulmonary toxicity (dry nonproductive cough, crackles, dyspnea, tachypnea) is an adverse affect of busulfan **(Myleran)**. It can lead to pulmonary fibrosis.

Chapter 9: Psychiatric Nursing Concepts

1. ③ Toddlers react very strongly to separation. Nurses frequently must act as surrogate mothers.
2. ② The child usually has a fairly accurate evaluation of a situation and the nurse needs to respond to his questions about dying in a way that allows him a chance to express his concerns.
3. ④ The dying of a child places an intense emotional strain on the parents and they may use the nurse as targets for their anger. The nurse can become an ally of the parents by allowing them to express their emotions and by assisting them in understanding what is happening.
4. ② The findings of studies of the behavior of terminally ill children is that they may experience anxiety in relationship to loneliness, separation, and death more frequently than children who are well.
5. ① Parents whose children are diagnosed with pyloric stenosis often feel that the problem was in some way related to inadequate parenting skills.
6. ② Continued presence of the same helping person enables the dying person to avoid experiencing a sense of abandonment and allows him/her and the family to establish the necessary trust for a comfortable working relationship.
7. ② A person with an inordinate attachment to the love object is unable to cope with life effectively when the attachment is disrupted, and as a result, experiences a grieving process that leads into a cycle of depression.
8. ② Obtaining informed consent for examination is a priority before any action is taken, including obtaining laboratory specimens and notifying police.
9. ② Although anxiety, fear, and guilt all play a part in abuse, the hostage response is when the victim assumes responsibility for the violence inflicted on themselves. Victims tend to blame the violence inflicted on themselves. Victims tend to blame themselves for the abuse and develop a sense of unworthiness.
10. ③ Indicators of neglect include: poor hygiene, poor nutrition, poor skin integrity, contractures, urine burns/excoriation, pressure ulcers, and dehydration. A hip fracture may be due to osteoporosis. Confusion and disorientation are associated with dementia.

Chapter 10: Psychiatric Disorders

1. ③ The client is at particular risk for suicide when she/he appears to be coming out of her/his depression because she/he may have the energy and opportunity to kill her/himself.
2. ① To protect the client, he should be moved into a quiet environment away from others. This will help him regain some control and will not produce unneeded stimuli.
3. ④ Affective changes in the schizophrenic are self-protective, because they enable the client to deny the painful emotional impact of the external world.
4. ③ In setting goals with self-destructive clients, the highest priority should be given to goals that are relevant to self-preservation of life.
5. ③ When the parents can verbalize the need to change the plans that they had made for their infant, it usually signifies that they are beginning to face reality.
6. ④ The nurse by his/her attitude and approach conveys interest and caring. If the nurse is repulsed by the client, this is conveyed nonverbally if not verbally.
7. ④ During the manic phase of manic-depression, all the body systems speed up, as described in the situation.

8. ③ Bizarre ideas that focus on the body being incapacitated are known as somatic delusions and are sometimes seen in schizophrenia.
9. ② Babies with Down's syndrome have a high incidence of congenital heart disease, especially atrial defects.
10. ① The withdrawn client maintains emotional distance until the barrier of fear of rejection can be broken through contact with another person in a therapeutic relationship.
11. ② One of the common side effects of antipsychotic medications is drowsiness. The effect diminishes usually after the client has taken the medication for a few days.
12. ③ Lithium toxicity is a serious problem for bipolar clients. Symptoms include: diarrhea, confusion, ataxia, slurred speech, hypotension, seizures, oliguria, coma, and death.
13. ② Cocaine has amphetamine-like affects on the body which are increased BP, pulse, along with paranoia and anxiety.

Chapter 11: Integumentary System

1. ② The burns are on the anterior trunk and do not involve extremities, hence the problem would be watching for infection, as the eschar makes it difficult to visually examine the healing skin. Removal of the eschar enhances healing and prevents infection which occurs due to the moist, enclosed area under the eschar.
2. ③ Impetigo is caused by the streptococcus or staphylococcus. Ointments are applied if the lesion is not on the face. For facial lesions, a systemic antibiotic is given.
3. ② Pediculosis capitis (head lice) is characterized by tiny white colored nits (eggs) which attach to the base of the hair shaft and are highly contagious. Scabies form burrows and the itching is often more intense at night. Acne is characterized by pustules. Tinea capitis is characterized by a red, scaly rash with central clearing in the well-defined margins.
4. ④ An allergic reaction to ampicillin would be the most life threatening, hence skin testing is often done prior to administration of the antibiotic for the first time.
5. ② Malignant melanoma is the most difficult to treat, involves extensive full thickness skin resections, and hence has the worst prognosis. Basal cell carcinoma and squamous cell are easier to treat and do not metastasize like melanoma. Oates cell is a tumor of the lung.
6. ④ This is Stage 4 pressure ulcer, as there is tissue necrosis with infection in underlying sinus tracts.
7. ③ Scaling, itching, and redness are common signs of tinea pedis or athlete's foot.
8. ① People with light to pale skin and who are excessively exposed to sunlight are most at risk to develop malignant melanoma.
9. ② Herpes zoster is considered infectious and the client must be placed in contact precautions. Antiviral medications would be given instead of antifungals. Lesions are usually along the sensory dermatomes (waist, neck, face) and not in the perineal area.
10. ③ Recognition of the signs and symptoms of infection are the highest priority. Pruritus creates an increased risk for infection, as the integrity of the skin may be traumatized.
11. ① Dry skin should be moisturized daily and prn, especially after client takes a bath which should be limited.
12. ② When there is evidence of burns around the face, the airway should be carefully assessed. Increased respiratory rate may be the first sign of respiratory complications.
13. ④ All of the skin is destroyed in a full thickness or 3rd degree burn. Often it has a dry appearance and may be white or charred, and usually requires skin grafting to repair. Option 1 is a first degree burn; option 2 is a fourth degree burn; and option 3 is second degree burn.

Chapter 12: Sensory

1. ① Atropine causes mydriasis or pupillary dilation, which can precipitate an attack of acute glaucoma. It should be questioned if it is ordered for a client with glaucoma. The other drugs would be safe for the client with glaucoma.
2. ③ Glaucoma has a strong hereditary tendency. Those with a family history of glaucoma should have intraocular pressure monitored yearly after the age of 30 instead of waiting until after 40 as with low-risk individuals. Client should not wait until eye problems occur to be tested.
3. ① Medications must be evaluated regarding increasing the intraocular pressure. Increase in the intraocular pressure could cause further damage to the eye in the client with glaucoma. The loss of vision is not reversible; glaucoma is painless, and is not correlated with the blood pressure.
4. ① The goal of a myringotomy is to promote drainage by making a surgical incision into the tympanic membrane, which also relieves the pressure and prevents eardrum perforation and reduces pain.
5. ② The use of a warm normal saline irrigation along with instillation of mineral oil would

soften the wax to assist in the removal of the cerumen from the ear canal.

6. ③ Penicillin and cephalosporin medications are not ototoxic. Aminoglycosides are ototoxic. The other three options all are risk factors for hearing loss.
7. ② The use of an ophthalmic anesthetic agent in the eye would necessitate the nurse to teach the client not to rub his eye until the "feeling" has returned (usually in 30min), to avoid additional trauma.
8. ④ Conjunctivitis is contagious through physical contact. The child should be directed not to touch the eye if at all possible. Handwashing should be stressed after contact and the child should not share any items which might be contaminated.
9. ④ Due to lymph fluid buildup in the ear, diuretics would be used to reduce inner ear pressure. Other medications given are **Valium**, **Antivert**, antiemetics, and antihistamines.
10. ③ The hearing aid amplifies sound, but does not change the overall ability to interpret incoming sound. It is used for conductive hearing loss clients.

Chapter 13: Endocrine System

1. ① When clients are sleeping, the only observable symptom of hypoglycemia is diaphoresis.
2. ③ If bleeding occurs, the blood will drain posteriorly.
3. ① Symptoms of acute pancreatitis are steatorrhea (fatty stools), hyperglycemia, elevated lipase and amylase, abdominal pain, and fever.
4. ② The unconscious, hypoglycemic client needs immediate treatment with intravenous glucose.
5. ① Calcium chloride or calcium gluconate should be available to treat tetany caused by accidental removal of the parathyroid glands during surgery.
6. ① Insulin acts to lower blood sugar primarily by improving the transport of glucose into the cells.
7. ① As carbohydrates are utilized for energy, insulin needs decrease. Therefore, during exercise, increase carbohydrate intake to cover needed energy requirements is needed..
8. ① Fluid and fat accumulation in the areas behind the eyeballs forces the eyes forward out of their sockets.
9. ① Diaphoresis and a shaky feeling are early signs of hypoglycemia. Severe thirst is a sign of hyperglycemia while drowsiness and coma are late symptoms of hypoglycemia.
10. ④ Glucose attaches to the hemoglobin molecule of the red blood cell. Glycosylated hemoglobin gives an average of blood glucose over the past three months and can be sampled at any time during the day.
11. ① Vasopressin alleviates polyuria by increasing ADH secretions. Urine specific gravity will return to normal level of 1.001 to 1.030.

Chapter 14: Hematologic System

1. ② In autosomal recessive traits, both parents are carriers. There is a 25% chance with each pregnancy that the child will have the disease.
2. ③ The other options can all be within normal limits for a two-year-old. Increased bruising is not normal.
3. ① Adequate hydration is critical during intrapartum for the client with sickle cell disease. Oxygen may or may not be ordered in low concentrations; a Foley catheter is contraindicated as a potential cause for infection.
4. ④ Infections are the most frequent predisposing factor for sickle cell crisis.
5. ② Tissue hypoxia occurs due to the decreased oxygen carrying capacity of the red cells. The sickled cells begin to clump together, which leads to vascular occlusion.
6. ② Iron deficiency anemia is characterized by fatigue, dizziness, weakness, increased pulse, palpitations, and increased sensitivity to cold. The adult female often becomes anemic due to a variety of reasons, such as poor nutrition and heavy menses.
7. ② Fresh fruits an vegetables harbor micro-organisms which can cause infections. Either peel or cook the vegetables and peel the fruit. Doctor is to be notified for a temperature over 100°.
8. ② The toddler will need to have a balanced diet. A diet based on milk products will not cover the nutritional needs of the toddler.
9. ④ First action is to apply ice and a compression dressing to reduce swelling and bleeding into the joint.
10. ② The whole blood must be given with in the first 30 minutes to prevent hemolysis and bacteria growth in the blood. Vital signs are to be checked after the first 50cc and first 15 minutes.
11. ② Stop the blood and disconnect the line to decrease the further infusion of red cells. Begin the normal saline with a new tubing.

Chapter 15: Respiratory System

1. ③ Retained secretions may cause hypoventilation; this results in an increase in the PCO_2.

2. ② A leak in the cuff would allow air to pass through the trachea and vocal cords, allowing the patient to make a noise—to speak.

3. ④ Use of oxygen may help to relieve shortness of breath but will not eliminate it. O_2 supports combustion but is not explosive; the major purpose of oxygen therapy is to decrease the workload of the heart in chronic pulmonary diseasesthus assisting to prevent right heart failure.

4. ① As croup causes upper airway obstruction, inspiratory stridor is a predominant symptom.

5. ④ Physical conditioning is important for clients with COPD; activity needs to be paced so that undue fatigue does not occur. Some increase in shortness of breath with exercise is to be expected, but will not damage the lung. If the client stops exercises before an increase in shortness of breath, he/she will not gain training effect.

6. ④ The catheter must be advanced to an adequate depth (to prevent secretion buildup at the end of the tube and to clear the airway as much as possible); to minimize trauma, suction is only applied during catheter withdrawal.

7. ③ There is specific information to convey to the client's husband regarding the bloody drainage in the chest tube bottle. After explaining the reason for the amount of drainage, then it may be appropriate to sit down and talk with her.

8. ② CPAP only works when the infant is breathing on his own. When the airway is opened for a breath, the CPAP increases the pressure in the airway, which increases airflow to the lungs and oxygenation.

9. ① An endotracheal tube which is inserted too far—beyond the carina—is most likely to enter the right mainstem bronchus. The volume of air from the ventilator is then only delivered to the right lung, breath sounds are decreased or absent over the left lung.

10. ④ Before the child is fully awake, she should be placed on her abdomen with her head turned to the side to facilitate the drainage of secretions and to prevent aspiration. When alert, she may sit up, or assume the position of comfort.

11. ① In an autosomal recessive inheritance pattern, the parents are not unaffected, but each parent carries the trait. There is a 255 chance with each pregnancy that a child will be born with the disease. If children do not have disease, there is a 50% chance they will be carriers, and a 25% chance they will not be a carrier or have the disease.

12. ② Tension pneumothorax occurs when air enters the pleural space with each inspiration, becomes trapped there, and is not expelled during expiration (i.e., one-way valve effect). Pressure builds in the chest as the accumulation of air in the pleural space increases. This can lead to a mediastinal shift.

13. ③ The wheezing is due to narrowing of the airway caused by bronchospasm. There is also increased mucus production that hinders the airway; this is results in trapping of air in the alveoli.

14. ① Diminished breath sounds are typically noted over the consolidated area. The cough is generally productive. The breathing is rapid and shallow without the use of accessory muscles. Hemoptysis may occur, but not hematemesis.

15. ① Pulse oximetry is the placement of a sensor on the finger or ear lobe, a beam of light passes through the tissue. Spriometry measures tidal volume and ventilation. Blood gases are an invasive measurement of arterial oxygen.

16. ③ In clients with chronic high pCO_2 levels (COPD), the administration of oxygen at too high of a liter flow will cause CO_2 narcosis which leads to apnea and the necessity of using an Ambu bag to ventilate the client.

17. ② Positioning over the bedside table allows the ribs to separate which assists the physician in positioning the needle into the pleural cavity. If unable to assume a sitting position, then the client is placed on affected side with head of bed slightly elevated. The area containing the fluid should be dependent.

18. ② Expectorants **(Robitussin)** stimulate secretions and reduce the viscosity of the mucus. Decongestants produce a vasoconstriction of dilated arterioles which leads to a reduction in the congestion. Antihistamines block the release of histamine and are used to treat mild allergic disorders.

19. ③ Decongestants should be avoided in clients with hypertension, as they often have pseudoephedrine and phenylephrine which causes CNS stimulation (anxiety, increased blood pressure, insomnia, etc.).

20. ④ Pulmonary embolus is the common complication of immobility (venous pooling of blood), estrogen therapy (increased incidence of embolism in high doses), and long bone fracture (fat embolus).

21. ④ Bronchitis is associated with coughing and excessive sputum production. Unless the client has an infection, their temperature is not elevated and they would not have a sore throat.

Their pulse and respiratory rate would both be elevated.

22. ③ The key to this answer is in the stem, "the nurse auscultates and hears a rubbing, friction sound," which is a pleuritic friction rub.

23. ② Most important assessment finding with a chronic bronchitis client is their history of productive cough and dyspnea. You might see peripheral edema, if they go into heart failure, but no hemoptysis (usually associated with pulmonary edema).

24. ① The respiratory rate is within normal limits at 18. The option for the pulse oximetry is too low. The pulse rate is too high and the productive cough with rapid breathing is not as significant as the decrease in respiratory rate.

25. ③ Bronchospasm is a medical emergency that can rapidly develop into a respiratory arrest. Client would more than likely have respiratory acidosis.

26. ② The ineffective clearing of secretions with resultant pooling can lead to an increased risk of infection. Their appetite is usually decreased and they have an increased A-P diameter of the chest.

27. ① Symptoms of tuberculosis include fatigue, cough, low grade fever, night sweats, shortness of breath, and weight loss. They usually do not have problems with rash, pleural edema, oliguria, or increased pulse.

28. ④ Interpreting a TB skin test for a non-high risk individual is 15mm raised area, however, in this situation the nurse is checking "a fellow employee's" skin test which would indicate a health care worker and the 11mm reaction indicates the person has been exposed to the TB bacillus.

29. ④ ARDS is a form of pulmonary edema that is characterized by labored respirations and low pO_2 in spite of a high FIO_2.

Chapter 16: Vascular System

1. ② The level of the right atrium must be determined and each successive reading be determined from the same point of reference on the client.

2. ④ Medication should be administered with a small gauge needle (25 gauge) into the subcutaneous tissue, without aspirating or massaging the area. Partial thromboplastin time (PTT) is utilized to monitor heparin.

3. ③ Noncompliance with blood pressure medications is a common problem in the treatment of hypertension. The client must understand that the only way to maintain her blood pressure under control is to stay on her medications.

4. ② The primary action of **Inderal** is to slow the cardiac rate. The medication is effective in the treatment of hypertension or dysrhythmias that result in tachycardia.

5. ① Early ambulation is the most effective and safe way to prevent thrombophlebitis with any type of client.

6. ③ Smoking causes vasoconstriction which increases the complications brought about by PVD.

7. ④ Immobility creates an environment for clotting due to venous stasis. Having the client ambulate as soon as possible stimulates circulation, reducing the possibility of clot formation.

8. ③ Reducing fat to less than 30 percent of total calories has been found to be the most effective way to loose and maintain weight loss. This approach is a non-pharmacological approach to blood pressure control.

9. ③ Occlusion to the aortic/femoral bypass graft is considered an immediate medical emergency and physician notification is imperative.

10. ④ With the head of the bed flat and having the client hold his breath during the tubing change causes an increase in thoracic pressure, this decreases the complication of an air embolus.

11. ④ Dopamine will support renal perfusion in the initial stages of shock, as the client becomes more decompensated, there is decreased effect of the dopamine on the renal perfusion.

12. ① The increased urine output indicates the kidneys are being perfused, therefore other vital organs are probably being perfused as well. The other measurements are improving, but are not indicative of tissue perfusion.

13. ① A low CVP reading would be associated with hypovolemia due to hemorrhage; this leads to decreased urine output that is associated with a decrease in renal perfusion.

14. ③ A complication of hypertension is CHF which may be first seen as dyspnea on exertion. The client should exercise as tolerated and stop when she gets tired or begins to have shortness of breath, regardless of the amount of time she has already exercised.

15. ④ Decongestants and cough over the counter medications frequently have pseudoephedrine in them. This medication will cause an increase in blood pressure.

16. ② **Nipride** is a very powerful, rapid vasodilator. The nurse should decrease the infusion first before the pressure drops further, then assess the client's response to the decreased rate.

17. ① A common side effect of a combination of antihypertensives and diuretics medications is

postural hypotension. It is important to teach the client how to deal with it.

18. ① **Aldactone** is a potassium sparing diuretic. The client's potassium level is high and the medication should be held and the doctor notified.

Chapter 17: Cardiac System

1. ③ By injecting contrast dye into the coronary arteries, cardiac catheterization with angiography allows visualization of the coronary arteries and provides information on their patency.
2. ① Jugular vein distention with the client in a sitting position, or with a 45 degree head elevation, is indicative of an increase in the central venous pressure. Many clients experience jugular vein distention when in a supine position and it is not indicative of an increase in the CVP.
3. ④ Nitroglycerin is a vasodilator. It dilates the coronary arteries, thereby increasing myocardial blood supply; vasodilation of the peripheral circulation decreases the pressure against which the heart has to pump, thereby decreasing the afterload.
4. ④ In order to decrease pulmonary congestion and dyspnea, it is desirable to decrease cardiac workload by encouraging bedrest.
5. ③ A low cardiac output decreases renal perfusion and results in oliguria and impaired renal function. Oliguria is less than 30 ml per hour.
6. ② **Nitro-dur** is used to prevent angina so that the client can perform the normal activities of daily living without chest pain. Sublingual nitroglycerin is used to treat immediate chest pain.
7. ① Compensatory mechanisms assist the failing heart to maintain an adequate cardiac output and blood flow to the tissues. These changes will initially maintain the blood flow in client's with decrease in cardiac output.
8. ③ Restlessness and diaphoresis may be indicative of decreased cardiac output, frequently originating from a dysrhythmia.
9. ① Nitroglycerin is a vasodilator and can cause orthostatic hypotension. For safety, the client should take it only while sitting or lying down.
10. ① It is important to have a thorough nursing assessment prior to the surgery for comparison after surgery.
11. ④ A low potassium can precipitate digitalis toxicity. The client has been taking her medications and not eating regularly. She also has an irregular heart beat, increased lethargy along with nausea, all of which can be signs of digitalis toxicity.
12. ③ A first degree block can only be evaluated with an EKG or monitor tracing because the distinguishing factor is a prolonged P-R interval, all beats are being conducted.
13. ② The treatment of choice is lidocaine IV push to attempt to convert the dysrhythmia before it progresses to ventricular fibrillation. Defibrillation and CPR are not done when there is cardiac output that is adequate enough to allow the client to stay conscious.
14. ④ Most demand pacemakers are set somewhere between 60-72, if the client's pulse rate falls below the preset pacemaker rate, the pacemaker should take over the pacing. With a bradycardia, the ventricular escape beats occur.
15. ④ The point of maximal impulse is the correct location to auscultate the apical pulse.
16. ① Atropine is administered for symptomatic bradycardia, an increase in pulse rate is the therapeutic response for this client.
17. ① Dyspnea on exertion is a classic sign of left ventricular problems, regardless of the precipitating cause.
18. ④ An echocardiogram provides information regarding flow of blood through the mitral valve and the left ventricular performance.
19. ③ Antibiotics (usually IVPB) are indicated for a bacterial endocarditis. The home care nurse will monitor this client's daily IVPBs. This is to prevent the vegetation growth on the valves.
20. ② Coronary artery bypass surgery is performed to revascularize the coronary blood vessels. This is accomplished by harvesting the client's own vessels (sapheneous vein, inframammary artery) for the grafts. This will promote increased blood flow to the heart muscle and eventually increase oxygenation.
21. ④ With left-sided heart failure, there is pulmonary problems. It would be important to decrease the venous return to the heart in order to improve the dyspnea which is due to congestion in the lungs.
22. ④ Nitroglycerin should be put under the tongue at the first onset of chest pain and repeated every 5 minutes for 3 doses. If after the 3rd tablet the pain is not relieved, the client should go to the hospital.
23. ① Digitalis slows the heart rate, strengthens the contraction, and improves cardiac output by decreasing the workload and heart rate.
24. ④ As the edema resolves in congestive heart failure, an increased urine output would be noted, primarily from the effects of diuretics.
25. ③ Jugular vein distension indicates increased venous pressure. This correlates with early indicators of right-sided congestive heart failure.

Chapter 18: Gastrointestinal System

1. ① Coffee ground material is old blood. This is a normal occurrence on the third postoperative day and should be correlated with the vital signs.
2. ① Nasogastric tubes are left in place several days postoperative gastric resection. It is important to prevent the stomach from becoming distended and putting pressure on the suture line.
3. ① Being NPO prior to a barium swallow and a gastroduodenoscopy and receiving a low residue diet the evening prior to the procedures are routine orders for these tests.
4. ③ Enemas or laxatives are not administered prior to surgery. If gastric motility is stimulated, there is an increased danger of appendiceal rupture; all other orders are appropriate preoperatively.
5. ② The characteristic position of comfort for the appendicitis client is on the side with the legs flexed against the abdomen; the head of the bed should remain slightly elevated to decrease the upward spread of infection in case the appendix ruptures.
6. ④ Chilling is normal after surgery because the temperature of the operating room is cool. Simply apply blankets to maintain the client's body temperature.
7. ② The syndrome is self-limiting. Decreasing fluid intake with and after meals, eating small meals, and decreasing carbohydrate and salt intake will decrease the dumping effect.
8. ① Rebound pain is elected by pressing firmly over the area known as McBurney's point. The rebound pain, decreased bowel sounds, fever, tender abdomen are all characteristic of the clinical picture of appendicitis.
9. ① Evaluate the nasogastric tube patency; it is very important to assess the client and determine the source of the nausea prior to calling the doctor.
10. ④ An upper GI will indicate delayed gastric emptying and an elongated pyloric channel.
11. ③ Duodenal ulcers are characterized by high gastric acid secretions and rapid gastric emptying. Food buffers the effect of the acid. Therefore, pain increases with stomach emptying.
12. ① The client's stoma may be catheterized on return from surgery, and the catheter left in place for about 2 weeks. The client is taught how to catheterize his stoma every 2-4 hours to remove any drainage. The potential for fluid and electrolyte imbalance is decreased. The stoma should not leak.
13. ② The primary problem with diverticula is food or undigestible fiber that gets caught in the pouches. The client should avoid this type of fibers.
14. ① Perforation is characterized by increasing distention and "board like" abdomen, other options may be seen with hemorrhage.

Chapter 19: Hepatic and Biliary System

1. ③ A T-tube is used after a common bile duct exploration to maintain patency of the duct until healing can occur. A T-tube should never be irrigated by the nurse. The purpose of the tube is to maintain bile drainage.
2. ② Semi-Fowler's position improves lung expansion. The incision for a cholecystectomy is high and may interfere with respiratory exchange. The other positions would probably interfere with respirations.
3. ④ Vitamin K is necessary for normal clotting. Cholecystitis can decrease the absorption of fat soluble vitamins (A, D, E, K,) by interfering with fat metabolism, which can lead to potential difficulties with clotting.
4. ③ T-tube drainage decreases after day 2 and may stop between day 3 and 5. T-tubes are not irrigated. Placement is not checked. Repositioning will not change the drainage.
5. ③ Clients with cirrhosis need increased Vitamin B especially B_6. **Thorazine** is hepatotoxic. Dietary intake should include adequate protein to build tissue. Daily weight is essential to monitor for volume overload.
6 ① HBV is spread by sexual contact. The client should not be sexually active until the HbsAB (antibodies to antigen) are present. There will be no bilirubin in the urine or stools; clay colored stools are expected so they would not be reported.
7. ① Vital signs must be assessed first if monitoring for bleeding or shock.
8 ③ IV Albumin is given to replace protein lost in the ascites fluid and to restore oncotic pressure in the vascular bed.
9. ③ Paper towels are utilized to create a clean area surface. Alcohol preps are not effective. The gown and gloves are not indicated for assessment.
10. ③ With end stage liver disease the liver cannot break down ammonia by products of protein metabolism. The increased ammonia levels in the serum cross the blood brain barrier causing uncontrolled drowsiness and confusion.

Chapter 20: Neurological System

1. ③ Recurrent headaches that increase in frequency and severity are frequently the first complaint of a client with a brain tumor.

2. ① The rehabilitation program for a stroke client includes actions that prevent deformity (passive range of motion on affected side and active on the unaffected side) as well as complications that may be associated with immobility. The client's affected side should be protected and food placed on the unaffected side so the client can control it.
3. ④ An electroencephalogram measures the brain's electrical activity and is often used to localize tumors.
4. ③ When a stroke occurs in the dominant hemisphere, the client experiences communication difficulties or aphasia. Speech retraining cannot begin until client understands and can follow directions.
5. ② Straining at defecation or the use of the Valsalva maneuver may aggravate increased intracranial pressure. The nurse promotes normal bowel movements that prevent straining.
6. ② The priority after a grand mal seizure is to maintain a patent airway.
7. ④ The first side effect to be noticed may be gastrointestinal problems. Taking medication with meals may alleviate these symptoms.
8. ① Bladder dysfunction may occur postoperatively due to impaired innervation to the bladder from the lumbar area. The client should be checked every 2 to 4 hours for bladder distention.
9. ② An early symptom of Parkinson's disease is slowness of movements in all normal activities of daily living.
10. ③ Due to the emotional stress of Parkinson's disease, mood disturbances often occur.
11. ③ Decreased mobility over an extended period of time leads to stasis of secretions.
12. ③ Irritability and vomiting are common signs of increased intracranial pressure in the infant; the symptoms are often delayed in the infant due to the open fontanels. Retinal hemorrhage, paresis, and papilledema are indications of more acute hematoma formation.
13. ④ Lowering the client's head increases intracranial pressure.
14. ② Because the motor fibers from one side of the brain cross to the opposite side before passing down the spinal cord, hemorrhage on the brain's left side causes right-sided hemiplegia and vice-versa.

Chapter 21: Musculoskeletal System

1. ② Following surgery, edema may cause compression of structures in the operative area, thus resulting in similar pain he experienced prior to surgery.
2. ② Green stick fracture refers to the splintering of the bone, not a complete fracture. The name comes from the splintering effect when trying to break a "green stick."
3. ④ In any client in traction, a nursing priority is to determine the correct amount of weight and to assess for effectiveness of countertraction. Weights must hang freely for countertraction to be effective.
4. ② Elevation of the stump in the initial postoperative period is used to prevent edema. The stump is wrapped from distal to proximal.
5. ③ The cast should be supported on a pillow that will not absorb the moisture and keep the cast wet. Palms of the hand should be used in turning the client. Heat should not be applied to a damp cast.
6. ④ Always check the weights and make sure they are not lodged against the bed or another area. There are no pin sites and the boot does not need to be removed that often.
7. ① Physical therapy helps relax muscles and relieves the aching and stiffness of the involved joints.
8. ① Osteoarthritis has a gradual onset and affects weight-bearing joints with pain that is more pronounced after exercise and morning stiffness.
9. ① Heparin is administered prophylactically to prevent thromboembolic complications in clients who are immobilized for prolonged periods of time.
10. ① Circulation and neurosensory status distal to the fracture is always a priority in clients with fractures.
11. ① The movement and sensation should be evaluated prior to surgery to have as base for evaluation post operative. Radiating leg pain is diagnostic of the condition and assessing it preoperatively is not as beneficial as determining movement and sensation.
12. ② Check the cast to make sure it is not too tight and constricting circulation. The child is not in traction; the arms are not part of the treatment; and the circulation is checked distal to the cast.
13. ② Check the status of circulation distal to the area of injury.
14. ② Compartmental syndrome is characterized by consistent pain and loss of sensation distal to the area of injury. The client can have an adequate peripheral pulse and still have a problem with compartmental syndrome. The client in balanced suspension traction has pins or wires exerting traction on the bone.
15. ① The callus is the network for new bone formation and an area of beginning mineral deposits.

It is more than blood cells and granulation tissue.

16 ① Balanced suspension traction with a Thomas splint requires checking the groin area where the thigh is supported. The leg of the affected side is suspended off the bed, the heel is usually not a problem.

17. ② Conservative treatment means without surgical intervention. The most common conservative therapy includes bedrest and a muscle relaxant.

18. ① Phantom limb pain is a real pain for the client and is common in amputees. Phantom pain can best be controlled by pain medication.

Chapter 22: Reproductive System

1. ① A Class IV Pap smear is highly suspicious for malignancy. A Class III is tissue dysplasia. A definitive diagnosis of malignancy would require a biopsy.
2. ① The herpes virus type II is concentrated in the vesicles, and therefore the infection is highly contagious when this fluid is released.
3. ① Prior to discharge, the client is instructed to avoid douching. On her post-operative visit to the doctor, he will evaluate the cervical area healing and will advise her regarding sexual intercourse.
4. ④ The client usually seeks treatment for a variety of symptoms, including painful intercourse.
5. ④ Low back pain and decreased urine output are serious symptoms that may indicate accidental intraoperative cutting of the ureter.
6. ③ Having the client void before the examination will make the procedure less painful and more accurate. Lubricant on the speculum may interfere with the Pap smear.
7. ④ Gonorrhea in men is the most symptomatic with urethritis, dysuria, and purulent drainage.
8. ④ Fluorescent Treponemal Antibody Absorption Test is used to recognize the spirochete treponema pallidum which causes syphilis.
9. ③ Up to 100cc of serosanguineous fluid would be an acceptable amount of drainage over a 24 hour period in a post mastectomy client.
10. ④ Elevating the affected arm promotes drainage of lymph from the extremity as well as decreases fluid from the wound site which reduces swelling.
11. ④ Flank pain may be indicative of an infection or a ureteral obstruction causing increased pressure on the renal pelvis. Other options are symptoms of BPH for which he is in the hospital to have treated.
12. ② Since she no longer has regular periods, she should perform SBE at the same time each month.
13. ② The examination should be done at the same time each month to order to develop a regular routine. After a shower when the scrotum is warm and the testicles are descended away from the body is a good time to perform the examination.
14. ① The primary complication is the obstruction of the urinary catheter with clots or tissue There should be a large amount of drainage from the catheter because the irrigating fluid is infusing into the bladder. The catheter drainage should be closer to 300-400cc per hour. It is not unusual for the drainage to be grossly bloody on the operative day, but it should begin to clear over next 24 hours.

Chapter 23: Urinary-Renal System

1. ④ Failure of the tube to drain freely can result in pain, trauma, wound dehiscence, and infection.
2. ③ Movement of the client will help disseminate the fluid throughout the abdomen.
3. ② A high fluid intake will help keep solutes diluted, thus preventing kidney stone formation.
4. ④ Each time, outflow should be about 100 to 200 ml more than inflow.
5. ② Urea is an end product of protein metabolism. In renal failure the kidneys cannot clear all of the urea from the blood and the BUN will be elevated.
6. ③ Protect the arm with the functioning shunt. No blood pressure should be taken on that arm, and there should be no needle sticks. The access is not irrigated.
7. ① Secondary infections are the cause of death in 50- 90 % of clients with acute renal failure.
8. ④ The goal in chronic renal failure is to prevent acute failure and maintain whatever function is left. This is best done by minimizing stress and the workload on the kidneys.
9. ③ Bladder neck strictures are common long-term problems of a TURP. Recurrent UTIs and spasms are unlikely. Reflux occurs primarily prior to the TURP.
10. ② The first specimen is discarded prior to the collection starting. Collection will continue until the completed time frame; the patient should void prior to the sample being completed.
11. ① The most characteristic symptom of renal colic is sudden, severe pain. The client may also exhibit nausea and vomiting, pallor, and be diaphoretic during the acute pain episode.

12. ④ The hemoglobin levels are not affected by the dialysis. the chemical components of the blood are altered by the dialysis.

Chapter 24: Antepartum

1. ③ Iron needs during pregnancy can most readily be met by taking iron supplements.
2. ③ False labor contractions decrease when walking, are not concentrated in one part of the uterus, do not increase in intensity and frequency, and do not result in cervical effacement or dilation.
3. ④ Striae gravidarum are caused by the stretching, rupture, and atrophy of the deep connective tissue of the skin. They are pink or reddish during pregnancy and become silvery white after delivery.
4. ③ An oxytocin challenge test, or stress test, is conducted by giving an infusion of oxytocin to the mother and evaluating the fetus's response to subsequent uterine contractions as plotted on a fetal monitor. The test is negative if there are no late decelerations and positive if there are late decelerations in more than one-half of the contractions.
5. ① Women can be advised in pregnancy to prevent back strain through measures such as good posture and body mechanics. Appropriate shoes worn during periods of activity may also be helpful.
6. ④ With bright vaginal bleeding, the nurse would anticipate that the client will have a cesarean section. It is critical that the client's stomach be empty prior to surgery or prior to delivery to decrease the incidence of aspiration.
7. ④ Home pregnancy tests are either the HAI or the ELISA type test. The are best when done on the first voided specimen and may be positive within the first few days following a missed period.
8. ③ When a woman indicates that she does not drink milk, it is important to pursue the reason for the avoidance or whether she is not able to tolerate milk. Remember to *assess* before you implement, i.e., gather information about her dislike.
9. ① Chorionic gonadotropin is a placental hormone which, when present, indicates the presence of pregnancy.
10. ④ Näegle's rule states that you count back three months from the date of the last menstrual period and add 7 days to determine the EDC. 35 percent of all women deliver within 5 days either before or after this date.
11. ① An L/S ratio (converts 2:1 at approximately 34-35 weeks) determines the relationship of two components of the fetal lung, lecithin and sphingomyelin, known as surfactant. Adequate surfactant must be present at birth in order for the alveoli to maintain expansion.

Chapter 25: Intrapartum and Postpartum

1. ① Hypotonic uterine motility can occur in the presence of various degrees of cephalopelvic disproportion. In the first stage of labor it is most often related to cephalopelvic disproportion due to the presence of pelvic contractions.
2. ① Mild, variable decelerations are evidence of cord compression. Fetal hypoxia and uteroplacental insufficiency are related to the development of late decelerations. Head compression is related to the development of early decelerations.
3. ④ Uterus palpated to right of umbilicus may indicate a full bladder. The fundus should be a the level of the midline. The temperature, lochia, and episiotomy assessment findings are within normal limits.
4. ④ The correct method of timing contractions is from the beginning of one contraction to the beginning of the next. When the contraction ends is only of concern when the nurse needs to know the duration of the contraction, not the frequency.
5. ③ When a woman does not want to view her infant at birth, the possibility of inadequate bonding may be occurring, which requires further evaluation by the nurse. Most mothers ask questions about their infant's bluish color and molding of the head.
6. ② The erratic pattern on the fetal monitor is due to faulty lead placement. Although positioning on the side is an excellent nursing measure, it does not address the rationale behind the erratic pattern. Options #3 & #4 would possibly be done after the leads were checked.
7. ① Oral contraceptives should be avoided when a woman is lactating, since the increased estrogen and progesterone tend to interfere with the peripheral action of prolactin, thus decreasing the supply of milk.
8. ③ Station refers to the relationship of the biparietal diameter of the fetal head to the ischial spines of the mother. When this diameter reaches the ischial spine, the station is known as zero. A -1 indicates that the fetus is one cm above the ischial spine.
9. ② The release of oxytocin from the posterior pituitary during the infant's suckling increases the contractions of the uterus and gives rise to afterpains.

10. ② The second stage of labor for a primigravida is about one hour and for a multipara as little as several minutes.
11. ③ It is important to be gentle, since the episiotomy is easily irritated and hemorrhoids are quite common.
12. ③ The definition of effacement is thinning of the cervix. Dilation refers to cervical opening, attitude to fetal posture, and transition to the last phase of the first stage of labor.
13. ② A mother's complaint of excruciating perineal pain following birth is frequently related to the development of a perineal hematoma.
14. ① When a laboring client is at +3, delivery is imminent. The +stations are noted after the neonate has engaged and is moving through the birth canal. The sequence is as follows: -4, -3, -2, -1, 0, +1, +2, +3, +4 then delivery.
15. ② If the entire areola is in the infant's mouth, the infant does not suck on the end of the nipple and traumatize it. Mothers should start out on the unaffected nipple for nursing to initiate the let-down reflex which needs stronger sucking to occur.

Chapter 26: Newborn

1. ② The priority here is the respiratory distress. The first nursing action is to increase the inspired oxygen; it would be appropriate to do a quick but thorough assessment of the infant and advise the supervisor or doctor regarding the infant's status.
2. ② To prevent regurgitation through the nose and sucking through the tube during the postoperative period, use a rubber-tipped Asepto syringe (Brecht feeder).
3. ② The premature infant's temperature-regulating mechanism is poorly developed at birth. Heat production is low and heat loss high because of the greater body surface relative to weight and the lack of subcutaneous fat.
4. ① Promoting lifesaving oxygen exchange is a priority measure at this time.
5. ④ The medication is given to prevent maternal sensitization to the Rh antibodies. It will not prevent nor treat the problem if it has already occurred; it is not given to the infant.
6. ③ It is important that the child be positioned in such a manner that he does not traumatize the incisional area and that the airway is maintained.
7. ④ Client has possible abruptio placentae and may require an emergency delivery via Cesearean, so it will be important to determine when she last ate. Placenta previa is painless, vaginal bleeding.
8. ③ The basis for the damage which occurs from RLF comes from the degree of immaturity, the concentration of oxygen, and the length of exposure to the oxygen.
9. ① Approximately 40 percent to 60 percent of all full-term babies develop jaundice between the second and fourth days of life. In the absence of disease or specific cause, it is referred to as physiologic jaundice.
10 ③ It is not necessary to cover the neonate's eyes with use of the fiberoptic blanket. Feedings and fluids should be encouraged to promote excretion of the bilirubin. The stool would be loose, rather than constipated, while the jaundice is resolving.

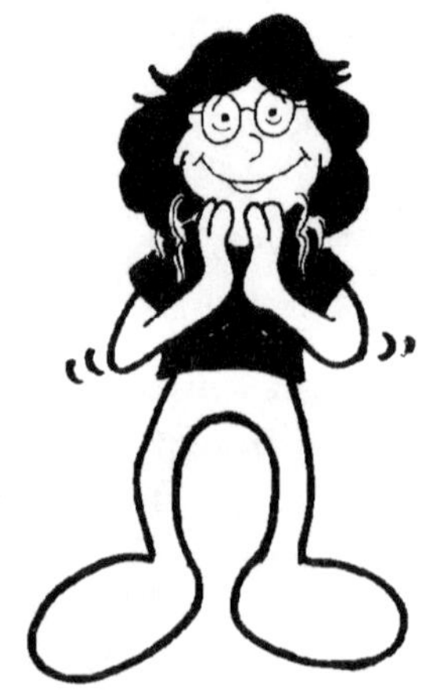

NCLEX-RN PRACTICE TEST

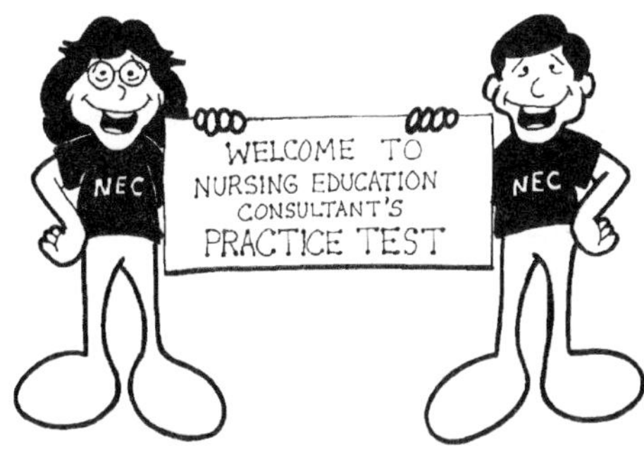

1. The nurse is administering Aminophylline IV drip. Which nursing observation would reflect the therapeutic response to the medication?

① Increased expectoration of purulent sputum.
② No dyspnea, sleeping at intervals.
③ Cardiac rate of 80 beats per minute.
④ Systolic blood pressure levels from 120 to 130 mm Hg.

2. The nurse is assessing a greenstick fracture of the ulna. She understands that:

① The bone is broken across the epiphyseal plate.
② There is a splintering of the bone on one side.
③ There is a separation of the bone at the fracture site.
④ The bone is broken into several fragments.

3. During the fourth stage of labor, where should the nurse be able to palpate the client's fundus?

① Two cm above the umbilicus.
② To the right of the umbilicus.
③ Two cm below the umbilicus.
④ At the level of the umbilicus.

4. The mother of an infant with cleft lip/cleft palate repair is concerned about spoiling him if she picks him up and holds him when he cries. Which response by the nurse would be most appropriate?

① It is important that he not be allowed to cry; therefore, spoiling him should not be the major concern.
② Crying is important; once his lip is healed, he should be allowed extra crying time.
③ Crying may put a strain on the suture line, and he needs extra holding and cuddling because he cannot suckle.
④ He should be allowed to cry, but she should try first to comfort him in the crib to avoid spoiling him.

5. The client is to receive chest physiotherapy four times a day. When is the best time to schedule the chest physiotherapy?

① One hour before each meal and at bedtime.
② Once each shift and once prn.
③ 4 AM, 10 AM, and 10 PM.
④ Whenever necessary to eliminate coughing.

6. How is the countertraction in Buck's traction is achieved?

① Applying a ten-pound counterweight at the knee.
② Placing shock blocks under the head of the bed.
③ Elevating the knee gatch and elevating the head of the bed about 30°.
④ Elevating the foot of the bed frame and allowing the weights to hang freely.

7. To effectively perform percussion and postural drainage to the apical segments of the lungs, the client is placed in which position?

① Sitting.
② Trendelenburg.
③ Side-lying.
④ Prone.

8. An elderly client is admitted in congestive heart failure. What observation by the nurse indicates the client's condition is getting worse?

① Arterial blood gases show a significant decrease in the pH and PCO_2.
② Blood pressure of 160/98, pulse of 110.
③ Urinary output is 60cc per hour and crackles are heard at the base bilaterally.
④ Increasing irritability and confusion.

9. A client had a long leg cast applied to his left leg about four hours ago after the reduction of a compound fracture. Which nursing observations would be of most concern?

① Client complains of the cast feeling warm on the inside.
② Complains of constant pain in the left leg an hour after being medicated with 75mg of Demerol (**Meperdine**).
③ The toes on the affected foot are pale, cool to touch and there is a decreased capillary refill.
④ The pulse distal to the cast is irregular, and palpable at a rate of 88.

10. Dumping syndrome is a common complication for the gastric resection client. What will the nurse assess to determine if the client is experiencing this problem?

① Complaints of nausea and vomiting following PO medications.
② Presence of bowel sounds and his ability to tolerate soft foods after the nasogastric tube is removed.
③ Anxiety, nausea, light-headedness, and tachycardia about 15 to 20 minutes after eating.
④ Decrease in blood pressure, increase in pulse rate about 20 to 30 minutes after ambulating.

11. The nurse is assessing a client who has been receiving aminophylline IV for three days. Which data or symptoms are of most concern to the nurse?

① Nausea.
② Drowsiness.
③ Decreased urinary output.
④ Constipation.

12. By the second day after an MVA, the client's chest x-ray reveals a lung contusion on the right side. Based on this diagnosis, the nurse expects what type of sputum?

① Copious amounts of yellow, thick sputum.
② Clear sputum with streaks of blood.
③ Sputum that layers in the sputum cup.
④ Sputum containing large clots of blood.

13. What is an important assessment information to obtain in a client with a fractured hip?

① Circulation and sensation distal to the fracture.
② Amount of swelling around the fracture site.
③ Degree of bone healing that has occurred.
④ Amount of pain that the fracture and healing are causing.

14. The nurse is concerned about compartmental syndrome in an 8 year old client with a greenstick fracture. What will the nurse teach the mother to observe for?

① Swelling and discoloration of the hand distal to the fracture site.
② Hematoma formation and pain in the upper arm and shoulders.
③ Severe pain radiating proximal to the cast and fracture area.
④ Decreased sensation and ability to move the fingers of the affected hand.

15. In performing the initial newborn assessment, which finding is associated with Down's syndrome?

① Asymmetry of the gluteal folds.
② Hypertonicity of the skeletal muscles.
③ A rounded occiput and high set ears.
④ Simian creases on the palms and soles.

16. A diabetic client asks the nurse about the glycosylated hemoglobin test. What is the nurse's best response regarding the purpose of this test?

① Determines how close the client is to having an insulin reaction.
② Assesses blood glucose control prior to the current status.
③ Determines how much glucose is excreted over a twenty-four hour control period.
④ Evaluates the exact amount of iron supplement the client will need to take.

17. A client is one day postoperative right lobectomy. The physician tells the nurse he wants the client positioned on his left side and back only. What is the rationale behind this order?

① By putting the client on the operative side, the thoracotomy incision is supported and is less likely to be damaged by coughing.
② Positioning on the left side facilitates the cough reflex and assists in clearing the mucus out of the major airways.
③ Drainage from the left thoracic area is accomplished by positioning the client on the left side, this also promotes full expansion of the right lung.
④ Pain from coughing will be decreased if the client is positioned on the operative side which promotes drainage of the right lung.

18. To encourage proper breathing exercises, what will the nurse teach the COPD client to do?

① Utilize pursed-lip breathing.
② Inhale two to three times longer then exhale.
③ Use high abdominal breathing with muscles of the diaphragm.
④ Inhale through the mouth and exhale through the nose.

19. The nurse is preparing a teaching plan for a client who is going to be discharged on Lithium. What will be included regarding the signs and symptoms of lithium toxicity?

① Paradoxical excitement, akathisia, rash.
② Confusion, ataxia, muscle weakness.
③ Photosensitivity, contact dermatitis.
④ Tremor, thirst, weight gain.

20. A client is to receive an IV of Lactated Ringer's, 1000 cc, to run for 8 hours. The drip factor is 10 gtt/cc. How many drops per minute is the IV regulated?

① 24 gtt/min.

② 12 gtt/min.
③ 21 gtt/min.
④ 30 gtt/min.

21. The nurse plans to explain preoperative procedures, the operating room, the recovery room, and postoperative procedures to a 6 year old. Which interventions is implemented first?

① Explain to the child the need for preoperative medications.
② Tell the child that her parents will be waiting in her room for her.
③ Describe the appearance of the recovery room and the operating room.
④ Ask the child to tell you what she knows about the operation.

22. A client is 4 days post gastrectomy. There is an order to clamp the nasogastric tube for 4 hours. About 2 hours after clamping, the client begins to complain of nausea. What is the best nursing action?

① Aspirate the stomach contents to prevent problems with vomiting.
② Unclamp the nasogastric tube and connect it back to the previous level of suction.
③ Call the doctor and advise him of the client's nausea.
④ Administer the antiemetic that is ordered on a PRN basis.

23. A mental health client reports to the nurse that the television is talking to her in a threatening manner. What is the nurses best response to the client's verbalization about the television?

① "That is not logically possible."
② "What leads you to believe that?"
③ "That is a strange idea. How do you know someone on the television was talking to you?"
④ "That seems unusual. Thoughts may seem confusing when one is upset or frightened."

24. The medical record is a legal document. The nurse writing in it should:

① Include any information she thinks is true.
② Cross out any mistake so thoroughly that it cannot be read.
③ Skip lines so she or other nurses can fill in more information later.
④ Include only facts pertinent to care, use opinions in assessment area of charting area only.

25. What are the nursing precautions during a tubing change of a CVP line?

① Flush the catheter with 3cc of normal saline and then heparin prior to disconnecting the line.
② Position the client on his right side and have him take a deep breath.
③ Elevate the head of the bed, disconnect the tubing from the fluid container prior to disconnecting from the client.
④ Position the client flat, have him take a deep breath and hold it while the line is disconnected and a new one connected.

26. What is important to evaluate when the admitting nurse is assessing an elderly man with a long history of congestive heart failure and symptoms of pulmonary edema?

① Increased BUN, confusion, and dysphagia.
② Orthopnea, anxiety, respirations wheezing, and bubbling on auscultation.
③ Slight dyspnea, cyanosis, and pursed lip breathing.
④ Low grade fever, hemoptysis, and bilateral rales in the lower lobes.

27. In considering long term rehabilitation goals and safety aspects, what are the nursing interventions to assist the postop above-the-knee amputation (AKA) client to ambulate?

① Emphasizing the importance of always using the walker.
② Encouraging use of the wheelchair until the prosthesis is comfortable.
③ Assisting to ambulate by supporting the affected side.
④ Teaching to lie in the supine position when in bed.

28. During the admission procedure for a client with a diagnosis of schizophrenia, catatonic type, the client demonstrates "waxy flexibility." How will the nurse identifies this in the client's behavior?

① Abandoning all voluntary forms of motor activity.
② Keeping the arm raised long after the nurse has finished taking the blood pressure.
③ Difficulty in maintaining thought processes and suddenly dashing about the room.
④ Mimicking the behavior of the nurse during the admission routine.

29. The nursing care plan for a client receiving external radiation therapy includes the administration of which medication prior to the treatment?

① Haloperidol (**Haldol**).
② Meperdine (**Demerol**).
③ Hydroxyzine (**Vistaril**).

④ Indomethacin (**Indocin**).

30. The client has diabetic neuropathy that requires an amputation of his right leg below the knee. In the immediate postoperative period, what is a priority nursing action?

① Check for bleeding from the incision.
② Keep the stump adducted from the hip.
③ Notify the prosthetist to prepare the artificial limb.
④ Have the physical therapist begin partial weight-bearing.

31. In planning nursing care for the client with a flail chest, what are important nursing actions to include?

① Turn side to side, cough and deep breathe.
② Percussion and postural drainage bilaterally.
③ Position supine to prevent pressure over flailed area.
④ Circumferential taping of the chest for stability.

32. The nurse is caring for a client with schizophrenia, catatonic type, The client refuses to eat, what is the best nursing action?

① Serve food in a more attractive setting.
② Gavage feed the client with nutritional liquids.
③ Force feed the client with a spoon.
④ Explore the client's feelings about not eating.

33. A client is converted to warfarin (Coumadin) after being on IV Heparin. What would the nurse caution to client to decrease in his diet?

① Whole grains and oats.
② All milk and milk products.
③ Eggs and red meat.
④ Leafy green vegetables.

34. What is important for the nurse to check while an IV oxytocin (Pitocin) drip is being administered to a laboring woman?

① The frequency and duration of contractions every 15 minutes.
② The FHT and vaginal discharge every hour.
③ The hypotensive and bradycardiac effects of oxytocin (**Pitocin**).
④ The client's respirations and potential for hypoxia.

35. A bone aspiration is done to assess the adequacy of treatment in a client with leukemia. Where is the site used for small children?

① Tibia.
② Iliac crest.
③ Sternum.
④ Radius.

36. A client is learning to inject his own insulin. The nurse knows that more teaching is needed when she observes what action by the client?

① Wipes the top of the insulin vial with alcohol.
② Withdraws the prescribed amount of insulin within 0.2 ml.
③ Refers to injection chart and chooses a previously unused site for injection.
④ Keeps the insulin in the refrigerator and prepares and injects it immediately.

37. Prior to initiating preoperative teaching plan for a craniotomy client, what is a priority nursing assessment?

① Level of consciousness.
② Educational background.
③ Age.
④ Health history.

38. Which nursing action helps to improve the respiratory status of a client with an acute asthmatic attack?

① Help the client to attain a slow, prolonged expiration.
② Have client forcefully exhale.
③ Provide rest by leaving client alone, and in supine position.
④ Have the client breath into a paper bag.

39. A 9 month old baby with otitis media is brought to the clinic by his mother. Nose drops have been ordered for nasal congestion. How will the nurse teach the mother to administer the drops to achieve the most therapeutic effect?

① Place the baby in Trendelenburg position after instillation of the nose drops.
② Suction the secretions in the baby's nasal passages after the drops are instilled.
③ Dilute the medication with saline prior to instilling it in the nose.
④ Give the medication about a half hour before the baby is fed.

40 The nurse is assessing a child with croup. What is an early indication of hypoxia?

① Cyanosis.
② Tachypnea.
③ Confusion.
④ Frequency of cough.

41. The COPD client complains of dyspnea after daily exercises. What is the best action by the nurse?

① Assist him to bed and put his oxygen on at 3 liters per minute.

② Have him lie down immediately, and administer an respiratory treatment.
③ Explain that the dyspnea is an anticipated response to the increased level of activity.
④ Discourage him from further exercising, since it is increasing his dyspnea.

42. The nurse is completing the assessment of a postpartum client the day after delivery. Where will she palpate the fundus?

① 2 fingerbreadths above the umbilicus.
② 1 to 2 fingerbreadths below the umbilicus.
③ Midline at the level of the umbilicus.
④ Deviated to the right of the umbilicus.

43. A client in a mental health unit has a persistent idea that he is the son of God. These symptoms indicate he is having what type of delusions?

① Persecution.
② Grandeur.
③ Reference.
④ Religiosity.

44. A 38 year old female is found to have Stage 0 carcinoma of the cervix and is scheduled for a vaginal hysterectomy. What is the interpretation of this terminology regarding the client's cancer?

① Has spread to the pelvic wall.
② Has metastasized to the bone.
③ Is confined to the epithelial cells of the cervix.
④ Is limited to the cervical tissue and vaginal mucosa.

45. What source of data provides the nurse with the most accurate assessment of the status of the water-sealed chest drainage therapy?

① Volume of fluid drained.
② Breath sounds.
③ Chest x-ray report.
④ Client's level of shortness of breath.

46. A client with a complete transverse fracture of the left femur is being stabilized with balanced suspension traction utilizing a Thomas splint and a Kirschner wire. What kind of traction is this?

① Intermittent skin traction.
② Continuous skeletal traction.
③ Intermittent skeletal traction.
④ Continuous skin traction.

47. As the dying process progresses, a client with metastatic cancer is experiencing severe weakness. What is a therapeutic nursing intervention?

① Administer pain medication more frequently.
② Determine the client's attitude toward death.
③ Place the client in a private room.
④ Institute comfort measures.

48. When developing a teaching plan for a client with genital herpes type II, which point is included?

① Sexual activity must be avoided entirely.
② Recurrent outbreaks are often less severe than initial outbreak.
③ Once treated, the infection will not recur.
④ There is no need for one's sexual partner to be treated.

49. The nurse is administering Diabinese (chlorpropamide) to a client. Which observation indicates the therapeutic response to this medication?

① Blood sugar maintained at 100 to 120 mg/dl.
② Decrease in the serum uric acid levels.
③ Urine output increased to 60cc's per hour.
④ Blood pressure increased to 120/80.

50. The labor monitor shows repeated variable decelerations. Which nursing action is a priority?

① Give client nasal oxygen.
② Change client's position.
③ Increase the rate of her IV infusion.
④ Call the physician.

51. The nurse is providing care to a client with closed chest drainage. What problems will occur if the closed chest drainage is disrupted?

① Hemorrhage will result, due to sudden decrease in pressure at the operative site.
② Air will enter the thoracic cavity and collapse the lung.
③ Air will escape the thoracic cavity and expand the lung too rapidly.
④ Water in the drainage bottle will flow into the pleural cavity.

52. While feeding a 4 month old client with cerebral palsy, the nurse observes that he has difficulty taking formula and rice cereal. What is the probable cause of this feeding problem?

① Weakness of the muscles used in sucking and swallowing.

② Delayed eruption of the lateral and central incisors.
③ Inability to relax completely during mealtime.
④ Decrease in appetite due to overexertion.

53. The COPD client's arterial blood gas results are PO_2 of 85, PCO_2 of 40, and HCO_3- of 24. What is the best nursing action based on these results?

① Administer oxygen at 2 L. to prevent the client from becoming hypoxic.
② No action is necessary, this is within normal range for a COPD client.
③ Anticipate the development of metabolic acidosis and administer $NaHCO_3$.
④ Position in high Fowler's and anticipate need for assisted ventilation.

54. What will the postoperative care for the client with a hip repair include?

① Keeping the client flat in bed for two days.
② Maintaining the Buck's traction with leg adducted.
③ Getting the client up in a chair, non-weight bearing, two days post op.
④ Keeping the client's leg slightly bent at the knee to prevent internal rotation.

55. A client is admitted with multiple rib fractures. The nurse notes than an area over the client's right clavicle is puffy and that there is a "crackling" noise with palpation. This observation indicates that the nurse should assess the client for what other data?

① Paradoxical respirations and flail chest.
② Development of a pneumothorax.
③ Infiltrated subclavian IV with fluid infusing.
④ Hypercapia with increasing level of hypoxia,

56. A client does not want to remove wedding band prior to surgery. What is the best nursing intervention?

① Wrap tape around it to secure it to the finger.
② Tell the client that the surgery cannot be done if he does not remove the ring.
③ Place a note on the chart stating that the client refused to remove it.
④ Remind the client that the hospital will not be liable for any loss.

57. Which nursing intervention best meets the client's mobility needs after a below-the-knee amputation of the right leg?

① Assisting the client to be out of bed and do full range of motion for the right hip.
② Continuous elevation of the residual right limb on a pillow.
③ Teaching the client to lift 5-pound weights with her arms to increase upper body strength.
④ Providing passive range-of-motion exercises to the unaffected leg.

58. The nurse is preparing a teaching plan regarding breast feeding. What is important information to include?

① Ovulation is suppressed and pregnancy is impossible while she is breast-feeding.
② Ovulation is not suppressed and pregnancy is possible even though she is breast-feeding.
③ The uterus will not return to a normal size while she is breast-feeding.
④ If she does not begin to menstruate in three months, she should stop breast-feeding.

59. Post-cardiac catheterization, the nurse tells the client to increase his fluid intake. What is the goal of this nursing intervention?

① Promote excretion of the contrast dye used during coronary angiography.
② Replace blood loss during the procedure.
③ Provide hydration so that blood clots will not form.
④ Provide intake because solid food is prohibited for 24 hours post catheterization.

60. What is the initial nursing care for the depressed client?

① Involve in group exercises to decrease depression and make her feel better.
② Put the client in the room with another client experiencing the same type of problem.
③ Schedule one nurse to consistently interact with the client; and focus on establishing rapport.
④ Involve the client in group activities including men so she can see not all are like her husband.

61. A client with chronic glomerulonephritis begins to suffer from some muscle twitching. What additional information is important for the nurse to determine?

① Other neurological changes.
② The need to increase oral intake.
③ The presence of circulatory changes.
④ An increase in the need for calcium.

62. The preoperative teaching plan for a client scheduled for a right lower lobe (RLL) lobectomy includes deep breathing and coughing. Which statement by the nurse to the client is accurate?

① If you practice, you'll be able to take just as deep a breath right after surgery as you can now.
② Before you take a deep breath, you should breathe out as far as possible.

③ After you take the deep breath, hold it in as long as you can.
④ Taking a deep breath will feel good.

63. What data would the nurse anticipate finding in the health history of a client with cervical cancer?

① Irregular menses.
② Increased menstrual flow.
③ Weight gain.
④ Postcoital bleeding.

64. What is the most important assessment for the nurse to make before a client goes for a cardiac catheterization?

① Verify whether the client has been NPO since midnight.
② Assess the pulses and temperature of his extremities.
③ Prepare the client for a preprocedure EKG.
④ Determine if the client understands the procedure.

65. Which dietary modification is included in the diet of a client with cystic fibrosis?

① Decreased salt intake.
② Increased fat intake.
③ Supplements of vitamins A, D, and E.
④ Decreased protein intake.

66. The nurse is caring for a client in pulmonary edema. What position is important for this client to avoid?

① Supine with legs elevated.
② Low Fowler's with legs dependent.
③ Sitting at bedside.
④ High Fowler's with legs straight in front.

67. In the complete assessment of a preterm infant, the nurse included the Dubowitz scale. The Dubowitz assessment scale or scoring system:

① Is used to determine an infant's general state of health at birth.
② Is inaccurate once the infant is over 24 to 48 hours of age.
③ Is only to be used on small-for-dates and less than 2,500 gm infants.
④ Is used to determine gestational age.

68. The nurse expects an infant to weigh how many pounds at the age of two months (based on birth weight of 7 lbs. and normal growth and development)?

① 11 pounds.
② 15 pounds.
③ 10 pounds.
④ 9 pounds.

69. A client is admitted to the critical care area about 4 hours after an auto accident. He has no voluntary movement in both lower extremities. What will the nurse anticipate occurring?

① Progression of the extent of the paralysis secondary to swelling and edema of the spinal column.
② Autonomic dysreflexia resulting from damage to the spinothalamic tracts.
③ Spasticity of the muscles of the affected extremities precipitating an increase in blood pressure.
④ Decrease in the sensation of the affected extremities and development of decubiti.

70. Discharge planning for a 6-year-old tonsillectomy client includes when to seek medical attention. Which postoperative conditions merits such attention?

① Development of a heavy, dirty gray membrane over the tonsillar area.
② Complaints of throat pain on the sixth postoperative day.
③ Complaints of an earache without fever.
④ Development of bleeding in the throat on the sixth postoperative day.

71. Which statement made by the parents of a 10 month old infant does the nurse identify as describing a clinical manifestation of cystic fibrosis?

① "He tastes salty when I kiss him."
② "This baby has more wet diapers than my first child."
③ "He still wakes up at night."
④ "The baby gets very upset whenever I leave him."

72. The nurse is assessing a woman who is receiving an epidural anesthetic for a normal term delivery. What is important for the nurse to monitor to determine the side effects of epidural anesthesia?

① The onset of tetanic uterine contractions.
② Significant decrease in blood pressure.
③ Decrease renal perfusion resulting in oliguria.
④ The onset of a severe frontal headache.

73. How should the nurse position a client to facilitate tracheal catheterization and nasotracheal suctioning?

① High-Fowler's, neck flexed.
② Semi-Fowler's, neck hyperextended.
③ Semi-Fowler's, head in "sniff" position.

④ Bed flat, neck hyperextended.

74. Which medication is most often utilized initially in the treatment of the rheumatoid arthritic client?

① Corticosteroids.
② Aspirin.
③ Indomethacin.
④ Gold salts.

75. Which nursing observation indicates that an asthma client's respiratory status is getting worse?

① Increased production of thin, white, copious amount of sputum.
② Wheezing only on expiration.
③ Decreased breath sounds with inspiratory and expiratory wheezing.
④ Audible wheezing after cough.

76. What is the best indication of the progress of a client with CHF?

① The medication schedule.
② Accurate intake record.
③ Record of daily weight loss.
④ Length of afternoon nap.

77. If a client were developing peritonitis, what information is noted on a nursing assessment?

① Abdominal pain in the area of the incision, pain increase with coughing.
② Temperature increases to 102° F., rigid abdomen, decreased or absent bowel sounds.
③ Purulent drainage from the surgical wound, nausea and vomiting after clear liquid intake.
④ Absent bowel sounds, decreased white cell count, low grade fever.

78. Prior to beginning a client's medication therapy with levodopa for Parkinson's disease, it is important for the nurse to determine if he takes what medication?

① Monoamine oxidase inhibitors.
② Corticosteroids.
③ Diuretics.
④ Hormonal preparations.

79. A client with a diagnosis of adult respiratory distress syndrome (ARDS) is receiving oxygen at 10 liters per minute via a face mask. The arterial blood gases are: PO_2 60mm Hg, PCO_2 30mm Hg, pH 7.5. What is a correct interpretation of these values?

① Hypoxemia with hyperventilation and respiratory alkalosis.
② Hypocapnia with metabolic alkalosis and hypoventilation.
③ Hypoventilation resulting in hypoxemia, and hypercapnia.
④ Hypoxemia with hyperventilation and respiratory acidosis.

80. When transporting a client to the x-ray department, how should the nurse provide for the water sealed chest drainage system?

① Hang the drainage apparatus on the head of the bed.
② Clamp the chest tube until the client reaches the x-ray department.
③ Keep the collection system below the level of the client's chest.
④ Disconnect chest tube from drainage collections chamber.

ANSWERS & RATIONALE PRACTICE TEST

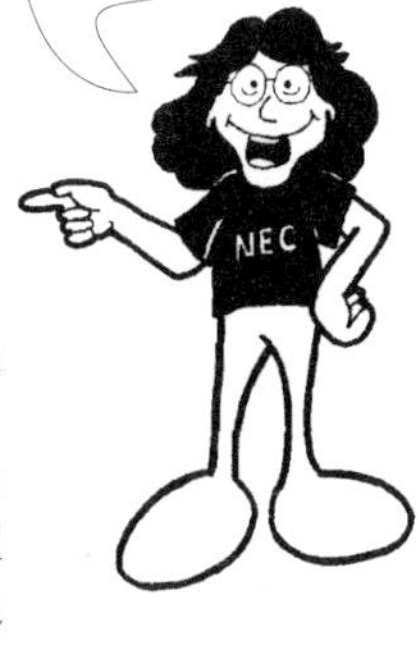

1. ② The primary action of aminophylline is bronchodilatation which results in decreased respiratory distress. Hypotension is a possible side effect, and increased production of sputum is the action of an expectorant.
2. ② Greenstick fracture occurs most often in children as a result of the flexibility of the bone. The bone bends and splinters on one side; there is no separation or fragmentation of the bone.
3. ④ The fourth stage of labor is the first one to four hours following birth when the fundus should be contracted at the umbilicus.
4. ③ Crying needs to be prevented to minimize undue stress to the suture line. Cuddling, holding, and other comfort methods are effective.
5. ① Respiratory toilet should normally be done one hour before each meal and before bedtime in order to clear the airway.
6. ④ Countertraction is best applied by using the client's own weight as the counterpull. This is best achieved by elevating the end of the bed frame to maintain the countertraction.
7. ① The sitting position will allow gravity to help drain the apical or upper segments of the lungs.
8. ④ Increasing irritation and confusion are early indications of hypoxia. The PCO2 usually goes up, and the bloodpressure and pulse are within expected levels. Crackles at the base of the lungs is a common finding in this client.
9. ② Constant pain unrelieved by medications is a concern regarding compartmental syndrome. The pale cool toes are common initially after application of the cast as is the warm feeling as well.
10. ③ Dumping syndrome is a physiological problem associated with too rapid movement of food through the stomach after a gastric resection. When this undigested hypertonic mass reaches the intestine, fluids are drawn to dilute it, which results in the symptoms characteristic of the problem.
11. ① Amiophylline acts as a CNS stimulant. Thus, nausea is often a central effect; in addition, theophylline causes increased heart rate, nervousness, diuresis, and often increased GI motility.
12. ② You would expect some blood streaking due to hemorrhage into alveoli, but not large clots of blood—that would be indicative of additional problems. Yellow sputum would be indicative of infection.
13. ① Circulation and sensation are the priority assessments that must be made after any fracture because of the possibility of nerve or circulatory involvement.
14. ④ Indications of compartmental syndrome include: decreased sensation and decreased mobility in the extremity distal to the fracture/cast, loss of pulse, skin cool to touch and blanched in color occurring in area distal to the fracture/cast.
15. ④ Simian creases are often found in babies with Down's syndrome.
16. ② Glycosylated hemoglobin provides information in clients who experience fluctuations in control. It measures the reaction when the glucose combines with the hemoglobin molecule and is indicative of the general blood sugar control the client has had over the past few days. It is not influenced by the type of treatment or the current level of blood sugar.
17. ③ Gravity will promote drainage from the operative site. It also allows for complete expansion of the unaffected lung to promote oxygenation.
18. ① Pursed-lip breathing slows or retards the flow rate of exhaled air; this keeps airways open and prevents alveolar collapse.
19. ② Confusion, ataxia, and GI distress are symptoms of lithium toxicity. Other symptoms include impaired coordination, dizziness, headache, blurred vision, and muscle weakness. It is very important to watch for these symptoms because lithium toxicity is a real potential problem.
20. ③ The calculation would be 1000/480 x 10 = 20-21 gtt/min.
21. ④ The first step in the teaching/learning process is to determine the child's present knowledge. Further explanations are then planned accordingly.
22. ② The nausea may lead to vomiting and should be addressed early. Opening the tube to drainage and suction will assist in preventing vomiting. Aspiration of gastric contents may damage the gastric incision area, and an antiemetic does not solve the problem.
23. ④ Incorporate reasonable doubt and connect the belief to the client's feelings when responding to persons who are experiencing delusions.
24. ④ The chart is a legal document which contains accurate notes which honestly record the events that occur during your care of the client.
25. ④ By positioning the client flat and having him take a breath and hold it, the intrathoracic pressure is increased and there is decreased possibility that the

client will experience an air emboli during the tubing change.

26. ② With the increase in the capillary pressure, fluid moves into the interstitial spaces causing severe dyspnea, frothy sputum, and wet breath sounds. As the client becomes hypoxic, he will become cyanotic and very anxious.

27. ③ The center of gravity changes when a lower limb is amputated. Assist the client from the affected side while letting him move the unaffected side.

28. ② The symptom of "waxy flexibility," consists of the client retaining, for a considerable length of time without apparent fatigue, an odd position in which his/her body has been placed.

29. ③ Many client's experience nausea and vomiting in accordance with radiation therapy. An antiemetic given prior to therapy can remedy this side effect.

30. ① Hemorrhage can be a postoperative complication for clients who are to undergo delayed prosthesis fitting.

31. ① Turning, coughing and deep breathing are appropriate airway care. Percussion could traumatize the chest wall, and circumferential taping would severely limit thoracic excursion.

32. ② The highest priority for a withdrawn client who is mute and immobile may be to meet biological needs. Gavage feeding may be necessary with an explanation to the client that the purpose is to maintain health and is not punitive.

33. ④ Leafy green vegetables are high in Vit. K, which is the antidote for Coumadin. He does not have to avoid all intake, but he should limit his intake of vegetables such as cabbage and spinach.

34. ① Oxytocin is given frequently to improve the quality of uterine contractions. Oxytocin should be considered a potentially dangerous drug. Overdose can cause hypertonias and possible rupture of the uterus.

35. ② The iliac crest is used in young children because it is easy to locate and permits easy restraint of the child.

36. ④ Cold insulin increases tissue hypertrophy. All extra bottles may be stored in the refrigerator, but the bottle currently being used should remain at room temperature, and the insulin be injected at room temperature. Insulin should not be subjected to extreme temperatures, but is stable at room temperature.

37. ① Although the client may have impaired cognition, preoperative teaching should be individualized according to the level of consciousness of the client.

38. ① Doing a slow, prolonged exhalation will allow the client to exhale a greater volume (a forced exhalation increases the airway obstruction)- then a pattern should also decrease the client's respiratory work.

39. ④ Because children naturally breathe through the nose, administration of nose drops before feeding promotes clearance of the nasal passages.

40. ② Studies have shown that the respiratory rate correlates with the degree of hypoxemia; cyanosis and confusion would be late signs of hypoxemia.

41. ③ The COPD client is always dyspneic. It is important that he exercise to prevent the detrimental effects of immobility.

42. ② Immediately after delivery, the fundus is at the level of the umbilicus, midline. Each day after that it descends 1 to 2 cm.

43. ② Persons with delusions of grandeur identify themselves with a famous or powerful person such as God, a political leader, or a sports hero. This delusion usually reflects low self-esteem and a poorly developed ego.

44. ③ Stage O or preinvasive cancer is defined as carcinoma in situ; it is limited to the epithelial cells of the cervix.

45. ③ Although all of the observations could help to assess the outcome, the best is the chest x-ray, which can visualize the air and fluid in the pleural space.

46. ② The placement of a Kirschner wire through the affected femur constitutes skeletal traction. Skeletal traction is continuous. Skin traction may be intermittent.

47. ④ When the client's condition weakens, there is decreased sensation and need for pain medication, however, other measures need to be instituted to keep the client as comfortable as possible.

48. ② The initial outbreak is usually the worse. The infection does tend to reoccur, and is very contagious when the vesicles are present. The sexual partner needs to be evaluated for the active form of the virus.

49. ① This is a hypoglycemic medication used for the control of adult onset diabetes, the desired response is a normal blood sugar.

50. ② The priority nursing measure to correct a variable deceleration is to change the mother's position in order to release pressure on the umbilical cord. The administration of nasal oxygen or increasing the rate of the IV infusion are measures that are appropriate to implement when late decelerations are present.

51. ② Negative pressure is needed to establish proper ventilation in the pulmonary system.

52. ① Children with cerebral palsy often have feeding difficulties due to poor sucking ability and persistent tongue thrust.

53. ② These are all normal blood gas values so no action is needed. The PCO_2 of 40 is within the high normal ranges, and the PO_2 is within an acceptable range.

54. ③ When the hip is pinned, early mobility is possible. There is no reason to keep the client flat since she would be turned while in bed.

55. ② Often, after trauma, air in the pleural space (pneumothorax) dissects through soft tissue, causing subcutaneous emphysema. It is the air in the tissues that causes the crackling noise.

56. ① Dislodging his wedding band during surgery is the primary risk. If a client refuses to remove a band, it must be safely and securely held in place with tape.

57. ① It is very important to prevent a flexion contracture in the right hip. If a flexion contracture occurs, it will be very difficult to have a functioning prosthesis.

58. ② Although menstruation usually does not occur, ovulation may occur, which means that lactation is not a reliable method of contraception.

59. ① Contrast dye used during coronary angiography is nephrotoxic. Therefore, fluids must be encouraged postcatheterization.

60. ③ With any client, one of the initial nursing goals is to establish trust. This is especially important in the psychiatric client.

61. ① As the toxic waste products build up in the blood, CNS changes can begin to occur. The nurse should monitor the client closely for neurological changes.

62. ③ With or without incentive spirometry devices, the postoperative deep breathing maneuver is called an SMI - sustained maximal inspiration - the client breathes out normally, takes a deep breath in and holds it.

63. ④ Postcoital bleeding is a common symptom of cervical cancer. Irregular menses and increased menstrual flow are more common with uterine cancer.

64. ② When a client is scheduled for an arteriogram, it is vital that the pulses and temperature distal to the insertion site be assessed prior to the procedure. The other assessments are important but not the priority.

65. ③ The lack of pancreatic enzymes leads to malabsorption of fats and therefore deficits of the fat soluble vitamins.

66. ① The problem with pulmonary edema is the heart cannot handle the venous return, by elevating the clients legs all of the venous blood is put back into the central system. The legs should remain straight or dependent.

67. ④ Because the problems of the preterm infant and the low-birth-weight infant may be different, it is important to assess gestational age. Dubowitz scoring is one method of assessing gestational age.

68. ① A newborn should gain 1½ - 2 pounds per month for the first 3-5 months.

69. ① The nurse should assess for an increase in the level of paralysis due to the edema of the spinal cord and plan appropriate nursing interventions.

70. ④ Bleeding from five to ten days postoperatively is a complication of a tonsillectomy and adenoidectomy. This is the time when there is tissue sloughing as healing occurs. The sign noted is frequent swallowing and it requires immediate medical attention.

71. ① Because of the high sodium and chloride content of the sweat, the child with cystic fibrosis will often taste "salty."

72. ② With the epidural anesthesia there is vasodilation which may precipitate hypotension, the relaxation of the uterus onto the aorta may also precipitate hypotension. The client must be carefully monitored for the above problems.

73. ③ Client should be positioned so as to maximize the anatomical opening into the larynx and lower airway.

74. ② Acetylsalicylic acid (aspirin) is the drug of choice and is the most effective.

75. ③ The decreased breath sounds indicate the client is moving less air, while the wheezing demonstrates both inspiratory and expiratory obstruction; with a lesser degree of obstruction, wheezing is heard only in expiration; sputum production often increases after some of the obstruction is relieved.

76. ③ Weight loss is used to evaluate the success of diuretic therapy in the CHF client.

77. ② Peritonitis, or an inflammation of the lining of the peritoneal cavity occurs if the appendix ruptures prior to removal. Symptoms include those associated with an acute infection, plus rigid guarding of the abdomen, shallow respirations, and absent bowel sounds.

78. ① Monoamine oxidase inhibitors and levodopa should not be administered together.

79. ① The PCO_2 is below normal, therefore, the client is hyperventilating; the pH is elevated—alkalotic. The change in pH can be explained by the decreased PCO_2, therefore, the client demonstrates respiratory alkalosis. These blood gases are typical of the early stages of ARDS.

80. ③ Fluid must not be returned to the pleural cavity, and negative pressure must be maintained. The incorrect options would inhibit the drainage of air and fluid from the pleural space.

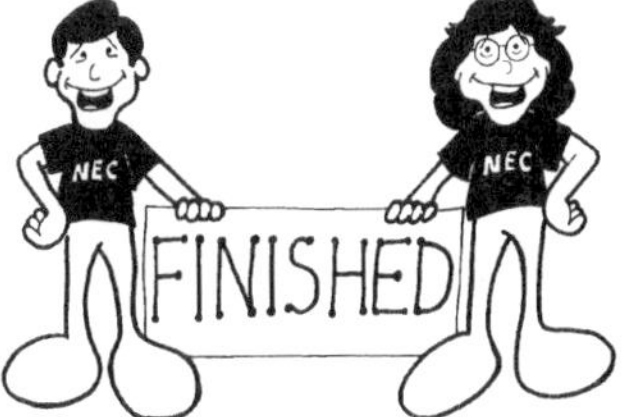

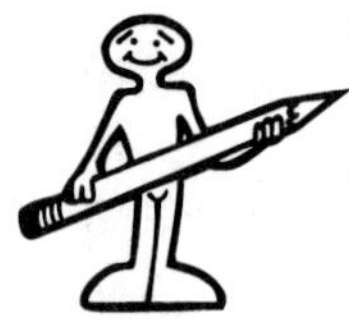

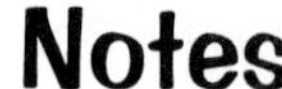

Notes

Appendix A NORMAL LABORATORY DATA

TEST	NORMAL ADULT VALUES
BLOOD SERUM VALUES	
Red cell count ($10^6/\mu L$)	Men: 4.6-6.2 Women: 4.2-5.4
Hemoglobin (g/dl)	Men: 14–18. Women: 12.–16.
Hematocrit (%)	Men: 40-50% Women: 37-47%
Complete white blood count (WBC)	4.5-11. 10^3ul
Differential WBC	Expressed as a percent of total WBC
Granulocytes	
Neutrophils	56%
Eosinophils	2.7%
TBasophils	0.3%
Nongranular leukocytes	
Monocytes	4%
Lymphocytes	34.0%
Sodium (serum or plasma)	136-145 mEq/L
Potassium (plasma)	3.5-5.1 mEq/L
Chloride (serum) 97-107 mEq/L	98-107 mEq/L
Magnesium (serum)	1.3-2.1 mEq/L
Iron serum	Men 65-175 μg/dl Women 50-170 μg/dl
Calcium (ionized) serum	44-55% of total serum calcium
Calcium, total serum	8.2-10.2 mg/dl
Phosphorus serum	2.5-4.5 mg/dl
Alkaline phosphatase	4.5-13 King-Armstrong units or 1.4-4.4 Bodansky units
Blood urea nitrogen (BUN)	5-20mg/dl
Creatinine (serum)	0.7-1.5 mg/dl
Uric acid (serum)	Adult males: 4.5-7.0 mg/dl Adult females: 2.5-6.5 mg/dl
Creatinine phosphokinase (CPK)	Male: 38-175 U/L Female:25-135 U/L
Alanine aminotransferase (ALT)	10-35 IU/L at 37° C.
Aspartate aminotransferase (AST)	8-20 U/L
C-reactive protein	<1mg/dl
Erythrocyte sedimentation rate (ESR):	Adult - Female: 0-20mm/hr Male: 1-10mm/hr

Appendix A NORMAL LABORATORY DATA

TEST	NORMAL ADULT VALUES
Blood platelets	150,000-450,000 cells µl
Serum osmolarity	285-319 mOsm/kg H_20
Prostate specific anitgen	0.81-0.89 ng/ml male >15yrs.
Prothrombin time	10-13 sec
Avtivated partial thromboplastin time (aPTT)	30-45 seconds
Bleeding time	Ivy: 2-7 min Duke: 1-3 min
Interanational normalizing ratio (INR)	2-3 prophylaxis for DVT 2.5-3.5 prosthetic cardiac valves
CO_2	Arterial:19-24 mEq/L Venous: 22-26 mEq/L
Fibrin split-products (FSP)	< 10µg/ml
Fibrinogen	Quantitative: 200-400 mg/dl
Lactic acid dehydrogenase (LDH)	70-200 IU/L
Serum albumin	3.5-5.5 gm/dl.
Glucose (baseline fasting)	70-110 mg/dl
Glycosylated hemoglobin assay	5-8% of total hemoglobin
Glucose 2 hour postprandial	<140mg/dl
Ammonia	15-45 µg/dl
Indirect bilirubin	0.2-0.8mg/dl
Direct bilirubin	up to 0.4 mg/dl
Total bilirubin	0.3-1.3 mg/dl
NORMAL ARTERIAL BLOOD GAS VALUES	
Acidity index (pH)	7.35-7.45
Partial pressure of dissolved 0_2 (PaO_2)	80-100 mm Hg
Percentage of Hgb saturated with 0_2 (0_2 saturation)	95% or above
Partial pressure of dissolved CO_2 ($PaCO_2$)	35-45 mm Hg
Bicarbonate (HCO_3)	22-28 mEq/L

Appendix A NORMAL LABORATORY DATA

TEST	NORMAL ADULT VALUES
URINE VALUES	
Urinalysis	
Albumin	Negative or < 20 mg/dl
Bilirubin	Negative
Color	Clear, golden yellow
Glucose	Negative
Hemoglobin	Negative
Ketones	Negative
Microscopic urinalysis	
Bacteria	Negative
Casts	0-4 hyaline casts per low-power field
Crystals	Few
Mucous threads	Negative
Red blood cells	0-5 per high-power field
Squamous epithelial cells	Seen on voided specimen in females; negative on voided specimen in males; negative for catheterized specimens
White blood cells	0-5 per high-power field
Uric acid (urine)	250-750 mg/24 hr
Urine electrolytes	40-220 mEq/24 hr (varies with dietary intake)
Sodium	110-250 mEq/24hrs
Chloride	Varies with diet; based on average calcium intake of 600-800 mg/24 hr, excretion
Calculated ionized calcium	may be 100-300 mg/24
Urine osomolarity	500-800 mOsm/kg H_20 (with normal fluid intake)
Urine specific gravity	1.003-1.030
Creatinine clearance (24 hour urine)	Adult male: 21-26 mg/kg/24hr Adult female: 16-22 mg/kg/24hr
NORMAL CEREBRAL SPINAL FLUID VALUES	
Blood	None; CSF should be clear
Leukocyte count	0-5 adult, 0-10 child
Enzymes (LDH)	10% of serum level
Glucose	50-80 mg/dl, should be 20 mg less than serum glucose level
Protein	15 to 45 mg/dl
Albumin	56-76%
IgG	1-4 mg/dl
Pressure	90-180 mm H_20

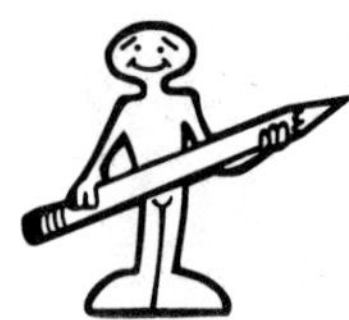

Notes

Appendix B State Boards of Nursing

For further information about NCLEX-RN™, write to the National Council of State Boards of Nursing, Inc.:

National Council of State Boards of Nursing, Inc.
676 North St. Clair Street, Suite 550
Chicago, IL 60611-2921
(312) 787-6555
(http://www.nscbn.org)

For information about the dates, requirements, and specifics of writing the examination in your state, contact the appropriate state board of nursing. The address and telephone number of each state board of nursing is listed below.

Alabama Board of Nursing
770 Washington Avenue
RSA Plaza, Ste 250
Montgomery, AL 36130-3900
Phone: (334) 242-4060
FAX: (334) 242-4360
Contact Person: N. Genell Lee, MSN, JD, RN, Exec. Officer
www.abn.state.al.us/

Alaska Board of Nursing
Dept. of Comm. & Econ. Development
Div. of Occupational Licensing
3601 C Street, Suite 722
Anchorage, AK 99503
Phone: (907) 269-8161
FAX: (907) 269-8196
Contact Person: Dorothy Fulton, MA, RN, Exec. Dir.
www.dced.state.ak.us/occ/pnur.htm

Arizona State Board of Nursing
1651 E. Morten Avenue, Suite 210
Phoenix, AZ 85020
Phone: (602) 331-8111
FAX: (602) 906-9365
Contact Person: Joey Ridenour, MN, RN, Exec. Dir.
www.azboardofnursing.org/

Arkansas State Board of Nursing
University Tower Building
1123 S. University, Suite 800
Little Rock, AR 72204-1619
Phone: (501) 686-2700
FAX: (501) 686-2714
Contact Person: Faith Fields, MSN, RN, Exec. Dir.
www.state.ar.us/nurse

California Board of Registered Nursing
400 R St., Ste. 4030
Sacramento, CA 95814-6239
Phone: (916) 322-3350
FAX: (916) 327-4402
Contact Person: Ruth Ann Terry, MPH, RN, Exec. Officer
Www.rn.ca.gov/

Colorado Board of Nursing
1560 Broadway, Suite 880
Denver, CO 80202
Phone: (303) 894-2430
FAX: (303) 894-2821
Contact Person: Patricia Uris, PhD, RN, Prog. Administrator
www.dora.state.co.us/nursing/

Connecticut Board of Examiners for Nursing
Dept. of Public Health
410 Capitol Avenue, MS# 13PHO
P.O. Box 340308
Hartford, CT 06134-0328
Phone: (860) 509-7624
FAX: (860) 509-7553
Contact Person: Jan Wojick , Board Liaison
www.state.ct.us/dph/

Delaware Board of Nursing
861 Silver Lake Blvd
Cannon Building, Suite 203
Dover, DE 19904
Phone: (302) 739-4522
FAX: (302) 739-2711
Contact Person: Iva Boardman, MSN, RN, Exec. Dir.

District of Columbia Board of Nursing
Department of Health
825 N. Capitol Street, N.E., 2nd Floor
Room 2224
Washington, DC 20002
Phone: (202) 442-4778
FAX: (202) 442-9431
Contact Person: Bonnie Rampersaud, Acting Prog. Manager for Program Licensing

Florida Board of Nursing
Capital Circle Officer Center
4052 Bald Cypress Way
Rm 120
Tallahassee, FL 32399-3252
Phone: (850) 488-0595
Contact Person: Dan Coble, RN, PhD, Exec. Dir.
www.doh.state.fl.us/mqa/

Georgia State Board of Licensed Practical Nurses
237 Coliseum Drive
Macon, GA 31217-3858
Phone: (478) 207-1300
FAX: (478) 207-1633
Contact Person: Jacqueline Hightower, JD, Exec. Director
www.sos.state.ga.us/ebd-lpn/

Georgia Board of Nursing
237 Coliseum Drive
Macon, GA 31217-3858
Phone: (478) 207-1640
FAX: (478) 207-1660
Contact Person: Shirley Camp, BSN, JD, RN, Exec. Dir.
www.sos.state.ga.us/ebd-rn/

Hawaii Board of Nursing
Professional & Vocational Licensing Division
P.O. Box 3469
Honolulu, HI 96801
Phone: (808) 586-3000
FAX: (808) 586-2689
Contact Person: Kathleen Yokouchi, MBA, BBA, BA, Exec. Officer
www.state.hi.us/dcca/pvl/areas_nurse.html

Idaho Board of Nursing
280 N. 8th Street, Suite 210
P.O. Box 83720
Boise, ID 83720
Phone: (208) 334-3110
FAX: (208) 334-3262
Contact Person: Sandra Evans, MA,Ed., RN, Exec. Dir.
www.state.id.us/ibn/ibnhome.htm

Illinois Department of Professional Regulation
James R. Thompson Center
100 West Randolph, Suite 9-300
Chicago, IL 60601
Phone: (312) 814-2715
FAX: (312) 814-3145
Contact Person: Deborah Taylor, RN, Ed.D Nursing Act Assistant Coordinator
www.dpr.state.il.us/

Illinois Department of Professional Regulation
320 W. Washington St.
3rd Floor
Springfield, IL 62786
Phone: (217) 782-8556
FAX: (217) 782-7645
Contact Person:
Web Site:

Indiana State Board of Nursing
Health Professions Bureau
402 W. Washington Street, Room W041
Indianapolis, IN 46204
Phone: (317) 232-2960
FAX: (317) 233-4236
Contact Person: Kristen Kelley , Dir. of Nursing of IN BON
www.state.in.us/hpb/boards/isbn/

Iowa Board of Nursing
RiverPoint Business Park
400 S.W. 8th Street
Suite B
Des Moines, IA 50309-4685
Phone: (515) 281-3255
FAX: (515) 281-4825
Contact Person: Lorinda Inman, MSN, RN, Exec. Dir.
www.state.ia.us/government/nursing/

Kansas State Board of Nursing
Landon State Office Building
900 S.W. Jackson, Suite 551-S
Topeka, KS 66612
Phone: (785) 296-4929
FAX: (785) 296-3929
Contact Person: Mary Blubaugh, MSN, RN, Exec. Administrator
www.ksbn.org

Kentucky Board of Nursing
312 Whittington Parkway, Suite 300
Louisville, KY 40222
Phone: (502) 329-7000
FAX: (502) 329-7011
Contact Person: Sharon Weisenbeck, MS, RN, Exec. Dir.
www.kbn.state.ky.us/

Louisiana State Board of Practical Nurse Examiners
3421 N. Causeway Boulevard, Suite 203
Metairie, LA 70002
Phone: (504) 838-5791
FAX: (504) 838-5279
Contact Person: Claire Glaviano, BSN, MN, RN, Exec. Dir.
www.lsbpne.com/

Louisiana State Board of Nursing
3510 N. Causeway Boulevard, Suite 501
Metairie, LA 70002
Phone: (504) 838-5332
FAX: (504) 838-5349
Contact Person: Barbara Morvant, MN, RN, Exec. Dir.
Www.lsbn.state.la.us/

Maine State Board of Nursing
158 State House Station
Augusta, ME 04333
Phone: (207) 287-1133
FAX: (207) 287-1149
Contact Person: Myra Broadway, JD, MS, RN, Exec. Dir.
www.state.me.us/boardofnursing

Maryland Board of Nursing
4140 Patterson Avenue
Baltimore, MD 21215
Phone: (410) 585-1900
FAX: (410) 358-3530
Contact Person: Donna Dorsey, MS, RN, Exec. Dir.
www.mbon.org

Massachusetts Board of Registration in Nursing
Commonwealth of Massachusetts
239 Causeway Street
Boston, MA 02114
Phone: (617) 727-9961
FAX: (617) 727-1630
Contact Person: Theresa Bonanno, MSN, RN, Exec. Dir.
www.state.ma.us/reg/boards/rn/

Michigan CIS/Office of Health Services
Ottawa Towers North
611 W. Ottawa, 4th Floor
Lansing, MI 48933
Phone: (517) 373-9102
FAX: (517) 373-2179
Contact Person: Diane Lewis, Policy Manager for Licensing Division
www.cis.state.mi.us/bhser/genover.htm

Minnesota Board of Nursing
2829 University Avenue SE
Suite 500
Minneapolis, MN 55414
Phone: (612) 617-2270
FAX: (612) 617-2190
Contact Person: Shirley Brekken, MS, RN, Exec. Dir.
www.nursingboard.state.mn.us/

Mississippi Board of Nursing
1935 Lakeland Drive, Suite B
Jackson, MS 39216-5014
Phone: (601) 987-4188
FAX: (601) 364-2352
Contact Person: Marcia Rachel, PhD, RN, Exec. Dir.
Www.msbn.state.ms.us/

Missouri State Board of Nursing
3605 Missouri Blvd.
P.O. Box 656
Jefferson City, MO 65102-0656
Phone: (573) 751-0681
FAX: (573) 751-0075
Contact Person: Lori Scheidt, BS, Acting Exec. Dir.
Www.ecodev.state.mo.us/pr/nursing/

Montana State Board of Nursing
301 South Park
PO Box 200513
Helena, MT 59620-0513
Phone: (406) 841-2340
FAX: (406) 841-2343
Contact Person: Barbara Swehla, MN, RN, Exec. Dir.
www.discoveringmontana.com/dli/bsd/license/bsd_boards/nur_board/board_page.htm

Nebraska Health and Human Services System
Dept. of Regulation & Licensure, Nursing Section
301 Centennial Mall South
Lincoln, NE 68509-4986
Phone: (402) 471-4376
FAX: (402) 471-3577
Contact Person: Charlene Kelly, PhD, RN, Exec. Dir.
Nursing and Nursing Support
www.hhs.state.ne.us/crl/nursingindex.htm
Nebraska Center of Nursing: http://www.center4nursing.org

Nevada State Board of Nursing
Administration, Discipline & Investigations
1755 East Plumb Lane
Suite 260
Reno, NV 89502
Phone: (775) 688-2620
FAX: (775) 688-2628
Contact Person: Debra Scott, MS, RN, Exec. Dir.
www.nursingboard.state.nv.us

Nevada State Board of Nursing
License Certification and Education
4330 S. Valley View Blvd.
Suite 106
Las Vegas, NV 89103
Phone: (702) 486-5800
FAX: (702)) 486-5803
Contact Person: Don Rennie MS, RN, Associate Exec. Dir. for Licensure & Certification
www.nursingboard.state.nv.us

New Hampshire Board of Nursing
P.O. Box 3898
78 Regional Drive, BLDG B
Concord, NH 03302
Phone: (603) 271-2323
FAX: (603) 271-6605
Contact Person: Cynthia Gray, MBA, BS, RN, CPN, Exec. Dir.
Www.state.nh.us/nursing/

New Jersey Board of Nursing
P.O. Box 45010
124 Halsey Street, 6th Floor
Newark, NJ 07101
Phone: (973) 504-6586
FAX: (973) 648-3481
Contact Person: Patricia Lynch Polansky, MS, RN, Exec. Dir.
Www.state.nj.us/lps/ca/medical.htm

New Mexico Board of Nursing
4206 Louisiana Boulevard, NE
Suite A
Albuquerque, NM 87109
Phone: (505) 841-8340
FAX: (505) 841-8347
Contact Person: Debra Brady, PhD, RN, Exec. Dir.
www.state.nm.us/clients/nursing

New York State Board of Nursing
Education Bldg.
89 Washington Avenue
2nd Floor West Wing
Albany, NY 12234
Phone: (518) 474-3817 Ext. 120
FAX: (518) 474-3706
Contact Person: Barbara Zittel, PhD, RN, Exec. Secretary
www.nysed.gov/prof/nurse.htm

North Carolina Board of Nursing
3724 National Drive, Suite 201
Raleigh, NC 27612
Phone: (919) 782-3211
FAX: (919) 781-9461
Contact Person: Polly Johnson, MSN, RN, Exec. Dir.
www.ncbon.com/

North Dakota Board of Nursing
919 South 7th Street, Suite 504
Bismarck, ND 58504
Phone: (701) 328-9777
FAX: (701) 328-9785
Contact Person: Constance Kalanek, PhD, RN, Exec. Dir.
www.ndbon.org/

Ohio Board of Nursing
17 South High Street, Suite 400
Columbus, OH 43215-3413
Phone: (614) 466-3947
FAX: (614) 466-0388
Contact Person: Janice Lanier, RN, JD, Interim Exec. Dir.
www.state.oh.us/nur/

Oklahoma Board of Nursing
2915 N. Classen Boulevard, Suite 524
Oklahoma City, OK 73106
Phone: (405) 962-1800
FAX: (405) 962-1821
Contact Person: Kimberly Glazier, M.Ed., RN, Exec. Dir.
www.youroklahoma.com/nursing

Oregon State Board of Nursing
800 NE Oregon Street, Box 25
Suite 465
Portland, OR 97232
Phone: (503) 731-4745
FAX: (503) 731-4755
Contact Person: Joan Bouchard, MN, RN, Exec. Dir.
www.osbn.state.or.us/

Pennsylvania State Board of Nursing
124 Pine Street
Harrisburg, PA 17101
Phone: (717) 783-7142
FAX: (717) 783-0822
Contact Person: Miriam Limo, MS, MSN, RN, Exec. Secretary
www.dos.state.pa.us/bpoa/nurbd/mainpage.htm

Rhode Island Board of Nurse
Registration and Nursing Education
105 Cannon Building
Three Capitol Hill
Providence, RI 02908
Phone: (401) 222-5700
FAX: (401) 222-3352
Contact Person: Charles Alexandre, MSN, RN, Exec. Officer
www.health.state.ri.us

South Carolina State Board of Nursing
110 Centerview Drive
Suite 202
Columbia, SC 29210
Phone: (803) 896-4550
FAX: (803) 896-4525
Contact Person: Martha Bursinger, RN, MSN, Exec. Dir.
www.llr.state.sc.us/pol/nursing

South Dakota Board of Nursing
4300 South Louise Ave., Suite C-1
Sioux Falls, SD 57106-3124
Phone: (605) 362-2760
FAX: (605) 362-2768
Contact Person: Diana Vander Woude, MS, RN, Exec. Sec.
www.state.sd.us/dcr/nursing/

Tennessee State Board of Nursing
426 Fifth Avenue North
1st Floor - Cordell Hull Building
Nashville, TN 37247
Phone: (615) 532-5166
FAX: (615) 741-7899
Contact Person: Elizabeth Lund, MSN, RN, Exec. Dir.
170.142.76.180/bmf-bin/BMFproflist.pl

Texas Board of Nurse Examiners
333 Guadalupe, Suite 3-460
Austin, TX 78701
Phone: (512) 305-7400
FAX: (512) 305-7401
Contact Person: Katherine Thomas, MN, RN, Exec. Dir.
www.bne.state.tx.us/

Utah State Board of Nursing
Heber M. Wells Bldg., 4th Floor
160 East 300 South
Salt Lake City, UT 84111
Phone: (801) 530-6628
FAX: (801) 530-6511
Contact Person: Laura Poe, MS, RN, Exec. Administrator
www.commerce.state.ut.us/

Vermont State Board of Nursing
109 State Street
Montpelier, VT 05609-1106
Phone: (802) 828-2396
FAX: (802) 828-2484
Contact Person: Anita Ristau, MS, RN, Exec. Dir.
vtprofessionals.org/nurses/

Virgin Islands Board of Nurse Licensure
Veterans Drive Station
St. Thomas, VI 00803
Phone: (340) 776-7397
FAX: (340) 777-4003
Contact Person: Winifred Garfield, CRNA, RN, Exec. Secretary

Virginia Board of Nursing
6606 W. Broad Street, 4th Floor
Richmond, VA 23230
Phone: (804) 662-9909
FAX: (804) 662-9512
Contact Person: Nancy Durrett, MSN, RN, Exec. Dir.
www.dhp.state.va.us/

Washington State Nursing Care Quality Assurance Commission
Department of Health
1300 Quince Street SE
Olympia, WA 98504-7864
Phone: (360) 236-4700
FAX: (360) 236-4738
Contact Person: Paula Meyer, MSN, RN, Exec. Dir.
www.doh.wa.gov/nursing/

West Virginia Board of Examiners for Licensed Practical Nurses
101 Dee Drive
Charleston, WV 25311
Phone: (304) 558-3572
FAX: (304) 558-4367
Contact Person: Lanette Anderson, RN, BSN, JD, Exec. Secretary
www.lpnboard.state.wv.us/

West Virginia Board of Examiners for Registered Professional Nurses
101 Dee Drive
Charleston, WV 25311
Phone: (304) 558-3596
FAX: (304) 558-3666
Contact Person: Laura Rhodes, MSN, RN, Exec. Dir.
www.state.wv.us/nurses/rn/

Wisconsin Department of Regulation and Licensing
1400 E. Washington Avenue
P.O. Box 8935
Madison, WI 53708
Phone: (608) 266-0145
FAX: (608) 261-7083
Contact Person: Kimberly Nania , Director, Bureau of Health Service Professions
www.drl.state.wi.us/

Wyoming State Board of Nursing
2020 Carey Avenue, Suite 110
Cheyenne, WY 82002
Phone: (307) 777-7601
FAX: (307) 777-3519
Contact Person: Cheryl Lynn Koski, MS, RN, CS, Exec. Dir.
nursing.state.wy.us/

Nursing Examination Boards Outside United States

Guam Board of Nurse Examiners
P.O. Box 2816
1304 East Sunset Boulevard
Barrgada, GU 96913
Phone: (671) 475-0251
FAX: (671) 477-4733

Commonwealth of Puerto Rico
Board of Nurse Examiners
800 Roberto H. Todd Avenue
Room 202, Stop 18
Santurce, PR 00908
Phone: (787) 725-7506
FAX: (787) 725-7903
Contact Person: Magda Bouet , Exec. Dir. of the Office of Regulations and Certifications of Health Care Professions

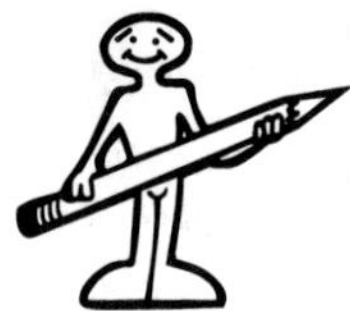

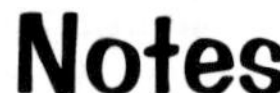

Notes

Index

A

B

C

D

E

F

G

H

I

J

K

L

M

N

O

P

R

S

T

U

V

W

X

Z

Notes

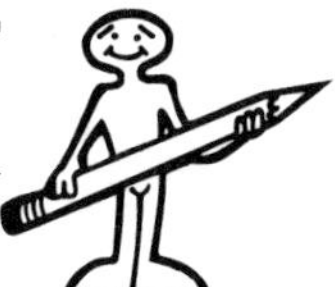

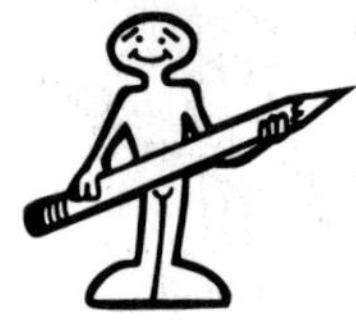
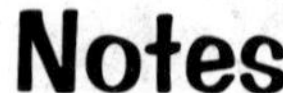

Notes

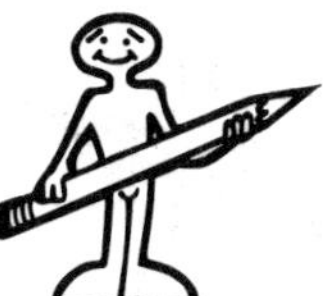

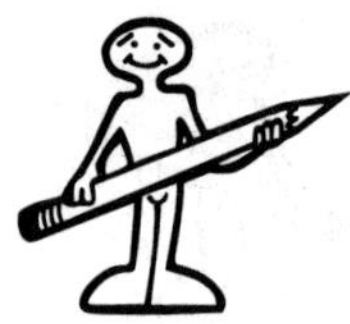
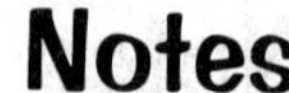

Notes